DRUGS
FOR THE
HEART

8TH EDITION

DRUGS
FOR THE
HEART

Lionel H. Opie, MD, DPhil, DSc, FRCP
Senior Scholar and Professor Emeritus
Hatter Institute for Cardiovascular Research in Africa
Department of Medicine and Groote Schuur Hospital
Faculty of Health Sciences
University of Cape Town
Cape Town, South Africa

CO-EDITOR

Bernard J. Gersh, MBChB, DPhil, FACC, FRCP
Professor of Medicine
Cardiovascular Diseases
Mayo Clinic
Rochester, Minnesota

FOREWORD BY
Eugene Braunwald, MD

ORIGINAL ARTWORK BY
Jeannie Walker

ELSEVIER
SAUNDERS

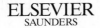

ELSEVIER
SAUNDERS

1600 John F. Kennedy Blvd.
Ste 1800
Philadelphia, PA 19103-2899

DRUGS FOR THE HEART   ISBN: 978-1-4557-3322-4

Notice

Knowledge and best practice in this field are constantly changing. As new research and experience broaden our understanding, changes in research methods, professional practices, or medical treatment may become necessary.

Practitioners and researchers must always rely on their own experience and knowledge in evaluating and using any information, methods, compounds, or experiments described herein. In using such information or methods they should be mindful of their own safety and the safety of others, including parties for whom they have a professional responsibility.

With respect to any drug or pharmaceutical products identified, readers are advised to check the most current information provided (i) on procedures featured or (ii) by the manufacturer of each product to be administered, to verify the recommended dose or formula, the method and duration of administration, and contraindications. It is the responsibility of practitioners, relying on their own experience and knowledge of their patients, to make diagnoses, to determine dosages and the best treatment for each individual patient, and to take all appropriate safety precautions.

To the fullest extent of the law, neither the Publisher nor the authors, contributors, or editors, assume any liability for any injury and/or damage to persons or property as a matter of products liability, negligence or otherwise, or from any use or operation of any methods, products, instructions, or ideas contained in the material herein.

Library of Congress Cataloging-in-Publication Data

Opie, Lionel H.
  Drugs for the heart / Lionel H. Opie ; co-editor, Bernard J. Gersh ; with the collaboration of
John P. DiMarco ... [et al.] ; foreword by Eugene Braunwald. – 8th ed.
      p. ; cm.
  Includes bibliographical references and index.
  ISBN 978-1-4557-3322-4 (pbk. : alk. paper)
  I. Gersh, Bernard J. II. Title.
  [DNLM: 1. Cardiovascular Agents–pharmacology. 2. Cardiovascular Agents–therapeutic use.
3. Cardiovascular Diseases–drug therapy. QV 150]

  615.7′1–dc23
                                                                                    2012044538

Content Strategist: Dolores Meloni
Content Development Specialist: Andrea Vosburgh
Publishing Services Manager: Jeffrey Patterson
Project Manager: Anita Somaroutu/Maria Bernard
Design Manager: Steve Stave
Marketing Manager: Helena Mutak

Printed in China

Last digit is the print number: 9   8   7   6   5   4

Contributors

Keith A.A. Fox, MBChB, FRCP, FmedSci
Professor of Cardiology
University of Edinburgh
Edinburgh, Scotland, UK
Chapter 9. Antithrombotic Agents

Bernard J. Gersh, MBChB, DPhil, FACC
Professor of Medicine
Cardiovascular Division
Mayo Clinic
Rochester, Minnesota
Chapter 8. Antiarrhythmic Drugs and Strategies; Chapter 9. Antithrombotic Agents; Chapter 12. Which Therapy for Which Condition?

Antonio M. Gotto, Jr., MD, DPhil
Dean Emeritus and Co-Chairman of the Board of Overseers
Lewis Thomas University Professor
Weill Cornell Medical College;
The Stephen and Suzanne Weiss Dean and Professor of Medicine
Weill Medical College of Cornell University
New York, New York;
Vice President and Provost for Medical Affairs Emeritus
Cornell University
New York, New York
Chapter 10. Lipid-Modifying and Antiatherosclerotic Drugs

John D. Horowitz, MBBS, PhD
Professor of Cardiology
Department of Medicine
University of Adelaide;
Director, Cardiology and Clinical Pharmacology Units
Queen Elizabeth Hospital
Adelaide, Australia
Chapter 2. Nitrates and Newer Antianginals

Norman M. Kaplan, MD
Clinical Professor of Medicine
Hypertension Division
University of Texas Southwestern Medical School
Dallas, Texas
Chapter 4. Diuretics; Chapter 7. Antihypertensive Therapies

Henry Krum, MBBS, PhD, FRACP, FESC
Professor of Medicine
CCRE Therapeutics
Monash University;
Director, Department of Clinical Pharmacology
Alfred Hospital
Melbourne, Victoria, Australia
Chapter 7. Antihypertensive Therapies

Juris J. Meier, MD
Professor of Medicine
Division of Diabetes and Gastrointestinal Endocrinology
University Hospital St. Josef-Hospital, Ruhr-University Bochum
Bochum, Germany
Chapter 11. Metabolic Syndrome, Hyperglycemia, and Type 2 Diabetes

Stanley Nattel, MD
Professor and Paul-David Chair in Cardiovascular Electrophysiology
Department of Medicine
University of Montreal;
Cardiologist and Director, Electrophysiology Research Program
Department of Medicine
Montreal Heart Institute
Montreal, Quebec, Canada
Chapter 8. Antiarrhythmic Drugs and Strategies

Lionel H. Opie, MD, DPhil, DSc, FRCP
Senior Scholar and Professor Emeritus
Hatter Institute for Cardiovascular Research in Africa
Department of Medicine and Groote Schuur Hospital
Faculty of Health Sciences
University of Cape Town
Cape Town, South Africa
Chapter 1. β-Blocking Agents; Chapter 2. Nitrates and Newer Antianginals; Chapter 3. Calcium Channel Blockers; Chapter 4. Diuretics; Chapter 5. Inhibitors of the Renin-Angiotensin-Aldosterone System; Chapter 6. Heart Failure; Chapter 7. Antihypertensive Therapies; Chapter 8. Antiarrhythmic Drugs and Strategies; Chapter 9. Antithrombotic Agents; Chapter 10. Lipid-Modifying and Antiatherosclerotic Drugs; Chapter 11. Metabolic Syndrome, Hyperglycemia, and Type 2 Diabetes; Chapter 12. Which Therapy for Which Condition?

Marc A. Pfeffer, MD, PhD
Dzau Professor of Medicine
Department of Medicine
Harvard Medical School;
Senior Physician
Cardiovascular Division
Brigham and Women's Hospital
Boston, Massachussetts
Chapter 5. Inhibitors of the Renin-Angiotensin-Aldosterone System

Karen Sliwa, MD, PhD, FESC, FACC
Professor, Hatter Institute for Cardiovascular Research in Africa and IIDMM
Cape Heart Centre
University of Cape Town;
Professor or Medicine and Cardiology
Groote Schuur Hospital
Cape Town, South Africa
Chapter 6. Heart Failure, chronic section

John R. Teerlink, MD, FACC, FAHA, FESC, FRCP(UK)
Professor of Medicine
School of Medicine
University of California, San Francisco;
Director, Heart Failure
Director, Echocardiography
Section of Cardiology
San Francisco Veterans Affairs Medical Center;
San Francisco, California
Chapter 6. Heart Failure, acute section

Ronald G. Victor, MD
George Burns and Gracie Allen Professor of Medicine
Director, Hypertension Center of Excellence
Co-Director, The Heart Institute
Associate Director of Clinical Research, The Heart Institute
Cedars-Sinai Medical Center
Los Angeles, California
Chapter 4. Diuretics; Chapter 7. Antihypertensive Therapies

Harvey D. White, DSc
Director of Coronary Care and Green Lane Cardiovascular
    Research Unit
Green Lane Cardiovascular Services, Cardiology Department
Auckland City Hospital
Auckland, New Zealand
Chapter 9. Antithrombotic Agents

Foreword

Cardiovascular disease is destined to become an even more important cause of morbidity and mortality as the population of the so-called developed world ages and the epidemic of ischemic heart disease in more affluent and more obese persons in the developing world sets in. Fortunately, an ever-growing array of drugs that act on the cardiovascular system continues to become available. These agents are more efficacious and better tolerated than their predecessors, not only in the management of established disease but also increasingly in prevention. However, both trainees and practitioners of medicine and cardiology have ever-increasing difficulty in deciding how to choose the proper therapies for their patients. The eighth edition of Professors Opie's and Gersh's important book provides a rational approach to help with these important decisions. *Drugs for the Heart* is a concise yet complete presentation of cardiac pharmacology and therapeutics. It presents, in a very readable and eminently understandable fashion, an extraordinary amount of important information on the effects of drugs on the heart and circulation. The editors and the talented authors they have enlisted have the unique ability to explain, in a straightforward manner and without oversimplification, the mechanism of action of drugs. This book also summarizes the results of important clinical trials that have shaped regulatory approval and practice guidelines. Finally, it provides important practical information for the clinician.

The eighth edition of this now well-established and admired book builds on the strengths of its predecessors. The excellent explanatory diagrams (an Opie trademark) are even better and more numerous than in previous editions, while the text and references in this rapidly moving field are as fresh as this week's journals. For example, since the publication of the seventh edition the care of patients with many cardiovascular disorders has advanced considerably, and to describe the new landscape the editors have added several distinguished clinical scientists to their author list. These include John R. Teerlink and Karen Sliwa (heart failure), Henry Krum and Ronald G. Victor (antihypertensive therapies), Stanley Nattel (antiarrhythmic drugs), Harvey White (antithrombotic and antiplatelet agents), as well as Juris Meier (metabolic syndrome and diabetes). When these new authors are added to the experts continuing from the earlier edition, this makes a truly outstanding global team.

I strongly recommend this concise volume, which will be of enormous value and interest to all clinicians—specialists and generalists, as well as trainees at all levels, teachers and scientists—who wish to gain a clear understanding of contemporary cardiovascular pharmacology and apply this information most effectively to the care of patients with cardiovascular disease.

Eugene Braunwald, MD

Distinguished Hersey Professor of Medicine

Harvard Medical School

Boston, Massachusetts

The Lancet

Editorial, 1980
Review, 2009

(An editorial from The Lancet, *March 29, 1980, to introduce a series of articles on Drugs and the Heart.)**

Cardiovascular times are changing. After a mere ten years' repose the medical Rip van Winkle would be thoroughly bewildered. For instance, there has been a big switch in attitudes to the failing heart. Experience with beta-blockers has shown the fundamental importance of sympathetic activity in regulating cardiac contraction, and this activity can now be adjusted readily in either direction. Likewise, from calcium antagonists much has been discovered about the function of this ion at the cellular level and its importance in the generation of necrosis and cardiac arrhythmia. Continuous ambulatory electrocardiography and special electrophysiological techniques have eased the assessment of arrhythmias, and, again, of drugs to stop or prevent them. Many new drugs have come on the scene, and they have been increasingly devised to act at specific points on pathways to cellular metabolism.

Dr. van Winkle apart, there may be one or two other physicians who regard the new flood of Cardioactive drugs with alarm. For doctors such as these, Professor Lionel Opie has written the series of articles which begin on the next page. As Professor Opie remarks, drugs should be given, not because they *ought* to work, but because they *do* work. We hope that this series will help stimulate the critical approach to cardiovascular pharmacology that will be much needed in the coming decade.

Review of *Drugs for the Heart,* 7th Edition, *Lancet*, 2009, 374:518.

Packed with useful information, this book is infinitely navigable in 12 lucid and straightforward chapters. Everything you need to know about drugs for the heart is here.

I know that the book is also available online—no doubt my residents and students will be delighted with that version—but I like the paper version.

The book has the clearest figures and tables that I have ever seen.

Most importantly, the section editors don't just opine on how one might go about treating cardiovascular conditions with drugs, *they tell you how to do it.* Those of us who take care of patients like to know how experts do it. Opie and Gersh, and their troupe of contributors, are all experts. They talk from both a science viewpoint and experience.

This book is great on dosing, side-effect profiles, drug interactions, and how to use the agents in care.

*(Kim Eagle is the Albion Walter Hewlett Professor of Internal Medicine and Director of the Cardiovascular Center at the University of Michigan Health System; keagle@med.umich.adu.)

Preface

Taking the profound advice of these two early authors, changes for this eight edition are the following:

1. To stay current, rapid access to new information and new references is mandatory. **We anticipate an increasing online use of this book, which will be relatively easy.** In addition, as shown on the cover, this edition is now available online on Expert Consult. The website contains our regular updates on the important new drug trials. References in the online version of the book can now be accessed by a simple click that will link the reader to the article abstract in PubMed, and then to the original article. Please refer to the inside front cover on how to register using your unique PIN code.

2. These steps promote our aim of providing a readily accessible guide to cardiovascular drugs in a unique style and format. This compact book, again in the widely acclaimed **unique format,** gives crucial information in an easily accessible format for residents, cardiology fellows, and senior students (and, of course, consultants). We believe that this new edition will be more in demand than ever as it will be kept even more current than the previous editions.

3. Many of the illustrations are either new or newly re-created with the aim of conveying maximum clarity, in keeping with the increasingly visual times in which we live. **In the *Lancet,* Kim Eagle stated that the book has the clearest figures that he has ever seen.** We owe our sincerest gratitude to Jeannie Walker for her artistic genius, skills, and patience.

Lionel H. Opie
Bernard J. Gersh

Acknowledgments

We remain incredibly grateful to our contributors, Doctors Fox, Gotto, Horowitz, Kaplan, Meier, Nattel, Pfeffer, Sliwa, Krum, Teerlink, Victor, and White, for their close cooperation and for sharing their expertise, knowledge, and judgments with us.

We thank Andrea Vosburgh and Anne Konopka and others of the staff at Elsevier for unstinting and patient help.

Lionel Opie thanks the Departments of Medicine that invited him to give Grand Rounds at Harvard Medical School–affiliated hospitals during 2011, thereby gaining valuable insights into many novel aspects of drugs for the heart. In Cape Town he thanks Jeannie Walker for her patience and ability to translate abstract concepts and transform hand-drawn figures into outstanding illustrations; Victor Claasen for his infallible memory and reference retrieval service; Professor Patrick Commerford and his colleagues in the Cardiac Clinic for many discussions over the years; and Karen Sliwa, Sandrine Lecour, and other members of the Hatter Institute for encouragement; and last but not least, Carol for bearing with me during those long sessions hunting up articles on the net.

Lionel H. Opie

Bernard J. Gersh

Contents

Contents

β-Blocking Agents

LIONEL H. OPIE

"The β-adrenergic-G-protein-adenylyl cyclase system is the most powerful mechanism to augment human cardiac performance. Chronic desensitization in heart failure must impair and weaken cardiac performance."

Brodde, 2007[1]

β-adrenergic receptor antagonist agents retain their dominant position in the therapy of all stages of ischemic heart disease, with the exception of Prinzmetal's vasospastic variant angina. β-blockade is still regarded as standard therapy for effort, mixed effort, rest, and unstable angina. β-blockers reduce mortality in the long term after myocardial infarction (MI), and exert a markedly beneficial effect on outcomes in patients with chronic congestive heart failure (CHF). β-blockers are antiarrhythmic agents and standard therapy to control the ventricular rate in chronic atrial fibrillation. Conversely, established approved indications in the United States (Table 1-1) include some examples of conditions such as hypertension for which β-blockade used to be, but no longer is, clear-cut "first-line" therapy. When correctly used, β-blockers are relatively safe. In older adults β-blockade risks include excess nodal inhibition and a decreased cardiac output, which in the senescent heart could more readily precipitate heart failure.

The extraordinary complexity of the β-adrenergic signaling system probably evolved millions of years ago when rapid activation was required for hunting and resisting animals, with the need for rapid inactivation during the period of rest recovery. These mechanisms are now analyzed.[2]

Mechanism

The β₁-adrenoceptor and signal transduction. Situated on the cardiac sarcolemma, the β_1-receptor is part of the adenylyl (= adenyl) cyclase system (Fig. 1-1) and is one of the group of G protein–coupled receptors. The G protein system links the receptor to adenylyl cyclase (AC) when the G protein is in the stimulatory configuration (G_s, also called $G\alpha s$). The link is interrupted by the inhibitory form (G_i or $G\alpha i$), the formation of which results from muscarinic stimulation following vagal activation. When activated, AC produces cyclic adenosine monophosphate (cAMP) from adenosine triphosphate (ATP). The intracellular second messenger of β_1-stimulation is cAMP; among its actions is the "opening" of calcium channels to increase the rate and force of myocardial contraction (the positive inotropic effect) and increased reuptake of cytosolic calcium into the sarcoplasmic reticulum (SR; relaxing or lusitropic effect, see Fig 1-1). In the sinus node the pacemaker

Table 1-1

Indications For β-Blockade and US FDA-Approved Drugs

Indications for β-Blockade	FDA-Approved Drugs
1. Ischemic Heart Disease	
Angina pectoris	Atenolol, metoprolol, nadolol, propranolol
Silent ischemia	None
AMI, early phase	Atenolol, metoprolol
AMI, follow-up	Propranolol, timolol, metoprolol, carvedilol
Perioperative ischemia	Bisoprolol,* atenolol*
2. Hypertension	
Hypertension, systemic	Acebutolol, atenolol, bisoprolol, labetalol, metoprolol, nadolol, nebivolol, pindolol, propranolol, timolol
Hypertension, severe, urgent	Labetalol
Hypertension with LVH	Prefer ARB
Hypertension, isolated systolic	No outcome studies, prefer diuretic, CCB
Pheochromocytoma (already receiving alpha-blockade)	Propranolol
Hypertension, severe perioperative	Esmolol
3. Arrhythmias	
Excess urgent sinus tachycardia	Esmolol
Tachycardias (sinus, SVT, and VT)	Propranolol
Supraventricular, perioperative	Esmolol
Recurrences of Afib, Afl	Sotalol
Control of ventricular rate in Afib, Afl	Propranolol
Digitalis-induced tachyarrhythmias	Propranolol
Anesthetic arrhythmias	Propranolol
PVC control	Acebutolol, propranolol
Serious ventricular tachycardia	Sotalol
4. Congestive heart failure	Carvedilol, metoprolol, bisoprolol*
5. Cardiomyopathy	
Hypertrophic obstructive cardiomyopathy	Propranolol
6. Other cardiovascular indications	
POTS	Propranolol low dose*
Aortic dissection, Marfan syndrome, mitral valve prolapse, congenital QT prolongation, tetralogy of Fallot, fetal tachycardia	All?* Only some tested*
7. Central indications	
Anxiety	Propranolol*
Essential tremor	Propranolol
Migraine prophylaxis	Propranolol, nadolol, timolol
Alcohol withdrawal	Propranolol,* atenolol*
8. Endocrine	
Thyrotoxicosis (arrhythmias)	Propranolol
9. Gastrointestinal	
Esophageal varices? (data not good)	Propranolol?* Timolol negative study*
10. Glaucoma (local use)	Timolol, betoxalol, carteolol, levobunolol, metipranolol

*Well tested but not FDA approved.

Afib, Atrial fibrillation; *Afl,* atrial flutter; *AMI,* acute myocardial infarction; *ARB,* angiotensin receptor blocker; *CCB,* calcium channel blocker; *FDA,* Food and Drug Administration; *LVH,* left ventricular hypertrophy; *POTS,* postural tachycardia syndrome; *PVC,* premature ventricular contraction; *SVT,* supraventricular tachycardia; *VT,* ventricular tachycardia.

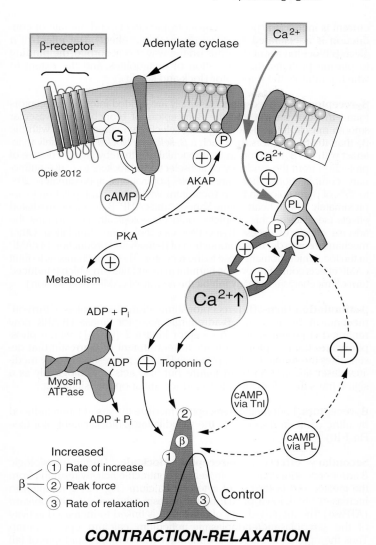

CONTRACTION-RELAXATION

Figure 1-1 β-adrenergic signal systems involved in positive inotropic and lusitropic (enhanced relaxation) effects. These can be explained in terms of changes in the cardiac calcium cycle. When the β-adrenergic agonist interacts with the β-receptor, a series of G protein-mediated changes lead to activation of adenylate cyclase and formation of the adrenergic second messenger, cyclic adenosine monophosphate (cAMP). The latter acts via protein kinase A to stimulate metabolism and to phosphorylate (P) the calcium channel protein, thus increasing the opening probability of this channel. More Ca^{2+} ions enter through the sarcolemmal channel, to release more Ca^{2+} ions from the sarcoplasmic reticulum (SR). Thus the cytosolic Ca^{2+} ions also increase the rate of breakdown of adenosine triphosphate (ATP) and to adenosine diphosphate (ADP) and inorganic phosphate (P_i). Enhanced myosin adenosine triphosphatase (ATPase) activity explains the increased rate of contraction, with increased activation of troponin-C explaining increased peak force development. An increased rate of relaxation (lusitropic effect) follows from phosphorylation of the protein phospholamban (PL), situated on the membrane of the SR, that controls the rate of calcium uptake into the SR. (Figure © L. H. Opie, 2012.)

current is increased (positive chronotropic effect), and the rate of conduction is accelerated (positive dromotropic effect). The effect of a given β-blocking agent depends on the way it is absorbed, the binding to plasma proteins, the generation of metabolites, and the extent to which it inhibits the β-receptor (lock-and-key fit).

β₂-receptors. The β-receptors classically are divided into the β_1-receptors found in heart muscle and the β_2-receptors of bronchial and vascular smooth muscle. If the β-blocking drug selectively interacts better with the β_1- than the β_2-receptors, then such a *β_1-selective blocker* is less likely to interact with the β_2-receptors in the bronchial tree, thereby giving a degree of protection from the tendency of nonselective β-blockers to cause pulmonary complications. There are sizable populations, approximately 20% to 25%, of β_2-receptors in the myocardium, with relative upregulation to approximately 50% in heart failure. Various "anti-cAMP" β_1-receptor–mediated effects (see later in this chapter) could physiologically help to limit the adverse effects of excess β_1-receptor catecholamine stimulation. Other mechanisms also decrease production of β_2-mediated production of cAMP in the local microdomain close to the receptor.[3] These mechanisms to limit cAMP effects could, however, be harmful in heart failure in which β-induced turn-off mechanisms already inhibit the activity of cAMP (next section).

β-stimulation turn-off. β-receptor stimulation also invokes a "turn-off" mechanism, by activating β-adrenergic receptor kinase (β-ARK now renamed G protein–coupled receptor kinase 2 [GRK₂]), which phosphorylates the receptor that leads to recruitment of β-arrestin that desensitizes the stimulated receptor (see Fig. 1-7). β-arrestin not only mediates desensitization in heart failure, but also acts physiologically as a signal transducer, for example to induce antiapoptotic signaling.[4]

β₃-receptors. Endothelial β_3-receptors mediate the vasodilation induced by nitric oxide in response to the vasodilating β-blocker nebivolol (see Fig. 1-10).[5,6]

Secondary effects of β-receptor blockade. During physiologic β-adrenergic stimulation, the increased contractile activity resulting from the greater and faster rise of cytosolic calcium (Fig. 1-2) is coupled to increased breakdown of ATP by the myosin adenosine triphosphatase (ATPase). The increased rate of relaxation is linked to increased activity of the sarcoplasmic/endoplasmic reticulum calcium uptake pump. Thus the uptake of calcium is enhanced with a more rapid rate of fall of cytosolic calcium, thereby accelerating relaxation. Increased cAMP also increases the phosphorylation of troponin-I, so that the interaction between the myosin heads and actin ends more rapidly. Therefore the β-blocked heart not only beats more slowly by inhibition of the depolarizing currents in the sinoatrial node, but has a decreased force of contraction and decreased rate of relaxation. Metabolically, β-blockade switches the heart from using oxygen-wasting fatty acids toward oxygen-conserving glucose.[7] All these *oxygen-conserving properties* are of special importance in the therapy of ischemic heart disease. Inhibition of lipolysis in adipose tissue explains why gain of body mass may be a side effect of chronic β-blocker therapy.

Receptor downregulation in human heart failure. Myocardial β-receptors respond to prolonged and excess β-adrenergic stimulation by internalization and downregulation, so that the β-adrenergic inotropic response is diminished. As outlined for β_2-receptors, there is an "endogenous antiadrenergic strategy," self-protective mechanism against the known adverse effects of excess adrenergic stimulation. However, the role of the β_2-receptor is still not fully clarified in advanced heart failure.[8] Regarding the β_1-receptor, the first step in internalization is the increased activity of β_1ARK, now renamed GRK₂ (see Fig. 1-7). GRK₂ then phosphorylates the β_1-receptor, which in the

BETA-RECEPTOR BLOCKADE

Opie 2012

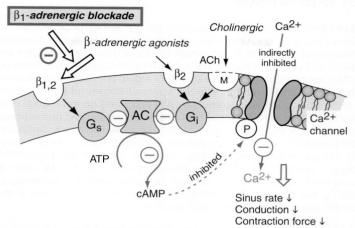

Figure 1-2 The β-adrenergic receptor is coupled to adenyl (= adenylyl) cyclase (AC) via the activated stimulatory G-protein, G_s. Consequent formation of the second messenger, cyclic adenosine monophosphate (cAMP) activates protein kinase A (PKA) to phosphorylate (P) the calcium channel to increase calcium ion entry. Activity of adenyl cyclase can be decreased by the inhibitory subunits of the acetylcholine (ACh)–associated inhibitory G-protein, G_i. cAMP is broken down by phosphodiesterase (PDE) so that PDE-inhibitor drugs have a sympathomimetic effect. The PDE is type 3 in contrast to the better known PDE type 5 that is inhibited by sildenafil (see Fig. 2-6). A current hypothesis is that the $β_2$–receptor stimulation additionally signals via the inhibitory G-protein, G_i, thereby modulating the harm of excess adrenergic activity. (Figure © L. H. Opie, 2012.)

presence of β-arrestin becomes uncoupled from G_s and internalizes. If the β-stimulation is sustained, then the internalized receptors may undergo lysosomal destruction with a true loss of receptor density or downregulation. However, *downregulation* is a term also often loosely applied to any step leading to loss of receptor response.

Clinical β-receptor downregulation occurs during prolonged β-agonist therapy. During continued infusion of dobutamine, a β-agonist, there may be a progressive loss or decrease of therapeutic efficacy, which is termed *tachyphylaxis*. The time taken and the extent of receptor downgrading depend on multiple factors, including the dose and rate of infusion, the age of the patient, and the degree of preexisting downgrading of receptors as a result of CHF. In CHF, the $β_1$-receptors are downregulated by the high circulating catecholamine levels, so that the response to $β_1$-stimulation is diminished. Cardiac $β_2$-receptors, not being downregulated to the same extent, are therefore increased in relative amounts; there are also some defects in the coupling mechanisms. Recent recognition of the dual signal path for the effects of $β_2$-receptor stimulation leads to the proposal that in CHF continued activity of the $β_2$-receptors may have beneficial consequences such as protection from programmed cell death or apoptosis. In practice, however, combined $β_1β_2$-receptor blockade by carvedilol is probably superior in the therapy of heart failure to $β_1$ selective blockade.

Receptor number upregulation. During sustained β-blocker therapy, the number of β-receptors increases.[9] This change in the receptor density could explain the striking effect of long-term β-blockade in heart failure, namely improved systolic function, in contrast to the short-term negative inotropic effect. This inotropic effect is not shared by other agents such as the angiotensin-converting enzyme (ACE) inhibitors that reduce mortality in heart failure.

Cardiovascular Effects of β-Blockade

β-blockers were originally designed by the Nobel prize winner Sir James Black to counteract the adverse cardiac effects of adrenergic stimulation. The latter, he reasoned, increased myocardial oxygen demand and worsened angina. His work led to the design of the prototype β-blocker, *propranolol*. By blocking the cardiac β-receptors, he showed that these agents could induce the now well-known inhibitory effects on the sinus node, atrioventricular (AV) node, and on myocardial contraction. These are respectively the negative chronotropic, dromotropic, and inotropic effects (Fig. 1-3). Of these, it is especially bradycardia and the negative inotropic effects that are relevant to the therapeutic effect in angina pectoris because these changes decrease the myocardial oxygen demand (Fig. 1-4). The inhibitory effect on the AV node is of special relevance in the therapy of supraventricular tachycardias (SVTs; see Chapter 8), or when β-blockade is used to control the ventricular response rate in atrial fibrillation.

Effects on coronary flow and myocardial perfusion. Enhanced β-adrenergic stimulation, as in exercise, leads to β-mediated coronary vasodilation. The signaling system in vascular smooth muscle again involves the formation of cAMP, but, whereas the latter agent increases cytosolic calcium in the heart, it paradoxically decreases calcium levels in vascular muscle cells (see Fig. 3-2). Thus during exercise the heart pumps faster and more forcefully and the coronary flow is increased—a logical combination. Conversely, β-blockade should have a coronary vasoconstrictive effect with a rise in coronary vascular resistance. However, the longer diastolic filling time, resulting from the decreased heart rate in exercise, leads to better diastolic myocardial perfusion, to give an overall therapeutic benefit.

Effects on systemic circulation. The effects previously described explain why β-blockers are antianginal as predicted by their developers. Antihypertensive effects are less well understood. In the absence of the peripheral dilatory actions of some β-blockers (see Fig. 1-11), it initially decrease the resting cardiac output by approximately 20% with a compensatory reflex rise in the peripheral vascular resistance. Thus within the first 24 hours of therapy, the arterial pressure is unchanged. The

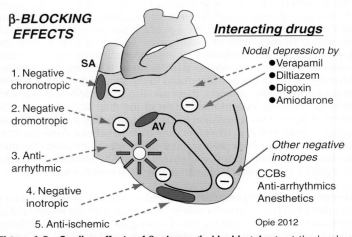

Figure 1-3 Cardiac effects of β-adrenergic blocking drugs at the levels of the sinoatrial (SA) node, atrioventricular (AV) node, conduction system, and myocardium. Major pharmacodynamic drug interactions are shown on the right. (Figure © L. H. Opie, 2012.)

ISCHEMIC OXYGEN BALANCE
Opie 2012

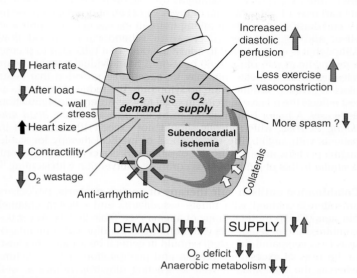

Figure 1-4   Effects of β-blockade on ischemic heart. β-blockade has a beneficial effect on the ischemic myocardium, unless there is vasospastic angina when spasm may be promoted in some patients. Note unexpected proposal that β-blockade diminishes exercise-induced vasoconstriction. (Figure © L. H. Opie, 2012.)

peripheral resistance then starts to fall after 1 to 2 days and the arterial pressure now starts to fall in response to decreased heart rate and cardiac output. Additional antihypertensive mechanisms may involve (1) inhibition of those β-receptors on the terminal neurons that facilitate the release of norepinephrine (prejunctional β-receptors), hence lessening adrenergic mediated vasoconstriction; (2) central nervous effects with reduction of adrenergic outflow; and (3) decreased activity of the renin-angiotensin system (RAS) because β-receptors mediate renin release (the latter mechanism may explain part of the benefit in heart failure).

Angina Pectoris

Symptomatic reversible myocardial ischemia often reflects classical effort angina. Here the fundamental problem is inadequacy of coronary vasodilation in the face of increased myocardial oxygen demand, typically resulting from exercise-induced tachycardia (see Fig. 2-1). However, in many patients, there is also a variable element of associated coronary (and possibly systemic) vasoconstriction that may account for the precipitation of symptoms by cold exposure combined with exercise in patients with "mixed-pattern" angina. The choice of prophylactic antianginal agents should reflect the presumptive mechanisms of precipitation of ischemia.

β-blockade reduces the oxygen demand of the heart (see Fig. 1-4) by reducing the double product (heart rate × blood pressure [BP]) and by limiting exercise-induced increases in contractility. Of these, the most important and easiest to measure is the reduction in heart rate. In addition, an aspect frequently neglected is the increased oxygen demand resulting from left ventricular (LV) dilation, so that any accompanying ventricular failure needs active therapy.

All β-blockers are potentially equally effective in angina pectoris (see Table 1-1) and the choice of drug matters little in those who do not have concomitant diseases. *But a minority of patients do not respond to any β-blocker* because of (1) underlying severe obstructive coronary artery disease, responsible for angina even at low levels of exertion and at heart rates of 100 beats/min or lower; or (2) an abnormal increase in LV end-diastolic pressure resulting from an excess negative inotropic effect and a consequent decrease in subendocardial blood flow. Although it is conventional to adjust the dose of a β-blocker to secure a resting heart rate of 55 to 60 beats/min, in individual patients heart rates less than 50 beats/min may be acceptable provided that heart block is avoided and there are no symptoms. The reduced heart rate at rest reflects the relative increase in vagal tone as adrenergic stimulation decreases. A major benefit is the restricted increase in the *heart rate during exercise*, which ideally should not exceed 100 beats/min in patients with angina. The effectiveness of medical therapy for stable angina pectoris, in which the use of β-blockers is a central component, is similar to that of percutaneous coronary intervention with stenting.[10]

Combination antiischemic therapy of angina pectoris. β-blockers are often combined with nitrate vasodilators and calcium channel blockers (CCBs) in the therapy of angina (see Table 2-4). However, the combined use of β-blockers with nondihydropyridine calcium antagonists (e.g., verapamil, diltiazem) should in general be avoided, because of the risks of excess bradycardia and precipitation of heart failure, whereas the combination with long-acting dihydropyridines is well documented.[11]

Co-therapy in angina. Angina is basically a vascular disease that needs specific therapy designed to give long-term vascular protection. The following agents should be considered for every patient with angina: (1) aspirin and/or clopidogrel for antiplatelet protection, (2) statins and a lipid-lowering diet to decrease lipid-induced vascular damage, and (3) an ACE inhibitor that has proven protection from MI and with the doses tested (see Chapter 5, p. 143). Combinations of prophylactic antianginal agents are necessary in some patients to suppress symptoms, but have less clearcut prognostic implications.

Prinzmetal's variant angina. β-blockade is commonly held to be ineffective and even harmful, because of lack of efficacy. On the other hand, there is excellent evidence for the benefit of CCB therapy, which is the standard treatment. In the case of *exercise-induced anginal attacks in patients with variant angina,* a small prospective randomized study in 20 patients showed that nifedipine was considerably more effective than propranolol.[12]

Cold intolerance and angina. During exposure to severe cold, effort angina may occur more easily (the phenomenon of mixed pattern angina). Conventional β-blockade by propranolol is not as good as vasodilatory therapy by a CCB[13] and may reflect failure to protect from regional coronary vasoconstriction in such patients.[14]

Silent myocardial ischemia. Episodes of myocardial ischemia, for example detected by continuous electrocardiographic recordings, may be precipitated by minor elevations of heart rate, probably explaining why β-blockers are very effective in reducing the frequency and number of episodes of silent ischemic attacks. In patients with silent ischemia and mild or no angina, atenolol given for 1 year lessened new events (angina aggravation, revascularization) and reduced combined end-points.[15]

β-blockade withdrawal. Chronic β-blockade increases β-receptor density. When β-blockers are suddenly withdrawn, angina may be exacerbated, sometimes resulting in MI. Treatment of the withdrawal syndrome is by reintroduction of β-blockade. Best therapy is to avoid this condition by gradual withdrawal.

Acute Coronary Syndrome

Acute coronary syndrome (ACS) is an all-purpose term, including unstable angina and acute myocardial infarction (AMI), so that management is based on risk stratification (see Fig. 12-3). Plaque fissuring in the wall of the coronary artery with partial coronary thrombosis or platelet aggregation on an area of endothelial disruption is the basic pathologic condition. Urgent antithrombotic therapy with heparin (unfractionated or low molecular weight) or other antithrombotics, plus aspirin is the basic treatment (see Chapter 9). Currently, early multiple platelet–receptor blockade is standard in high-risk patients.

  β-blockade is a part of conventional in-hospital quadruple therapy, the other three agents being statins, antiplatelet agents, and ACE inhibitors, a combination that reduces 6-month mortality by 90% compared with treatment by none of these.[16] β-blockade is usually started early, especially in patients with elevated BP and heart rate, to reduce the myocardial oxygen demand and to lessen ischemia (see Fig. 1-4). The major argument for early β-blockade is that threatened infarction, into which unstable angina merges, may be prevented from becoming overt.[17] Logically, the lower the heart rate, the less the risk of recurrent ischemia. However, the actual objective evidence favoring the use of β-blockers in unstable angina itself is limited to borderline results in one placebo-controlled trial,[18] plus only indirect evidence from two observational studies.[16,19]

Acute ST-Elevation Myocardial Infarction

Early ST-elevation myocardial infarction. There are no good trial data on the early use of β-blockade in the reperfusion era. Logically, β-blockade should be of most use in the presence of ongoing pain,[20] inappropriate tachycardia, hypertension, or ventricular rhythm instability.[21] In the COMMIT trial early intravenous metoprolol given to more than 45,000 Asiatic patients, about half of whom were treated by lytic agents and without primary percutaneous coronary intervention, followed by oral dosing, led to 5 fewer reinfarctions and 5 fewer ventricular fibrillations per 1000 treated.[22] The cost was increased cardiogenic shock, heart failure, persistent hypotension and bradycardia (in total, 88 serious adverse events). In the United States, metoprolol and atenolol are the only β-blockers licensed for intravenous use in AMI. Overall, however, no convincing data emerge for routine early intravenous β-blockade.[23] With selected and carefully monitored exceptions, it is simpler to introduce oral β-blockade later when the hemodynamic situation has stabilized. The current American College of Cardiology (ACC)–American Heart Association (AHA) guidelines recommend starting half-dose oral β-blockade on day 2 (assuming hemodynamic stability) followed by dose increase to the full or the maximum tolerated dose, followed by long-term postinfarct β-blockade.[24]

AHA postinfarct recommendations 2011. (1) Administer β-blockade for all postinfarct patients with an ejection fraction (EF) of 40% or less unless contraindicated, with use limited to carvedilol, metoprolol succinate, or bisoprolol, which reduce mortality *(Class 1, Level of Evidence A)*; (2) administer β-blockade for 3 years in patients with normal LV function after AMI or ACS; *(Class 1, Level B)*. It is also reasonable to continue β-blockade beyond 3 years *(Class IIa, Level B)*.[25]

Benefits of postinfarct β-blockade. In the postinfarct phase, β-blockade reduces mortality by 23% according to trial data[26] and by 35% to 40% in an observational study on a spectrum of patients including diabetics.[27] Timolol, propranolol, metoprolol, and atenolol are all effective and licensed for this purpose. Metoprolol has excellent long-term data.[28] Carvedilol is the only β-blocker studied in the reperfusion era and in a population also receiving ACE inhibitors.[29] As the LV dysfunction was an entry point, the carvedilol dose was gradually uptitrated, and all-cause mortality was reduced. The mechanisms concerned are multiple and include decreased ventricular arrhythmias[30] and decreased reinfarction.[31] β-Blockers with partial agonist activity are relatively ineffective, perhaps because of the higher heart rates.

The only outstanding questions are (1) whether low-risk patients really benefit from β-blockade (there is an increasing trend to omit β-blockade especially in patients with borderline hyperglycemic values); (2) when to start (this is flexible and, as data for early β-blockade are not strong,[26] oral β-blocker may be started when the patient's condition allows, for example from 3 days onward[29] or even later at about 1 to 3 weeks); and (3) how long β-blockade should be continued. Bearing in mind the risk of β-blockade withdrawal in patients with angina, many clinicians continue β-blockade administration for the long term once a seemingly successful result has been obtained. The benefit in high-risk groups such as older adults or those with low EFs increases progressively over 24 months.[27]

The *high-risk patients* who should benefit most are those often thought to have contraindications to β-blockade.[27] Although CHF was previously regarded as a contraindication to β-blockade, postinfarct patients with heart failure benefited more than others from β-blockade.[27] Today this category of patient would be given a β-blocker after treatment of fluid retention cautiously with gradually increasing doses of carvedilol, metoprolol, or bisoprolol. The SAVE trial[31] showed that ACE inhibitors and β-blockade are additive reducing postinfarct mortality, at least in patients with reduced EFs. The benefit of β-blockade when added to co-therapy by ACE inhibitors is a mortality reduction of 23% to 40%.[27,29] Concurrent therapy by CCBs or aspirin does not diminish the benefits of postinfarct β-blockade.

Despite all these strong arguments and numerous recommendations, β-blockers are *still underused in postinfarct patients* at the expense of many lives lost. In the long term, 42 patients have to be treated for 2 years to avoid one death, which compares favorably with other treatments.[26]

Lack of Outcome Studies in Angina

Solid evidence for a decrease in mortality in postinfarct follow-up achieved by β-blockade has led to the assumption that this type of treatment must also improve the outcome in effort angina or unstable angina. Regretfully, there are no convincing outcome studies to support this proposal. In unstable angina, the short-term benefits of metoprolol were borderline.[18] In effort angina, a metaanalysis of 90 studies showed that β-blockers and CCBs had equal efficacy and safety, but that β-blockers were better tolerated[32] probably because of short-acting nifedipine capsules which were then often used. In angina plus hypertension, direct comparison has favored the CCB verapamil (see next section).

β-Blockers for Hypertension

β-blockers are no longer recommended as first-line treatment for hypertension by the Joint National Council (JNC) of the USA and have been relegated to fourth- or even fifth-line choices by the National Institute of Clinical Excellence of the UK.[33] β-blockers are the least effective of the standard antihypertensive drug classes at preventing major cardiovascular events, especially stroke.[34] β-blockers are more likely to predispose to new diabetes[35] and they are the least cost-effective of the major classes of antihypertensive agents (the costs of hospitalization, clinical events, and therapy of new diabetes).[36] The crucial study was ASCOT, in which the much better cardiovascular outcomes of amlodipine with or without perindopril compared with the atenolol with or without diuretic[34] could be explained by the lower central aortic pressures with amlopidine.[37] In 2003 JNC 7 listed the following as "compelling indications" for the use of β-blockers: heart failure with hypertension, post-MI hypertension, high coronary risk, and diabetes.[38] JNC 8 is due to appear this year and its view of β-blockers will elicit great interest. The exact mechanism of BP lowering by β-blockers remains an open question (see Fig. 7-10). A sustained fall of cardiac output and a late decrease in peripheral vascular resistance (after an initial rise) are important. Inhibition of renin release also contributes, especially to the late vasodilation. Of the large number of β-blockers now available, all are antihypertensive agents but few have outcome studies.[39]

For **patients at high risk of coronary artery disease,** such as those with diabetes, chronic renal disease, or a 10-year Framingham risk score of 10% or more, first-line antihypertensive choices should exclude β-blockers, according to the AHA.[40]

Hypertension plus effort angina: risk of new diabetes. In the INVEST study, in 6391 patients with hypertension and coronary artery disease followed for more than 2 years, the β-blocker atenolol gave similar major cardiovascular outcomes to the nondihydropyridine CCB verapamil, and yet the β-blocker group had more anginal episodes, new diabetes, and psychological depression.[41,42] More new diabetes in the atenolol group could be explained by (1) the greater use of add-on diuretics and (2) the greater use of an ACE inhibitor, trandolapril, in the verapamil group.

Older adult patients. In certain hypertension subgroups such as older adults, especially those with left ventricular hypertrophy (LVH), comparative studies show better outcome data with the other agents such as diuretics[43] and the angiotensin receptor blocker (ARB) losartan.[44] One possible reason is that at equivalent brachial artery pressures, β-blockade reduces the central aortic pressure less than other agents.[45]

Black patients. In black older adults, atenolol was only marginally more antihypertensive than placebo.[46] Unexpectedly, in younger blacks (age less than 60 years), atenolol was the second most effective agent, following diltiazem, and more effective than the diuretic hydrochlorothiazide.[46]

Diabetic hypertensives. BP-reducing therapy based on atenolol versus captopril showed no major differences nor even trends, although the β-blocker group had gained weight and more often needed additional glucose-lowering treatment to control the blood sugar.[47]

Combination antihypertensive therapy. To reduce the BP, β-blockers may be combined with CCBs, α-blockers, centrally active agents, and cautiously with diuretics. Because β-blockers reduce renin levels, combination with ACE inhibitors or an ARB is not so logical. Increased new diabetes is a risk during β-blocker-thiazide cotherapy.[35,48] Much less well tested is the use of carvedilol that may increase insulin sensitivity.[49] *Ziac* is bisoprolol (2.5 to 10 mg) with a very low dose of hydrochlorothiazide (6.25 mg). This drug combination has been approved as first-line therapy (starting with bisoprolol 2.5 mg plus thiazide 6.25 mg) for systemic hypertension by the Food and Drug Administration, an approval rarely given to a combination product. Metabolic side effects of higher thiazide doses were minimized and there was only a small increase in fatigue and dizziness. In the United States, atenolol and chlorthalidone (Tenoretic) and metoprolol tartrate and hydrochlorothiazide (Lopressor

HCT) are combinations widely used, yet they often contain diuretic doses that are higher than desirable (e.g., chlorthalidone 25 mg; see Chapter 7). Combinations of such prodiabetic doses of diuretics with β-blockade, in itself a risk for new diabetes,[50] is clearly undesirable. Note that standard doses of β-blocker or diuretic even separately predispose to new diabetes.[35] In the ASCOT hypertension study, amlodipine with or without perindopril gave better outcomes than atenolol with or without bendroflumethiazide, including less new diabetes (see Chapter 7).

β-Blockers for Arrhythmias

β-blockers have multiple antiarrhythmic mechanisms (Fig. 1-5) and are effective against many supraventricular and ventricular arrhythmias. Basic studies show that they counter the arrhythmogenic effects of excess catecholamine stimulation by countering the proarrhythmic effects of increased cAMP and calcium-dependent triggered arrhythmias.[51,52] Logically, β-blockers should be particularly effective in arrhythmias caused by increased adrenergic drive (early phase AMI, heart failure, pheochromocytoma, anxiety, anesthesia, postoperative states, and some exercise-related arrhythmias, as well as mitral valve prolapse) or by increased cardiac sensitivity to catecholamines (thyrotoxicosis). β-blockade may help in the prophylaxis of SVTs by inhibiting the initiating atrial ectopic beats and in the treatment of SVT by slowing the AV node and lessening the ventricular response rate. Perhaps surprisingly, in sustained ventricular tachyarrhythmias the empirical use of metoprolol was as effective as electrophysiologically guided antiarrhythmic therapy.[53] Likewise, in ventricular tachyarrhythmias, the ESVEM study showed that sotalol, a β-blocker with added Class III activity (Fig. 1-5), was more effective than a variety of Class I antiarrhythmics.[54]

In patients with atrial fibrillation, current management practices often aim at control of ventricular rate ("rate control") rather than restoration and maintenance of sinus rhythm ("rhythm control"). β-blockers, together with low-dose digoxin, play an important role in rate control in such patients.

In postinfarct patients, β-blockers outperformed other antiarrhythmics[26] and decreased arrhythmic cardiac deaths.[55] In postinfarct patients with depressed LV function and ventricular arrhythmias,

ANTI-ARRYTHMIC EFFECTS OF β-BLOCKERS

Opie 2012

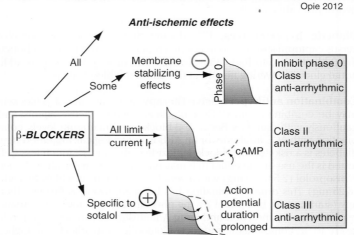

Figure 1-5 Antiarrhythmic properties of β-blockers. Antiischemic effects indirectly lessen arrhythmias. Note that only sotalol has added Class-III antiarrhythmic effects. It is questionable whether the membrane stabilizing effects of propranolol confer additional antiarrhythmic properties. (Figure © L. H. Opie, 2012.)

a retrospective analysis of data from the CAST study shows that β-blockade reduced all-cause mortality and arrhythmia deaths.[56] Although the mechanism of benefit extends beyond antiarrhythmic protection,[57] it is very unlikely that β-blockers can match the striking results obtained with an implantable defibrillator (23% mortality reduction in Class 2-3 heart failure).[57,58] In *perioperative patients,* β-blockade protects from atrial fibrillation.[59]

Intravenous esmolol is an ultrashort-acting agent esmolol that has challenged the previously standard use of verapamil or diltiazem in the perioperative period in acute SVT, although in the apparently healthy person with SVT, adenosine is still preferred (see Chapter 8). Intravenous esmolol may also be used acutely in atrial fibrillation or flutter to reduce the rapid ventricular response rate (see later).

β-Blockers in Heart Failure

That β-blockers, with their negative inotropic effects, could increase cardiac contraction and decrease mortality in heart failure is certainly counterintuitive, especially bearing in mind that the β_1-receptor is downregulated (Fig. 1-6). Not only does the cardiac output increase, but

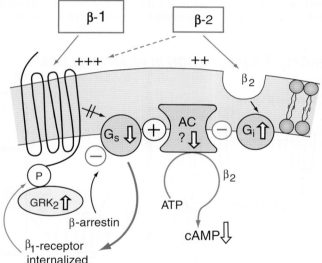

Figure 1-6   β-adrenergic receptors in advanced heart failure. Downregulation and uncoupling of β-adrenergic receptor signal systems results in depressed levels of cyclic adenosine monophosphate (cAMP) and decreased contractility, which may be viewed as an autoprotective from the adverse effects of cAMP. Note: (1) β-receptor downregulation starts as a result of inhibitory phosphorylation of the receptor mediated by G protein–coupled receptor kinase (GRK$_2$; previously β_1 adrenergic receptor kinase [β_1ARK]), GRK$_2$ increases in response to excess β-adrenergic stimulation of the receptor, (2) β-receptor uncoupling from G$_s$ results from β-arrestin activity, (3) β-receptor downregulation is a result of internalization, (4) increased G$_i$ is a result of increased messenger ribonucleic acid activity, (5) β_2 receptors are relatively upregulated and appear to exert an inhibitory effect on contractile via enhanced G$_i$. (For details see Opie LH, *Heart Physiology from Cell to Circulation.* Lippincott Williams and Wilkins, Philadelphia, 2004:508.) (Figure © L. H. Opie, 2012.)

abnormal patterns of gene expression revert toward normal.[60] Several mechanisms are proposed, of which the first three are well-studied.

1. *Improved β-adrenergic signaling.* Myocardial β-receptors respond to prolonged and excess β-adrenergic stimulation by internalization and downregulation (see Fig. 1-6), so that the β-adrenergic inotropic response is diminished. This is a self-protective mechanism against the known adverse effects of excess adrenergic stimulation. The first step in β_1-receptor internalization is the increased activity of β_1ARK, now renamed GRK_2. GRK_2 then phosphorylates the β_1-receptor, which in the presence of β-arrestin becomes uncoupled from G_s and internalizes (Fig. 1-7).[4] If the β-stimulation is sustained, then the internalized receptors may undergo lysosomal destruction with true loss of receptor density or downregulation. However, *downregulation* is a term also often loosely applied to any step leading to loss of receptor response. Experimental β-blockade decreases the expression of GRK_2 and increases the activity of AC, thereby improving contractile function. *Relative upregulation of the β2-receptor* may have inhibitory effects (see Fig. 1-6), including continued excessive formation of G_i and hyperphosphorylated SR (see Fig. 1-7). However, the role of the β_2-receptor in advanced heart failure is still not fully clarified.[8] Thus not surprisingly in clinical heart failure studies carvedilol with its blockade of β_1, β_2, and β_3 receptors is superior to the β_1-selective blocker metoprolol.[61,62]

2. *Self-regulation.* There is a potent and rapid physiologic switch-off feedback mechanism that mutes β-adrenergic receptor stimulation and avoids perpetuated activation of this receptor (see Fig. 1-7).

EXCESS β-STIMULATION IN HEART FAILURE
Opie 2012

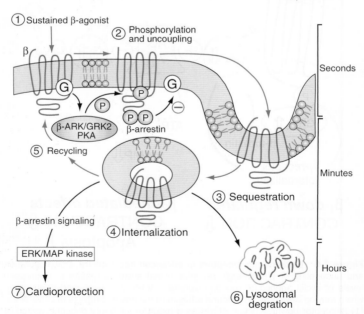

Figure 1-7 Mechanisms of β-adrenergic receptor desensitization and internalization. Note the internalized receptor complex with growth stimulation via mitogen-activated protein (MAP) kinase. *β-ARK,* β-agonist receptor kinase; *ERK,* extracellular signal-regulated kinase; *GRK2,* G protein–coupled receptor kinase; *PKA,* protein kinase A. (Adapted from Hein L, Kobilka BK: Adrenergic receptors. From molecular structures in vivo function. *Trends Cardiovasc Med* 1997;7:137.) (Figure © L. H. Opie, 2012.)

Physiologically, this very rapid *desensitization of the β-receptor* occurs within minutes to seconds. Sustained β-agonist stimulation rapidly induces the activity of the GRK_2, thereby increasing the affinity of the β-receptor for another protein family, the *arrestins* that dissociate the agonist-receptor complex. β-arrestin not only lessens the activation of AC, thereby inhibiting is activity,[63] but furthermore switches the agonist coupling from G_s to inhibitory G_i.[64]

Resensitization of the receptor occurs if the phosphate group is split off by a phosphatase so that the receptor may then more readily be linked to G_s. β-arrestin signaling can also evoke an alternative counterbalancing protective path by activating the epidermal growth factor receptor that leads to the protective ERK/MAP kinase path (see item 7 in Fig. 1-7).[65] β-blocker drugs may have complex effects by β-arrestin agonism.[66] Although receptor-arrestin effects are best described for the $β_2$-receptor, they also occur to a lesser extent with the $β_1$-receptor.[63]

In heart failure, prolonged hyperadrenergic β-receptor stimulation is linked to adverse end results, both impairing contractile function and enhancing adverse signaling. There is long-term compensatory desensitization of the β-adrenergic receptor in chronic heart failure.[67] Conversely, transgenic mice with GRK_2 (previously Beta-adrenergic receptor kinase, BARK) overexpression are protected from heart failure.[67] Of note, the desensitization process is reversible as occurs during experimental cardiac resynchronization therapy, when specific suppressors of the inhibitor G protein (see G_i in Fig. 1-6) are much increased in activity so that β-adrenergic signaling becomes more normal.[68]

3. *The hyperphosphorylation hypothesis.* The proposal is that continued excess adrenergic stimulation leads to hyperphosphorylation of the calcium-release channels (also known as the *ryanodine receptor*) on the SR. This causes defective functioning of these channels with excess calcium leak from the SR, with cytosolic calcium overload. Because the calcium pump that regulates calcium uptake into the SR is simultaneously downregulated, the pattern of rise and fall of calcium ions in the cytosol is impaired with poor contraction and delayed relaxation. These abnormalities are reverted toward normal with β-blockade,[69,70] which also normalizes the function of the calcium release channel.[71]

4. *Bradycardia.* β-blockade may act at least in part by reduction of the heart rate (Fig. 1-8). Multiple studies have suggested that a high resting heart rate is an independent risk factor for cardiovascular disease,[72] which could reflect the role of excess adrenergic tone. Bradycardia may improve coronary blood flow and decrease the myocardial oxygen demand. Experimentally, long-term heart rate reduction lessens extracellular matrix collagen, besides improving the LV EF.[73] To achieve adequate bradycardia, the addition of ivabradine may be required (see Chapter 6, p. 195).

5. *Protection from catecholamine myocyte toxicity.* The circulating concentrations of norepinephrine found in severe heart failure are high enough to be directly toxic to the myocardium, experimentally damaging the membranes and promoting subcellular destruction, acting at least in part through cytosolic calcium overload.[74]

6. *Antiarrhythmic effects.* In experimental heart failure, ventricular arrhythmias are promoted via increased formation of cAMP and calcium-mediated afterpotentials.[52]

7. *Antiapoptosis.* Coupling of the $β_2$-receptor to the inhibitory G-protein, G_1, may be antiapoptotic.[75]

8. *Renin-angiotensin inhibition.* When added to prior ACE inhibitor or ARB therapy, β-blockade by metoprolol increases the blockade of the RAS.[62]

β-BLOCKADE IN HEART FAILURE

Opie 2012

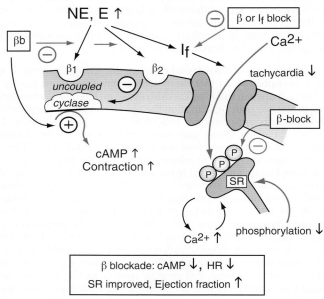

Figure 1-8 Proposed mechanisms of action of β-blockade in heart failure. By inhibiting the effects of norepinephrine (NE) and epinephrine (E), β-blockade lessens the feedback mechanism whereby G protein–receptor kinase inhibits receptor activity (see Fig. 1-6). β-blockade therefore indirectly increases formation of cyclic adenosine monophosphate (cAMP) and improves contractions. β-blockade, by reducing the heart rate, lessens calcium entry into failing myocytes to decrease cytosolic calcium overload. This bradycardia is achieved by inhibition of the current I_f and other nonspecific pacemaking currents. Thirdly, β-blockade inhibits the phosphorylation of the sarcoplasmic reticulum (SR) and therefore facilitates calcium ion release and, indirectly, uptake of calcium by the SR (see Fig. 1-7). (Figure © L. H. Opie, 2012.)

How to Apply β-Blockers in Heart Failure

β-blockers are now recognized as an integral part of anti–heart failure therapy based on neurohumoral antagonism[76] with coherent molecular mechanisms (see Fig. 1-8).[76] They benefit a wide range of patients with stable systolic heart failure, including women, diabetics, older adults as in the nebivolol study (SENIORS), and, in several studies, black patients.[77] The principles are the following: (1) Select patients with stable heart failure; start slowly and uptitrate gradually (Table 1-2),[78] while watching for adverse effects. If necessary cut back on the dose or titrate more slowly. (2) The usual procedure is to add β-blockade to existing therapy, including ACE inhibition and diuretics, and, optionally in some studies, digoxin, when the patient is hemodynamically stable and not in Class IV or severe Class III failure. (3) However, in several recent studies,[79,80] β-blockers were also given before ACE inhibitors, which is logical, considering that excess baroreflex-mediated adrenergic activation may be an important initial event in heart failure (see Fig. 5-8). (4) Never stop the β-blocker abruptly (risk of ischemia and infarction). (5) Use only β-blockers with doses that are well understood and clearly delineated, and with proven benefit, notably carvedilol, metoprolol, bisoprolol, and nebivolol (see Table 1-2). The first three of these drugs have *reduced mortality* in large trials by approximately one third. Of these, only carvedilol and long-acting metoprolol are approved in the United States. However, data for carvedilol are strongest in

Table 1-2

β-Blocker	First Dose	Third Week	Fifth-Sixth Week	Final Dose

Heart Failure: A Firm Indication for β-Blockade—Titration and Doses of Drugs*

β-Blocker	First Dose	Third Week	Fifth-Sixth Week	Final Dose
Carvedilol	3.125	6.25 × 2	12.5 × 2	25 × 2
Metoprolol SR	25[†]	50	100	200
Bisoprolol	1.25	3.75	5	10
Nebivolol	1.25	2.5	5	10

*All doses in milligrams. Data from placebo-controlled large trials, adapted from McMurray, Heart, 1999, 82 (suppl IV), 14-22. For exact nebivolol dosage in older adults, here modified, see reference 78. Forced titration in all studies, assuming preceding dose tolerated. Dose once daily for metoprolol and bisoprolol and twice daily for carvedilol. Carvedilol doses from US package insert. Doses taken with food to slow absorption; target dose may be increased to 50 mg bid for patients > 85 kg.

[†]Slow-release metoprolol (CR/XL formulation), reduce initial dose to 12.5 mg in severe heart failure.

the COMET trial[61]; carvedilol reduced mortality more than metoprolol. Thus far there is no evidence that diastolic heart failure improves.[78]

For every heart rate reduction of 5 beats/min with β-blockade, there is an 18% reduction (cardiac index, 6%-29%) in the risk for death as occurred in the 23 β-blocker trials in 19,209 patients, of whom more than 95% had systolic dysfunction.[81] Perhaps unexpectedly, the dose of β-blocker did not relate to any benefit. The initiation of β-blockade is a slow process that requires careful supervision and may temporarily worsen the heart failure; we strongly advise that only the proven β-blockers be used in the exact dose regimens that have been tested (see Table 1-2). Propranolol, the original gold-standard β-blocker, and atenolol, two commonly used agents, have not been well studied in heart failure.

Other Cardiac Indications

In *hypertrophic obstructive cardiomyopathy,* high-dose propranolol is standard therapy although verapamil and disopyramide are effective alternatives.

In *catecholaminergic polymorphic ventricular tachycardia* high-dose β-blockers prevent exercise-induced ventricular tachycardia (VT), although most patients continue to have ventricular ectopy during exercise, so that heart rate–reducing calcium blockers may give added benefit.[82]

In *mitral stenosis with sinus rhythm,* β-blockade benefits by decreasing resting and exercise heart rates, thereby allowing longer diastolic filling and improved exercise tolerance. In mitral stenosis with chronic atrial fibrillation, β-blockade may have to be added to digoxin to obtain sufficient ventricular slowing during exercise. Occasionally β-blockers, verapamil, and digoxin are all combined. Heart block is a risk during co-therapy of β-blockers with verapamil.

In *mitral valve prolapse,* β-blockade is the standard procedure for control of associated arrhythmias.

In *dissecting aneurysms,* in the hyperacute phase, intravenous propranolol has been standard, although it could be replaced by esmolol. Thereafter, oral β-blockade is continued.

In *Marfan syndrome* with aortic root involvement, β-blockade is likewise used against aortic dilation and possible dissection.

In *neurocardiogenic (vasovagal) syncope,* β-blockade should help to control the episodic adrenergic reflex discharge believed to contribute to symptoms. However, a detailed study on 208 patients showed that metoprolol did not work.[83]

In *Fallot's tetralogy,* propranolol 2 mg/kg twice daily is usually effective against the cyanotic spells, probably acting by inhibition of right ventricular contractility.

Congenital QT-prolongation syndromes are now classified both on the basis of genotype and phenotype. β-blocker therapy is theoretically most effective when the underlying mutation affects K^+ channel–modulated outward currents. β-blockers reduce the overall frequency of major and minor cardiac events by approximately 60%, thus not eliminating the need for implantable defibrillator insertion in high-risk patients.[84] In the related condition of *catecholaminergic polymorphic VT*, β-blockers are also moderately effective.[85]

In postural tachycardia syndrome (POTS), both low-dose propranolol (20 mg)[86] and exercise training are better than high-dose propranolol (80 mg daily).[87]

Noncardiac Indications for β-Blockade

Stroke. In an early trial the nonselective blocker propranolol was only modestly beneficial in reducing stroke (although ineffective in reducing coronary artery disease [CAD]).[88] The β_1 selective agents are more effective in stroke reduction.[89]

Vascular and noncardiac surgery. β-blockade exerts an important protective effect in selected patients. Perioperative death from cardiac causes and MI were reduced by bisoprolol in high-risk patients undergoing vascular surgery.[90] A risk-based approach to noncardiac surgery is proposed by a very large observational study on 782,969 patients. In those at no or very low cardiac risk, β-blockers were without benefit and in fact were associated with more adverse events, including mortality. In those at very high cardiac risk, mortality decreased by 42%, with a number needed to treat of only 33.[91] Thus risk factor assessment is vital (see original article for revised cardiac risk index). In patients undergoing vascular surgery, but otherwise not at very high risk, perioperative metoprolol gave no benefit yet increased intraoperative bradycardia and hypotension.[92]

Impact of POISE study. In the major prospective POISE (Peri-Operative ISchemic Evaluation) study on a total of 8,351 patients, perioperative slow-release metoprolol decreased the incidence of nonfatal MI from 5.1% to 3.6% ($p < 0.001$), yet increased total perioperative mortality from 2.3% to 3.1% ($p < 0.05$), with increased stroke rates and markedly increased significant hypotension and bradycardia. *Thus routine perioperative inception of metoprolol therapy is not justified.* As metoprolol exerts markedly heterogenous cardiovascular effects according to metabolic genotype, involving subtypes of cytochrome P450 2D6,[93] genetic differences may have accounted for part of the adverse cardiovascular findings in POISE and another study.[92]

In an important focused update given by ACC-AHA,[94] the major recommendations are the following: (1) Class I indication for perioperative β-blocker use in patients already taking the drug; (2) Class IIa recommendations for patients with inducible ischemia, coronary artery disease, or multiple clinical risk factors who are undergoing vascular (i.e., high-risk) surgery and for patients with coronary artery disease or multiple clinical risk factors who are undergoing intermediate-risk surgery; (3) Initiation of therapy, particularly in lower-risk groups, requires careful consideration of the risk/benefit ratio; (4) If initiation is selected, it should be started well before the planned procedure with careful perioperative titration to achieve adequate heart rate control while avoiding frank bradycardia or hypotension. In the light of the POISE results, routine administration of perioperative β-blockers, particularly in higher fixed-dose regimens begun on the day of surgery, cannot be advocated.

Thyrotoxicosis. Together with antithyroid drugs or radioiodine, or as the sole agent before surgery, β-blockade is commonly used in thyrotoxicosis to control symptoms, although the hypermetabolic state is not decreased. β-blockade controls tachycardia, palpitations, tremor, and nervousness and reduces the vascularity of the thyroid gland, thereby facilitating operation. In thyroid storm, intravenous propranolol can be given at a rate of 1 mg/min (to a total of 5 mg at a time); circulatory collapse is a risk, so that β-blockade should only be used in thyroid storm if LV function is normal as shown by conventional noninvasive tests.

Anxiety states. Although propranolol is most widely used in anxiety (and is licensed for this purpose in several countries, including the United States), probably all β-blockers are effective, acting not centrally but by a reduction of peripheral manifestations of anxiety such as tremor and tachycardia.

Glaucoma. The use of local β-blocker eye solutions is now established for open-angle glaucoma; care needs to be exerted with occasional systemic side effects such as sexual dysfunction, bronchospasm, and cardiac depression. Among the agents approved for treatment of glaucoma in the United States are the nonselective agents timolol (Timoptic), carteolol, levobunolol, and metipranolol. The cardioselective betaxolol may be an advantage in avoiding side effects in patients with bronchospasm.

Migraine. Propranolol (80 to 240 mg daily, licensed in the United States) acts prophylactically to reduce the incidence of migraine attacks in 60% of patients. The mechanism is presumably by beneficial vasoconstriction. The antimigraine effect is prophylactic and not for attacks once they have occurred. If there is no benefit within 4 to 6 weeks, the drug should be discontinued.

Esophageal varices. β-blockade has been thought to prevent bleeding by reducing portal pressure. No benefit was found in a randomized study.[95]

Pharmacologic Properties of Various β-Blockers

β-blocker "generations." *First-generation nonselective agents,* such as propranolol, block all the β-receptors (both β_1 and β_2). *Second-generation cardioselective agents,* such as atenolol, metoprolol, acebutolol, bisoprolol, and others, have, when given in low doses, relative selectivity for the β_1 (largely cardiac) receptors (Fig. 1-9). *Third-generation vasodilatory* agents have added properties (Fig. 1-10), acting chiefly through two mechanisms: first, direct vasodilation, possibly mediated by release of nitric oxide as for carvedilol (see Fig. 1-10) and nebivolol,[6] and, second, added α-adrenergic blockade, as in labetalol and carvedilol. A third vasodilatory mechanism, as in pindolol and acebutolol, acts via β_2-intrinsic sympathomimetic activity (ISA), which stimulates arterioles to relax; however, these agents are less used at present and do not neatly fit into the division of the three "generations." Acebutolol is a cardioselective agent with less ISA than pindolol that was very well tolerated in a 4-year antihypertensive study.[96]

Nonselective agents (combined β_1-β_2-blockers). The prototype β-blocker is propranolol, which is still often used worldwide and is a World Health Organization essential drug. By blocking β_1-receptors, it affects heart rate, conduction, and contractility, yet by blocking β_2-receptors, it tends to cause smooth muscle contraction with risk of bronchospasm in predisposed individuals. This same quality might, however, explain the benefit in migraine when vasoconstriction could inhibit the attack. Among the nonselective blockers, nadolol and sotalol are much longer acting and lipid-insoluble.

β₁ VS β₂ SELECTIVITY
Opie 2012

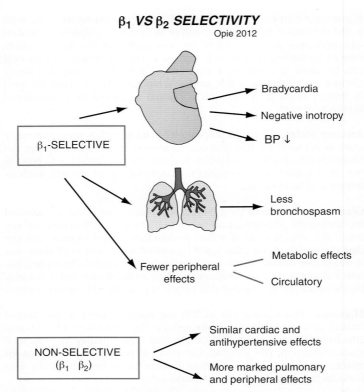

Figure 1-9   β₁- versus β₂-cardioselectivity. In general, note several advantages of cardioselective β-blockers (exception: heart failure). Cardioselectivity is greatest at low drug doses. (Figure © L. H. Opie, 2012.)

Combined β₁–β₂–α-blocker. Carvedilol is very well supported for preferential use in heart failure, in which this combination of receptor blockade should theoretically be ideal, as shown by better outcomes than with metoprolol in the COMET study.[97]

Cardioselective agents (β₁-selectivity). Cardioselective agents (acebutolol, atenolol, betaxolol, bisoprolol, celiprolol, and metoprolol) are as antihypertensive as the nonselective ones (see Fig. 1-9). Selective agents are preferable in patients with chronic lung disease or chronic smoking, insulin-requiring diabetes mellitus, and in stroke prevention.[89] Cardioselectivity varies between agents, but is always greater at lower doses. Bisoprolol is among the most selective. Cardioselectivity declines or is lost at high doses. No β-blocker is completely safe in the presence of asthma; low-dose cardioselective agents can be used with care in patients with bronchospasm or chronic lung disease or chronic smoking. In angina and hypertension, cardioselective agents are just as effective as noncardioselective agents. In AMI complicated by stress-induced hypokalemia, nonselective blockers theoretically should be better antiarrhythmics than β₁-selective blockers.

Vasodilating β-blockers. Carvedilol and nebivolol are the prototypes (see Fig. 1-10). These agents could have added value in the therapy of hypertension by achieving vasodilation and, in the case of nebivolol, better reduction of LVH is claimed.[98]

Antiarrhythmic β-blockers. All β-blockers are potentially antiarrhythmic by virtue of Class II activity (see Fig. 1-6). Sotalol is a unique β-blocker with prominent added Class III antiarrhythmic activity (see Fig. 1-6; Chapter 8).

VASODILATORY β-BLOCKERS

Opie 2012

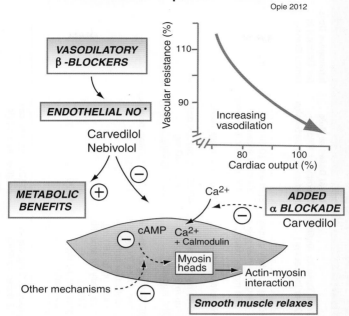

Figure 1-10 Vasodilatory mechanisms and effects. Vasodilatory β-blockers tend to decrease the cardiac output less as the systemic vascular resistance falls. Vasodilatory mechanisms include α-blockade (carvedilol), formation of nitric oxide (nebivolol and carvedilol), and intrinsic sympathomimetic activity (ISA). ISA, as in pindolol, has a specific effect in increasing sympathetic tone when it is low, as at night, and increasing nocturnal heart rate, which might be disadvantageous in nocturnal angina or unstable angina. (Figure © L. H. Opie, 2012.)

Pharmacokinetic Properties of β-Blockers

Plasma half-lives. Esmolol, given intravenously, has the shortest of all half-lives at only 9 min. Esmolol may therefore be preferable in unstable angina and threatened infarction when hemodynamic changes may call for withdrawal of β-blockade. The half-life of propranolol (Table 1-3) is only 3 hours, but continued administration saturates the hepatic process that removes propranolol from the circulation; the active metabolite 4-hydroxypropranolol is formed, and the effective half-life then becomes longer. The biological half-life of propranolol and metoprolol (and all other β-blockers) exceeds the plasma half-life considerably, so that twice-daily dosages of standard propranolol are effective even in angina pectoris. Clearly, the higher the dose of any β-blocker, the longer the biologic effects. Longer-acting compounds such as nadolol, sotalol, atenolol, and slow-release propranolol (Inderal-LA) or extended-release metoprolol (Toprol-XL) should be better for hypertension and effort angina.

Protein binding. Propranolol is highly bound, as are pindolol, labetalol, and bisoprolol. Hypoproteinemia calls for lower doses of such compounds.

First-pass liver metabolism. First-pass liver metabolism is found especially with the highly lipid-soluble compounds, such as propranolol, labetalol, and oxprenolol. Major hepatic clearance is also found with acebutolol, nebivolol, metoprolol, and timolol. First-pass metabolism varies greatly among patients and alters the dose required. In liver

Table 1-3

Properties of Various β-Adrenoceptor Antagonist Agents, Nonselective Versus Cardioselective and Vasodilatory Agents

Generic Name (Trade Name)	Extra Mechanism	Plasma Half-Life (h)	Lipid Solubility	First-Pass Effect	Loss by Liver or Kidney	Plasma Protein Binding (%)	Usual Dose for Angina (Other Indications)	Usual Doses as Sole Therapy for Mild or Moderate Hypertension	Intravenous Dose (as Licensed In United States)
Noncardioselective									
Propranolol*† (Inderal)	—	1-6	+++	++	Liver	90	80 mg 2× daily usually adequate (may give 160 mg 2× daily)	Start with 10-40 mg 2× daily. Mean 160-320 mg/day, 1-2 doses	1-6 mg
(Inderal-LA)	—	8-11	+++	++	Liver	90	80-320 mg 1× daily	80-320 mg 1× daily	—
Carteolol* (Cartrol)	ISA +	5-6	0/+	0	Kidney	20-30	(Not evaluated)	2.5-10 mg single dose	—
Nadolol*† (Corgard)	—	20-24	0	0	Kidney	30	40-80 mg 1× daily; up to 240 mg	40-80 mg/day 1× daily; up to 320 mg	—
Penbutolol (Levatol)	ISA +	20-25	+++	++	Liver	98	(Not studied)	10-20 mg daily	—
Sotalol† (Betapace; Betapace AF)	—	7-18 (mean 12)	0	0	Kidney	5	(80-240 mg 2× daily in two doses for serious ventricular arrhythmias; up to 160 mg 2× daily for atrial fib, flutter)	80-320 mg/day; mean 190 mg	—
Timolol† (Blocadren)	—	4-5	+	+	L, K	60	(post-AMI 10 mg 2× daily)	10-20 mg 2× daily	—
Cardioselective									
Acebutolol* (Sectral)	ISA ++	8-13 (diacetolol)	0 (diacetolol)	++	L, K	15	(400-1200 mg/day in 2 doses for PVC)	400-1200 mg/day; can be given as a single dose	—

Drug (Trade)		Half-life (h)	§[1]	§[2]	Elimination	%	Indication	Dose	IV dose
Atenolol*† (Tenormin)	—	6-7	0	0	Kidney	10	50-200 mg 1× daily	50-100 mg/day 1× daily	5 mg over 5 min; repeat 5 min later
Betaxolol* (Kerlone)	—	14-22	++	++	L, then K	50	—	10-20 mg 1× daily	—
Bisoprolol* (Zebeta)	—	9-12	0	+	L, K	30	10 mg 1× daily (not in US) (HF, see Table 1-2)	2.5-40 mg 1× daily (see also Ziac)	—
Metoprolol*† (Lopressor)	—	3-7	++	+	Liver	12	50-200 mg 2× daily (HF, see Table 1-2)	50-400 mg/day in 1 or 2 doses	5 mg 3× at 2 min intervals
Vasodilatory β-Blockers, Nonselective									
Labetalol* (Trandate) (Normodyne)	—	6-8	++	+++	L, some K	90	As for hypertension	300-600 mg/day in 3 doses; top dose 2400 mg/day	Up to 2 mg/min, up to 300 mg for severe HT
Pindolol* (Visken)	ISA +++	4	+	+	L, K	55	2.5-7.5 mg 3× daily (in UK, not US)	5-30 mg/day 2× daily	—
Carvedilol* (Coreg)	β₁, β₂; α-block; metabolic	6	++	+	Liver	95	(US, UK for heart failure) Angina in UK: up to 25 mg 2× daily	12.5-25 mg 2× daily	
Vasodilatory β-Blockers, Selective									
Nebivolol (Bistolic in USA; Nebilet in UK)	NO-vasodilation; metabolic	10 (24 h, metabolites)	+++ (genetic variation)	+++	L, K	98	Not in UK or US (in UK, heart failure, adjunct in older adults)	5 mg once daily; 2.5 mg in renal disease or older adults	—

§Octanol-water distribution coefficient (pH 7.4, 37° C) where 0 = <0.5; + = 0.5-2; ++ = 2-10; +++ = >10

*Approved by FDA for hypertension.

†Approved for angina pectoris.

‡Approved for life-threatening ventricular tachyarrhythmias.

§Metabolic, insulin sensitivity increased.

AMI, Acute myocardial infarction; FDA, Food and Drug Administration; fib, fibrillation; HF, heart failure; HT, hypertension; ISA, intrinsic sympathomimetic activity; K, kidney; L, liver; NO, nitric oxide; PVC, premature ventricular contractions.

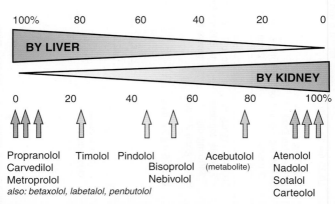

ROUTE OF ELIMINATION
Opie 2012

Figure 1-11 Comparative routes of elimination of β-blockers. Those most hydrophilic and least lipid-soluble are excreted unchanged by the kidneys. Those most lipophilic and least water-soluble are largely metabolized by the liver. Note that the metabolite of acebutolol, diacetolol, is largely excreted by the kidney, in contrast to the parent compound. (For derivation of data in figure, see third edition. Estimated data points for acebutolol and newer agents added.) (Figure © L. H. Opie, 2012.)

disease or low-output states the dose should be decreased. First-pass metabolism produces active metabolites with, in the case of propranolol, properties different from those of the parent compound. Metabolism of metoprolol occurs predominantly via cytochrome P450 2D6–mediated hydroxylation and is subject to marked genetic variability.[93] Acebutolol produces large amounts of diacetolol, and is also cardioselective with ISA, but with a longer half-life and chiefly excreted by the kidneys (Fig. 1-11). Lipid-insoluble hydrophilic compounds (atenolol, sotalol, nadolol) are excreted only by the kidneys (see Fig. 1-11) and have low brain penetration. In patients with renal or liver disease, the simpler pharmacokinetic patterns of lipid-insoluble agents make dosage easier. As a group, these agents have low protein binding (see Table 1-3).

Pharmacokinetic interactions. Those drugs metabolized by the liver and hence prone to hepatic interactions are metoprolol, carvedilol, labetalol, and propranolol, of which metoprolol and carvedilol are more frequently used. Both are metabolized by the hepatic CYP2D6 system that is inhibited by paroxetine, a widely used antidepressant that is a selective serotonin reuptake inhibitor. To avoid such hepatic interactions, it is simpler to use those β-blockers not metabolized by the liver (see Fig. 1-11). β-blockers, in turn, depress hepatic blood flow so that the blood levels of lidocaine increase with greater risk of lidocaine toxicity.

Concomitant Diseases and Choice of β-blocker

Respiratory disease. Cardioselective β₁-blockers in low doses are best for patients with reversible bronchospasm. In patients with a history of asthma, no β-blocker can be considered safe.

Associated cardiovascular disease. For *hypertension plus effort angina*, see "β-blockers for hypertension" earlier in this chapter. In patients with *sick sinus syndrome,* pure β-blockade can be dangerous. Added ISA may be best. In patients with *Raynaud phenomenon,* propranolol with its peripheral vasoconstrictive effects is best avoided. In active *peripheral vascular disease,* β-blockers are generally contraindicated, although the evidence is not firm.

Renal disease. The logical choice should be a β-blocker eliminated by the liver rather than the kidney (see Fig. 1-11). Of those, the vasodilating β-blocker nebivolol conserved the estimated glomerular filtration rate in patients with heart failure better than did metoprolol.[99]

Diabetes mellitus. In diabetes mellitus, the risk of β-blockade in insulin-requiring diabetics is that the symptoms of hypoglycemia might be masked. There is a lesser risk with the cardioselective agents. In type 2 diabetics with hypertension, initial β-blocker therapy by atenolol was as effective as the ACE inhibitor, captopril, in reducing macrovascular end points at the cost of weight gain and more antidiabetic medication.[47] Whether *diabetic nephropathy* benefits as much from treatment with β-blockade is not clear. ARBs and ACE inhibitors have now established themselves as agents of first choice in diabetic nephropathy (see Chapter 5, p. 136). Carvedilol combined with RAS blocker therapy in diabetic patients with hypertension results in better glycemic control and less insulin resistance than combination therapy that includes metoprolol.[100] Although better glycemic control should theoretically translate into fewer cardiovascular events and other adverse outcomes, the short-term nature of this study does not allow conclusions on outcomes.

Those at risk of new diabetes. The β-blocker and diuretics pose a risk of new diabetes,[35] which should be lessened by a truly low dose of the diuretic or by using another combination. Regular blood glucose checks are desirable.

Side Effects of β-Blockers

The *four major mechanisms for β-blocker side effects* are (1) smooth muscle spasm (bronchospasm and cold extremities), (2) exaggeration of the cardiac therapeutic actions (bradycardia, heart block, excess negative inotropic effect), (3) central nervous system penetration (insomnia, depression), and (4) adverse metabolic side effects. The *mechanism of fatigue* is not clear. When compared with propranolol, however, it is reduced by use of either a cardioselective β-blocker or a vasodilatory agent, so that both central and peripheral hemodynamic effects may be involved. When patients are appropriately selected, double-blind studies show no differences between a cardioselective agent such as atenolol and placebo. This may be because atenolol is not lipid soluble and should have lesser effects on bronchial and vascular smooth muscle than propranolol. When *propranolol* is given for hypertension, the rate of serious side effects (bronchospasm, cold extremities, worsening of claudication) leading to withdrawal of therapy is approximately 10%.[101] The rate of withdrawal with atenolol is considerably lower (approximately 2%), but when it comes to dose-limiting side effects, both agents can cause cold extremities, fatigue, dreams, worsening claudication, and bronchospasm. Increasing heart failure remains a potential hazard when β-blockade therapy is abruptly started at normal doses in a susceptible patient and not tailored in.

Central side effects. An attractive hypothesis is that the lipid-soluble β-blockers (epitomized by propranolol) with their high brain penetration are more likely to cause central side effects. An extremely detailed comparison of propranolol and atenolol showed that the latter, which is not lipid soluble, causes far fewer central side effects than does propranolol.[102] However, depression remains an atenolol risk.[42] The lipid-solubility hypothesis also does not explain why metoprolol, which is moderately lipid soluble, appears to interfere less with some complex psychological functions than does atenolol and may even enhance certain aspects of psychological performance.[103]

Quality of life and sex life. In the first quality-of-life study reported in patients with hypertension, propranolol induced considerably more central effects than did the ACE inhibitor captopril.[104] More modern β-blockers, with different fundamental properties, all leave the quality of life largely intact in hypertensives. However, there are a number of negatives. First, *weight gain* is undesirable and contrary to the lifestyle pattern required to limit cardiovascular diseases, including the metabolic syndrome and hypertension. Second, β-blockade may precipitate *diabetes*,[50] a disease that severely limits the quality of life. Third, during *exercise*, β-blockade reduces the total work possible by approximately 15% and increases the sense of fatigue. Vasodilatory β-blockers may be exceptions but lack outcome studies in hypertension. *Erectile dysfunction* is an age-dependent complication of β-blockade. In a large group with mean age 48 years, erectile problems took place in 11% given a β-blocker, compared with 26% with a diuretic and 3% with placebo.[105] β-blockers have consistently impaired sexual intercourse more than an ACE inhibitor or ARB, the latter improving sexual output.[106] Changing to nebivolol may improve erections.[107] Sildenafil (Viagra) or similar agents should also help, but are relatively contraindicated if the β-blocker is used for angina (because of the adverse interaction with nitrates, almost always used in those with angina).

Adverse metabolic side effects and new diabetes. The capacity of β-blockers to increase new diabetes, whether given for hypertension or postinfarct,[35] comes at a time when diabetes is increasingly recognized as major cardiovascular hazard (see Chapters 7 and 11). A wise precaution is to obtain fasting blood glucose levels and, if indicated, a glucose tolerance curve before the onset of chronic β-blockade and at annual intervals during therapy. Note that the vasodilatory β-blockers carvedilol and nebivolol both promote formation of nitric oxide and both have a better metabolic profile than comparator cardioselective agents, without, however, long-term outcome data in hypertension (see "Specific β-Blockers" later in this chapter).

Contraindications to β-Blockade

The absolute contraindications to β-blockade can be deduced from the profile of pharmacologic effects and side effects (Table 1-4). Cardiac absolute contraindications include severe bradycardia, preexisting high-degree heart block, sick sinus syndrome, and overt LV failure unless already conventionally treated and stable (Fig. 1-12). Pulmonary contraindications are overt asthma or severe bronchospasm; depending on the severity of the disease and the cardioselectivity of the β-blocker used, these may be absolute or relative contraindications. The central nervous system contraindication is severe depression (especially for propranolol). Active peripheral vascular disease with rest ischemia is another contraindication. The metabolic syndrome suggests caution.

Overdose of β-Blockers

Bradycardia may be countered by intravenous atropine 1 to 2 mg; if serious, temporary transvenous pacing may be required. When an infusion is required, glucagon (2.5 to 7.5 mg/h) is logical because it stimulates formation of cAMP by bypassing the occupied β-receptor. However, evidence is only anecdotal.[108] Logically an infusion of a phosphodiesterase inhibitor,

Table 1-4

β-Blockade: Contraindications and Cautions

(Note: cautions may be overridden by the imperative to treat, as in postinfarct patients)

Cardiac

Absolute: Severe bradycardia, high-degree heart block, cardiogenic shock, overt untreated left ventricular failure (versus major use in early or stabilized heart failure).
Relative: Prinzmetal's angina (unopposed α-spasm), high doses of other agents depressing SA or AV nodes (verapamil, diltiazem, digoxin, antiarrhythmic agents); in angina, *avoid sudden withdrawal.*

Pulmonary

Absolute: Severe asthma or bronchospasm. Must question for past or present asthma. Risk of fatalities.
Relative: Mild asthma or bronchospasm or chronic airways disease. Use agents with cardioselectivity plus β$_2$-stimulants (by inhalation).

Central Nervous

Absolute: Severe depression (especially avoid propranolol).
Relative: Vivid dreams: avoid highly lipid-soluble agents (see Fig. 1-11) and pindolol; avoid evening dose. Visual hallucinations: change from propranolol. Fatigue (all agents). If low cardiac output is cause of fatigue, try vasodilatory β-blockers. Erectile dysfunction may occur (check for diuretic use; consider change to nebivolol and/or ACE inhibitor/ARB). Psychotropic drugs (with adrenergic augmentation) may adversely interact.

Peripheral Vascular, Raynaud Phenomenon

Absolute: Active disease: gangrene, skin necrosis, severe or worsening claudication, rest pain.
Relative: Cold extremities, absent pulses, Raynaud phenomenon. Avoid nonselective agents (propranolol, sotalol, nadolol); prefer vasodilatory agents.

Diabetes Mellitus

Relative: Insulin-requiring diabetes: nonselective agents decrease reaction to hypoglycemia; use selective agents. Note successful use of atenolol in type 2 diabetes in prolonged UK trial at cost of weight gain and more antidiabetic drug usage.

Metabolic Syndrome or Prediabetes

β-blockers may increase blood sugar by 1-1.5 mmol/L and impair insulin sensitivity especially with diuretic co-therapy; consider use of carvedilol or nebivolol.

Renal Failure

Relative: As renal blood flow falls, reduce doses of agents eliminated by kidney (see Fig. 1-11).

Liver Disease

Relative: Avoid agents with high hepatic clearance (propranolol, carvedilol, timolol, acebutolol, metoprolol). Use agents with low clearance (atenolol, nadolol, sotalol). See Fig 1-11. If plasma proteins low, reduce dose of highly bound agents (propranolol, pindolol, bisoprolol).

Pregnancy Hypertension

β-blockade increasingly used but may depress vital signs in neonate and cause uterine vasoconstriction. Labetalol and atenolol best tested. Preferred drug: methyldopa.

Surgical Operations

β-blockade may be maintained throughout, provided indication is not trivial; otherwise stop 24 to 48 hours beforehand. May protect against anesthetic arrhythmias and perioperative ischemia. Preferred intravenous drug: esmolol. Use atropine for bradycardia, β-agonist for severe hypotension.

Age

β-blockade often helps to reduce BP, but lacks positive outcome data. Watch pharmacokinetics and side effects in all older adult patients.

Continued

Table 1-4

β-Blockade: Contraindications and Cautions (Continued)
Smoking
In hypertension, β-blockade is less effective in reducing coronary events in smoking men.
Hyperlipidemia
β-blockers may have unfavorable effects on the blood lipid profile, especially nonselective agents. Triglycerides increase and HDL-cholesterol falls. Clinical significance unknown, but may worsen metabolic syndrome. Vasodilatory agents, with intrinsic sympathomimetic activity or α-blocking activity, may have mildly favorable effects.

ACE, Angiotensin-converting enzyme; *AV,* atrioventricular; *ARB,* angiotensin receptor blocker; *BP,* blood pressure; *HDL,* high-density lipoprotein; *SA,* sinoatrial.
Adapted from Kjeldssen, LIFE elderly substudy, *JAMA* 2002;288:1491.

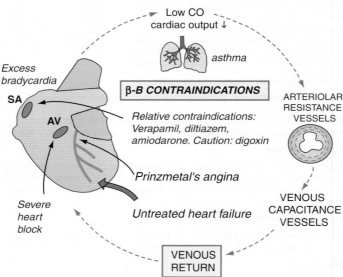

Figure 1-12   Contraindications to β-blockade. Metabolic syndrome (not shown) is a relative contraindication to β-blockade for hypertension. (Figure © L. H. Opie, 2012.)

such as amrinone or milrinone, should help cAMP to accumulate. Alternatively, dobutamine is given in doses high enough to overcome the competitive β-blockade (15 mcg/kg/min). In patients without ischemic heart disease, an infusion (up to 0.10 mcg/kg/min) of isoproterenol may be used.

Specific β-Blockers

Of the large number of β-blockers, the ideal agent for hypertension or angina might have (1) advantageous pharmacokinetics (simplicity, agents not metabolized in liver); (2) a high degree of cardioselectivity (bisoprolol); (3) long duration of action (several); and (4) a favorable metabolic profile, especially when associated with vasodilatory properties (carvedilol and nebivolol).

   Propranolol *(Inderal)* is the historical gold standard because it is licensed for so many different indications, including angina, acute-stage

MI, postinfarct follow-up, hypertension, arrhythmias, migraine prophylaxis, anxiety states, and essential tremor. However, propranolol is not β_1-selective. Being lipid soluble, it has a high brain penetration and undergoes extensive hepatic first-pass metabolism. Central side effects may explain its poor performance in quality-of-life studies. Propranolol also has a short half-life so that it must be given twice daily unless long-acting preparations are used. The chief of the other agents are dealt with alphabetically.

Acebutolol *(Sectral)* is the cardioselective agent with ISA that gave a good quality of life in the 4-year TOMH study in mild hypertension. In particular, the incidence of impotence was not increased.[109]

Atenolol *(Tenormin)* was one of the first of the cardioselective agents and now in generic form is one of the most widely used drugs in angina, in postinfarct protection, and in hypertension. However, its use as first-line agent in hypertension is falling into disfavor,[110] with poor outcomes, including increased all-cause mortality when compared with the CCB amlodipine in ASCOT.[34] There are very few trials with outcome data for atenolol in other conditions, with two exceptions: the ASIST study in silent ischemia[15] and INVEST in hypertensives with coronary artery disease. Here atenolol had equality of major clinical outcomes with verapamil at the cost of more episodes of angina, more new diabetes, and more psychological depression.[41,111] Note that atenolol was often combined with a diuretic and verapamil with an ACE inhibitor. In the British Medical Research Council trial of hypertension in older adults, atenolol did not reduce coronary events.[88] More recently, atenolol was inferior to the ARB losartan in the therapy of hypertensives with LVH.[112]

Bisoprolol *(Zebeta in the United States, Cardicor or Emcor in the United Kingdom)* is a highly β_1-selective agent, more so than atenolol, licensed for hypertension, angina heart failure in the United Kingdom but only for hypertension in the United States. It was the drug used in the large and successful CIBIS-2 study in heart failure, in which there was a large reduction not only in total mortality but also in sudden death.[113] In CIBIS-3, bisoprolol compared well with enalapril as first-line agent in heart failure.[80] A combination of low-dose bisoprolol and low-dose hydrochlorothiazide (Ziac) is available in the United States (see Combination Therapy on page 11).

Carvedilol *(Coreg in the United States, Eucardic in the United Kingdom)* is a nonselective vasodilator α-β-blocker with multimechanism vasodilatory properties mediated by antioxidant activity, formation of nitric oxide, stimulation β-arrestin-MAP-kinase[65] and α-receptors, that has been extensively studied in CHF[61] and in postinfarct LV dysfunction.[29] Metabolically, carvedilol may increase insulin sensitivity.[49] In the United States, it is registered for hypertension, for CHF (mild to severe), and for post-MI LV dysfunction (EF ≤ 40%), but not for angina.

Labetalol *(Trandate, Normodyne)* is a combined α- and β-blocking antihypertensive agent that has now largely been supplanted by carvedilol except for acute intravenous use as in hypertensive crises (see Table 7-4 on page 261).

Metoprolol *(Toprol-XL)* is cardioselective and particularly well studied in AMI and in postinfarct protection. Toprol-XL is approved in the United States for stable symptomatic Class 2 or 3 heart failure.[114] It is also registered for hypertension and angina. *Lopressor, shorter acting,* is licensed for angina and MI.

Nadolol *(Corgard)* is very long acting and water soluble, although it is nonselective. It is particularly useful when prolonged antianginal activity is required.

Nebivolol *(Nebilet in the United Kingdom, Bystolic in the United States)* is a highly cardioselective agent with peripheral vasodilating properties mediated by nitric oxide.[6] Hepatic metabolites probably account for the vasodilation[115] and the long biological half-life.[116] Nebivolol reverses endothelial dysfunction in hypertension, which may explain its use for erectile dysfunction in hypertensives.[107] There are also metabolic benefits. In a 6-month study, nebivolol, in contrast to atenolol and at equal BP levels, increased insulin sensitivity and adiponectin levels in hypertensives.[117] Nebivolol given in the SENIORS trial to older adult patients with a history of heart failure or an EF of 35% or less reduced the primary composite end-point of all-cause mortality and cardiovascular hospitalizations, also increasing the EF and reducing heart size.[78]

Penbutolol *(Levatol)* has a modest ISA, similar to acebutolol, but is nonselective. It is highly lipid-soluble and is metabolized by the liver.

Sotalol *(Betapace, Betapace AF)* is a unique nonselective β-blocker that has Class 3 antiarrhythmic activity. It is licensed for life-threatening ventricular arrhythmias as Betapace, and now also as Betapace AF for maintenance of sinus rhythm in patients with symptomatic atrial fibrillation or atrial flutter. Sotalol is a water-soluble drug, excreted only by the kidneys, so that Betapace AF is contraindicated in patients with a creatinine clearance of less than 40 mL/min.

Timolol *(Blocarden)* was the first β-blocker shown to give postinfarct protection and it is one of the few licensed for this purpose in the United States. Other approved uses are for hypertension and in migraine prophylaxis.

Ultrashort-Acting Intravenous β-Blockade

Esmolol *(Brevibloc)* is an ultrashort-acting β_1-blocker with a half-life of 9 minutes, rapidly converting to inactive metabolites by blood esterases. Full recovery from β-blockade occurs within 30 minutes in patients with a normal cardiovascular system. *Indications* are situations in which on-off control of β-blockade is desired, as in SVT in the perioperative period, or sinus tachycardia (noncompensatory), or emergency hypertension in the perioperative period (all registered uses in the United States). Other logical indications are emergency hypertension (pheochromocytoma excluded) or in unstable angina.[118] *Doses* are as follows: For *SVT,* loading by 500 mcg/kg/min over 1 minute, followed by a 4-minute infusion of 50 mcg/kg/min (US package insert). If this fails, repeat loading dose and increase infusion to 100 mcg/kg/min (over 4 minutes). If this fails, repeat loading dose and then infuse at rates up to 300 mcg/kg/min. Thereafter, to maintain control, infuse at adjusted rate for up to 24 hours. For *urgent perioperative hypertension,* give 80 mg (approximately 1 mg/kg) over 30 seconds and infuse at 150 to 300 mcg/kg/min if needed. For more gradual control of BP, follow routine for SVT. Higher doses are usually required for BP control than for arrhythmias. After the emergency, replace with conventional antiarrhythmic or antihypertensive drugs. For *older adult patients with non-ST elevation MI* requiring acute β-blockade despite symptoms of heart failure, a cautious infusion of 50-200 mcg/kg/min may be tried.[119] *Cautions* include extravasation of the acid solution with risk of skin necrosis.

From the Past, into the Future

Predictions are often wrong. Nonetheless, trends can be identified, looking both backward and forward (Fig. 1-13). Originally, β-blockers were created by Sir James Black in 1962 to counter adrenergic stimulation in effort angina, for which he later received the Nobel Prize. In 1964 Brian Prichard discovered the antihypertensive properties. In 1975 Waagstein and Hjalmarson showed clinical improvement following β-blockade in seven patients with advanced congestive cardiomyopathy. In 1981 the Norwegian Study Group reported a major benefit for β-blockade in postinfarct patients. In 1986 in ISIS-1, a ground-breaking mega-trial on AMI, the Oxford group of Peter Sleight found that acute

CHANGING PATTERNS OF
β-BLOCKER USE
Opie 2012

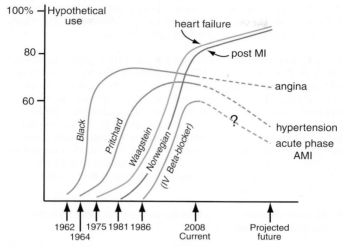

Figure 1-13 Hypothetical patterns of change of β-blocker use over time.
See text for details. (Dr. J. D. Horowitz is thanked for discussions leading to
this figure. Figure © J. D. Horowitz.)

β-blockade diminished postinfarct mortality. Currently, use in uncomplicated hypertension as first-line agent is under challenge. Projecting into
the future, evidence-based use of β-blockade will be optimal in heart
failure and in postinfarct patients, with a slight decline in angina as
metabolic agents come into greater use. There already is and there will
be a greater trend away from β-blockers as agents of first choice in
uncomplicated hypertension.

SUMMARY

1. *Despite some setbacks in recent hypertension trials,*
β-blockers still come closest to providing all-purpose cardiovascular therapy with the conspicuous absence of any benefit for lipid
problems. Licensed indications include angina, hypertension, AMI,
postinfarct follow-up, arrhythmias, and now heart failure. Data for
postinfarct protection and for mortality reduction in CHF are
particularly impressive. Other data are less compelling (Table 1-5).

2. *In heart failure,* solid data support the essential and earlier
use of β-blockers in stable systolic heart failure, to counter the
excessive adrenergic drive. Only three agents have been studied in
detail, namely carvedilol, metoprolol, and bisoprolol, of which only
the first two are approved for heart failure in the United States. In
older adults, nebivolol improved EF in systolic but not diastolic
heart failure. Following the recommended protocol with slow,
incremental doses of the chosen agent is essential.

3. *For coronary heart disease,* β-blockade is very effective
symptomatic treatment, alone or combined with other drugs, in 70%
to 80% of patients with classic effort angina. However, atenolol-based

therapy was no better at lessening major outcomes than verapamil-based therapy, and worse for some minor outcomes. β-blockers are part of the essential postinfarct protection armamentarium. For ACSs, indirect evidence suggests a quadruple follow-up regime of aspirin, statin, ACE inhibitor, and β-blockade, but there are no compelling outcome trials. Overall, there is no clinical evidence that β-blockers slow the development of coronary artery disease.

4. *In hypertension* β-blockers have lost their prime position, although they reduce the BP effectively in 50% to 70% of those with mild to moderate hypertension. The crucial study showed that for equal brachial pressures, the aortic pressure was less reduced with atenolol than with the CCB amlodipine, which could explain why β-blockers reduce stroke less than several other agents. Older adults with hypertension, especially those of the black ethnic group, respond less well to β-blocker monotherapy. The previously recommended combination of β-blockers and diuretics may provoke new diabetes, with lesser risk if the diuretic dose is truly low.

5. *In arrhythmias* β-blockers are among the more effective ventricular antiarrhythmics.

6. *Metabolic side-effects,* including new diabetes, have come to the fore. β-blockers can be diabetogenic even without diuretics. The vasodilatory β-blockers carvedilol and nebivolol appear to be exceptions and have outcome studies only in heart failure.

7. *Is there still a role for propranolol?* There is no particular advantage for this original "gold standard" drug, with its poor quality-of-life outcomes, unless hypertension or angina with some other condition in which experience with propranolol is greater than with other β-blockers (e.g., POTS, hypertrophic cardiomyopathy, migraine prophylaxis, anxiety, or essential tremor) is also occurring.

8. *Other β-blockers* are increasingly used because of specific attractive properties: cardioselectivity (acebutolol, atenolol, bisoprolol, metoprolol), vasodilatory capacity and possible metabolic superiority (carvedilol and nebivolol), positive data in heart failure (carvedilol, metoprolol, bisoprolol, nebivolol) or postinfarct protection (metoprolol, carvedilol, timolol), lipid insolubility and no hepatic metabolism (atenolol, nadolol, sotalol), long action (nadolol) or long-acting formulations, ISA in selected patients to help avoid bradycardia (pindolol, acebutolol), and well-studied antiarrhythmic properties (sotalol). Esmolol is the best agent for intravenous use in the perioperative period because of its extremely short half-life.

9. *Evidence-based use* directs the use of those agents established in large trials because of the known doses and clearly expected benefits. For example, for postinfarct protection propranolol, metoprolol, carvedilol, and timolol are the best studied, of which only carvedilol has been studied in the reperfusion era. For stabilized heart failure, carvedilol, metoprolol, and bisoprolol have impressive data from large trials. Carvedilol especially merits attention, being licensed for a wide clinical range, from hypertension to LV dysfunction to severe heart failure, and having best trial data in heart failure. For arrhythmias, sotalol with its class III properties stands out.

Table 1-5

Conditions	Must Use* (Level A)	May Use (Level B)	Don't Use (Data Poor)
Summary of use of β-Blockers in Cardiovascular Disease			
Heart failure	✓✓		
Post-MI	✓✓		
Arrhythmias (ventricular, post-MI)	✓✓		
Arrhythmias (others)		✓	
ACS, unstable angina (NSTE)		✓	
ACS, acute-phase MI		✓	
Stable angina without MI		✓	
Hypertension (initial choice)			Selective
Hypertension (selected)		✓	
Metabolic syndrome			Careful

Note: "Must use" can override "Don't use."
   *Unless contraindicated.
   ✓✓ = strongly indicated; ✓ = indicated.
   ACS, Acute coronary syndrome; *MI,* myocardial infarction; *NSTE,* non-ST elevation.
   For concepts, see reference 110.

References

1. Brodde OE. Beta-adrenoceptor blocker treatment and the cardiac beta-adrenoceptor-G-protein(s)-adenylyl cyclase system in chronic heart failure. *Naunyn Schmiedebergs Arch Pharmacol* 2007;374:361–372.
2. Opie LH, et al. Cardiac survival strategies: an evolutionary hypothesis with rationale for metabolic therapy of acute heart failure. *Transact Royal Soc South Africa* 2010:65:185–189.
3. DiPilato LM, et al. FRETting mice shed light on cardiac adrenergic signaling. *Circ Res* 2006;99:1021–1023.
4. Lefkowitz RJ, et al. Transduction of receptor signals by beta-arrestins. *Science* 2005;308:512–517.
5. Dessy C, et al. Endothelial beta-3-adrenoreceptors mediate nitric oxide-dependent vasorelaxation of coronary microvessels in response to the third-generation beta-blocker nebivolol. *Circulation* 2005;112:1198–1205.
6. Heusch G. Beta(3)-adrenoceptor activation just says NO to myocardial reperfusion injury. *J Am Coll Cardiol* 2011;58:2692–2694.
7. Wallhaus TR, et al. Myocardial free fatty acid and glucose use after carvedilol treatment in patients with congestive heart failure. *Circulation* 2001;103:2441–2446.
8. Brodde OE, et al. Cardiac adrenoceptors: physiological and pathophysiological relevance. *J Pharmacol Sci* 2006;100:323–337.
9. Heilbrunn SM, et al. Increased beta-receptor density and improved hemodynamic response to catecholamine stimulation during long-term metoprolol therapy in heart failure from dilated cardiomyopathy. *Circulation* 1989;79:483–490.
10. Boden WE, et al. Optimal medical therapy with or without PCI for stable coronary disease. *N Engl J Med* 2007;356:1503–1516.
11. Poole-Wilson PA, et al. Effect of long-acting nifedipine on mortality and cardiovascular morbidity in patients with stable angina requiring treatment (ACTION trial): randomised controlled trial. *Lancet* 2004;364:849–857.
12. Kugiyama K, et al. Effects of propranolol and nifedipine on exercise-induced attack in patients with variant angina: assessment by exercise thallium-201 myocardial scintigraphy with quantitative rotational tomography. *Circulation* 1986;74:374–380.
13. Peart I, et al. Cold intolerance in patients with angina pectoris: effect of nifedipine and propranolol. *Br Heart J* 1989;61:521–528.
14. Kern MJ, et al. Potentiation of coronary vasoconstriction by beta-adrenergic blockade in patients with coronary artery disease. *Circulation* 1983;67:1178–1185.
15. ASIST study, Pepine C, et al. Effects of treatment on outcome in mildly symptomatic patients with ischemia during daily life. The Atenolol Silent Ischemia Study (ASIST). *Circulation* 1994;90:762–768.
16. Mukherjee D, et al. Impact of combination evidence-based medical therapy on mortality in patients with acute coronary syndromes. *Circulation* 2004;109:745–749.
17. Yusuf S, et al. Reduction in infarct size, arrhythmias and chest pain by early intravenous beta blockade in suspected acute myocardial infarction. *Circulation* 1983;67 (Suppl I): I32–I41.
18. HINT Study. Early treatment of unstable angina in the coronary care unit, a randomised, double-blind placebo controlled comparison of recurrent ischemia in patients treated with nifedipine or metoprolol or both. Holland Inter-university Nifedipine Trial. *Br Heart J* 1986;56:400–413.

19. Miller CD, et al. Impact of acute beta-blocker therapy for patients with non-ST-segment elevation myocardial infarction. *Am J Med* 2007;120:685–692.

20. Ryden L, et al. A double-blind trial of metoprolol in acute myocardial infarction. *N Engl J Med* 1983;308:614–618.

21. Norris RM, et al. Prevention of ventricular fibrillation during acute myocardial infarction by intravenous propranolol. *Lancet* 1984;883–886.

22. Chen ZM, et al. Early intravenous then oral metoprolol in 45,852 patients with acute myocardial infarction: randomised placebo-controlled trial. *Lancet* 2005;366:1622–1632.

23. Bates ER. Role of intravenous beta-blockers in the treatment of ST-elevation myocardial infarction: of mice (dogs, pigs) and men. *Circulation* 2007;115:2904–2906.

24. Antman EM, et al. 2007 Focused update of the ACC/AHA 2004 guidelines for the management of patients with ST-elevation myocardial infarction. *Circulation* 2008;117:296–329.

25. Smith Jr SC. Secondary prevention and risk reduction therapy for patients with coronary and other atherosclerotic vascular disease: 2011 update: a guideline from the AHA and ACC Foundation. *Circulation* 2011;124:2458–2473.

26. Freemantle N, et al. β-blockade after myocardial infarction: systemic review and meta regression analysis. *Br Med J* 1999;318:1730–1737.

27. Gottlieb SS, et al. Effect of beta-blockade on mortality among high-risk and low-risk patients after myocardial infarction. *N Engl J Med* 1998;339:489–497.

28. Olsson G, et al. Long-term treatment with metoprolol after myocardial infarction: effect on 3-year mortality and morbidity. *J Am Coll Cardiol* 1985;5:1428–1437.

29. CAPRICORN Investigators. Effect of carvedilol on outcome after myocardial infarction in patients with left-ventricular dysfunction: the CAPRICORN randomised trial. *Lancet* 2001;357:1385–1390.

30. Teo KK, et al. Effects of prophylactic antiarrhythmic drug therapy in acute myocardial infarction: an overview of results from randomized controlled trials. *JAMA* 1993; 270:1589–1595.

31. SAVE Study, Pfeffer MA, et al. Effect of captopril on mortality and morbidity in patients with left ventricular dysfunction after myocardial infarction: results of the Survival and Ventricular Enlargement trial. *N Eng J Med* 1992;327:669–677.

32. Heidenreich PA, et al. Meta-analysis of trials comparing β-blockers, calcium antagonists, and nitrates for stable angina. *JAMA* 1999;281:1927–1936.

33. Krause T, et al for the Guideline Development Group. Management of hypertension: summary of NICE guidance. *Br Med J* 2011 Aug 25;343:d4891.

34. Dahlöf B, et al. Prevention of cardiovascular events with an antihypertensive regimen of amlodipine adding perindopril as required versus atenolol adding bendroflumethiazide as required, in the Anglo-Scandinavian Cardiac Outcomes Trial-Blood Pressure Lowering Arm (ASCOT-BPLA): a multicentre randomised controlled trial. *Lancet* 2005;366:895–906.

35. Lam SK. Incident diabetes in clinical trials of antihypertensive drugs. *Lancet* 2007;369:1514–1515.

36. Williams B. Beta-blockers and the treatment of hypertension. *J Hypertens* 2007;25: 1351–1353.

37. Williams B, et al. Differential impact of blood pressure-lowering drugs on central aortic pressure and clinical outcomes: principal results of the Conduit Artery Function Evaluation (CAFE) study. *Circulation* 2006;113:1213–1225.

38. Chobanian AV, et al. The seventh report of the Joint National Committee on Prevention, Detection, Evaluation and Treatment of High Blood Pressure. *JAMA* 2003;289:2560–2572.

39. Psaty BM, et al. Health outcomes associated with antihypertensive therapies used as first-line agents: a systemic review and meta-analysis. *JAMA* 1997;277:739–745.

40. Rosendorff C, et al. Treatment of hypertension in the prevention and management of ischemic heart disease: a scientific statement from the American Heart Association Council for High Blood Pressure Research and the Councils on Clinical Cardiology and Epidemiology and Prevention. *Circulation* 2007;115:2761–2788.

41. Pepine CJ, et al. A calcium antagonist vs a non-calcium antagonist hypertension treatment strategy for patients with coronary artery disease. The International Verapamil-Trandolapril Study (INVEST): a randomized controlled trial. *JAMA* 2003;290:2805–2816.

42. Ried LD, et al. A Study of Antihypertensive Drugs and Depressive Symptoms (SADD-Sx) in patients treated with a calcium antagonist versus an atenolol hypertension treatment strategy in the International Verapamil SR-Trandolapril Study (INVEST). *Psychosom Med* 2005;67:398–406.

43. Messerli FH, et al. Are beta-blockers efficacious as first-line therapy for hypertension in the elderly? A systematic review. *JAMA* 1998;279:1903–1907.

44. Kjeldsen SE, et al. For the LIFE Study Group. Effects of losartan on cardiovascular morbidity and mortality in patients with isolated systolic hypertension and left ventricular hypertrophy. *JAMA* 2002;288:1491–1498.

45. Morgan T, et al. Effect of different antihypertensive drug classes on central aortic pressure. *Am J Hypertens* 2004;17:118–123.

46. Materson BJ, et al. Single-drug therapy for hypertension in men: a comparison of six antihypertensive agents with placebo. The Department of Veterans Affairs Cooperative Study Group on Antihypertensive Agents. *N Engl J Med* 1993;328:914–921.

47. UKPDS 39. UK Prospective Diabetes Study Group. Efficacy of atenolol and captopril in reducing risk of macrovascular and microvascular complications in type 2 diabetes: UKPDS 39. *Br Med J* 1998;317:713–720.

48. Dunder K, et al. Increase in blood glucose concentration during antihypertensive treatment as a predictor of myocardial infarction: population based cohort study. *Br Med J* 2003;326:681–685.

49. Lithell H, et al. Metabolic effects of carvedilol in hypertensive patients. *Eur J Clin Pharmacol* 1997;52:13–17.

50. Gress TW, et al. For the Atherosclerosis Risk in Communities Study. Hypertension and antihypertensives therapy as risk factors for type 2 diabetes mellitus. *N Engl J Med* 2000;342:905–912.

51. Lubbe WH, et al. Potential arrhythmogenic role of cyclic adenosine monophosphate (AMP) and cytosolic calcium overload: implications for prophylactic effects of beta-blockers in myocardial infarction and proarrhythmic effects of phosphodiesterase inhibitors. *J Am Coll Cardiol* 1992;19:1622–1633.

52. Pogwizd SM, et al. Arrhythmogenesis and contractile dysfunction in heart failure. *Circ Res* 2001;88:1159–1167.

53. Steinbeck G, et al. A comparison of electrophysiologically guided antiarrhythmic drug therapy with beta-blocker therapy in patients with symptomatic, sustained ventricular tachyarrhythmias. *N Engl J Med* 1992;327:987–992.

54. ESVEM Study, Mason JW. A comparison of seven antiarrhythmic drugs in patients with ventricular tachyarrhythmias. Electrophysiologic Study versus Electrocardiographic Monitoring Investigators. *N Engl J Med* 1993;329:452–458.

55. Boutitie F, et al. Amiodarone interactions with beta-blockers. Analysis of the merged EMIAT (European Myocardial Infarct Trial) and CAMIAT (Canadian Amiodarone Myocardial Infarct Trial) databases. *Circulation* 1999;99:2268–2275.

56. Kennedy HL, et al. β-blocker therapy in the cardiac arrhythmia suppression trial. *Am J Cardiol* 1994;74:674–680.

57. Ellison KE, et al. Effect of beta-blocking therapy on outcome in the Multicenter UnSustained Tachycardia Trial (MUSTT). *Circulation* 2002;106:2694–2699.

58. Bardy GH, et al. Sudden cardiac death in heart failure trial (SCD-HeFT) investigators. *N Engl J Med* 2005;352:225–237. Erratum in *N Engl J Med* 2005;352:2146.

59. Bradley D, et al. Pharmacologic prophylaxis: American College of Chest Physicians guidelines for the prevention and management of postoperative atrial fibrillation after cardiac surgery. *Chest* 2005;128:39S-47S.

60. Lowes BD, et al. Myocardial gene expression in dilated cardiomyopathy treated with beta-blocking agents. *N Engl J Med* 2002;346:1357–1365.

61. Poole-Wilson PA, et al. Comparison of carvedilol and metoprolol on clinical outcomes in patients with chronic heart failure in the Carvedilol Or Metoprolol European Trial (COMET): randomised controlled trial. *Lancet* 2003;362:7–13.

62. RESOLVD Investigators. Effects of metoprolol CR in patients with ischemic and dilated cardiomyopathy. The Randomized Evaluation of Strategies for Left Ventricular Dysfunction Pilot Study. *Circulation* 2000;101:378–384.

63. Opie LH, et al. Mechanisms of cardiac contraction and relaxation. In: Bonow RO, et al., eds. *Braunwald's heart disease: a textbook of cardiovascular medicine,* 9th edition. Philadelphia: Elsevier Saunders, 2011:459–486.

64. Baillie GS, et al. Beta-arrestin-mediated PDE4 cAMP phosphodiesterase recruitment regulates beta-adrenoceptor switching from Gs to Gi. *Proc Natl Acad Sci U S A* 2003;100:940–945.

65. Engelhardt S. Alternative signaling: cardiomyocyte beta1-adrenergic receptors signal through EGFRs. *J Clin Invest* 2007;117:2396–2398.

66. Tzingounis AV, et al. Beta-blocker drugs mediate calcium signaling in native central nervous system neurons by beta-arrestin-biased agonism. *Proc Natl Acad Sci U S A* 2010;107:21028–21033.

67. Penela P, et al. Mechanisms of regulation of G protein-coupled receptor kinases (GRKs) and cardiovascular disease. *Cardiovasc Res* 2006; 69:46–56.

68. Chakir K, et al. Mechanisms of enhanced beta-adrenergic reserve from cardiac resynchronization therapy. *Circulation* 2009;119:1231–1240.

69. Doi M, et al. Propranolol prevents the development of heart failure by restoring FKBP 12.6-mediated stabilization of ryanodine receptor. *Circulation* 2002;105:1374–1379.

70. Kubo H, et al. Patients with end-stage congestive heart failure treated with beta-adrenergic receptor antagonists have improved ventricular myocyte calcium regulatory protein abundance. *Circulation* 2001;104:1012–1018.

71. Reiken S, et al. β-blockers restore calcium release channel function and improve cardiac muscle performance in human heart failure. *Circulation* 2003;107:2459–2466.

72. Cook S, et al. High heart rate: a cardiovascular risk factor? *Eur Heart J* 2006;27: 2387–2393.

73. Mulder P, et al. Long-term heart rate reduction induced by the selective I_f current inhibitor ivabradine improves left ventricular function and intrinsic myocardial structure in congestive heart failure. 2004;109:1674–1679.

74. Engelhardt S, et al. Altered calcium handling is critically involved in the cardiotoxic effects of chronic beta-adrenergic stimulation. *Circulation* 2004;109:1154–1160.

75. Communal C, et al. Opposing effects of β_1- and β_2-adrenergic receptors on cardiac myocyte apoptosis: role of a pertussis toxin-sensitive G protein. *Circulation* 1999;100: 2210–2212.

76. Packer M, et al. Consensus recommendations for the management of chronic heart failure. *Am J Cardiol* 1999;83(2A):1A-38A.

77. Shekelle PG, et al. Efficacy of angiotensin-converting enzyme inhibitors and beta-blockers in the management of left ventricular systolic dysfunction according to race, gender, and diabetic status: a meta-analysis of major clinical trials. *J Am Coll Cardiol* 2003;41:1529–1538.

78. Ghio S, et al. Effects of nebivolol in elderly heart failure patients with or without systolic left ventricular dysfunction: results of the SENIORS echocardiographic substudy. *Eur Heart J* 2006;27:562–568.

79. Sliwa K, et al. Impact of initiating carvedilol before angiotensin-converting enzyme inhibitor therapy on cardiac function in newly diagnosed heart failure. *J Am Coll Cardiol* 2004;44:1825–1830.

80. Willenheimer R, et al. Effect on survival and hospitalization of initiating treatment for chronic heart failure with bisoprolol followed by enalapril, as compared with the opposite sequence: results of the randomized Cardiac Insufficiency Bisoprolol Study (CIBIS) III. *Circulation* 2005;112:2426–2435.

81. McAlister FA, et al. Meta-analysis: beta-blocker dose, heart rate reduction, and death in patients with heart failure. *Ann Intern Med* 2009;150:784–794.

82. Rosso R, et al. Calcium channel blockers and beta-blockers versus beta-blockers alone for preventing exercise-induced arrhythmias in catecholaminergic polymorphic ventricular tachycardia. *Heart Rhythm* 2007;4:1149–1154.

83. Sheldon R, et al. Prevention of Syncope Trial (POST): a randomized, placebo-controlled study of metoprolol in the prevention of vasovagal syncope. *Circulation* 2006;113:1164–1170.

84. Sauer AJ, et al. Long QT syndrome in adults. *J Am Coll Cardiol* 2007;49:329–337.

85. Liu N, et al. Catecholaminergic polymorphic ventricular tachycardia. *Herz* 2007;32: 212–217.

86. Raj SR, et al. Propranolol decreases tachycardia and improves symptoms in the Postural Tachycardia Syndrome (POTS): less is more. *Circulation* 2009;120:725–734.

87. Fu Q, et al. Exercise training versus propranolol in the treatment of the postural orthostatic tachycardia syndrome. *Hypertension* 2011;58:167–175.

88. MRC Working Party. Medical Research Council trial of treatment of hypertension in older adults: principal results. *Br Med J* 1992;304:405–412.

89. Webb AJ, et al. Effects of β-blocker selectivity on blood pressure variability and stroke: a systematic review. *Neurology* 2011;77:731–737.

90. Poldermans D, et al. The effect of bisoprolol on perioperative mortality and myocardial infarction in high-risk patients undergoing vascular surgery. *N Engl J Med* 1999;341: 1789–1794.

91. Lindenauer PK, et al. Perioperative beta-blocker therapy and mortality after major non-cardiac surgery. *N Engl J Med* 2005;353:349–361.

92. Yang H, et al. The effects of perioperative beta-blockade: results of the Metoprolol after Vascular Surgery (MaVS) study, a randomized controlled trial. *Am Heart J* 2006;152: 983–990.

93. Ismail R, et al. The relevance of CYP2D6 genetic polymorphism on chronic metoprolol therapy in cardiovascular patients. *J Clin Pharm Ther* 2006;31:99–109.

94. Fleischmann KE, et al. 2009 ACCF/AHA focused update on perioperative beta blockade: a report of the American College of Cardiology Foundation/American Heart Association task force on practice guidelines. *Circulation* 2009;120:2123–2151.

95. Groszmann RJ, et al. Beta-blockers to prevent gastroesophageal varices in patients with cirrhosis. *N Engl J Med* 2005;353:2254–2261.

96. TOMH Study, Neaton JD, et al. Treatment of Mild Hypertension study (TOMH). Final results. *JAMA* 1993;270:713–724.

97. Metra M, et al. Influence of heart rate, blood pressure, and beta-blocker dose on outcome and the differences in outcome between carvedilol and metoprolol tartrate in patients with chronic heart failure: results from the COMET trial. *Eur Heart J* 2005; 26:2259–2268.

98. Kampus P, et al. Differential effects of nebivolol and metoprolol on central aortic pressure and left ventricular wall thickness. *Hypertension* 2011;57:1122–1128.

99. Ito H, et al. Differential effects of carvedilol and metoprolol on renal function in patients with heart failure. *Circ J* 2010;74:1578–1583.

100. Bakris GL, et al. Metabolic effects of carvedilol vs metoprolol in patients with type 2 diabetes mellitus and hypertension: a randomized controlled trial. *JAMA* 2004;292: 2227–2236.

101. Simpson WT. Nature and incidence of unwanted effects with atenolol. *Postgrad Med J* 1977;53:162–167.

102. Conant J, et al. Central nervous system side effects of beta-adrenergic blocking agents with high and low lipid solubility. *J Cardiovasc Pharmacol* 1989;13:656–661.

103. Streufert S, et al. Impact of β-adrenergic blockers on complex cognitive functioning. *Am Heart J* 1988;116:311–315.

104. Croog S, et al. The effects of antihypertensive therapy on the quality of life. *N Eng J Med* 1986;314:1657–1664.

105. TAIM Study, Wassertheil-Smoller S, et al. The Trial of Antihypertensive Interventions and Management (TAIM) Study. Final results with regard to blood pressure, cardiovascular risk and quality of life. *Am J Hypertens* 1992;5:37–44.

106. Fogari R, et al. Sexual activity in hypertensive men treated with valsartan or carvedilol: a crossover study. *Am J Hypertens* 2001;14:27–31.

107. Brixius K, et al. Nitric oxide, erectile dysfunction and beta-blocker treatment (MR NOED study): benefit of nebivolol versus metoprolol in hypertensive men. *Clin Exp Pharmacol Physiol* 2007;34:327–331.

108. Boyd R, et al. Towards evidence based emergency medicine: best BETs from the Manchester Royal Infirmary. Glucagon for the treatment of symptomatic beta blocker overdose. *Emerg Med J* 2003;20:266–267.

109. Grimm RH, et al. Long-term effects on sexual function of five antihypertensive drugs and nutritional hygienic treatment in hypertensive men and women. Treatment of Mild Hypertension Study (TOMHS). *Hypertension* 1997;29:8–14.

110. Bangalore S, et al. Cardiovascular protection using beta blockers. *JACC* 2007; 50.

111. Jandeleit-Dahm KA, et al. Why blockade of the renin-angiotensin system reduces the incidence of new-onset diabetes. *J Hypertens* 2005;23:463–473.

112. Dahlöf B, et al. For the LIFE Study Group. Cardiovascular morbidity and mortality in the Losartan Intervention For Endpoint reduction in hypertension study (LIFE): a randomised trial against atenolol. *Lancet* 2002;359:995–1003.
113. Lechat P, et al. Heart rate and cardiac rhythm relationships with bisoprolol benefit in chronic heart failure in CIBIS II Trial. *Circulation* 2001;103:1428–1433.
114. MERIT-HF Study Group. Effect of metoprolol CR/XL in chronic heart failure: Metoprolol CR/XL Randomized Trial in Congestive Heart Failure (MERIT-HF). *Lancet* 1999;353: 2001–2007.
115. Broeders MA, et al. Nebivolol: a third-generation beta-blocker that augments vascular nitric oxide release: endothelial beta(2)-adrenergic receptor-mediated nitric oxide production. *Circulation* 2000;102:677–684.
116. Van de Water A, et al. Pharmacological and hemodynamic profile of nebivolol, a chemically novel, potent, and selective beta 1-adrenergic antagonist. *J Cardiovasc Pharmacol* 1988;11:552–563.
117. Celik T, et al. Comparative effects of nebivolol and metoprolol on oxidative stress, insulin resistance, plasma adiponectin and soluble P-selectin levels in hypertensive patients. *J Hypertens* 2006;24:591–596.
118. Hohnloser SH, et al. For the European Esmolol Study Group. Usefulness of esmolol in unstable angina pectoris. *Am J Cardiol* 1991;67:1319–1323.
119. Koutouzis M, et al. Intravenous esmolol is well tolerated in elderly patients with heart failure in the early phase of non-ST elevation myocardial infarction. *Drugs Aging* 2006;23:673–680.

2

Nitrates and Newer Antianginals

LIONEL H. OPIE · JOHN D. HOROWITZ

"When the remedy is used for a long time, the dose requires to be increased before the effect is produced."

Brunton, 1867[1]

The Nature of Angina of Effort

Besides the classic and well-described constricting chest pain with its characteristic radiation that is brought on by effort in those with symptomatic coronary artery disease (CAD), and its diagnostic relief by cessation of effort, there are a series of crescendo and decrescendo events that precede and follow the anginal pain (Fig. 2-1). The crescendo events constitute the ischemic cascade of Nesto,[2] to which must be added postischemic stunning,[3] often ignored.

The initial imbalance between the oxygen supply and demand leads to inadequate myocardial blood flow (myocardial ischemia) that, in turn, sets off a series of metabolic changes. A deficit of high-energy phosphates leads to loss of potassium, gain of sodium and calcium, with rapid onset of diastolic dysfunction. A little later this is followed by systolic dysfunction, electrocardiogram (ECG) changes, shortness of breath, and then the onset of anginal chest pain that stops the effort. In the recovery period the ECG reverts to normal shortly after pain relief, but systolic recovery can be delayed for at least 30 minutes (stunning).

This chapter focuses on the antianginal effects of nitrates, one of *four major classes of antianginals,* including β-blockers and calcium channel blockers (CCBs) (Fig. 2-2). Mechanistically, nitrates and CCBs are coronary vasodilators, with nitrates also reducing the preload and CCBs the afterload. β-blockers reduce oxygen demand by slowing the heart and by a negative inotropic effect. Metabolic antianginals constitute the new fourth class acting by metabolic modulation without major hemodynamic effects. Recent therapeutic developments have somewhat extended this classification, with the development of several agents with multiple effects or with totally novel mechanisms of action, such as the sinus node inhibitor ivabradine.

This chapter reviews (1) the organic nitrates, both as regards their anitanginal effects and also their other therapeutic agents, and (2) recently developed novel agents with antianginal properties, including the metabolic modulators, ivabradine, allopurinol, and ranolazine. In this context, it is important to consider prophylactic antianginal therapy as only a component of therapy for patients with symptomatic myocardial ischemia, with other key considerations being the use of other agents that are both cardioprotective and antiatherosclerotic (aspirin, statins, angiotensin-converting enzyme [ACE] inhibitors, and

EFFORT ANGINA

Opie 2012

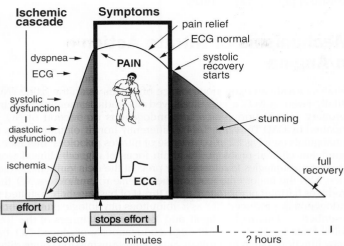

Figure 2-1 **The ischemic cascade** leading to the chest pain of effort angina followed by the period of mechanical stunning with slow recovery of full function. For basic concepts see Nesto.[2] *ECG*, Electrocardiogram. (Figure © L. H. Opie, 2012.)

ACTION OF ANTIANGINALS

Opie 2012

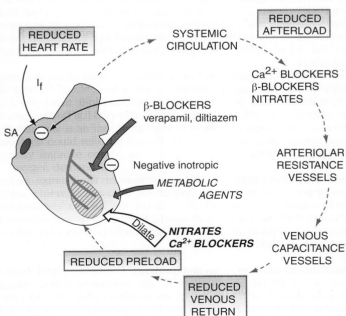

Figure 2-2 **Proposed antianginal mechanisms** for the major four classes of antianginal agents: nitrates, β-blockers, calcium channel blockers, and metabolic agents (for details of metabolic agents, see Figure 2-7). *SA*, Sinoatrial. (Figure © L. H. Opie, 2012.)

angiotensin receptor blockers [ARBs]) and the use of anti–heart failure drugs when necessary, whereas for some selected patients a considered invasive approach is appropriate.

Mechanisms of Nitrate Action in Angina

Nitrates provide an exogenous source of vasodilator nitric oxide (NO˙, usually given as NO), a very short-lived free radical, thereby inducing coronary vasodilation even when endogenous production of NO˙ is impaired by CAD. Thus nitrates act differently from the other classes of antianginals (see Fig. 2-2). Chronic use of nitrates produces tolerance, a significant clinical problem. The main focus of current clinical work remains on strategies to minimize or prevent the development of tolerance, with the major emphasis on the adverse role of excess NO˙ that produces harmful peroxynitrite.[4] The thrust of basic work has shifted to endogenously produced NO˙ as a ubiquitous physiologic messenger, as described by Ignarro, Furchgott, and Murad,[5] the winners of the 1998 Nobel Prize for Medicine. Although endogenously produced NO˙ has many functions (such as a role in vagal neurotransmission) quite different from the NO˙ derived from exogenous nitrates, there are important shared vasodilatory effects.

Coronary and peripheral Vasodilatory effects. A distinction must be made between antianginal and coronary vasodilator properties. Nitrates preferentially dilate large coronary arteries and arterioles greater than 100 mcm in diameter[6] to (1) redistribute blood flow along collateral channels and from epicardial to endocardial regions and (2) relieve coronary spasm and dynamic stenosis, especially at epicardial sites, including the coronary arterial constriction induced by exercise. Thereby exercise-induced myocardial ischemia is relieved. Thus nitrates are "effective" vasodilators for angina; dipyridamole and other vasodilators acting more distally in the arterial tree are not, but rather have the risk of diverting blood from the ischemic area—a "coronary steal" effect.

The additional peripheral hemodynamic effects of nitrates, originally observed by Lauder Brunton,[1] cannot be ignored. Nitrates do reduce the afterload, in addition to the preload of the heart (Fig. 2-3). The arterial wave reflection from the periphery back to the aorta is altered in such a way that there is "true" afterload reduction, with the aortic systolic pressure falling even though the brachial artery pressure does not change.[7]

Reduced oxygen demand. Nitrates increase the venous capacitance, causing pooling of blood in the peripheral veins and thereby a reduction in venous return and in ventricular volume. There is less mechanical stress on the myocardial wall and the myocardial oxygen demand is reduced. Furthermore, a fall in the aortic systolic pressure also reduces the oxygen demand.

Endothelium and vascular mechanisms. The fundamental mechanism of nitrate biological effect is the enzyme-mediated release of highly unstable NO˙ from the nitrate molecule (Fig. 2-4).[8] An intact vascular endothelium is required for the vasodilatory effects of some vascular active agents (thus acetylcholine physiologically vasodilates but constricts when the endothelium is damaged). Nitrates vasodilate whether or not the endothelium is physically intact or functional. Prolonged nitrate therapy with formation of peroxynitrite may, however, inhibit endothelial nitric oxide synthase (NOS), which is one of several postulated mechanisms of nitrate tolerance. Similarly, long-term use of long-acting nitrates may cause endothelial dysfunction mediated by

ACTION OF NITRATES ON CIRCULATION
Opie 2012

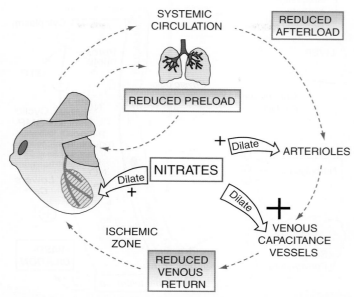

Figure 2-3   Schematic diagram of effects of nitrate on the circulation. The major effect is on the venous capacitance vessels with additional coronary and peripheral arteriolar vasodilatory benefits.(Figure © L. H. Opie, 2012.)

free radicals (see later, Fig. 2-5).[4,9] Whether this problem extends to aggravation of preexisting endothelial dysfunction is uncertain. Thus nitrate tolerance and endothelial dysfunction have partially shared pathogenetic mechanisms.

Nitrates, after entering the vessel wall, are bioconverted to release NO˙, which stimulates guanylate cyclase to produce cyclic guanosine monophosphate (GMP; see Fig. 2-4). In addition, NO˙ acts potentially via direct S-nitrosylation of a number of proteins, altering their physiologic properties via a posttranslational modification step. NO˙ may also be "scavenged" by the superoxide (O_2^-) radical, generating peroxynitrate ($ONOO^-$), which in high concentrations contributes to nitrate toxicity (Fig. 2-5) and the induction of nitrate tolerance. Conversely, low concentrations enhance the vasodilator effects of NO˙.

Overall the best known mechanism linked to clinical practice is that calcium in the vascular myocyte falls, and vasodilation results (see Fig. 2-4). Sulfhydryl (SH) groups are required for such formation of NO˙ and the stimulation of guanylate cyclase. Nitroglycerin powerfully dilates when injected into an artery, an effect that is probably limited in humans by reflex adrenergic-mediated vasoconstriction. Hence (1) nitrates are better venous than arteriolar dilators, and (2) there is an associated adrenergic reflex tachycardia[10] that can be attenuated by concurrent β-blockade.

Effects of NO˙ on myocardial relaxation and contractile proteins. NO˙ has a fundamental role as a modulator of myocardial relaxation, mediated at least in part by cyclic GMP (see Fig. 2-4).[11] This effect is independent of the restoration of coronary blood flow that in turn can reverse ischemic diastolic dysfunction. Furthermore, NO˙ improves diastolic function in human heart muscle where it acts on the contractile proteins by increasing troponin I phosphorylation of the springlike cytoskeletal protein titin.[12] In long-term therapy, NO˙ donors may limit or

NITRATE MECHANISMS
Opie 2012

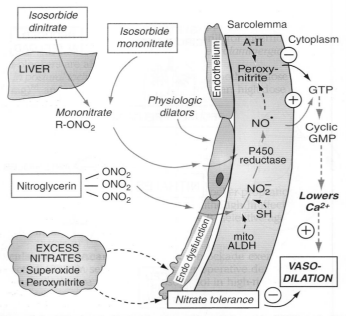

Figure 2-4   Effects of nitrates in generating nitric oxide (NO·) and stimulating guanylate cyclase to cause vasodilation. Nitrate tolerance is multifactorial in origin, including the endothelial effects of peroxynitrite and superoxide that ultimately inhibit the conversion of guanosine triphosphate (GTP) to cyclic guanosine monophosphate (GMP). Note that mononitrates bypass hepatic metabolism and the mitochondrial aldehyde dehydrogenase-2 (mito ALDH) step required for bioactivation of nitroglycerin. Hence reduced or genetic lack of ALDH-2 may also be a cause of nitrate tolerance.[8] *SH,* Sulfhydryl. (Figure © L. H. Opie, 2008.)

reverse left ventricular hypertrophy (LVH).[13] These studies raise the possibility that organic nitrates may exert a role in the management of systemic hypertension, in which LVH is a marker and modulator of long-term cardiovascular risk. However, to date, there have been only sporadic clinical investigations.

Antiaggregatory effects. Organic nitrates mimic the effects of endogenous NO· in inhibiting and potentially reversing platelet aggregation.[3,14,15] These effects are mediated primarily via the classical pathway of stimulation of activation of soluble guanylate cyclase (see Fig. 2-4).

Pharmacokinetics of Nitrates

Bioavailability and half-lives. The various preparations differ so much that each needs to be considered separately. As a group, nitrates are absorbed from the mucous membranes, the skin, and the gastrointestinal (GI) tract. The prototype agent, nitroglycerin, has pharmacokinetics that are not well understood. It rapidly disappears from the blood with a half-life of only a few minutes, largely by extrahepatic mechanisms that convert the parent molecule to longer acting and active dinitrates.[16] Isosorbide dinitrate, on the other hand, must first be converted in the liver to active mononitrates (see Fig. 2-4) that have half-lives of approximately 4 to 6 hours with ultimate renal excretion. The mononitrates are completely bioavailable without any hepatic metabolism,

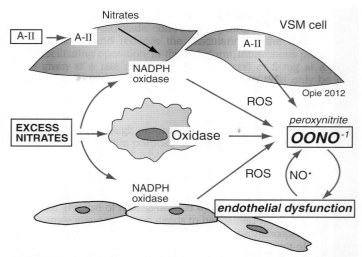

Figure 2-5   The formation of peroxynitrite and the role of oxidases in the process. Excess nitrate administration leads to stimulation of the oxidase system. The end result is increased endothelial dysfunction. Angiotensin II stimulates the vascular smooth muscle (VSM) cells to form peroxynitrite. Some of the procedures that diminish these processes, leading to endothelial dysfunction, include administration of carvedilol (strong data), high doses of atorvastatin (human volunteer data), and the angiotensin receptor blocker telmisartan (experimental data). *NADPH,* Nicotinamide adenine dinucleotide phosphate; *NO·,* nitric oxide; *OONO,* peroxynitrite; *ROS,* reactive oxygen species.

with half-lives of 4-6 hours. In reality, knowledge of pharmacokinetics is of limited interest because of the highly variable relationship between the plasma concentrations of the nitrates, the levels of their active metabolites, and the onset and duration of pharmacologic action that matter most to the clinician.[16] Of the many nitrate preparations (Table 2-1), sublingual nitroglycerin remains the gold standard for acute anginal attacks.[17] In practice, patients are often also given long-acting nitrates. "No matter which long-acting preparation is used, physicians should prescribe the drug in a manner to decrease the likelihood of nitrate tolerance. This involves an on-off strategy of at least a 10-hour nitrate free interval each day."[17] This policy does, however, entertain the risk of precipitation of angina during the nitrate-free interval, which is often at night.

Nitrate Interactions with Other Drugs

Many of the proposed interactions of nitrates are pharmacodynamic, involving potentiation of vasodilatory effects, as with the CCBs. However, the chief example of vasodilator interactions is with the selective phosphodiesterase-5 (PDE-5) inhibitors such as sildenafil as used for erectile dysfunction. PDE-5 inhibitors are increasingly used for the therapy of pulmonary hypertension (see Chapter 5) and their benefits in heart failure are being explored. As a group, these agents can cause serious hypotensive reactions when combined with nitrates (see Fig. 2-5). Hence the package insert of each agent forbids co-administration to patients taking nitrates in any form either regularly or intermittently. For example, sildenafil decreases the blood pressure (BP) by approximately 8.4/5.5 mm Hg, and by much more in those taking nitrates. The exertion of sexual intercourse also stresses the cardiovascular system further. As a group, these

Table 2-1

Nitrate Preparations: Doses, Preparations, and Duration of Effects

Compound	Route	Preparation and Dose	Duration of Effects and Comments
Amyl nitrite	Inhalation	2-5 mg	10 sec-10 min; for diagnosis of LV outflow obstruction in hypertrophic cardiomyopathy.
Nitroglycerin (trinitrin, GTN)	(a) Sublingual tablets	0.3-0.6 mg up to 1.5 mg	Peak blood levels at 2 min; t½ approximately 7 min; for acute therapy of effort or rest angina. Keep tightly capped.
	(b) Spray	0.4 mg/metered dose	Similar to tablets at same dose.
	(c) Ointment	2%; 6 × 6 ins or 15 × 15 cm or 7.5-40 mg	Apply 2× daily; 6-h intervals; effect up to 7 h after first dose. No efficacy data for chronic use.
	(d) Transdermal patches	0.2-0.8 mg/h patch on for 12 h, patch off for 12 h	Effects start within minutes and last 3-5 h. No efficacy data for second or third doses during chronic therapy.
	(e) Oral; sustained release	2.5-13 mg 1-2 tablets 3× daily	4-8 h after first dose; no efficacy data for chronic therapy.
	(f) Buccal	1-3 mg tablets 3× daily	Effects start within minutes and last 3-5 h. No efficacy data for second or third doses during chronic therapy.
	(g) Intravenous infusion (discontinued in US)	5-200 mcg/min (care with PVC); Tridil 0.5 mg/mL or 5 mg/mL; Nitro bid IV 5 mg/mL	In unstable angina, increasing doses are often needed to overcome tolerance. High-concentration solutions contain propylene glycol; crossreacts with heparin.
Isosorbide dinitrate (sorbide nitrate) Isordil	(a) Sublingual	2.5-15 mg	Onset 5-10 min, effect up to 60 min or longer.
	(b) Oral tablets	5-80 mg 2-3× daily	Up to 8 h (first dose; then tolerance) with 3× or 4× daily doses; 2× daily 7 h apart may be effective but data inadequate.
	(c) Spray	1.25 mg on tongue	Rapid action 2-3 min.
	(d) Chewable	5 mg as single dose	Exercise time increased for 2 min-2.5 h.
	(e) Oral; slow-release	40 mg once or 2× daily	Up to 8 h (first dose; 2× daily not superior to placebo).
	(f) Intravenous infusion	1.25-5 mg/h (care with PVC)	May need increasing doses for unstable angina at rest.
	(g) Ointment	100 mg/24 h	Not effective during continuous therapy.
Isosorbide 5-mononitrate	Oral tablets	20 mg 2× day (7 h apart); 120-240 mg 1× daily (slow release)	12-14 h after chronic dosing for 2 weeks. Efficacy up to 12 h after 6 weeks.
Pentaerythritol tetranitrate (not in US)	Sublingual	10 mg as needed	No efficacy data.

GTN, glyceryl trinitrate; IV, Intravenous; LV, left ventricular; PVC, polyvinylchloride tubing; t½, half-life.
Long acting, available in the United States: Nitroglycerin Extended Release, nitroglycerin transdermal patch.
Available in the United States: Extended Release Isosorbide dinitrate, Isosorbide mononitrate.

drugs should also not be given with α-adrenergic blockers. In case of inadvertent *PDE-5-nitrate combinations*, administration of an α-adrenergic agonist or even of norepinephrine may be needed.

An essential question for men with acute coronary syndrome (Fig. 2-6). Whenever a male patient presents with an anginal attack or acute coronary syndrome (ACS), whether or not precipitated by sexual intercourse, one essential question is whether the patient has recently taken sildenafil (Viagra), vardenafil (Levitra) or tadalafil (Cialis)? If so, how soon can a nitrate be given? In clinical practice nitrates may be started 24 hours after sildenafil.[17] A 24-hour interval for vardenafil can also be inferred from data in the package insert. For the longer-acting tadalafil the corresponding interval is 48 hours.[18]

Beneficial combination with hydralazine. There is a beneficial interaction between nitrates and hydralazine whereby the latter helps to lessen nitrate tolerance,[19] probably acting through inhibition of free radical formation. This may explain why the combination of nitrates and hydralazine is effective in heart failure[20] and is now approved for use in the United States as BiDil (Nitromed, Inc) for patients with heart failure who self-identify as black (see Chapter 6, page 198). Approval was based in part on results of the African-American Heart Failure Trial (A-HeFT) showing that BiDil gave a 43% reduction in death and a 39% reduction in hospitalizations.[21] The combination used was isosorbide dinitrate 20 mg and hydralazine 37.5 mg, both given three times daily.

Despite the proven efficacy of this combination in African Americans, much remains to be understood about the precise mechanism of interaction between isosorbide dinitrate and hydralazine, as well as understanding the optimal patient population. There could

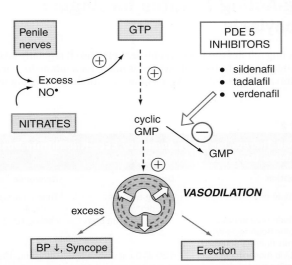

Figure 2-6 A serious nitrate drug interaction. The mechanism of normal erection involves penile vasodilation mediated by guanosine triphosphate (GTP) and cyclic guanosine monophosphate (GMP). The phosphodiesterase-5 inhibitors (PDE 5) such as sildenafil (Viagra) act by inhibiting the enzymatic breakdown of penile cyclic GMP to GMP with increased vasodilation. This is not confined to the penis and peripheral vasodilation added to that caused by nitrates, gives rise to an excess fall of blood pressure (BP) and possible syncope. Hence the use of PDE 5 inhibitors in any patient taking nitrates is contraindicated. *NO•*, Nitric oxide. (Figure © L. H. Opie, 2012.)

be a potentially incremental role of such combination therapy in other ethnic groups of patients with severe heart failure in whom other forms of pharmacotherapy are relatively contraindicated, for example, on the basis of renal dysfunction.

Short-Acting Nitrates for Acute Effort Angina

Sublingual nitroglycerin is very well established in the initial therapy of angina of effort, yet may be ineffective, frequently because the patient has not received proper instruction or because of severe headaches. When angina starts, the patient should rest in the sitting position (standing promotes syncope, lying enhances venous return and heart work) and take sublingual nitroglycerin (0.3 to 0.6 mg) every 5 minutes until the pain goes or a maximum of four to five tablets have been taken. *Nitroglycerin spray* is an alternative mode of oral administration, which is more acceptable to some patients. It vasodilates sooner than does the tablet, which might be of special importance in those with dryness of the mouth.[22]

    Isosorbide dinitrate may be given *sublingually* (5 mg) to abort an anginal attack and then exerts antianginal effects for approximately 1 hour. Because the dinitrate requires hepatic conversion to the mononitrate, the onset of antianginal action (mean time: 3.4 minutes) is slower than with nitroglycerin (mean time: 1.9 minutes), so that the manufacturers of the dinitrate recommend sublingual administration of this drug only if the patient is unresponsive to or intolerant of sublingual nitroglycerin. After oral ingestion, hemodynamic and antianginal effects persist for several hours. Single doses of isosorbide dinitrate confer longer protection against angina than can single doses of sublingual nitroglycerin (see Table 2-1).

Long-Acting Nitrates for Angina Prophylaxis

Long-acting nitrates are not continuously effective if regularly taken over a prolonged period, unless allowance is made for a nitrate-free or nitrate-low interval (Table 2-2).[23-26] Worsening of endothelial dysfunction is a

Table 2-2

Interval Therapy for Effort Angina by Eccentric Nitrate Dosage Schedules Designed to Avoid Tolerance		
Preparation	**Dose**	**Reference**
Isosorbide dinitrate	30 mg at 7 am, 1 pm*	Thadani & Lipicky, 1994[23]
Isosorbide mononitrate (Robins-Boehringer-Wyeth-Ayerst; Pharma-Schwartz)	20 mg at 8 am and 3 pm	Parker, 1993[24]
Isosorbide mononitrate, Extended-release (Key-Astra)	120-240 mg daily	Chrysant, 1993[25]
Transdermal nitrate patches	7.5-10 mg per 12 h; patches removed after 12 h	DeMots, 1989[26]
Phasic release nitroglycerin patch	15 mg, most released in first 12 h†	Parker, 1989†

*Efficacy of second dose not established; no data for other doses.
  †No data for other doses.
  †*Eur Heart J* 1989;10(Suppl. A):43-49.

potential complication of long-acting nitrates that should be avoided.[27] Hence the common practice of routine use of long-acting nitrates for patients with effort angina[28] may have to be reevaluated.

Isosorbide dinitrate (oral preparation) is frequently given for the prophylaxis of angina. An important question is whether regular therapy with isosorbide dinitrate gives long-lasting protection (3-5 hours) against angina. In a crucial placebo-controlled study, exercise duration improved significantly for 6 to 8 hours after single oral doses of 15 to 120 mg isosorbide dinitrate, but for only 2 hours when the same doses were given repetitively four times daily.[29] Marked tolerance develops during sustained therapy, despite much higher plasma isosorbide dinitrate concentrations during sustained than during acute therapy.[29] With the extended-release formulation of isosorbide dinitrate *(Tembids)*, eccentric twice-daily treatment with a 40-mg dose administered in the morning and 7 hours later was not superior to placebo in a large multicenter study.[23] Nonetheless eccentric dosing schedules of isosorbide dinitrate are still often used in an effort to avoid tolerance.

Mononitrates have similar dosage and effects to those of isosorbide dinitrate. Nitrate tolerance, likewise a potential problem, can be prevented or minimized when rapid-release preparations *(Monoket, Ismo)* are given twice daily in an eccentric pattern with doses spaced by 7 hours.[24] Using the slow-release preparation *(Imdur)*, the dose range 30-240 mg once daily was tested for antianginal activity. Only 120 and 240 mg daily improved exercise times at 4 and 12 hours after administration, even after 42 days of daily use.[25] These high doses were reached by titration over 7 days. A daily dose of 60 mg, still often used, was ineffective.

Transdermal nitroglycerin patches are designed to permit the timed release of nitroglycerin over a 24-hour period. Despite initial claims of 24-hour efficacy, major studies have failed to show prolonged improvement.

Pentaerythritol tetranitrate may have the advantage of provoking less nitrate tolerance than other nitrates[30] but this drug is not widely available (also see section on "Prevention and Limitation of Nitrate Tolerance" page 52).

Limitations: Side Effects and Nitrate Failure

Side Effects

Hypotension is the most serious and headache the most common side effect (Table 2-3). Headache characteristically occurs with sublingual nitroglycerin, and at the start of therapy with long-acting nitrates.[17] Often the headaches pass over while antianginal efficacy is maintained; yet headaches may lead to loss of compliance. Concomitant aspirin may protect from the headaches and from coronary events. In chronic lung disease, arterial hypoxemia may result from vasodilation and increased venous admixture. Occasionally, prolonged high-dose therapy can cause *methemoglobinemia* (see Table 2-3), which reduces the oxygen-carrying capacity of the blood and the rate of delivery of oxygen to the tissues. Treatment is by intravenous methylene blue (1-2 mg/kg over 5 min).

Failure of Nitrate Therapy

In contrast to the marked beneficial effects of sublingual nitroglycerin in reversing attacks of angina pectoris, long-acting nitrates are only moderately effective in reducing frequency of angina pectoris or in relieving symptoms in patients with heart failure. Apart from issues of noncompliance, the principal reason for limitation of therapeutic

Table 2-3

Nitrate Precautions and Side Effects

Precautions

Need airtight containers.
Nitrate sprays are inflammable.

Common Side Effects

Headaches *initially* frequently limit dose; often respond to aspirin.
Facial flushing may occur.
Sublingual nitrates may cause halitosis.

Serious Side Effects

Syncope and hypotension may occur.
Hypotension risks cerebral ischemia.
Alcohol or other vasodilators may augment hypotension.
Tachycardia frequent.
Methemoglobinemia: with prolonged high doses. Give IV methylene blue
   (1-2 mg/kg)

Contraindications

In **hypertrophic obstructive cardiomyopathy,** nitrates may exaggerate
   outflow obstruction.
Sildenafil (or similar agents): risk of hypotension or even acute MI.

Relative Contraindications

Cor pulmonale: decreased arterial pO_2.
Reduced venous return risky in constrictive pericarditis, tight mitral stenosis.

Tolerance

Continuous high doses lead to tolerance that eccentric dosage may avoid.
Cross-tolerance between formulations.

Withdrawal Symptoms

Gradually discontinue long-term nitrates.

IV, Intravenous; *MI,* myocardial infarction.

response to nitrates can be categorized as NO˙ resistance, "true" nitrate tolerance and nitrate "pseudo"-tolerance, alone, or in combination (Table 2-4).

Management of apparent failure of nitrate therapy. After exclusion of tolerance and poor compliance (headaches), therapy is stepped up (Table 2-5)[31] while excluding aggravating factors such as hypertension, thyrotoxicosis, atrial fibrillation, or anemia.

Table 2-4

Factors Limiting Responsiveness to Organic Nitrates		
Anomaly	**Principal Mechanisms**	**Effects**
NO resistance	"**Scavenging**" of NO Dysfunction of soluble guanylate cyclase	De novo hyporesponsiveness
"True" nitrate tolerance	(1) Impaired bioactivation of nitrates	Progressive attenuation of nitrate effect
	(2) Increased clearance of NO by O_2	Worsening of endothelial dysfunction
Nitrate pseudotolerance	Increased release of vasoconstrictors (angiotensin II catechol-amines, endothelin)	"Rebound" during nitrate-free periods

NO, Nitric oxide; *O_2,* oxygen.

Table 2-5

Proposed Step-Care for Angina of Effort

1. **General:** History and physical examination to exclude valvular disease, anemia, hypertension, thromboembolic disease, thyrotoxicosis, and heart failure. Check risk factors for coronary artery disease (smoking, hypertension, blood lipids, diabetes, obesity). Must stop smoking. Check diet.
2. **Prophylactic drugs.** Give aspirin, statins and ACE inhibitors. Control BP.
3. **Start-up.** *First-line therapy.* Short-acting nitrates are regarded as the basis of therapy, to which is added either a β-blocker or CCB (heart-rate lowering or DHP) β-blocker if prior infarct or heart failure. Otherwise level of evidence only C.[31] May use CCB (preferably verapamil as in INVEST[80] or diltiazem or long-acting dihydropyridine).
4. **Second-line therapy** is the combination of a short acting nitrate with a β-blocker plus a CCB (DHP).
5. **Third-line therapy.** The add-on choice is between long-acting nitrates, ivabradine, nicorandil, ranolazine, perhexiline (Australia and New Zealand), or trimetazidine (Europe). The European Guidelines, under review (2012), are expected to allow for any of these third-line drugs, except for long-acting nitrates, to be chosen as first-line agents.
6. **PCI with stenting** may be attempted at any stage in selected patients, especially for highly symptomatic single vessel disease.
7. **Consider bypass surgery** after failure to respond to medical therapy or for left main stem lesion or for triple vessel disease, especially if reduced LV function. Even response to medical therapy does not eliminate need for investigation.
8. **Nitrate failure** may occur at any of these steps. Consider nitrate tolerance or worsening disease or poor compliance.

ACE, Angiotensin-converting enzyme; *BP,* blood pressure; *DHP,* dihydropyridine; *LV,* left ventricular; *PCI,* percutaneous coronary intervention.

Nitrates for Acute Coronary Syndromes

Large trials have failed to show a consistent reduction in mortality in either unstable angina and non-ST elevation myocardial infarction (MI) or in ST-elevation MI. Therefore the goal of nitrate therapy is pain relief or management of associated acute heart failure[32] or severe hypertension.

Intravenous nitroglycerin is widely regarded as being effective in the management of pain in patients with ACS, although without properly controlled trials. Nitroglycerin should be infused at an initial rate of 5 mcg/min (or even 2.5 mcg/min in patients with borderline hypotension), using nonadsorptive delivery systems. Although earlier studies used progressive uptitration of infusion rates to relief of pain (with eventual rates of >1000 mcg/min in some patients), this strategy should be limited in general because of the risks of tolerance induction and subsequent "rebound." Given that even 10 mcg/min nitroglycerin induces some degree of tolerance within 24 hours,[33] a maximal infusion rate of 16 mcg/min is recommended in most cases.[34] Nitrate patches and nitroglycerin ointment should not be used. Intravenous therapy, which can be titrated upward as needed, is far better for control of pain.

Percutaneous coronary intervention. Intracoronary nitroglycerin is often used to minimize ischemia, for example, caused by coronary spasm. Some nitrate solutions contain high potassium that may precipitate ventricular fibrillation.

Nitrate contraindications. With right ventricular involvement in acute myocardial infarction (AMI), a nitrate-induced fall in left ventricular (LV) filling pressure may aggravate hypotension. A systolic BP of less than 90 mm Hg is a contraindication. Recent ingestion of sildenafil or its equivalent means that nitrate therapy must be delayed or avoided (see "Nitrate Interactions with Other Drugs," page 43).

Acute Heart Failure and Acute Pulmonary Edema

No clear guidelines exist regarding management of *acute decompensated heart failure*. In an observational study of more than 65,000 patients, intravenous nitroglycerin gave similar outcomes to the more modern and expensive intravenous nesiritide and better results than dobutamine.[35] However, the patients were not equally matched for BP at entry, so that randomized controlled trials are needed to develop practice guidelines.

In *acute pulmonary edema* from various causes, including AMI, nitroglycerin can be strikingly effective, with some risk of precipitous falls in BP and of tachycardia or bradycardia. Sublingual nitroglycerin in repeated doses of 0.8 to 2.4 mg every 5 to 10 minutes can relieve dyspnea within 15 to 20 minutes, with a fall of LV filling pressure and a rise in cardiac output.[36] Intravenous nitroglycerin, however, is usually a better method to administer nitroglycerin because the dose can be rapidly adjusted upward or downward depending on the clinical and hemodynamic response. Infusion rates required may be higher than the maximal use for AMI (i.e., above 200 mcg/min), but this is based on the idea of brief infusion when pulmonary edema is present without systemic hypotension. A similar approach has been validated with intravenously infused isosorbide dinitrate.[37]

On the other hand, the infusion rate of nitroglycerin at lower rates, in combination with N-acetylcysteine (NAC), was as effective as a diuretic-based treatment regimen in unselected patients with acute pulmonary edema.[38]

Congestive Heart Failure

Both short- and long-acting nitrates are used as unloading agents in the relief of symptoms in acute and chronic heart failure. Their dilating effects are more pronounced on veins than on arterioles, so they are best suited to patients with raised pulmonary wedge pressure and clinical features of pulmonary congestion. The combination of high-dose isosorbide dinitrate (60 mg four times daily) plus hydralazine was better than placebo in decreasing mortality, yet nonetheless inferior to an ACE inhibitor in severe congestive heart failure (CHF).[39] Dinitrate-hydralazine may therefore be chosen when a patient cannot tolerate an ACE inhibitor or it may be added to the therapy of heart failure, the latter indication being well validated in black patients.[21]

Nitrate tolerance remains a problem. Intermittent dosing designed to counter periods of expected dyspnea (at night, anticipated exercise) is one sensible policy.[40] Escalating doses of nitrates provide only a short-term solution and should be avoided in general. A third possible option is co-therapy with ACE inhibitors or hydralazine or both, which might blunt nitrate tolerance. *Nitrate patches* have given variable results in CHF.

Nitrate Tolerance and Nitric Oxide Resistance

Nitrate Tolerance

Nitrate tolerance often limits nitrate efficacy. Thus longer-acting nitrates, although providing higher and better-sustained blood nitrate levels, paradoxically often seem to lose their efficacy with time. This is the phenomenon of nitrate tolerance (see Fig. 2-4). A number of hypotheses have been proposed to account for development of nitrate tolerance. These may be summarized as follows:

1. *Impaired nitrate bioactivation.* Several investigators have demonstrated that the induction of tolerance to nitroglycerin and to other organic nitrates is relatively nitrate-specific, with minimal cross-tolerance to more direct activators of soluble guanylate cyclase, including NO· itself.[41,42] Infusion of nitroglycerin for 24 hours in patients with stable angina induced nitrate-specific tolerance, with simultaneous evidence of impaired bioactivation, via the enzymatic denitration of nitroglycerin and release of NO·.[42] As organic nitrate bioactivation is an enzymatic process, catalyzed by a large number of nitrate reductases, these findings have led to a search for a potential key "tolerance-inducing enzyme." Such an enzyme would be potentially inhibited after prolonged nitrate exposure.

2. *Aldehyde dehydrogenase (ALDH).* ALDH is an example of such an enzyme (see Fig. 2-4). Aldehydes are highly toxic compounds that generate reactive oxidative stress in the form of reactive oxygen species (ROS). Aldehydes physiologically result from numerous processes including the actions of catecholamines and are ubiquitously present in the environment. Normally their potentially noxious effects are kept at bay by the activity of the mitochondrial aldehyde dehydrogenase (ALDH$_2$). Inhibition of ALDH$_2$ by organic nitrates may remove a protective mechanism against oxidative stress.[43,44] ALDH$_2$ is dysfunctional in up to 30% of Chinese and Japanese; this anomaly is thus estimated to involve at least 0.5 billion persons worldwide.[8] This enzyme modulates bioactivation of some organic nitrates, including nitroglycerin (see mito ALDH in Fig. 2-4). Conversely, nitroglycerin can potently and rapidly inactivate ALDH, including ALDH$_2$,[45] an effect that appears to occur prior to onset of nitrate tolerance. Moreover, induction of nitrate tolerance occurs more readily in ALDH$_2$-knockout mice.[8] Furthermore, pentaerythritol tetranitrate that is less reliant on ALDH$_2$ for bioactivation is consequently less subject to tolerance induction,[46,47] in contrast to the endothelial dysfunction linked in normal subjects to the prolonged use of isosorbide-5-mononitrate.[9] However, it should also be noted that, apart from wide variability in the interactions between organic nitrates and various ALDH subtypes,[48] there are many other nitrate reductases: it therefore seems unlikely that inhibition of ALDH$_2$ is the single key mechanism underlying nitrate tolerance induction.[9]

3. *Free radical hypothesis: induction of oxidative stress and endothelial dysfunction.* A number of studies have linked the development of nitrate tolerance with increases in free radical release, oxidative stress and resultant induction of endothelial dysfunction.[49] Similarly, a number of studies in normal animal models and in normal humans[9] have demonstrated that induction of nitrate tolerance *may* be associated with the induction of vascular endothelial dysfunction. Based on the crucial role of ALDH$_2$ in limiting the harm of prolonged excess generation of ROS, any product that limits the generation of ROS may lessen the risk of nitrate tolerance. For example, agents stimulating guanylyl cyclase or the PDE 5 inhibitors with increased formation of vasodilatory cyclic GMP experimentally promote the activity of NO· (see Fig. 2-4).[50] Such mechanistic experimental data should not directly be translated into clinical practice because of the danger of excess vasodilation (see Fig. 2-4).

The problems with the free radical hypothesis include (1) the paucity of supporting data in tolerance occurring in the presence of preexistent coronary disease and thus of endothelial dysfunction,[33] (2) the finding that some nitrates may reduce oxidative stress,[51] and (3) the preservation of endothelial function in some models of tolerance.[52] Nevertheless, the free radical hypothesis would explain why nitrate tolerance can be lessened acutely in some models by concurrent therapy by vitamin[9,53,54] or hydralazine.[55-57] Other agents that reduce oxidative stress include statins, ACE inhibitors, and ARBs.[55]

Prevention and Limitation of Nitrate Tolerance

In effort angina, many studies now show that symptomatic tolerance can be lessened by interval dosing. Eccentric twice-daily doses of isosorbide mononitrate (Monoket, Ismo) or once-daily treatment with 120 or 240 mg of the extended-release formulation of mononitrate (Imdur) maintain clinical activity but may nonetheless lead to endothelial dysfunction.[9] There is considerable evidence that nitrate effects on blood vessels and platelets are SH-dependent.[58-60] Concomitant therapy with SH donors such as NAC potentiates nitroglycerin effects, both hemodynamically[61] and on platelet aggregation.[62] Concomitant nitroglycerin-NAC therapy may also limit tolerance induction clinically[63] while improving outcomes in unstable angina pectoris.[64] Simple procedures that might be tried are folic acid supplementation, supplemental L-arginine,[65] and vitamin C.[9] Rapidly increasing blood nitrate levels may overcome tolerance. Although there is strong evidence that nitrate-free intervals limit tolerance, they may be associated with "rebound" or the "zero-hour phenomenon."

Concomitant Cardiovascular Co-therapy (Fig. 2-7): *Carvedilol* has strong experimental and clinical support. It can attenuate nitrate tolerance induced in rodents by preventing free-radical generation and CYP depletion, and therefore maintaining the activity of the NO–cyclic GMP pathway (see Fig. 2-4).[66] Clinically, carvedilol prevents nitrate tolerance

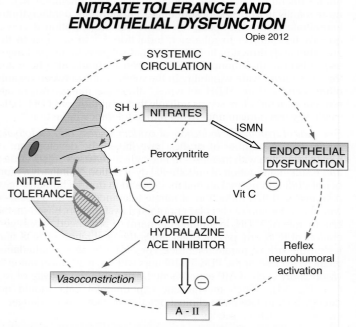

NITRATE TOLERANCE AND ENDOTHELIAL DYSFUNCTION
Opie 2012

Figure 2-7   Current proposals for therapy of nitrate tolerance. For cellular mechanisms of peroxynitrite, see Figure 2-3. Carvedilol, vitamin C, and hydralazine may all lessen free radical formation. Isosorbide dinitrate and hydralazine have proven long-term effects in heart failure patients. Angiotensin-converting enzyme inhibitors oppose the neurohumoral activation that is thought to occur as a result of nitrate-induced vasodilation, possibly involving reflex arterial constriction and impaired renal blood flow. *ISMN,* Isosorbide mononitrate; *SH,* sulfhydryl. (Figure © L. H. Opie, 2012.)

better than a β-blocker. As β-blockade is commonly used in effort angina, carvedilol may be the β-blocker that is preferred. To be sure would require more high-quality comparative trials in the modern era.

Nebivolol is a β-blocker that somewhat paradoxically, is also a $β_3$-adrenoceptor *agonist,* whereby it activates NOS, thus releasing NO·.[67] This unusual property should theoretically help to limit nitrate tolerance.

Hydralazine is logical, especially in CHF because (1) there are strong trial data favoring the nitrate-hydrazine combination, and (2) the hydralazine may overcome the effect of free radical formation.

Experimental nitroglycerin-induced endothelial dysfunction in humans can be prevented by high-dose *atorvastatin* (80 mg/day) for 7 days.[48] The proposed mechanism is statin-induced decrease of the nitroglycerin-induced oxidative stress.

Experimentally, telmisartan, an *ARB,* counters nitrate-induced vascular dysfunction.[68]

Choice of nitrate medication. Pentaerythritol tetranitrate (not in the United States) is relatively resistant to tolerance induction.[30] Experimentally, pentaerythritol tetranitrate improves angiotensin II–induced vascular dysfunction caused by stimulation of nicotinamide adenine dinucleotide phosphate oxidase activity (see Fig. 2-4) and formation of ROS (see Fig. 2-5).[47] Likewise, in experimental diabetes, vascular function is maintained.[69] In a small study on patients with CAD, treatment for 8 weeks with oral pentaerythritol tetranitrate 80 mg three times daily did not induce endothelial dysfunction.[70] Taken together, these observations suggest that pentaerythritol tetranitrate could be used more often (where it still is available). Decisive evidence from a prospective double-blinded clinical trial versus a standard nitrate is still required for proof of concept.

Nitrate Cross-Tolerance

Short- and long-acting nitrates are frequently combined. In patients already receiving isosorbide dinitrate, addition of sublingual nitroglycerin may give a further therapeutic effect, albeit diminished. Logically, as discussed in previous editions of this book, tolerance to long-acting nitrates should also cause cross-tolerance to short-acting nitrates, as shown for the capacitance vessels of the forearm, coronary artery diameter, and on exercise tolerance during intravenous nitroglycerin therapy.

Nitrate Pseudotolerance and Rebound

Rebound is the abrupt increase in anginal frequency during accidental nitrate withdrawal (e.g., displacement of an intravenous infusion) or during nitrate-free periods.[71,72] Nitrate pseudotolerance probably accounts for the "zero-hour phenomenon," whereby patients receiving long-acting nitrate therapy experience worsening of angina just prior to routine administration of medication.[26] The underlying mechanisms are unopposed vasoconstriction (angiotensin II, catecholamines, and endothelin) during nitrate withdrawal with attenuation of net vasodilator effect of NO·.[56]

Nitric Oxide Resistance

NO· resistance may be defined as *de novo* hyporesponsiveness to NO· effects, whether vascular or antiaggregatory. It also occurs with other "direct" donors of NO·, such as sodium nitroprusside. The occurrence of NO· resistance accounts for the finding that some patients with heart failure respond poorly to infused NO· donors, irrespective of prior nitrate exposure.[73] The mechanisms of NO· resistance in platelets relate primarily to incremental redox stress mediated by superoxide anion release.[74] There is a close association between NO· resistance and endothelial dysfunction as in ACS.[75] Platelet resistance to NO˙ is an adverse prognostic marker.[76]

Step-Care for Angina of Effort

The National Institute for Clinical Excellence (NICE) in the United Kingdom is an impartial body of experts drawn from the United Kingdom who aim to produce an impartial and high-quality document. Their full-length document on the management of stable angina, comprising 489 pages, is summarized in abridged format.[77] Each of the recommendations is supported by a table of all the relevant studies, which are graded into low, medium, and high quality. For example, comparison between β-blockers and CCBs covers 18 analyses.

First-line therapy. Short-acting nitrates are regarded as the basis of therapy, to which either a β-blocker or CCB is added.

Second-line therapy. Second-line therapy is the combination of a short acting nitrate with a β-blocker plus a CCB (dihydropyridine [DHP]) such as long-acting nifedipine, amlodipine, or felodipine. The NICE investigation could find no evidence of the difference in cardiac mortality or rate of nonfatal MI between patients treated with this combination compared with either of the two agents alone. However, there was objective evidence that during exercise testing the combination increased exercise time and time to ST depression in the short term when compared with one of the two agents alone. This beneficial effect of combination treatment was not matched by improved symptom control, as assessed by the frequency of episodes of angina and use of nitroglycerin. The short-term improvement in exercise tolerance would, however, translate to a subjective benefit for the patient.

Third-line therapy. The add-on choice is between long-acting nitrates, ivabradine, nicorandil, and ranolazine. We add perhexiline (Australia and New Zealand) and trimetazidine (Europe). The European Task Force for the management of stable angina, presently preparing its report for the European Guidelines, will also allow for any of these third-line drugs, except for long-acting nitrates, to be chosen as first-line agents according to the judgment and experience of the practicing physician or cardiologist.

Overall care. A full history and physical examination is required to exclude all remediable factors (see Table 2-5), not forgetting aortic stenosis that may be occult in older adults. Risk factors such as hypertension and lifestyle must be vigorously managed and aspirin, statins, and an ACE inhibitor given if there are no contraindications.[78] Percutaneous coronary intervention (PCI) and bypass surgery are increasingly taken as escape routes when coronary anatomy is appropriate. However, conservative management gives outcome results as good as PCI.[79] There are no long-term outcome studies on the benefits of nitrates alone in angina pectoris.

Combination Therapy for Angina

Existing data are inadequate to evaluate the overall efficacy of combinations of nitrates plus β-blockers and CCBs when compared with optimal therapy by each other or by any one agent alone. The COURAGE study reflects current American practice.[79] Almost all received a statin and aspirin, 86% to 89% a β-blocker, and 65% to 78% an ACE inhibitor or ARB. Nitrate use declined from 72% at the start to 57% at 5 years. However, only 43% to 49% were given a CCB, even though first-line therapy in those with effort angina or prior infarction by the CCB verapamil was identical in outcome with β-blockade by atenolol.[80]

β-blockade and long-acting nitrates are often combined in the therapy of angina (see Table 2-5). Both β-blockers and nitrates decrease the oxygen demand, and nitrates increase the oxygen supply; β-blockers block the tachycardia caused by nitrates. β-blockade tends to increase heart size and nitrates to decrease it.

CCBs and short-acting nitroglycerin are often combined. In a double-blind trial of 47 patients with effort angina, verapamil 80 mg three times daily decreased the use of nitroglycerin tablets by 25% and prolonged exercise time by 20%.[81] No outcome data have been reported. *CCBs and long-acting nitrates* are also often given together, however, again without support from outcome trial data.

Nitrates, β-blockers, and CCBs may also be combined as triple therapy. The ACTION study was a very large outcome study in which long-acting nifedipine gastrointestinal therapeutic system (GITS; Procardia XL, Adalat CC) was added to preexisting antianginal therapy, mostly β-blockers (80%) and nitrates (57% nitrates as needed, and 38% daily nitrates).[28] The CCB reduced the need for coronary angiography or bypass surgery, and reduced new heart failure. In hypertensive patients added nifedipine gave similar but more marked benefits plus stroke reduction.[82] There are two lessons. First, dual medical therapy by β-blockers and nitrates is inferior to triple therapy (added DHP CCBs); and second, hypertension in stable angina needs vigorous antihypertensive therapy as in triple therapy. However, we argue that "optimal medical therapy" should consider a metabolically active agent.

Metabolic and Other Newer Antianginal Agents

The metabolic antianginal agents and ranolazine have antianginal activity not mediated by nor associated with hemodynamic changes (Fig. 2-8). Their protective mechanisms oppose the basic metabolic

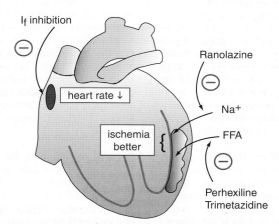

NOVEL ANTIANGINALS
Opie 2012

Figure 2-8   Novel antianginal agents work in different ways. I_f inhibition by ivabradine increases myocardial oxygen demand by decreasing the heart rate. Ranolazine decreases the inflow of sodium by the slow sodium current during ischemia and thereby lessens the intracellular sodium and calcium load. Perhexiline inhibits free fatty acid (FFA) oxidation at the level of the enzyme CPT-1. Trimetazidine inhibits fatty acid oxidation at the level of the mitochondrial long-chain oxidation and, in addition, improves whole-body insulin sensitivity. (Figure © L. H. Opie, 2012.)

mechanisms operative in the myocardial ischemia that is the basis of angina.

Ranolazine (Ranexa). Ranolazine is approved by the Food and Drug Administration for chronic effort angina, and may be used in combination with amlodipine, β-blockers, or nitrates. It is a metabolically active antianginal, originally thought to act by inhibition of oxygen-wasting fatty acid metabolism, thereby increasing the metabolism of protective glucose.[83] Currently, however, the favored mechanism is inhibition of the slow inward sodium current whereby sodium enters the ischemic cells, then dragging in calcium ions by sodium-calcium exchange with their proischemic effects. Controversy continues as to whether the antianginal effects of ranolazine, including a possibly beneficial effect in suppressing atrial fibrillation, might partially depend on improvement in myocardial energetics.[84] A metabolic mechanism is particularly relevant because of the recent findings that ranolazine lowers fasting plasma glucose and hemoglobin A1c in patients with non-ST elevation ACS and hyperglycemia.[85] Ranolazine helps in poorly controlled diabetes and may also improve symptomatic status in systolic heart failure by reducing calcium overload.[86]

Ranolazine cautions. Although the US packet insert warns about prolongation of the QT_c interval, in a recent large trial on patients with ACS no proarrhythmic effects were noted.[87] However, ranolazine should still be avoided in those with prior QT prolongation, or with other drugs that prolong the QT interval (see Fig. 8-6). Because it is metabolized by the hepatic enzyme CYP3A, drugs inhibiting this enzyme (ketoconazole, diltiazem, verapamil, macrolide antibiotics, human immunodeficiency virus protease inhibitors, and grapefruit juice) and chronic liver disease may all increase ranolazine blood levels and hence QT prolongation.

Trimetazidine. Trimetazidine is widely used as an antianginal drug in Europe but not in the United States or United Kingdom. It is a partial inhibitor of fatty acid oxidation without hemodynamic effects. Short-term clinical studies have demonstrated significant benefits including a reduction in weekly angina episodes and improved exercise time, but large, long-term trials are needed.[88] In diabetic patients with CAD trimetazidine decreased blood glucose, increased forearm glucose uptake, and improved endothelial function.[89] An interesting proposal is that, because it acts independently of any BP reduction, it could be used as an antianginal in those with erectile dysfunction in place of nitrates to allow free use of sildenafil and similar agents.

There is increasingly strong evidence that trimetazidine may also be useful in the treatment of chronic systolic heart failure[90] secondary to improvements in myocardial energetics. In heart failure added trimetazidine gives benefit to conventional therapy including β-blockades and RAS inhibition.[91] In a small series of neurologic patients, treatment with trimetazidine worsened previously diagnosed Parkinson disease,[92] which should become a contraindication to its use.

Perhexiline. Perhexiline inhibits fatty acid oxidation at the level of CPT-1, the enzyme that transports activated long-chain fatty acids into the mitochondria. Once widely used, hepatotoxicity and peripheral neuropathy became limitations in the 1980s. The subsequent realization that these side effects resulted mainly from slow hepatic hydroxylation and that their incidence could be reduced by measuring blood levels and lowering doses if needed, has led to a resurgence for use in refractory angina in Australia and New Zealand.[7,93-96] Elsewhere, perhexilene is not widely used. It should theoretically be ideal for the combination of angina and heart failure.[93]

Use in heart failure. Perhexiline improves symptoms and energetics in moderate systolic heart failure refractory to other therapy.[97] Perhexiline also improves nonobstructive hypertrophic cardiomyopathy.[98] The latter major finding, it must be emphasized, represents the first demonstration by a controlled trial that symptoms in heart failure caused by this condition are amenable to pharmacologic therapy.

Other Newer Antianginal Agents

Ivabradine. Ivabradine (Procoralan) is a blocker of the pacemaker current I_f, and hence does not act directly on the metabolism but indirectly by decreasing the heart rate and thus the metabolic demand of the heart. Its antianginal potency is similar to that of β-blockade[99] and amlodipine.[100] There is no negative inotropic effect nor BP reduction as with β-blockers, nor any rebound on cessation of therapy.[94] Ivabradine is licensed in the United Kingdom and other European countries for use in angina when β-blockers are not tolerated or are contradicted. In practice, it may be combined with β-blockade with clinical benefit,[101] but in this study the β-blocker was not upwardly titrated to achieve maximal heart rate reduction. Theoretically there is less risk of severe sinus node depression than with β-blockade because only one of several pacemaker currents is blocked, whereas β-blockade affects all. The downside is that the current I_f is also found in the retina, so that there may be disturbance of nocturnal vision with flashing lights (phosphenes)[102] that could impair driving at night and is often transient.

Use in heart failure. The SHIFT study established the clinical benefits of ivabradine in a group of patients with moderate systolic heart failure whose heart rates remained elevated despite β-blockade.[103] Ivabradine reduced cardiovascular mortality and hospital admissions, and also substantially improved quality of life. However, the findings of SHIFT have been challenged. In the *Lancet* editorial accompanying the SHIFT study, Teerlink questioned whether adequate β-blocker doses had been used.[104] Only 23% of the patients were at trial-established target doses and only half were receiving 50% or more of the targeted β-blocker dose (also see Chapter 6, page 196).

European approval. In December 2011 The European Medicines Agency's Committee for Medicinal Products for Human Use (CHMP) recommended the approval of the license of ivabradine. The license now includes the treatment of chronic heart failure New York Heart Association level II to IV with systolic dysfunction in patients in sinus rhythm and whose heart rate is 75 bpm or more, in combination with standard therapy including b-blocker therapy or when b-blocker therapy is contraindicated or not tolerated. The CHMP contraindications to use in heart failure are unstable or acute heart failure or pacemaker-dependent heart failure (heart rate imposed exclusively by the pacemaker).

Nicorandil. Nicorandil (not in the United States) has a double cellular mechanism of action, acting both as a potassium channel activator and having a nitratelike effect, which may explain why experimentally it causes less tolerance than nitrates. It is a nicotinamide nitrate, acting chiefly by dilation of the large coronary arteries, as well as by reduction of pre- and afterload. It is widely used as an antianginal agent in Japan. In the IONA study, 5126 patients with stable angina were followed for a mean of 1.6 years. Major coronary events including ACS were reduced.[105]

Allopurinol. Allopurinol may have a double energy-conserving mechanism. First, it might reduce myocardial oxygen consumption via inhibition of xanthine oxidase. Second, in heart failure allopurinol may act by promoting transfer of high-energy phosphate from creatine phosphate to adenosine triphosphate.[106] In keeping with these energy-enhancing concepts, Norman et al.[107] performed a double-blind placebo crossover study of high-dose allopurinol (600 mg/day) in patients with stable angina pectoris. They found a moderate increase in time to chest pain and to significant ST depression, thereby establishing an antianginal effect of high-dose allopurinol. Furthermore, this dose of allopurinol reduced vascular oxidative stress and improved endothelial function in patients with CAD.[108]

Despite the considerable interest arising from these findings, a number of important issues remain unclear. First, the mechanism of action is not clear. Favorable effects on myocardial energetics might underlie the increases in exercise tolerance.[106,109] Second, little information is currently available as to the dose-response characteristics of allopurinol in angina, its potency in otherwise refractory cases, or its long-term safety in the high dose used in the study performed by Norman et al.[107]

Are Nitrates Really Safe?

In contrast to the reasonable data for the safety of β-blockers and CCBs in effort angina,[110] logic would say that nitrate therapy that leads to excess production of free radicals, endothelial dysfunction, tachycardia, and renin-angiotensin activation may not be safe.[111] Analyses of two large databases showed that nitrate use was associated with increased mortality with hazard ratios of 1.6 and 3.8.[112] Prolonged nitrate therapy given to Japanese patients for vasospastic angina increased serious cardiac events in a descriptive study.[113] At present the best policy may lie in adding short-acting nitrates to β-blockers or CCBs plus the standard cardioprotective drugs such as aspirin, ACE inhibitors, and statins,[57] as in the EUROPA study (see Chapter 5).

SUMMARY

1. *Mechanisms of action.* Nitrates act by venodilation and relief of coronary vasoconstriction (including that induced by exercise) to ameliorate anginal attacks. They are also arterial dilators, and reduce aortic systolic pressure. Their unloading effects also benefit patients with CHF with high LV filling pressures.

2. *Intermittent nitrates for effort angina.* Sublingual nitroglycerin remains the basic therapy, usually combined with a β-blocker, a CCB, or both with careful assessment of lifestyle, BP, and blood lipid profile. As the duration of action lasts for minutes, nitrate tolerance is unusual because of the relatively long nitrate-free intervals between attacks. Intermittent isosorbide dinitrate has a delayed onset of action because of the need for hepatic transformation to active metabolites, yet the duration of action is longer than with nitroglycerin.

3. *For anginal prophylaxis.* Some newer nitrate preparations are not substantial advances over the old. We support the NICE recommendations for initial use of a short-acting nitrate plus either a β-blocker or CCB, then adding both the β-blocker and a DHP CCB, then adding a third-line agent, with some latitude in allowing the "third-line" agent (ivabradine, nicorandil, ranolazine, trimetazidine; or perhexiline in Australia and New Zealand) to be used as the initial combination with short-acting nitrates.

4. *Nitrate tolerance.* The longer the duration of nitrate action, the more tolerance is likely to develop. Thus it effectively turns into a balancing act between duration of action and avoidance of tolerance. Down-grading long-acting nitrates to a third-line choice as recommended by NICE, instead of a first-line choice as it is still often used, should lessen the risk of tolerance. Increasing data show that endothelial dysfunction, in which aldehyde formation plays a role, is incriminated in nitrate tolerance. Co-therapy with carvedilol or possibly nebivolol as the β-blockers of choice should help to prevent or delay tolerance, yet prospective clinical trials are lacking.

5. *For unstable angina at rest.* A nitrate-free interval is not possible, and short-term treatment for 24 to 48 hours with intravenous nitroglycerin is frequently effective; however, escalating doses are often required to overcome tolerance.

6. *Early phase AMI.* We suggest that intravenous nitrates be specifically reserved for more complicated patients.

7. *Treatment of CHF.* Tolerance also develops during treatment of CHF, so that nitrates are often reserved for specific problems such as acute LV failure, nocturnal dyspnea, or anticipated exercise. However, isosorbide dinitrate combined with hydralazine is now licensed for heart failure in self-defined black subjects.

8. *Acute pulmonary edema.* Nitrates are an important part of the overall therapy, acting chiefly by preload reduction.

9. *Nitrate tolerance.* The current understanding of the mechanism tolerance focuses on free radical formation (superoxide and peroxynitrite) with impaired bioconversion of nitrate to active NO⋅. During the treatment of effort angina by isosorbide dinitrate or mononitrate, substantial evidence suggests that eccentric doses with a nitrate-free interval largely avoid clinical tolerance, but endothelial dysfunction remains a long-term hazard. Besides addition of hydralazine (see previous discussion) other less well-tested measures include administration of antioxidants, statins, ACE inhibitors, and folic acid.

10. *Serious interaction with sildenafil-like agents.* Nitrates can interact very adversely with such agents, which are now often used to alleviate erectile dysfunction. The latter is common in those with cardiovascular disease, being a manifestation of endothelial dysfunction. The co-administration of these PDE-5 inhibitors with nitrates is therefore contraindicated. Every man presenting with ACS should be questioned about recent use of these agents (trade names: Viagra, Levitra, and Cialis). If any of these agents has been used, there has to be an interval of 24-48 hours (the longer interval for Cialis) before nitrates can be given therapeutically with reasonable safety but still with great care.

11. *Newer antianginal agents.* Newer antianginal agents other than nitrates are being increasingly tested and used. These include ivabradine, ranolazine, trimetazidine, perhexiline, and allopurinol. These directly or indirectly help to preserve the myocardial energy balance. There are relatively few significant side effects.

References

1. Brunton TL. On the use of nitrite of amyl in angina pectoris. *Lancet* 1867;2:97–98.
2. Nesto RW, et al. The ischemic cascade: temporal sequence of hemodynamic, electrocardiographic and symptomatic expressions of ischemia. *Am J Cardiol* 1987;57:23C–30C.
3. Rinaldi CA, et al. Randomized, double-blind crossover study to investigate the effects of amlodipine and isosorbide mononitrate on the time course and severity of exercise-induced myocardial stunning. *Circulation* 1998;98:749–756.
4. Parker JD. Therapy with nitrates: increasing evidence of vascular toxicity. *J Am Coll Cardiol* 2003;42:1835–1837.
5. Ignarro LJ, et al. Nitric oxide donors and cardiovascular agents modulating the bioactivity of nitric oxide: an overview. *Circ Res* 2002;90:21–28.
6. Harrison DG, et al. The nitrovasodilators: new ideas about old drugs. *Circulation* 1993; 87:1461–1467.
7. Kelly RP, et al. Nitroglycerin has more favourable effects on left ventricular afterload than apparent from measurement of pressure in a peripheral artery. *Eur Heart J* 1990;11: 138–144.

8. Chen CH et al. Mitochondrial aldehyde dehydrogenase and cardiac diseases. *Cardiovasc Res* 2010;88:51–57.

9. Thomas GR, et al. Once daily therapy with Isosorbide-5-mononitrate causes endothelial dysfunction in humans: evidence of a free radical mediated mechanism. *J Am Coll Cardiol* 2007;49:1289–1295.

10. Noll G, et al. Differential effects of captopril and nitrates on muscle sympathetic nerve activity in volunteers. *Circulation* 1997;95:2286–2292.

11. Ritchie RH, et al. Exploiting cGMP-based therapies for the prevention of left ventricular hypertrophy: NO˙ and beyond. *Pharmacol Ther* 2009;124:279–300.

12. Kruger M, et al. Protein kinase G modulates human myocardial passive stiffness by phosphorylation of the titin springs. *Circ Res* 2009;104:87–94.

13. Bronzwaer JGF, et al. Nitric oxide: the missing lusitrope in failing myocardium. *Eur Heart J* 2008;29:2453–2455.

14. Chirkov YY, et al. Antiplatelet effects of nitroglycerin in healthy subjects and in patients with stable angina pectoris. *J Cardiovasc Pharmacol* 1993;21:384–389.

15. Diodati J, et al. Effects of nitroglycerin at therapeutic doses on platelet aggregation in unstable angina pectoris and acute myocardial infarction. *Am J Cardiol* 1990;66: 683–688.

16. Bogaert MG. Clinical pharmacokinetics of nitrates. *Cardiovasc Drugs Ther* 1994;8:693–699.

17. Abrams J. How to use nitrates. *Cardiovasc Drugs Ther* 2002;16:511–514.

18. Kloner RA, et al. Time course of the interaction between tadalafil and nitrates. *J Am Coll Cardiol* 2003;42:1855–1860.

19. Gogia H, et al. Prevention of tolerance to hemodynamic effects of nitrates with concomitant use of hydralazine in patients with chronic heart failure. *J Am Coll Cardiol* 1995;26:1575–1580.

20. Cole RT, et al. Hydralazine and isosorbide dinitrate in heart failure: historical perspective, mechanisms and future directions. *Circulation* 2011;123:2414–2422.

21. Taylor AL, et al. Combination of isosorbide dinitrate and hydralazine in blacks with heart failure. *N Engl J Med* 2004;351:2049–2057.

22. Ducharme A, et al. Comparison of nitroglycerin lingual spray and sublingual tablet on time of onset and duration of brachial artery vasodilation in normal subjects. *Am J Cardiol* 1999;84:952–954.

23. Thadani U, et al. Short and long-acting oral nitrates for stable angina pectoris. *Cardiovasc Drugs Ther* 1994;8:611–623.

24. Parker JO. Eccentric dosing with isosorbide-5-mononitrate in angina pectoris. *Am J Cardiol* 1993;72:871–876.

25. Chrysant SG, et al. Efficacy and safety of extended-release isosorbide mononitrate for stable effort angina pectoris. *Am J Cardiol* 1993;72:1249–1256.

26. DeMots H, et al. Intermittent transdermal nitroglycerin therapy in the treatment of chronic stable angina. *J Am Coll Cardiol* 1989;13:786–795.

27. Thomas GR, et al. Once daily therapy with isosorbide-5-mononitrate causes endothelial dysfunction in humans: evidence of a free-radical-mediated mechanism. *J Am Coll Cardiol* 2007;49:1289–1295.

28. Poole-Wilson PA, et al. Effect of long-acting nifedipine on mortality and cardiovascular morbidity in patients with stable angina requiring treatment (ACTION trial): randomised controlled trial. *Lancet* 2004;364:849–857.

29. Thadani U, et al. Oral isosorbide dinitrate in angina pectoris: comparison of duration of action on dose-response relation during acute and sustained therapy. *Am J Cardiol* 1982;49:411–419.

30. Jurt U, et al. Differential effects of pentaerythritol tetranitrate and nitroglycerin on the development of tolerance and evidence of lipid peroxidation: a human in vivo study. *J Am Coll Cardiol* 2001;38:854–859.

31. Gibbons RJ, et al. ACC/AHA 2002 guideline update for the management of patients with chronic stable angina—summary article: a report of the American College of Cardiology/American Heart Association Task Force on practice guidelines (Committee on the Management of Patients With Chronic Stable Angina). *J Am Coll Cardiol* 2003;41:159–168.

32. GISSI-3 Study Group. GISSI-3: effects of lisinopril and transdermal glyceryl trinitrate singly and together on 6-week mortality and ventricular function after acute myocardial infarction. *Lancet* 1994;343:1115–1122.

33. Sage PR, et al. Nitroglycerin tolerance in human vessels: evidence for impaired nitroglycerin bioconversion. *Circulation* 2000;102:2810–2815.

34. Horowitz JD. Role of nitrates in unstable angina pectoris. *Am J Cardiol* 1992;70:64B–71B.

35. Abraham WT, et al. In-hospital mortality in patients with acute decompensated heart failure requiring intravenous vasoactive medications: an analysis from the Acute Decompensated Heart Failure National Registry (ADHERE). *J Am Coll Cardiol* 2005;46:57–64.

36. Bussmann WD, et al. [Effect of sublingual nitroglycerin in emergency treatment of classic pulmonary edema]. *Minerva Cardioangiol* 1978;26:623–632.

37. Cotter G, et al. Randomized trial of high-dose isosorbide dinitrate plus low-dose furosemide versus high-dose furosemide plus low-dose isosorbide dinitrate in severe pulmonary edema. *Lancet* 1998;351:389–393.

38. Beltrame JF, et al. Nitrate therapy is an alternative to furosemide/morphine therapy in the management of acute cardiogenic pulmonary edema. *J Card Fail* 1998;4:271–279.

39. V-HeFT II Study, Cohn JN, et al. A comparison of enalapril with hydralazine-isosorbide dinitrate in the treatment of chronic congestive cardiac failure. *N Engl J Med* 1991; 325:303–310.

40. Elkayam U, et al. Double-blind, placebo-controlled study to evaluate the effect of organic nitrates in patients with chronic heart failure treated with angiotensin-converting enzyme inhibition. *Circulation* 1999;99:2652–2657.

41. Agvald P, et al. Nitric oxide generation, tachyphylaxis and cross-tachyphylaxis from nitro-vasodilators in vivo. *Eur J Pharmacol* 1999;385:137–145.

42. Sage PR, et al. Nitroglycerin tolerance in human vessels: evidence for impaired nitroglycerin bioconversion. *Circulation* 2000;102:2810–2815.

43. Munzel T, et al. Nitrate therapy: new aspects concerning molecular action and tolerance. *Circulation* 2011;123:2132–2144.

44. Daiber A, et al. Nitrate reductase activity of mitochondrial aldehyde dehydrogenase (ALDH-2) as a redox sensor for cardiovascular oxidative stress. *Methods Mol Biol* 2011:594:43–55.

45. Tsou PS, et al. Differential metabolism of organic nitrates by aldehyde dehydrogenase 1a1 and 2: substrate selectivity, enzyme inactivation, and active cysteine sites. *AAPS J* 2011;13:548–555.

46. D'Souza Y, et al. Changes in aldehyde dehydrogenase 2 expression in rat blood vessels during glyceryl trinitrate tolerance development and reversal. *Br J Pharmacol* 2011;164:632–643.

47. Schuhmacher S, et al. Pentaerythritol tetranitrate improves angiotensin II-induced vascular dysfunction via induction of heme oxygenase-1. *Hypertension* 2010;55:897–904.

48. Liuni A, et al. Coadministration of atorvastatin prevents nitroglycerin-induced endothelial dysfunction and nitrate tolerance in healthy humans. *J Am Coll Cardiol* 2011;57:93–98.

49. Daiber A, et al. Nitrate tolerance as a model of vascular dysfunction: roles for mitochondrial aldehyde dehydrogenase and mitochondrial oxidative stress. *Pharmacol Rep* 2009; 61:33–48.

50. Milano G, et al. Phosphodiesterase-5 inhibition mimics intermittent reoxygenation and improves cardioprotection in the hypoxic myocardium. *PLoS One* 2011;6(11):e27910.

51. Muller S, et al. Inhibition of vascular oxidative stress in hypercholesterolemia by eccentric isosorbide mononitrate. *J Am Coll Cardiol* 2004;44:624–631.

52. Muller S, et al. Preserved endothelial function after long term eccentric isosorbide mononitrate despite moderate nitrate tolerance. *J Am Coll Cardiol* 2003;41:1994–2000.

53. Fink B, et al. Tolerance to nitrates with enhanced radical formation suppressed by carvedilol. *J Cardiovasc Pharmacol* 1999;34:800–805.

54. Fleming JW, et al. Muscarinic cholinergic-receptor stimulation of specific GTP hydrolysis related to adenylate cyclase activity in canine cardiac sarcolemma. *Circ Res* 1988; 64:340–350.

55. Munzel T, et al. Explaining the phenomenon of nitrate tolerance. *Circ Res* 2005;97:618–628.

56. Munzel T, et al. New insights into mechanisms underlying nitrate tolerance. *Am J Cardiol* 1996;77:24C–30C.

57. Munzel T, et al. Do we still need organic nitrates? *J Am Coll Cardiol* 2007;49:1296–1298.

58. Needleman P, et al. Mechanism of tolerance development to organic nitrates. *J Pharmacol Exp Ther* 1973;184:709–715.

59. Ignarro LJ. After 130 years, the molecular mechanism of action of nitroglycerin is revealed. *Proc Natl Acad Sci U S A* 2002;99:7816–7817.

60. Horowitz JD. Amelioration of nitrate tolerance: matching strategies with mechanisms. *J Am Coll Cardiol* 2003;41:2001–2003.

61. Horowitz JD, et al. Potentiation of the cardiovascular effects of nitroglycerin by N-acetylcysteine. *Circulation* 1983;68:1247–1253.

62. Loscalzo J. N-Acetylcysteine potentiates inhibition of platelet aggregation by nitroglycerin. *J Clin Invest* 1985;76:703–708.

63. Packer M, et al. Prevention and reversal of nitrate tolerance in patients with congestive heart failure. *N Engl J Med* 1987;317:799–804.

64. Horowitz JD, et al. Combined use of nitroglycerin and N-acetylcysteine in the management of unstable angina pectoris. *Circulation* 1988;77:787–794.

65. Parker JO, et al. The effect of supplemental L-arginine on tolerance development during continuous transdermal nitroglycerin therapy. *J Am Coll Cardiol* 2002;39:1199–1203.

66. Nakahira A, et al. Co-administration of carvedilol attenuates nitrate tolerance by preventing cytochrome P 450 depletion. *Circ J* 2010;74:1711–1717.

67. Heusch G. Beta(3)-adrenoceptor activation—just say NO to myocardial reperfusion injury. *J Am Coll Cardiol* 2011;58:2692–2694.

68. Knorr M, et al. Nitroglycerin-induced endothelial dysfunction and tolerance involve adverse phosphorylation and S-Glutathionylation of endothelial nitric oxide synthase: beneficial effects of therapy with the AT1 receptor blocker telmisartan. *Arterioscler Thromb Vasc Biol* 2011;31:2223–2231.

69. Schuhmacher S, et al. Vascular dysfunction in experimental diabetes is improved by pentaerithrity ltetranitrate but not isosorbide-5-mononitrate therapy. *Diabetes* 2011;60: 2608–2616.

70. Schnorbus B, et al. Effects of pentaerythritol tetranitrate on endothelial function in coronary artery disease: results of the PENTA study. *Clin Res Cardiol* 2010;99:115–124.

71. Ferratini M, et al. Intermittent transdermal nitroglycerin monotherapy in stable exercise-induced angina: a comparison with a continuous schedule. *Eur Heart J* 1989;10: 998–1002.

72. Figueras J, et al. Rebound myocardial ischaemia following abrupt interruption of intravenous nitroglycerin infusion in patients with unstable angina at rest. *Eur Heart J* 1991; 12:405–411.

73. Armstrong PW, et al. Pharmacokinetic-hemodynamic studies of intravenous nitroglycerin in congestive cardiac failure. *Circulation* 1980;62:160–166.

74. Chirkov YY, et al. Impaired tissue responsiveness to organic nitrates and nitric oxide: a new therapeutic frontier? *Pharmacol Ther* 2007;116:287–305.

75. Chirkov YY, et al. Stable angina and acute coronary syndromes are associated with nitric oxide resistance in platelets. *J Am Coll Cardiol* 2001;37:1851–1857.

76. Willoughby SR, et al. Platelet nitric oxide responsiveness: a novel prognostic marker in acute coronary syndromes. *Arterioscler Thromb Vasc Biol* 2005;25:2661–2666.
77. Henderson RA et al. Management of stable angina: summary of NICE guidance. *Heart* 2012;98:500–507.
78. Fraker Jr TD, et al. 2007 chronic angina focused update of the ACC/AHA 2002 Guidelines for the management of patients with chronic stable angina: a report of the American College of Cardiology/American Heart Association Task Force on Practice Guidelines Writing Group to develop the focused update of the 2002 Guidelines for the management of patients with chronic stable angina. *Circulation* 2007;116: 2762–2772.
79. Boden WE, et al. Optimal medical therapy with or without PCI for stable coronary disease. *N Engl J Med* 2007;356:1503–1516.
80. Pepine CJ, et al. A calcium antagonist vs a non-calcium antagonist hypertension treatment strategy for patients with coronary artery disease. The International Verapamil-Trandolapril Study (INVEST): a randomized controlled trial. *JAMA* 2003;290: 2805–2816.
81. Andreasen F, et al. Assessment of verapamil in the treatment of angina pectoris. *Eur J Cardiol* 1975;2:443–452.
82. Lubsen J, et al. Effect of long-acting nifedipine on mortality and cardiovascular morbidity in patients with symptomatic stable angina and hypertension: the ACTION trial. *J Hypertens* 2005;23:641–648.
83. Chaitman BR, et al. Effects of ranolazine with atenolol, amlodipine, or diltiazem on exercise tolerance and angina frequency in patients with severe chronic angina: a randomized controlled trial. *JAMA* 2004;291:309–316.
84. Cingolani E, et al. The electrophysiological properties of ranolazine: a metabolic anti-ischemic drug or an energy-efficient antiarrhythmic agent? *Rev Cardiovasc Med* 2011; 12:136–422.
85. Chisholm JW, et al. Effect of ranolazine on A1c and glucose levels in hyperglycemic patients with non-ST elevation acute coronary syndrome. *Diabetes Care* 2010;33: 1163–1168.
86. Sossalla S, et al. Role of ranolazine in angina, heart failure, arrhythmias, and diabetes. *Pharmacol Ther* Nov 26, 2012;133:311–323.
87. Scirica BM, et al. Effect of ranolazine, an antianginal agent with novel electrophysiological properties, on the incidence of arrhythmias in patients with non ST-segment elevation acute coronary syndrome: results from the Metabolic Efficiency With Ranolazine for Less Ischemia in Non ST-Elevation Acute Coronary Syndrome Thrombolysis in Myocardial Infarction 36 (MERLIN-TIMI 36) randomized controlled trial. *Circulation* 2007;116:1647–1652.
88. Ciapboni A, et al. Trimetazidine for stable angina. *Cochrane Database SYST REB* 2005;CD003614.
89. Fragasso G, et al. Short- and long-term beneficial effects of trimetazidine in patients with diabetes and ischemic cardiomyopathy. *Am Heart J* 2003;146:E18.
90. Tuunanen H, et al. Trimetazidine, a metabolic modulator, has cardiac and extracardiac benefits in idiopathic dilated cardiomyopathy. *Circulation* 2008;118:125–128.
91. Fragasso G, et al. Effect of partial inhibition of fatty acid oxidation by trimetazidine on whole body energy metabolism in patients with chronic heart failure. *Heart* 2011;97: 1495–1500.
92. Martí Massó JF, et al. Trimetazidine induces Parkinsonism, gait disorders and tremor. *Therapie* 2005;60:419–422.
93. Ashrafian H, et al. Perhexiline. *Cardiovasc Drug Rev* 2007;25:76–97.
94. Borer J, et al. Antianginal and anti-ischemic effects of ivabradine, an If inhibitor, in stable angina. *Circulation* 2003;107:817–823.
95. Cole PL, et al. Efficacy and safety of perhexiline maleate in refractory angina. A double-blind placebo-controlled clinical trial of a novel antianginal agent. *Circulation* 1990;81:1260–1270.
96. Lee L, et al. Metabolic manipulation in ischaemic heart disease, a novel approach to treatment. *Eur Heart J* 2004;25:634–641.
97. Lee L, et al. Metabolic modulation with perhexiline in chronic heart failure: a randomized controlled trial of short-term use of a novel treatment. *Circulation* 2005;112: 3280–3288.
98. Abozguia K, et al. Metabolic modulator perhexiline corrects energy deficiency and improves exercise capacity in symptomatic hypertrophic cardiomyopathy. *Circulation* 2010;122:1562–1569.
99. Tardif JC, et al. Efficacy of ivabradine, a new selective I(f) inhibitor, compared with atenolol in patients with chronic stable angina. *Eur Heart J* 2005;26:2529–2536.
100. Ruzyllo W, et al. Antianginal efficacy and safety of ivabradine compared with amlodipine in patients with stable effort angina pectoris: a 3-month randomised, double-blind, multicentre, noninferiority trial. *Drugs* 2007;67:393–405.
101. Werdan K, et al. Ivabradine in combination with beta-blocker improves symptoms and quality of life in patients with stable angina pectoris: results from the ADDITIONS study. *Clin Res Cardiol* 2012;101:365–373.
102. Cervetto L, et al. Cellular mechanisms underlying the pharmacological induction of phosphenes. *Br J Pharmacol* 2007;150:383–390.
103. Swedberg K, et al. Ivabradine and outcomes in chronic heart failure (SHIFT): a randomised placebo-controlled study. *Lancet* 2010;376:875–885.
104. Teerlink JR. Ivabradine in heart failure—no paradigm SHIFT yet. *Lancet* 2010;376: 847–849.

105. IONA Study Group. Effect of nicorandil on coronary events in patients with stable angina: The Impact Of Nicorandil in Angina (IONA) Randomized Trial. *Lancet* 2002;359: 1269–1275.
106. Opie LH. Allopurinol for heart failure: novel mechanisms. *J Am Coll Cardiol* 2012 [in press].
107. Norman A, et al. Effect of high-dose allopurinol on exercise in patients with chronic stable angina: a randomised, placebo controlled crossover trial. *Lancet*, 2010;375: 2161–2167.
108. Rajendra NS, et al. Mechanistic insights into the therapeutic use of high-dose allopurinol in angina pectoris. *J Am Coll Cardiol* 2011;58:820–828.
109. Lee J, et al. Effect of acute xanthine oxidase inhibition on myocardial energetics during basal and very high cardiac workstates. *J Cardiovasc Trans Res* 2011;4:504–513.
110. Heidenreich PA, et al. Meta-analysis of trials comparing β-blockers, calcium antagonists, and nitrates for stable angina. *JAMA* 1999;281:1927–1936.
111. Parker JD. Nitrate tolerance, oxidative stress, and mitochondrial function: another worrisome chapter on the effects of organic nitrates. *J Clin Invest* 2004;113:352–354.
112. Scherbel U, et al. Differential acute and chronic responses of tumor necrosis factor–deficient mice to experimental brain injury. *Proc Natl Acad Sci U S A* 1999;96:8721–8726.
113. Kosugi M, et al. Effect of long-term nitrate treatment on cardiac events in patients with vasospastic angina. *Circ J* 2011;75:2196–2205.

3

Calcium Channel Blockers

LIONEL H. OPIE

"Calcium antagonists have assumed a major role in the treatment of patients with hypertension or coronary heart disease."

Abernethy and Schwartz, 1999[1]

"There are none of the widely trumpeted dangers from dihydropyridine calcium channel blockers."

Kaplan, 2003, commenting on the results of ALLHAT[2]

Calcium channel blockers (CCBs; calcium antagonists) act chiefly by vasodilation and reduction of the peripheral vascular resistance. They remain among the most commonly used agents for hypertension and angina. Their major role in these conditions is now well understood, based on the results of a series of large trials. CCBs are a heterogeneous group of drugs that can chemically be classified into the dihydropyridines (DHPs) and the non-DHPs (Table 3-1), their common pharmacologic property being selective inhibition of L-type channel opening in vascular smooth muscle and in the myocardium (Fig. 3-1). Distinctions between the DHPs and non-DHPs are reflected in different binding sites on the calcium channel pores, and in the greater vascular selectivity of the DHP agents.[3] In addition, the non-DHPs, by virtue of nodal inhibition, reduce the heart rate (heart rate–lowering [HRL] agents). Thus verapamil and diltiazem more closely resemble the β-blockers in their therapeutic spectrum with, however, one major difference: CCBs are contraindicated in heart failure.

Pharmacologic Properties

Calcium Channels: L and T Types

The most important property of all CCBs is selectively to inhibit the inward flow of charge-bearing calcium ions when the calcium channel becomes permeable or is "open." Previously, the term *slow channel* was used, but now it is realized that the calcium current travels much faster than previously believed, and that there are at least two types of calcium channels, the L and T. The conventional long-lasting opening calcium channel is termed the *L-type channel,* which is blocked by CCBs and increased in activity by catecholamines. The function of the L-type is to admit the substantial amount of calcium ions required for initiation of contraction via calcium-induced calcium release from the sarcoplasmic reticulum (see Fig. 3-1). The T-type (*T* for transient) channel opens at more negative potentials than the L-type. It plays an important role in the initial depolarization of sinus and

Table 3-1

Binding Sites for CCBs, Tissue Specificity, Clinical Uses, and Safety Concerns

Site	Tissue Specificity	Clinical Uses	Contraindications	Safety Concerns
DHP Binding				
Prototype: nifedipine Site 1	Vessels > myocardium > nodes Vascular selectivity 10× N, A 100× Nic, I, F 1000× Nis	Effort angina (N, A) Hypertension (N,* A, Nic, I, F, Nis) Vasospastic angina (N, A) Raynaud phenomenon	Unstable angina, early phase AMI, systolic heart failure (possible exception: amlodipine)	Nifedipine capsules: excess BP fall especially in older adults; adrenergic activation in ACS Longer acting forms: safe in hypertension, no studies on ACS
Non-DHP Binding				
"Heart rate lowering" Site 1B, D Site 1C, V	SA and AV nodes > myocardium = vessels	Angina: effort (V, D), unstable (V), vasospastic (V, D) Hypertension (D,*V) Arrhythmias, supraventricular (D,† V) Verapamil: postinfarct patients (no US license)	Systolic heart failure; sinus bradycardia or SSS; AV nodal block; WPW syndrome; acute myocardial infarction (early phase)	Systolic heart failure, especially diltiazem. Safety record of verapamil may equal that of β-blockade in older adult patients with hypertension

FDA-approved drugs for listed indications in parentheses.
A, Amlodipine; ACS, acute coronary syndrome; AMI, acute myocardial infarction; AV, atrioventricular; BP, blood pressure; CCB, calcium channel blocker; D, diltiazem; DHP, dihydropyridine; F, felodipine; FDA, Food and Drug Administration; I, isradipine; N, nifedipine; Nic, nicardipine; Nis, nisoldipine; SA, sinoatrial; SSS, sick sinus syndrome; V, verapamil; WPW, Wolff-Parkinson-White syndrome.
*Long-acting forms only.
†Intravenous forms only.

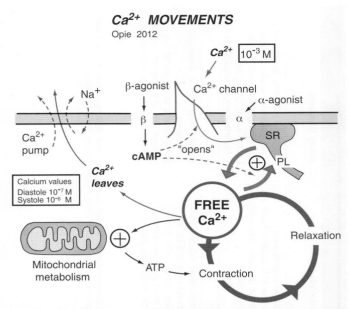

Figure 3-1   Role of calcium channel in regulating myocardial cytosolic calcium ion movements. α, alpha-adrenergic receptor; β, beta-adrenergic receptor; *cAMP,* cyclic adenosine monophosphate; *P,* phospholamban; *SR,* sarcoplasmic reticulum. (Figure © L.H. Opie, 2012.)

atrioventricular (AV) nodal tissue and is relatively upregulated in the failing myocardium. Currently there are no specific T-type blockers clinically available.

Cellular Mechanisms: β-Blockade versus CCBs

Both these categories of agents are used for angina and hypertension, yet there are important differences in their subcellular mode of action. Both have a negative inotropic effect, whereas only CCBs relax vascular and (to a much lesser extent) other smooth muscle (Fig. 3-2). CCBs "block" the entry of calcium through the calcium channel in both smooth muscle and myocardium, so that less calcium is available to the contractile apparatus. The result is vasodilation and a negative inotropic effect, which in the case of the DHPs is usually modest because of the unloading effect of peripheral vasodilation.

CCBs inhibit vascular contraction. In smooth muscle (see Fig. 3-2), calcium ions regulate the contractile mechanism independently of troponin C. Interaction of calcium with calmodulin forms calcium-calmodulin, which then stimulates myosin light chain kinase (MLCK) to phosphorylate the myosin light chains to allow actin-myosin interaction and, hence, contraction. Cyclic adenosine monophosphate (AMP) inhibits the MLCK. In contrast, β-blockade, by lessening the formation of cyclic AMP, removes the inhibition on MLCK activity and therefore promotes contraction in smooth muscle, which explains why asthma may be precipitated, and why the peripheral vascular resistance often rises at the start of β-blocker therapy (Fig. 3-3).

CCBs versus β-blockers. CCBs and β-blockers have hemodynamic and neurohumoral differences. Hemodynamic differences are well

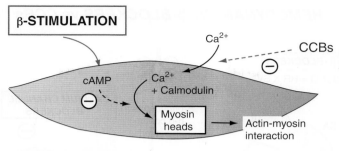

SMOOTH MUSCLE
β-blockade promotes contraction

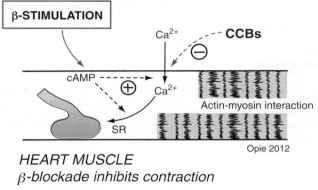

HEART MUSCLE
β-blockade inhibits contraction

Figure 3-2   Proposed comparative effects of β-blockade and calcium channel blockers (CCBs) on smooth muscle and myocardium. The opposing effects on vascular smooth muscle are of critical therapeutic importance. *cAMP,* Cyclic adenosine monophosphate; *SR,* sarcoplasmic reticulum. (Figure © L.H. Opie, 2012.)

defined (see Fig. 3-3). Whereas β-blockers inhibit the renin-angiotensin system by decreasing renin release and oppose the hyperadrenergic state in heart failure, CCBs as a group have no such inhibitory effects.[4] This difference could explain why β-blockers but not CCBs are an important component of the therapy of heart failure.

CCBs and carotid vascular protection. Experimentally, both nifedipine and amlodipine give endothelial protection and promote formation of nitric oxide. Furthermore, several CCBs including amlodipine, nifedipine, and lacidipine have inhibitory effects on carotid atheromatous disease.[5,6] Similar protective effects have not consistently been found with β-blockers. There is increasing evidence that such vascular protection may be associated with improved clinical outcomes.

Classification of Calcium Channel Blockers

Dihydropyridines

The DHPs all bind to the same sites on the α_1-subunit (the N sites), thereby establishing their common property of calcium channel antagonism (Fig. 3-4). To a different degree, they exert a greater inhibitory

HEMODYNAMICS: β-BLOCKERS vs CCBs

Opie 2012

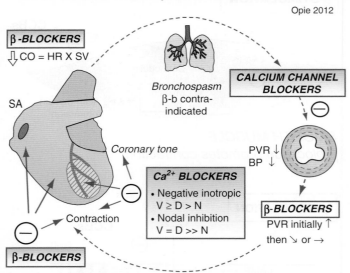

Figure 3-3 Comparison of hemodynamic effects of β-blockers and of CCBs, showing possibilities for combination therapy. *BP,* blood pressure; *CO,* cardiac output; *D,* diltiazem; *HR,* heart rate; *N,* nifedipine as an example of dihydropyridines; *PVR,* peripheral vascular resistance; *SA,* sinoatrial node; *SV,* stroke volume; *V,* verapamil. (Figure © L.H. Opie, 2012.)

CALCIUM CHANNEL MODEL

Opie 2012

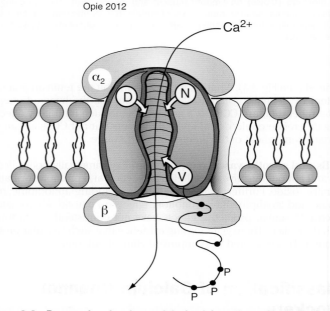

Figure 3-4   Proposed molecular model of calcium channel α_1-subunit with binding sites for nifedipine (N), diltiazem (D), and verapamil (V). It is thought that all dihydropyridines bind to the same site as nifedipine. Amlodipine has additional subsidiary binding to the V and D sites. *P* indicates sites of phosphorylation in response to cyclic adenosine monophosphate (see Fig. 3-1), which acts to increase the opening probability of the calcium channel. (Figure © L.H. Opie, 2012.)

effect on vascular smooth muscle than on the myocardium, conferring the property of vascular selectivity (see Table 3-1, Fig. 3-5). There is nonetheless still the potential for myocardial depression, particularly in the case of agents with less selectivity and in the presence of prior myocardial disease or β-blockade. For practical purposes, effects of DHPs on the sinoatrial (SA) and AV nodes can be ignored.

Nifedipine was the first of the DHPs. In the short-acting capsule form, originally available, it rapidly vasodilates to relieve severe hypertension and to terminate attacks of coronary spasm. The peripheral vasodilation and a rapid drop in blood pressure (BP) led to rapid reflex adrenergic activation with tachycardia (Fig. 3-6). Such proischemic effects probably explain why the short-acting DHPs in high doses have precipitated serious adverse events in unstable angina. The inappropriate use of short-acting nifedipine can explain much of the adverse publicity that once surrounded the CCBs as a group,[7] so that the focus has now changed to the long-acting DHPs, which are free of such dangers.[2]

Hence, the introduction of truly long-acting compounds, such as amlodipine or the extended-release formulations of nifedipine (GITS, XL, CC) and of others such as felodipine and isradipine, has led to substantially fewer symptomatic side effects. Two residual side effects of note are headache, as for all arteriolar dilators, and ankle edema, caused by precapillary dilation. There is now much greater attention to the appropriate use of the DHPs, with established safety and new trials in hypertension such as ACCOMPLISH suggesting a preeminent place for initial dual therapy by DHP and CCBs with an angiotensin-converting enzyme (ACE) inhibitor.[8,9]

Nondihydropyridines: Heart Rate–Lowering Agents

Verapamil and diltiazem bind to two different sites on the α_1-subunit of the calcium channel (see Fig. 3-4), yet have many properties in common with each other. The first and most obvious distinction from the DHPs is that verapamil and diltiazem both act on nodal tissue, being therapeutically effective in supraventricular tachycardias. Both tend to decrease the sinus rate. Both inhibit myocardial contraction more than

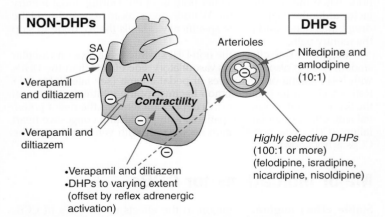

CARDIAC VS VASCULAR SELECTIVITY
Opie 2012

Figure 3-5 As a group, the dihydropyridines (DHPs) are more vascular selective, whereas the non-DHPs verapamil and diltiazem act equally on the heart and on the arterioles. *AV,* Atrioventricular; *SA,* sinoatrial. (Figure © L.H. Opie, 2012.)

ISCHEMIC HEART: CCB EFFECT

Opie 2012

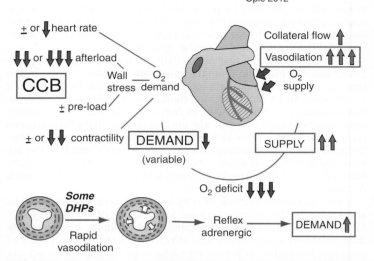

Figure 3-6   Mechanisms of antiischemic effects of calcium channel blockers. Note that the rapid arteriolar vasodilation resulting from the action of some short-acting dihydropyridines (DHPs) may increase myocardial oxygen demand by reflex adrenergic stimulation. *CCB,* Calcium channel blocker. (Figure © L.H. Opie, 2012.)

the DHPs or, put differently, are less vascular selective (see Fig. 3-5). These properties, added to peripheral vasodilation, lead to substantial reduction in the myocardial oxygen demand. Such "oxygen conservation" makes the HRL agents much closer than the DHPs to the β-blockers, with which they share some similarities of therapeutic activity. Two important exceptions are (1) the almost total lack of effect of verapamil and diltiazem on standard types of ventricular tachycardia, which rather is a contraindication to their use; and (2) the benefits of β-blockade in heart failure, against which the HRL agents are also clearly contraindicated. The salient features for the clinical use of these agents is shown in Table 3-2.

For supraventricular tachycardias, a frequency-dependent effect is important, so that there is better access to the binding sites of the AV node when the calcium channel pore is "open." During nodal reentry tachycardia, the channel of the AV node opens more frequently and the drug binds better, and hence specifically inhibits the AV node to stop the reentry path.

Regarding side effects, the non-DHPs, being less active on vascular smooth muscle, also have less vasodilatory side effects than the DHPs, with less flushing or headaches or pedal edema (see later, Table 3-4). Reflex tachycardia is uncommon because of the inhibitory effects on the SA node. Left ventricular (LV) depression remains the major potential side effect, especially in patients with preexisting congestive heart failure (CHF). Why constipation occurs only with verapamil of all the CCBs is not known.

Major Indications for CCBs

Stable effort angina. Common to the effects of all types of CCBs is the inhibition of the L-calcium current in arterial smooth muscle, occurring at relatively low concentrations (see Table 3-2). Hence coronary vasodilation is a major common property (see Fig. 3-3). Although the antianginal mechanisms are many and varied, the shared effects are

Table 3-2

Oral Heart Rate–Lowering CCBs: Salient Features for Cardiovascular Use

Agent	Dose	Pharmacokinetics and Metabolism	Side Effects and Contraindications	Kinetic and Dynamic Interactions
Verapamil				
Tablets (for IV use, see p. 78)	180-480 mg daily in two or three doses (titrated)	Peak plasma levels with 1-2 h. Low bioavailability (10%-20%), high first-pass metabolism to long-acting norverapamil. Excretion: 75% renal; 25% GI; t½ 3-7 h	Constipation; depression of SA, AV nodes, and LV; CI sick sinus syndrome, digoxin toxicity, excess β-blockade, LV failure; obstructive cardiomyopathy	Levels ↑ in liver or renal disease. Hepatic interactions; inhibits CYP3A4, thus decreases breakdown of atorvastatin, simvastatin, lovastatin/St. John's wort reduces plasma verapamil. Digoxin levels increased.
Slow release (SR) Verelan (Ver) Covera-HS (timed)	As above, two doses (SR) Single dose (Ver) Single bedtime dose	Peak effects: SR 1-2h, Ver 7-9h, t½ 5-12 h Co-delayed 4- to 6-h release	As above	As above
Diltiazem				
Tablets (for IV use see p. 79)	120-360 mg daily in three or four doses	Onset: 15-30 min. Peak: 1-2 h; t½ 5 h. Bioavailable 45% (hepatic). Active metabolites. 65% GI loss.	As for verapamil, but no constipation	As for verapamil, except little or no effect on digoxin levels, liver interactions less prominent. Cimetidine and liver disease increase blood levels. Propranolol levels increased.
Prolonged SR, CD, XR Tiazac	As above, 1 (XR, CD, Tiazac) or 2 doses	Slower onset, longer t½, otherwise similar	As above	As above

AV, Atrioventricular; CCB, calcium channel blocker; CI, confidence intervals; GI, gastrointestinal; IV, intravenous; LV, left ventricular; SA, sinoatrial; SR, slow release; t½, plasma elimination half-life; Ver, Verelan.

(1) coronary vasodilation and relief of exercise-induced vasoconstriction, and (2) afterload reduction resulting from BP reduction (see Fig. 3-6). In addition, in the case of verapamil and diltiazem, slowing of the sinus node with a decrease in exercise heart rate and a negative inotropic effect probably contribute (Fig. 3-7).

Unstable angina at rest. Of the major CCBs, *only verapamil* has a license for unstable angina, although intravenous diltiazem has one good supporting study.[10] Importantly the DHPs should not be used without concurrent β-blockade (risk of reflex adrenergic activation, see Fig. 3-6).

Coronary spasm. The role of spasm as a major cause of the anginal syndromes has undergone revision. Once seen as a major contributor to transient ischemic pain at rest, coronary spasm is now relatively discounted because β-blockade was more effective than nifedipine in several studies.[11] The role of coronary spasm in unstable angina has also been downplayed because nifedipine, in the absence of concurrent β-blockade, appeared to be harmful.[12] Coronary spasm remains important as a cause of angina precipitated by cold or hyperventilation, and in Prinzmetal's variant angina. All CCBs should be effective. Among those specifically licensed are verapamil and amlodipine.

Hypertension. *CCBs are excellent antihypertensive agents,* among the best for older adult and black patients (see Chapter 7). Overall, they are at least as effective as other antihypertensive classes in treating CHD and more effective than others in preventing stroke.[13] Furthermore, they are almost as good as other classes in preventing heart failure. Their effect is largely independent both of sodium intake, possibly because of their mild diuretic effect, and of the concurrent use of antiinflammatory agents such as nonsteroidal antiinflammatory drugs. In hypertension with nephropathy, both DHPs and non-DHPs reduce the

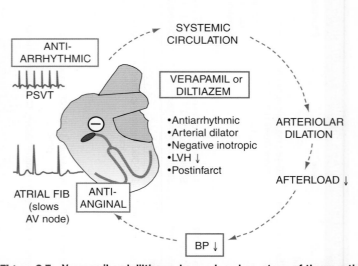

VERAPAMIL OR DILTIAZEM, MULTIPLE EFFECTS

Opie 2012

Figure 3-7   Verapamil and diltiazem have a broad spectrum of therapeutic effects. *Atrial fib,* Atrial fibrillation; *AV,* atrioventricular; *BP,* blood pressure; *LVH,* left ventricular hypertrophy; *PSVT,* paroxysmal supraventricular tachycardia. (Figure © L.H. Opie, 2012.)

BP, which is the primary aim, but non-DHPs reduce proteinuria better.[14]

Supraventricular tachycardia. Verapamil and diltiazem inhibit the AV node, which explains their effect in supraventricular tachycardias. Nifedipine and other DHPs are clinically ineffective.

Postinfarct protection. Although β-blockers are drugs of choice, both verapamil and diltiazem give some protection in the absence of prior LV failure. Verapamil is better documented.[15,16]

Vascular protection. Increased nitric oxide formation in cultured endothelial cells[17] and improved endothelial function in patients[18] may explain why CCBs slow down carotid atherosclerosis,[6] which in turn may be explain decreased stroke.[19] In CAMELOT, amlodipine slowed coronary atheroma and reduced cardiovascular events more than enalapril.[20]

Safety and Efficacy

The ideal cardiovascular drug is both efficacious in reducing hard end points, such as mortality, stroke, and myocardial infarction (MI), and safe. Safety, which is not generally well defined, may be regarded as the absence of significant adverse effects when the drug is used with due regard for its known contraindications. In the case of CCBs, previous controversy regarding both efficacy and safety has been laid to rest by new studies that strongly and beyond doubt support the safety of long-acting CCBs.[21-25]

Safety and efficacy in ischemic heart disease. In stable effort angina, imperfect evidence based on randomized controlled trials and a meta-analysis suggests equivalent safety and efficacy of CCBs (other than short-acting nifedipine) to β-blockers. Nonetheless, CCBs remain underused in stable effort angina, especially in the United States.[26] The largest angina trial, ACTION, found that adding long-acting nifedipine to existing β-blocker therapy in effort angina decreased new heart failure and the need for coronary angiography.[27] In unstable angina, a small trial supports the use of diltiazem.[10] There are no data to back the use of DHPs in un-stable angina.[12] In postinfarct follow-up, β-blockers remain the agents of choice, with the non-DHP HRL agents (especially verapamil) the second choice if β-blockers are contraindicated or not tolerated. DHPs lack good evidence for safety and efficacy in post-MI patients.

In hypertension, seven large outcome trials in which more than 50,000 patients received long-acting DHPs, often amlodipine, provide overwhelming proof of the safety and efficacy of these CCBs. Verapamil-based therapy had similar effects on coronary disease with hypertension to therapy based on atenolol in the INVEST trial, the primary end-points being all-cause deaths, nonfatal MI, or nonfatal stroke.[25] In diabetic hypertensives long-acting DHPs are also able to improve outcome.[28,29] In ALLHAT, amlodipine gave similar results in the diabetic and nondiabetic subgroups.[30] These findings make it difficult to agree with the view that CCBs have adverse effects in diabetics, in whom the major issue is adequate BP reduction. In fact, diabetes may rather be a positive indication for preferential use of a CCB.[31] Cancer, bleeding, and increased all-cause mortality, once incorrectly proposed as serious and unexpected side effects of the CCBs, are now all discounted.[2,30]

Verapamil

Verapamil (Isoptin, Calan, Verelan), the prototype non-DHP agent, remains the CCB with the most licensed indications. Both verapamil and diltiazem have multiple cardiovascular effects (see Fig. 3-7).

Electrophysiology. Verapamil inhibits the action potential of the upper and middle regions of the AV node where depolarization is calcium mediated. Verapamil thus inhibits one limb of the reentry circuit, believed to underlie most paroxysmal supraventricular tachycardias (see Fig. 8-4). Increased AV block and the increase in effective refractory period of the AV node explain the reduction of the ventricular rate in atrial flutter and fibrillation. Verapamil is ineffective and harmful in the treatment of ventricular tachycardias except in certain uncommon forms. Hemodynamically, verapamil combines arteriolar dilation with a direct negative inotropic effect (see Table 3-2). The cardiac output and LV ejection fraction do not increase as expected following peripheral vasodilation, which may be an expression of the negative inotropic effect. At rest, the heart only drops modestly with a greater inhibition of exercise-induced tachycardia.

Pharmacokinetics and interactions. Oral verapamil takes 2 hours to act and peaks at 3 hours. Therapeutic blood levels (80 to 400 ng/mL) are seldom measured. The elimination half-life is usually 3 to 7 hours, but increases significantly during chronic administration and in patients with liver or advanced renal insufficiency. Despite nearly complete absorption of oral doses, bioavailability is only 10% to 20%. There is a high first-pass liver metabolism by multiple components of the P-450 system, including CYP 3A4, the latter explaining why verapamil increases blood levels of several statins such as atorvastatin, simvastatin, and lovastatin, as well as ketoconazole. Because of the hepatic CYP3A4 interaction, the Food and Drug Administration (FDA) warns that the10-mg dose of simvastatin should not be exceeded in patients taking verapamil. Ultimate excretion of the parent compound, as well as the active hepatic metabolite norverapamil, is 75% by the kidneys and 25% by the gastrointestinal (GI) tract. Verapamil is 87% to 93% protein bound, but no interaction with warfarin has been reported. When both verapamil and digoxin are given together, their interaction causes digoxin levels to rise, probably as a result of a reduction in the renal clearance of digoxin. Norverapamil is the long-acting hepatic metabolite of verapamil, which appears rapidly in the plasma after oral administration of verapamil and in concentrations similar to those of the parent compound; like verapamil, norverapamil undergoes delayed clearance during chronic dosing.

Verapamil doses. The usual total oral daily dose is 180-360 mg daily, no more than 480 mg given once or twice daily (long-acting formulations) or three times daily for standard short-acting preparations (see Table 3-2). Large differences of pharmacokinetics among individuals mean that dose titration is required, so that 120 mg daily may be adequate for those with hepatic impairment or for older adults. During chronic oral dosing, the formation of norverapamil metabolites and altered rates of hepatic metabolism suggest that less frequent or smaller daily doses of short-acting verapamil may be used.[32] For example, if verapamil has been given at a dose of 80 mg three times daily, then 120 mg twice daily should be as good. Lower doses are required in older adult patients or those with advanced renal or hepatic disease or when there is concurrent β-blockade. Intravenous verapamil is much less used for supraventricular arrhythmias since the advent of adenosine and the ultra–short acting β-blocker, esmolol.

Slow-release preparations. Calan SR or Isoptin SR releases the drug from a matrix at a rate that responds to food, whereas Verelan releases the drug from a rate-controlling polymer at a rate not sensitive to food intake. The usual doses are 240 to 480 mg daily. The SR preparations are given once or twice daily and Verelan once daily. A controlled-onset, extended-release tablet (Covera-HS; COER-24; 180 or 240 mg tablets) is taken once daily at bed time, with the (unproven) aim of lessening adverse cardiovascular events early next morning.

Outcome studies. Verapamil was the antihypertensive equivalent of atenolol in hypertension, with coronary artery disease (CAD) regarding major outcomes with three extra benefits: less new diabetes, less angina, and less psychological depression.[25]

Side effects. Class side effects are those of vasodilation causing headaches, facial flushing, and dizziness. These may be lessened by the long-acting preparations, so that in practice they are often not troublesome. Tachycardia is not a side effect. Constipation is specific and causes most trouble, especially in older adult patients. Rare side effects may include pain in the gums, facial pain, epigastric pain, hepatotoxicity, and transient mental confusion. In older adults, verapamil may predispose to GI bleeding.[21]

Contraindications to verapamil (Fig. 3-8, Table 3-3). Contraindications, especially in the intravenous therapy of supraventricular tachycardias are sick sinus syndrome; preexisting AV nodal disease; excess therapy with β-blockade, digitalis, quinidine, or disopyramide; or myocardial depression. In the Wolff-Parkinson-White (WPW) syndrome complicated by atrial fibrillation, intravenous verapamil is contraindicated because of the risk of anterograde conduction through the bypass tract (see Fig. 8-14). Verapamil is also contraindicated in ventricular tachycardia (wide QRS-complex) because of excess myocardial depression, which may be lethal. An exception to this rule is exercise-induced ventricular tachycardia. Myocardial depression, if secondary to the supraventricular tachycardia, is not a contraindication, whereas preexisting LV systolic failure is. Dose reduction may be required in hepatic or renal disease (see "Pharmacokinetics and Interactions" earlier in this chapter).

Drug Interactions with Verapamil

β-blockers. Verapamil by intravenous injection is now seldom given, so that the potentially serious interaction with preexisting β-adrenergic

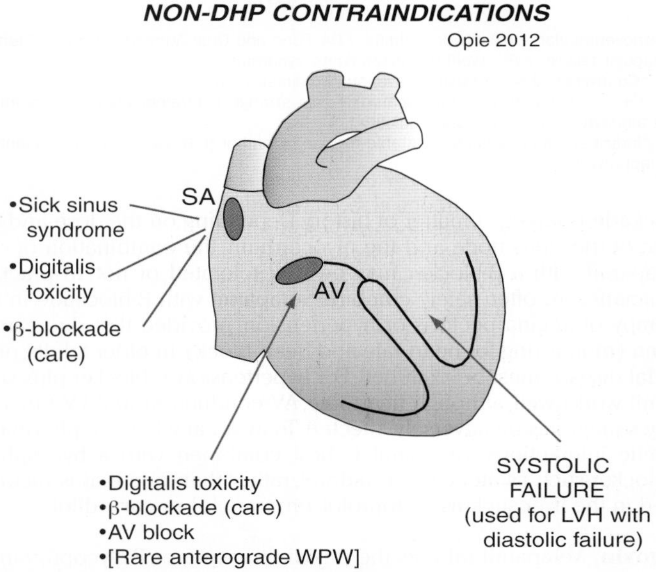

NON-DHP CONTRAINDICATIONS
Opie 2012

•Sick sinus syndrome
•Digitalis toxicity
•β-blockade (care)

SA

AV

•Digitalis toxicity
•β-blockade (care)
•AV block
•[Rare anterograde WPW]

SYSTOLIC FAILURE
(used for LVH with diastolic failure)

Figure 3-8 Contraindications to verapamil or diltiazem. For use of verapamil and diltiazem in patients already receiving β-blockers, see text. *AV,* Atrioventricular; *LVH,* left ventricular hypertrophy; *SA,* sinoatrial; *WPW,* Wolff-Parkinson-White preexcitation syndrome. (Figure © L.H. Opie, 2012.)

Table 3-3

Comparative Contraindications of Verapamil, Diltiazem, Dihydropyridines, and β-Adrenergic Blocking Agents

Contraindications	Verapamil	Diltiazem	DHPs	β-Blockade
Absolute				
Severe sinus bradycardia	0/+	0/+	0	++
Sick sinus syndrome	++	++	0	++
AV conduction defects	++	++	0	++
WPW syndrome	++	++	0	++
Digoxin toxicity, AV block*	++	++	0	++
Asthma	0	0	0	+++
Bronchospasm	0	0	0	0/++
Heart failure	+++	+++	++	Indicated
Hypotension	+	+	++	+
Coronary artery spasm	0	0	0	+
Raynaud and active peripheral vascular disease	0	0	0	+
Severe mental depression	0	0	0	+
Severe aortic stenosis	+	+	++	+
Obstructive cardiomyopathy	0/+	0/+	++	Indicated
Relative				
Insulin resistance	0	0	0	Care
Adverse blood lipid profile	0	0	0	Care
Digoxin nodal effects	Care	Care	0	Care
β-blockade	Care	Care	BP↓	—
Disopyramide therapy	Care	Care	0	Care
Unstable angina	Care	Care	++	0
Postinfarct protection	May protect	0 (+ if no LVF)	++	Indicated

AV, Atrioventricular; DHP, dihydropyridine; FDA, Food and Drug Administration; LVF, left ventricular failure; WPW, Wolff-Parkinson-White syndrome.

*Contraindication to rapid intravenous administration

+++ = Absolutely contraindicated; ++ = strongly contraindicated; + = relative contraindication; 0 = not contraindicated.

"Indicated" means judged suitable for use by author (L.H. Opie), not necessarily FDA approved.

blockade is largely a matter of history. Depending on the dose and the state of the sinus node and the myocardium, the combination of oral verapamil with a β-blocker may be well tolerated or not. In practice, clinicians can often safely combine verapamil with β-blockade in the therapy of angina pectoris or hypertension, provided that due care is taken (monitoring for heart rate and heart block). In older adults, prior nodal disease must be excluded. For hypertension, β-blocker plus verapamil works well, although heart rate, AV conduction, and LV function may sometimes be adversely affected. To avoid any hepatic pharmacokinetic interactions, verapamil is best combined with a hydrophilic β-blocker such as atenolol or nadolol, rather than one that is metabolized in the liver, such as metoprolol, propranolol, or carvedilol.

Digoxin. Verapamil inhibits the digoxin transporter, P-glycoprotein, to increase blood digoxin levels, which is of special relevance when both are used chronically to inhibit AV nodal conduction. In digitalis toxicity, rapid intravenous verapamil is absolutely contraindicated because it can lethally exaggerate AV block. There is no reason why, in the absence of digitalis toxicity or AV block, oral verapamil and digoxin should not be combined (checking the digoxin level).Whereas digoxin can be used for heart failure with atrial fibrillation, verapamil is negatively inotropic and should not be used.

Antiarrhythmics. The combined negative inotropic potential of verapamil and disopyramide is considerable. Co-therapy with flecainide may also give added negative inotropic and dromotropic effects.

Statins. Verapamil inhibits the hepatic CYP3A isoenzyme, and therefore potentially increases the blood levels of atorvastatin, simvastatin, and lovastatin, which are all metabolized by this isoenzyme.[21]

Other agents. Phenobarbital, phenytoin, and rifampin induce the cytochrome systems metabolizing verapamil so that its blood levels fall. Conversely, verapamil inhibits hepatic CYP3A to increase blood levels of cyclosporin, carbamazepine (Tegretol) and theophylline, as mentioned in the package insert.This inhibition is also expected to increase blood levels of ketoconazole and sildenafil. Cimetidine has variable effects.Alcohol levels increase.Verapamil may sensitize to neuromuscular blocking agents, and to the effects of lithium (neurotoxicity).

Therapy of verapamil toxicity. There are few clinical reports on management of verapamil toxicity.Intravenous calcium gluconate (1 to 2 g) or half that dose of calcium chloride, given over 5 minutes, helps when heart failure or excess hypotension is present.If there is an inadequate response, positive inotropic or vasoconstrictory catecholamines (see Chapter 5, p. 180) are given, or else glucagon. An alternative is hyperinsulinemic-euglycemic therapy.[33] Intravenous atropine (1 mg) or isoproterenol is used to shorten AV conduction.A pacemaker may be needed.

Clinical Indications for Verapamil

Angina. In chronic stable effort angina, verapamil acts by a combination of afterload reduction and a mild negative inotropic effect, plus reduction of exercise-induced tachycardia and coronary vasoconstriction.The heart rate usually stays the same or falls modestly. In a major outcome study in patients with CAD with hypertension, INVEST, verapamil-based therapy was compared with atenolol-based therapy, the former supplemented by the ACE inhibitor trandolapril, and the latter by a thiazide if required to reach the BP goal.[25] Major outcomes were very similar but verapamil-based therapy gave less angina and new diabetes.Verapamil doses of 240 to 360 mg daily were the approximate equivalent of atenolol 50-100 mg daily. In unstable angina at rest with threat of infarction, verapamil has not been tested against placebo, although licensed for this purpose in the United States. In Prinzmetal's variant angina therapy is based on CCBs, including verapamil, and high does may be needed.[34] Abrupt withdrawal of verapamil may precipitate rebound angina.

Hypertension. Verapamil is approved for mild to moderate hypertension in the United States.Besides the outcome study in CAD with hypertension (preceding section), in a long-term, double-blind comparative trial, mild to moderate hypertension was adequately controlled in 45% of patients given verapamil 240 mg daily,[35] versus 25% for hydrochlorothiazide 25 mg daily, versus 60% for the combination. Higher doses of verapamil might have done even better. Combinations can be with diuretics, β-blockers, ACE inhibitors, angiotensin receptor blockers (ARBs), or centrally acting agents. During combination with α-blockers, a hepatic interaction may lead to excess hypotension.

Verapamil for supraventricular arrhythmias. Verapamil is licensed for the prophylaxis of repetitive supraventricular tachycardias, and for rate control in chronic atrial fibrillation when given with digoxin (note interaction). For acute attacks of supraventricular tachycardias, when there is no myocardial depression, a bolus dose of 5 to 10 mg (0.1 to 0.15 mg/kg) given over 2 minutes restores sinus rhythm within 10 minutes in 60% of cases (package insert). However, this use is now largely supplanted by intravenous adenosine (see Fig. 8-7). When used for uncontrolled atrial fibrillation but with caution if there is a compromised LV failure, verapamil may safely be given (0.005 mg/kg/min, increasing) or as an intravenous bolus of 5 mg (0.075 mg/kg) followed by double the dose if needed. In atrial flutter, AV block is increased. In all supraventricular tachycardias, including atrial flutter and fibrillation, the presence of a bypass tract (WPW syndrome) contraindicates verapamil.

Other uses for verapamil. In hypertrophic cardiomyopathy, verapamil has been the CCB best evaluated. It is licensed for this purpose in Canada. When given acutely, it lessens symptoms, reduces the outflow tract gradient, improves diastolic function, and enhances exercise performance by 20% to 25%. Verapamil should not be given to patients with resting outflow tract obstruction. No long-term, placebo-controlled studies with verapamil are available. In retrospective comparisons with propranolol, verapamil appeared to decrease sudden death and gave better 10-year survival.[36] The best results were obtained by a combination of septal myectomy and verapamil. A significant number of patients on long-term verapamil develop severe side effects, including SA and AV nodal dysfunction, and occasionally overt heart failure.

Atypical ventricular tachycardia. Some patients with exercise-induced ventricular tachycardia caused by triggered automaticity may respond well to verapamil, as may young patients with idiopathic right ventricular outflow tract ventricular tachycardia (right bundle branch block and left axis deviation). However, verapamil can be lethal for standard wide complex ventricular tachycardia, especially when given intravenously. Therefore, unless the diagnosis is sure, verapamil must be avoided in ventricular tachycardia.

For postinfarct protection, verapamil is approved in the United Kingdom and in Scandinavian countries when β-blockade is contraindicated. Verapamil 120 mg three times daily, started 7 to 15 days after the acute phase in patients without a history of heart failure and no signs of CHF (but with digoxin and diuretic therapy allowed) was protective and decreased reinfarction and mortality by approximately 25% over 18 months.[15]

In intermittent claudication, carefully titrated verapamil increased maximum walking ability.[37]

Summary. Among CCBs, verapamil has the widest range of approved indications, including all varieties of angina (effort, vasospastic, unstable), supraventricular tachycardias, and hypertension. Indirect evidence suggests good safety, but nonetheless with risks of heart block and heart failure. Compared with atenolol in hypertension with CAD, there was less new diabetes, fewer anginas, and less psychological depression. Verapamil combined with β-blockade runs the risk of heart block; thus a DHP with β-blockade is much better.

Diltiazem

Although molecular studies show different channel binding sites for diltiazem and verapamil (see Fig. 3-4), in clinical practice they have somewhat similar therapeutic spectra and contraindications, so that they are often classified as the non-DHPs or HRL agents (see Fig. 3-5). Clinically, diltiazem is used for the same spectrum of disease as is verapamil: angina pectoris, hypertension, supraventricular arrhythmias, and rate control in atrial fibrillation or flutter (see Fig. 3-7). Of these, diltiazem is approved in the United States to treat angina (effort and vasospastic) and hypertension, with only the intravenous form approved for supraventricular tachycardias and for acute rate control. Diltiazem has a low side-effect profile, similar to or possibly better than that of verapamil; specifically the incidence of constipation is much lower (Table 3-4). On the other hand, verapamil is registered for more indications. Is diltiazem less a cardiodepressant than verapamil? There are no strictly comparable clinical studies to support this clinical impression.

Pharmacokinetics. Following oral administration of diltiazem, more than 90% is absorbed, but bioavailability is approximately 45% (first-pass hepatic metabolism). The onset of action of short-acting diltiazem is within 15 to 30 minutes (oral), with a peak at 1 to 2 hours. The elimination half-life is 4 to 7 hours; hence, dosage every 6 to 8 hours of the short-acting preparation is required for sustained therapeutic effect. The therapeutic plasma concentration range is 50 to 300 ng/mL. Protein binding is 80% to 86%. Diltiazem is acetylated in the liver to deacyldiltiazem (40% of the activity of the parent compound), which accumulates with chronic therapy. Unlike verapamil and nifedipine, only 35% of diltiazem is excreted by the kidneys (65% by the GI tract). Because of the hepatic CYP3A4 interaction, the FDA warns that the 10-mg dose of simvastatin should not be exceeded in patients taking diltiazem.

Diltiazem doses. The dose of diltiazem is 120 to 360 mg, given in four daily doses of the short-acting formulation or once or twice a day with slow-release preparations. Cardizem SR permits twice-daily doses. For once-daily use, Dilacor XR is licensed in the United States for hypertension and Cardizem CD and Tiazac for hypertension and angina. Intravenous diltiazem (Cardizem injectable) is approved for arrhythmias but not for acute hypertension. For acute conversion of paroxysmal supraventricular tachycardia, after exclusion of WPW syndrome (see Fig. 8-14) or for slowing the ventricular response rate in atrial fibrillation or flutter, it is given as 0.25 mg/kg over 2 minutes with electrocardiogram and BP monitoring. If the response is inadequate, the dose is repeated as 0.35 mg/kg over 2 minutes. Acute therapy is usually followed by an infusion of 5 to 15 mg/hr for up to 24 hrs. Diltiazem overdose is treated as for verapamil (see p. 77).

Side effects. Normally side effects of the standard preparation are few and limited to headaches, dizziness, and ankle edema in approximately 6% to 10% of patients (see Table 3-4). With high-dose diltiazem (360 mg daily), constipation may also occur. When the extended-release preparation is used for hypertension, the side-effect profile resembles placebo. Nonetheless, bradycardia and first-degree AV block may occur with all diltiazem preparations. In the case of intravenous diltiazem, side effects resemble those of intravenous verapamil, including hypotension and the possible risk of asystole and high-degree AV block when there is preexisting nodal disease. In postinfarct patients with preexisting poor LV function, mortality is increased by diltiazem, not decreased. Occasionally, severe skin rashes such as exfoliative dermatitis are found.

Contraindications. Contraindications resemble those of verapamil (see Fig. 3-8, Table 3-3): preexisting marked depression of the sinus or AV node, hypotension, myocardial failure, and WPW syndrome. Postinfarct LV failure with an ejection fraction of less than 40% is a clear contraindication.[38]

Drug interactions and combinations. Unlike verapamil, the effect of diltiazem on the blood digoxin level is often slight or negligible. As in the case of verapamil, there are the expected hemodynamic interactions with β-blockers. Nonetheless, diltiazem plus β-blocker may be used with care for angina watching for excess bradycardia or AV block or hypotension. Diltiazem may increase the bioavailability of oral

Table 3-4

Reported Side Effects of the Three Prototypical CCBs and Long-Acting Dihydropyridines

	Verapamil Covera-HS (%)	Diltiazem Short-Acting (%)	Diltiazem XR or CD (%)	Nifedipine Capsules* (%)	Nifedipine XL, CC, GITS (%)	Amlodipine 10 mg (%)	Felodipine ER 10 mg (%)
Facial flushing	<1	0-3	0-1	6-25	0-4	3	5
Headaches	< placebo	4-9	< placebo	3-34	6	< placebo	4
Palpitation	0	0	0	Low-25	0	4	1
Lightheadedness, dizziness	5	6-7	0	12	2-4	2	4
Constipation	12	4	1-2	0	1	0	0
Ankle edema, swelling	0	6-10	2-3	6	10-30	10	14
Provocation of angina	0	0	0	Low-14	0	0	0

CCB, Calcium channel blocker.

*No longer used in the United States.

Data from Opie LH. *Clinical use of calcium antagonist drugs.* Boston: Kluwer; 1990, p. 197, and from package inserts.

Side effects are dose related; no strict direct comparisons between the CCBs. Percentages are placebo-corrected.

propranolol perhaps by displacing it from its binding sites (package insert). Occasionally diltiazem plus a DHP is used for refractory coronary artery spasm, the rationale being that two different binding sites on the calcium channel are involved (see Fig. 3-4). Diltiazem plus long-acting nitrates may lead to excess hypotension. As in the case of verapamil, but probably less so, diltiazem may inhibit CYP3A cytochrome, which is expected to increase blood levels of cyclosporin, ketoconazole, carbamazepine (Tegretol), and sildenafil.[21] Conversely, cimetidine inhibits the hepatic cytochrome system breaking down diltiazem to increase circulating levels.

Clinical Uses of Diltiazem

Ischemic syndromes. The efficacy of diltiazem in chronic stable angina is at least as good as propranolol, and the dose is titrated from 120 to 360 mg daily (see Table 3-2). In unstable angina at rest, there is one good albeit small study showing that intravenous diltiazem (not licensed for this purpose in the United States) gives better pain relief than does intravenous nitrate, with improved 1-year follow up.[10] In Prinzmetal's variant angina, diltiazem 240 to 360 mg/day reduces the number of episodes of pain.

Diltiazem for hypertension. In the major long-term outcome study on more than 10,000 patients, the Nordic Diltiazem (NORDIL) trial, diltiazem followed by an ACE inhibitor if needed to reach BP goals was as effective in preventing the primary combined cardiovascular endpoint as treatment based on a diuretic, a β-blocker, or both.[39] In the smaller multicenter VA study, diltiazem was the best among five agents (atenolol, thiazide, doxazosin, and captopril) in reducing BP, and was especially effective in older adult white patients and in black patients.[40] Nonetheless, reduction of LV hypertrophy was poor at 1 year of follow-up, possibly because a short-acting diltiazem formulation was used.[41]

Antiarrhythmic properties of diltiazem. The main electrophysiologic effect is a depressant one on the AV node; the functional and effective refractory periods are prolonged by diltiazem, so that diltiazem is licensed for termination of an attack of supraventricular tachyarrhythmia and for rapid decrease of the ventricular response rate in atrial flutter or fibrillation. Only intravenous diltiazem is approved for this purpose in the United States (see "Diltiazem Doses" earlier in this chapter). Oral diltiazem can be used for the elective as well as prophylactic control (90 mg three times daily) of most supraventricular tachyarrhythmias (oral diltiazem is not approved for this use in the United States or United Kingdom). WPW syndrome is a contraindication to diltiazem.

Cardiac transplantation. Diltiazem acts prophylactically to limit the development of posttransplant coronary atheroma, independently of any BP reduction.[42]

Summary. Diltiazem, with its low side-effect profile, has advantages in the therapy of angina pectoris, acting by peripheral vasodilation, relief of exercise-induced coronary constriction, a modest negative inotropic effect, and sinus node inhibition. There are no outcome studies comparing diltiazem and verapamil. As in the case of verapamil, combination with β-blockade is generally not advised.

Nifedipine, The First DHP

The major actions of the DHPs can be simplified to one: arteriolar dilation (see Fig. 3-5). The direct negative inotropic effect is usually outweighed by arteriolar unloading effects and by reflex adrenergic stimulation (see Fig. 3-6), except in patients with heart failure.

Short-acting capsular nifedipine was first introduced in Europe and Japan as Adalat, and then became the best-selling Procardia in the United States. In angina, it was especially used for coronary spasm, which at that time was thought to be the basis of unstable angina. Unfortunately not enough attention was paid to three important negative studies,[12,43,44] which led to warnings against use in unstable angina in previous editions of this book. Capsular nifedipine is now only the treatment of choice when taken intermittently for conditions such as attacks of vasospastic angina or Raynaud phenomenon.

Long-Acting Nifedipine Formulations

The rest of this section largely focuses on long-acting nifedipine formulations (Procardia XL in the United States, Adalat LA elsewhere; Adalat CC) that are now widely used in the treatment of hypertension, in effort angina, and in vasospastic angina.

Pharmacokinetics. Almost all circulating nifedipine is broken down by hepatic metabolism by the cytochrome P-450 system to inactive metabolites (high first-pass metabolism) that are largely excreted in the urine. The long-acting, osmotically sensitive tablet (nifedipine GITS, marketed as Procardia XL or Adalat LA) releases nifedipine from the inner core as water enters the tablet from the GI tract (see Table 3-2). This process results in stable blood therapeutic levels of approximately 20 to 30 ng/mL over 24 hours. With a core-coat system (Adalat CC), the blood levels over 24 hours are more variable, with the trough-peak ratios of 41% to 91%.

Doses of nifedipine. In effort angina, the usual daily dose 30 to 90 mg of Procardia XL or Adalat LA (Adalat CC is not licensed in the United States for angina). Dose titration is important to avoid precipitation of ischemic pain in some patients. In cold-induced angina or in coronary spasm, the doses are similar and capsules (in similar total daily doses) allow the most rapid onset of action. In hypertension, standard doses are 30 to 90 mg once daily of Procardia XL or Adalat CC. In older adults or in patients with severe liver disease, doses should be reduced.

Contraindications and cautions (Fig. 3-9, Table 3-5). These are tight aortic stenosis or obstructive hypertrophic cardiomyopathy (danger of

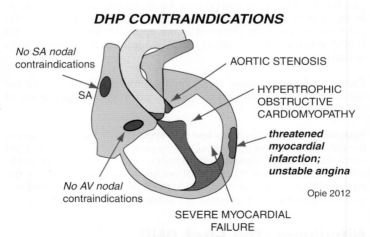

DHP CONTRAINDICATIONS

No SA nodal contraindications

SA

AORTIC STENOSIS

HYPERTROPHIC OBSTRUCTIVE CARDIOMYOPATHY

threatened myocardial infarction; unstable angina

No AV nodal contraindications

Opie 2012

SEVERE MYOCARDIAL FAILURE

Figure 3-9   Contraindications to dihydropyridines (DHPs) are chiefly obstructive lesions such as aortic stenosis or hypertrophic obstructive cardiomyopathy, and heart failure. Unstable angina (threatened infarction) is a contraindication unless combined nifedipine plus β-blockade therapy is used or unless (rarely) coronary spasm is suspected. *AV,* Atrioventricular; *SA,* sinoatrial. (Figure © L.H. Opie, 2012.)

Table 3-5

Long-Acting Dihydropyridines for Oral Use

Agent	Dose and Major Trials	Pharmacokinetics and Metabolism	Side Effects and Contraindications	Interactions and Precautions
Amlodipine (Norvasc, Istin)	5-10 mg once daily (ALLHAT, VALUE, ASCOT)	t_{max} 6-12 h. Extensive but slow hepatic metabolism, 90% inactive metabolites; 60% renal; $t\frac{1}{2}$ 35-50 h. Steady state in 7-8 days	Edema, dizziness, flushing, palpitation. CI: severe aortic stenosis, obstructive cardiomyopathy, LVF, unstable angina AMI. May use amlodipine in CHF class 2 or 3, but best avoided.	Prolonged $t\frac{1}{2}$ up to 56 h in liver failure. Reduce dose, also in older adults and in patients with heart failure. Hepatic metabolism via CYP3A4, interaction with simvastatin (do not exceed 20 mg simvastatin, FDA recommendation), atorvastatin and lovastatin. Grapefruit juice: caution, interaction not established.
Nifedipine prolonged release XL, LA, GITS, Adalat CC; Procardia XL	30-90 mg once daily (INSIGHT, ACTION)	Stable 24-h blood levels. Slow onset, approximately 6 h.	S/E: headache, ankle edema. CI: severe aortic stenosis, obstructive cardiomyopathy, LVF. Unstable angina if no β-blockade	Added LV depression with β-blockade. Avoid in unstable angina without β-blockade. Nifedipine via CYP 3A4 interacts with simvastatin (limit simvastatin to 20 mg) and probably atorvastatin, lovastatin. Cimetidine and liver disease increase blood levels.
Felodipine ER (Plendil)	5-10 mg once daily (HOT)	t_{max} 3-5 h. Complete hepatic metabolism (P-450) to inactive metabolites 75% renal loss, $t\frac{1}{2}$ 22-27 h	Edema, headache, flushing. CI as above except for CHF class 2 and 3 (mortality neutral).	Reduce dose with cimetidine, age, liver disease. Anticonvulsants enhance hepatic metabolism; grapefruit juice decreases CYP3A4 and markedly increases blood felodipine.

AMI, Acute myocardial infarction; *CHF,* congestive heart failure; *CI,* confidence intervals; *FDA,* Food and Drug Administration; *LV,* left ventricular; *LVF,* left ventricular failure; *S/E,* side effect; $t\frac{1}{2}$, plasma elimination half-life; t_{max}, time to peak blood level.

exaggerated pressure gradient), clinically evident heart failure or LV dysfunction (added negative inotropic effect), unstable angina with threat of infarction (in the absence of concurrent β-blockade), and preexisting hypotension. Relative contraindications are subjective intolerance to nifedipine and previous adverse reactions. In pregnancy, nifedipine should only be used if the benefits are thought to outweigh the risk of embryopathy (experimental; pregnancy category C, see Table 12-10).

Minor side effects. The bilateral ankle edema caused by nifedipine is distressing to patients but is not due to cardiac failure; if required, it can be treated by dose reduction, by conventional diuretics, or by an ACE inhibitor. Nifedipine itself has a mild diuretic effect. With extended-release nifedipine preparations (Procardia XL), the manufacturers claim that side effects are restricted to headache (nearly double that found in controls) and ankle edema (dose-dependent, 10% with 30 mg daily, 30% with 180 mg daily). The low incidence of acute vasodilatory side effects, such as flushing and tachycardia, is because of the slow rate of rise of blood DHP levels.

Severe or rare side effects. In patients with LV dysfunction, the direct negative inotropic effect can be a serious problem. Rarely, side effects are compatible with the effects of excess hypotension and organ under-perfusion, namely myocardial ischemia or even infarction, retinal and cerebral ischemia, and renal failure. Other unusual side effects include muscle cramps, myalgia, hypokalemia (via diuretic effect), and gingival swelling.

Drug interactions. Cimetidine and grape fruit juice (large amounts) inhibit the hepatic CYP3A4 P-450 enzyme system breaking down nifedipine, thereby substantially increasing its blood levels. Phenobarbital, phenytoin, and rifampin induce this system metabolizing so that nifedipine blood levels should fall (not mentioned in package insert). In some reports, blood digoxin levels rise. Volatile anesthetics interfere with the myocardial calcium regulation and have inhibitory effects additional to those of nifedipine.

Rebound after cessation of nifedipine therapy. In patients with vasospastic angina, the manufacturers recommend that the dose be tailed off.

Nifedipine poisoning. In one case there was hypotension, SA and AV nodal block, and hyperglycemia. Treatment was by infusions of calcium and dopamine (see also "Amlodipine: The First of the Second-Generation DHPs" later in this chapter).

Combination with β-blockers and other drugs. In patients with reasonable LV function, nifedipine may be freely combined with β-blockade (Fig. 3-10), provided that excess hypotension is guarded against. In LV dysfunction, the added negative inotropic effects may precipitate overt heart failure. In the therapy of effort or vasospastic angina, nifedipine is often combined with nitrates. In the therapy of hypertension, nifedipine may be combined with diuretics, β-blockers, methyldopa, ACE inhibitors, or ARBs. Combination with prazosin or (by extrapolation) other α-blockers may lead to adverse hypotensive interactions.

Clinical Uses of Long-Acting Nifedipine

Effort angina. In the United States only Procardia XL and not Adalat CC is licensed for effort angina, when β-blockade and nitrates are ineffective or not tolerated. Whereas capsular nifedipine modestly increases the heart rate (that may aggravate angina), the extended-release preparations leave the heart rate unchanged.[45] Their antianginal activity and safety approximates that of the β-blockers, albeit the cost of more subjective symptoms.[46] In the ACTION study on patients with stable

CCBs VERSUS β-BLOCKADE, CV EFFECTS
Opie 2012

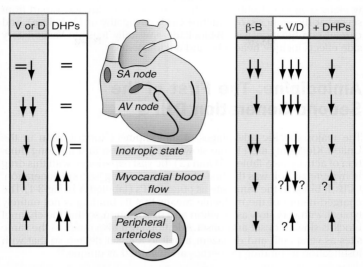

Figure 3-10   Proposed hemodynamic effects of calcium channel blockers (CCB), singly or in combination with β-blockade (β2B). Note that some of these effects are based on animal data and extrapolation to humans needs to be made with caution. *AV,* Atrioventricular; *D,* diltiazem; *DHP,* dihydropyridines; *SA,* sinoatrial; *V,* verapamil. (Figure © L.H. Opie, 2012.)

coronary disease, one of the largest studies on effort angina (N ≈7,800), 80% already receiving β-blockade, the major benefits of added long-acting nifedipine were less new heart failure, less coronary angiography and less bypass surgery.[27] In the retrospective substudy on hypertensives (mean initial 151/85 mm Hg falling to 136/78 mm Hg) new heart failure decreased by 38% and major stroke by 32%, without altering cardiovascular death.[24]

Acute coronary syndromes. In Prinzmetal's vasospastic angina, nifedipine gives consistent relief. In other acute coronary syndromes, nifedipine should not be used.

Systemic hypertension. Long-acting nifedipine and other DHPs are increasingly used. The major outcome study with nifedipine GITS, the INSIGHT study, showed equivalence in mortality and other major outcomes to the diuretic, with less new diabetes or gout or peripheral vascular disease and more heart failure.[5] Capsular forms are not licensed for hypertension in the United States because of intermittent vasodilation and reflex adrenergic discharge, as well as the short duration of action. Procardia XL and Adalat CC are, however, approved and the dose is initially 30 mg once daily up to 90 mg daily.

Vascular protection. Intriguing basic and clinical work suggests that nifedipine and other CCBs have vascular protective qualities, especially in the carotid vessels.[47]

Summary. Long-acting nifedipine is widely used as a powerful arterial vasodilator with few serious side effects and is now part of the accepted therapy of hypertension and of effort or Prinzmetal's vasospastic angina. In hypertension, it gives equivalent outcomes to a diuretic. Long-acting nifedipine is especially well-tested in hypertensive anginal patients when added to β-blockade, as in the ACTION study. However, in unstable angina at rest, nifedipine in any formulation should not be used as monotherapy, unless vasospastic angina is the working diagnosis. Contraindications to nifedipine are few (apart from severe aortic stenosis, obstructive cardiomyopathy, or LV failure), and careful combination with β-blockade is usually feasible. Vasodilatory side effects include headache and ankle edema.

Amlodipine: The First of the Second-Generation DHPs

The major specific advantages of amlodipine (Norvasc; Istin in the United Kingdom) are (1) the slow onset of action and the long duration of activity (see Table 3-5) and (2) the vast experience with this drug in hypertension. It was the first of the longer-acting "second-generation" CCBs. It binds to the same site as other DHPs (labeled *N* in Fig. 3-4). The charged nature of the molecule means that its binding is not entirely typical, with very slow association and dissociation, so that the channel block is slow in onset and offset. Additionally, it also binds to the same sites as verapamil and diltiazem, albeit to a lesser degree, so that with justification its binding properties are regarded as unique.[48]

Pharmacokinetics. Peak blood levels are reached after 6 to 12 hours, followed by extensive hepatic metabolism to inactive metabolites. The plasma levels increase during chronic dosage probably because of the very long half-life. The elimination half-life is 35 to 48 hours, increasing slightly with chronic dosage. In older adults, the clearance is reduced and the dose may need reduction. Regarding drug interactions, no effect on digoxin levels has been found, nor is there any interaction with cimetidine (in contrast to verapamil and nifedipine). Because of the hepatic CYP3A4 interaction, the FDA warns that the 20-mg dose of simvastatin should not be exceeded in patients taking amlodipine. There is no known effect of grapefruit juice.

Hypertension. Amlodipine has an outstanding record in major BP trials (Table 3-6).[49] As initial monotherapy, a common starting dose is 5 mg daily going up to 10 mg. In a large trial on mild hypertension in a middle-aged group over 4 years, amlodipine 5 mg daily was the best tolerated of the agents compared with an α-blocker, a β-blocker, a diuretic, and an ACE inhibitor.[50] In the largest outcome study, ALLHAT, amlodipine had the same primary outcome (fatal and nonfatal coronary heart disease) as the diuretic and ACE-inhibitor groups, but with modestly increased heart failure while decreasing new diabetes.[30] In another mega-trial, ASCOT-BP Lowering Arm, amlodipine usually in combination with the ACE inhibitor perindopril gave much better outcomes than a β-blocker usually combined with a diuretic.[23] Specifically, all cardiovascular events were decreased including heart failure, new diabetes was less, and decreased mortality led to premature termination of the trial.

The decisive ACCOMPLISH study, comparing initial antihypertensive treatment with benazepril plus amlodipine versus benazepril plus hydrochlorothiazide, was terminated early as the CCB–ACE inhibitor combination was clearly superior to the ACE inhibitor-diuretic.[8] Both primary and secondary end-points were reduced by approximately 20%. For cardiovascular deaths, nonfatal MI, and nonfatal stroke, heart rate was 0.79 (95% cardiac index, 0.67-0.92; P = 0.002).[8] When matching the BP reductions exactly, the benefits were the same.[9] The progression of nephropathy was slowed to a greater extent with this combination.[51]

In diabetic type 2 hypertensives, ALLHAT showed that amlodipine was as effective as the diuretic in the relative risk of cardiovascular disease.[52] In advanced diabetic nephropathy, amlodipine compared

Table 3-6

Amlodipine: Major Outcome Trials in Hypertension			
Acronym	Numbers and Duration	Comparison	End Points
ALLHAT[30]	9048 in amlodipine arm	Amlodipine vs others (diuretic, ACE inhibitor, α-blocker)	Equal CHD, stroke, all-cause mortality, at same BP target; more HF, less new diabetes
ASCOT[23]	18,000 patients, 5 years, BP > 160/100 or 140/90 on drug; age 40-80; 3+ risk factors for CHD	Amlodipine vs atenolol 2nd: A + perindopril vs atenolol + thiazide	Mortality reduced, major fall in all CV events
VALUE, Amlodipine[49]	15,245 patients, age 50+, initial BP 155/87 mm Hg	Amlodipine vs valsartan ± thiazide	Equal cardiac and mortality outcomes
ACCOMPLISH[8,9]	11,506 patients, at high risk for events	Benazepril + amlodipine vs benazepril + hydrochlorothiazide	Hazard ratio 0.79 for CV death, nonfatal MI, and nonfatal stroke (CI, 0.67-0.92; P=0.002)

ACCOMPLISH, Avoiding Cardiovascular Events through Combination Therapy in Patients Living with Systolic Hypertension; *ACE,* angiotensin-converting enzyme; *ALLHAT,* Antihypertensive and Lipid-Lowering treatment to prevent Heart Attack Trial; *ASCOT,* Anglo Scandinavian Cardiac Outcomes Trial; *BP,* blood pressure; *CHD,* coronary heart disease; *CI,* confidence intervals; *CV,* cardiovascular; *HF,* heart failure; *MI,* myocardial infarction; *VALUE,* Valsartan Antihypertensive Long-term Use Evaluation Trial.

with irbesartan protected from MI, whereas irbesartan decreased the heart failure and the progression of nephropathy.[53]

Effort angina and coronary artery disease. Amlodipine is well tested in effort angina, with an antianginal effect for 24 hours, and often better tolerated than β-blockers. In CAMELOT amlodipine was given for 2 years to 663 patients with angiographic CAD; amlodipine decreased cardiovascular events by 31% versus enalapril despite similar BP reduction.[20,54] Although atheroma volume fell in this trial, arterial lumen dimensions were unchanged. In PREVENT, amlodipine given to patients with coronary angiographic disease had reduced outcome measures after 3 years.[55] Exercise-induced ischemia was more effectively reduced by amlodipine than by the β-blocker atenolol, whereas ambulatory ischemia was better reduced by atenolol, and for both settings the combination was the best.[56] However, the CCB–β-blocker combination is often underused, even in "optimally treated" stable effort angina, as incorrectly claimed in COURAGE.[26] Exercise-induced ischemia is at the basis of effort angina. After the anginal pain is relieved by nitrates, the ejection fraction takes approximately 30 min to recover, a manifestation of postischemic stunning. Amlodipine markedly attenuates such stunning,[57] hypothetically because cellular calcium overload underlies stunning. In Prinzmetal's vasospastic angina, another licensed indication, amlodipine 5 mg daily lessens symptoms and ST changes. For cardiovascular protection in hypertension, amlodipine was the major drug in the notable ASCOT study reducing strokes, total major events, and mortality.[23]

Contraindications, cautions, and side effects. Amlodipine has the same contraindications as other DHPs (see Fig. 3-9). It is untested in unstable angina, acute myocardial infarction and follow-up. First principles strongly suggest that it should not be used in the absence of concurrent β-blockade. In heart failure CCBs as a group are best avoided but amlodipine may be added, for example, for better control of angina. In liver disease the dose should be reduced. Of the side effects, peripheral edema is most troublesome, occurring in approximately 10% of patients at 10 mg daily (see Table 3-4). In women there is more edema (15%) than in men (6%). Next in significance are dizziness (3% to 4%) and flushing (2% to 3%). Compared with verapamil, edema is more common but headache and constipation are less common. Compared with placebo, headache is not increased (package insert). Amlodipine gave an excellent quality of life compared with other agents in the TOMH study.[50]

Summary. The very long half-life of amlodipine, good tolerability, and virtual absence of drug interactions (exception: high-dose simvastatin) makes it an effective once-a-day antianginal and antihypertensive agent, setting it apart from agents that are either twice or thrice daily. Side effects are few; ankle edema is the chief side effect. Exercise-induced ischemia is more effectively reduced by amlodipine than by the β-blocker atenolol, and the combination is even better. However, the CCB–β-blocker combination is often underused, even in some studies reporting "optimally treated" stable effort angina. Amlodipine-based therapy in the notable ASCOT study in hypertension gave widespread cardiovascular protection, thereby dispelling the once-held belief that CCBs had some adverse outcome effects.

Felodipine

Felodipine (Plendil ER) shares the standard properties of other long-acting DHPs. In the United States, it is only licensed for hypertension in a starting dose of 5 mg once daily, then increasing to 10 mg or decreasing to 2.5 mg as needed. As monotherapy, it is approximately as effective as nifedipine. Initial felodipine monotherapy was the basis of a very large outcome study (Height of Hypertension [HOT]) in Scandinavia in which the aim was to compare BP reduction to different diastolic levels, 90, 85, or 80 mm Hg.[28] Combination with other agents such as ACE inhibitors and β-blockers was often required to attain the goals. Best results were found with the lowest BP group in diabetics, in whom hard end points such as cardiovascular mortality were reduced. Felodipine, like other DHPs, combines well with β-blockers.[58] There are two drug interactions of note: cimetidine, which increases blood felodipine levels, and anticonvulsants, which markedly decrease levels, both probably acting at the level of the hepatic enzymes. Grapefruit juice markedly inhibits the metabolism. The high vascular selectivity of felodipine led to extensive testing in heart failure, yet achieving no sustained benefit in the large Ve-HeFT-III trial in which it was added to conventional therapy.[59]

Other Second-Generation Dihydropyridines

Other second-generation DHPs include, in alphabetical order, benidipine, cilnidipine, isradipine, lacidipine, lercanidipine, nicardipine, and nisoldipine. There appears to be no particular reason for choosing any of these instead of the much better studied agents with outcome results such as amlodipine, nifedipine, and felodipine except that (1) cilnidipine was more renoprotective than amlodipine in a small study that should be extended[60] and (2) use of lacidipine is strengthened by a large scale study with long-term follow up. *Lacidipine* (2-6mg daily, only in Europe and the United Kingdom) is highly lipophilic and may therefore exert vascular protection. In the ELSA trial the progression of carotid atherosclerosis was slowed when compared with atenolol, even though the ambulatory BP reduction of −7/−5 mm Hg was less than with the β-blocker (−10/−9 mm Hg).[6] Lacidipine also limited the development of new metabolic syndrome and new diabetes.[61] Lacidipine caused less ankle edema in a small direct comparison with amlodipine. *Benidipine,* well-studied in Japan, counters cardiac remodeling partially through nitric oxide,[62] and in hypertension (dose 4 mg/day) when combined with an ARB, β-blocker, or thiazide diuretic was similarly effective for the prevention of the major cardiovascular events and the achievement of target BP[63] In a small post-MI trial, benidipine was as effective as β-blockade in reducing cardiovascular events.[64]

Third-Generation Dihydropyridines

Third-generation DHP CCBs inhibit T-type calcium channels on vascular muscular cells such as those localized on postglomerular arterioles. Sadly, they had a somewhat rocky start when the prototype agent, mibefradil, had to be withdrawn after a series of successful studies because of hepatic side effects. Now there is interest in a newer agent, *manidipine.*[65] In the DEMAND study on 380 subjects for a mean of 3.8 years, combined manidipine and ACE-inhibitor therapy reduced both macrovascular events and albuminuria in hypertensive patients with type 2 diabetes mellitus, whereas the ACE inhibitor did not. The proposed mechanism was reduced postglomerular resistance and decreased intraglomerular pressure. Cardioprotective effects extended beyond improved BP and metabolic control. Worsening of insulin resistance was almost fully prevented in those on combination therapy, which suggested additional effects possibly manidipine-mediated activation of adipocyte peroxisome proliferator-activated receptor-γ. The authors estimated that approximately 16 subjects had to be treated with the combined therapy to prevent one major cardiovascular event. Much larger trials are required to place the third-generation CCBs firmly on the therapeutic map.

SUMMARY

1. *Spectrum of use.* CCBs (calcium antagonists) are widely used in the therapy of hypertension and underused in effort angina. The major mechanism of action is by calcium channel blockade in the arterioles, with peripheral or coronary vasodilation thereby explaining the major effects in hypertension and in effort angina. The HRL CCBs have a prominent negative inotropic effect, and inhibit the sinus and the AV nodes. These inhibitory cardiac effects are absent or muted in the DHPs, of which nifedipine is the prototype, now joined by amlodipine, felodipine, and others. Of these, amlodipine is very widely used in hypertension with proven outcome benefit. As a group, the DHPs are more vascular selective and more often used in hypertension than the HRL agents, also called the non-DHPs. Only the non-DHPs, verapamil and diltiazem, have antiarrhythmic properties by inhibiting the AV node. Both DHPs and non-DHPs are used against effort angina, albeit acting through different mechanisms and often underused especially in the United States.

2. *Safety and efficacy.* Previous serious concerns about the long-term safety of the CCBs as a group have been annulled by seven large outcome studies in hypertension, with one in angina pectoris. Nonetheless, as with all drugs, cautions and contraindications need to be honored.

3. *Ischemic heart disease.* All the CCBs work against effort angina, with efficacy and safety rather similar to β-blockers. The largest angina outcome study, ACTION, showed the benefits of adding a long acting DHP to prior β-blockade. In unstable angina the DHPs are specifically contraindicated in the absence of β-blockade because of their tendency to vasodilation-induced reflex adrenergic activation. Although the use of the HRL non-DHPs in unstable angina is relatively well supported by data, they have in practice been supplanted by β-blockers. In postinfarct patients, verapamil may be used if β-blockade is not tolerated or contraindicated, provided that there is no heart failure, although it is not licensed for this purpose in the United States. DHPs do not have good postinfarct data.

4. *Hypertension.* Strong overall evidence from a series of large outcome studies favors the safety and efficacy on hard end points, including coronary heart disease, of longer-acting DHPs. One large outcome study on coronary heart disease shows that the non-DHP verapamil gives results overall as good as atenolol with less new diabetes.

5. *Diabetic hypertension.* ALLHAT showed that amlodipine was as effective as the diuretic or the ACE inhibitor in the relative risk of cardiovascular disease. Other data suggest that initial antihypertensive therapy in diabetics should be based on an ACE inhibitor or ARB, especially in those with nephropathy. To achieve current BP goals in diabetics, it is almost always necessary to use combination therapy, which would usually include an ACE inhibitor or ARB, and a CCB besides a diuretic or β-blocker.

6. *Heart failure.* Heart failure remains a class contraindication to the use of all CCBs, with two exceptions: diastolic dysfunction based on LV hypertrophy, and otherwise well-treated systolic heart failure when amlodipine may be cautiously added if essential, for example, for control of angina

References

1. Abernethy DR, et al. Calcium-antagonist drugs. *New Engl J Med* 1999;341:1447–1455.
2. Kaplan NM. The meaning of ALLHAT. *J Hypertens* 2003;21:233–234.
3. Opie LH. Calcium channel antagonists in the treatment of coronary artery disease: fundamental pharmacological properties relevant to clinical use. *Prog Cardiovasc Dis* 1996;38:273–290.
4. Binggeli C, et al. Effects of chronic calcium channel blockade on sympathetic nerve activity in hypertension. *Hypertension* 2002;39:892–896.
5. Brown MJ, et al. Morbidity and mortality in patients randomised to double-blind treatment with a long-acting calcium-channel blocker or diuretic in the International Nifedipine GITS study: intervention as a goal in hypertension treatment. *Lancet* 2000;356:366–372.
6. Zanchetti A, et al. On behalf of the ELSA Investigators. Calcium antagonist lacidipine slows down progression of asymptomatic carotid atherosclerosis: principal results of the European Lacidipine Study on Atherosclerosis (ELSA), a randomized, double-blind, long-term trial. *Circulation* 2002;106:2422–2427.
7. Opie LH, et al. Nifedipine and mortality: grave defects in the dossier. *Circulation* 1995;92:1068–1073.
8. Jamerson K, et al. ACCOMPLISH Trial Investigators Benazepril plus amlodipine or hydrochlorothiazide for hypertension in high-risk patients. *N Engl J Med* 2008;359:2417–2428.
9. Jamerson KA, et al. Efficacy and duration of benazepril plus amlodipine or hydrochlorothiazide on 24-hour ambulatory systolic blood pressure control. *Hypertension* 2011;57: 174–179.
10. Göbel EJ, et al. Long-term follow-up after early intervention with intravenous diltiazem or intravenous nitroglycerin for unstable angina pectoris. *Eur Heart J* 1998;19:1208–1213.
11. Ardissino D, et al. Transient myocardial ischemia during daily life in rest and exertional angina pectoris and comparison of effectiveness of metoprolol versus nifedipine. *Am J Cardiol* 1991;6:946–952.
12. HINT Study. Early treatment of unstable angina in the coronary care unit, a randomised, double-blind placebo controlled comparison of recurrent ischemia in patients treated

with nifedipine or metoprolol or both. Holland Inter-university Nifedipine Trial. *Br Heart J* 1986;56:400–413.

13. Law MR, et al. Use of blood pressure lowering drugs in the prevention of cardiovascular disease: meta-analysis of 147 randomised trials in the context of expectations from prospective epidemiological studies. *Brit Med J* 2009;338:b1665.

14. Bakris GL, et al. Differential effects of calcium antagonist subclasses on markers of nephropathy progression. *Kidney Int* 2004;65;1991–2002.

15. Fischer Hansen J, The Danish Study Group on Verapamil in Myocardial Infarction. Treatment with verapamil during and after an acute myocardial infarction: a review based on the Danish verapamil infarction trials I and II. *J Cardiovasc Pharmacol* 1991;18(Suppl 6): S20–S25.

16. Pepine CJ, et al. Verapamil use in patients with cardiovascular disease: an overview of randomized trials. *Clin Cardiol* 1998;21:633–641.

17. Brovkovych V, et al. Synergistic antihypertensive effects of nifedipine on endothelium. *Hypertension* 2001;37:34–39.

18. ENCORE Investigators. Effect of nifedipine and cerivastatin on coronary endothelial function in patients with coronary artery disease: the ENCORE I Study (evaluation of nifedipine and cerivastatin on recovery of coronary endothelial function). *Circulation* 2003;107:422–428.

19. Verdecchia P, et al. Asymptomatic left ventricular systolic dysfunction in essential hypertension: prevalence, determinants, and prognostic value. *Hypertension* 2005;45:412–418.

20. Nissen SE, et al. Effect of intensive compared with moderate lipid-lowering therapy on progression of coronary atherosclerosis: a randomized controlled trial. *JAMA* 2004;291:1071–1080.

21. Opie LH, et al. Current status of safety and efficacy of calcium channel blockers in cardiovascular diseases. A critical analysis based on 100 studies. *Prog Cardiovasc Dis* 2000;43:171–196.

22. BP Trialists. Effects of different blood-pressure-lowering regimens on major cardiovascular events: results of prospectively-designed overviews of randomised trials. *Lancet* 2003;362:1527–1535.

23. Dalhöf B, et al. Prevention of cardiovascular events with an antihypertensive regimen of amlodipine adding perindopril as required versus atenolol adding bendroflumethiazide as required, in the Anglo-Scandinavian Cardiac Outcomes Trial-Blood Pressure Lowering Arm (ASCOT-BPLA): a multicentre randomised controlled trial. *Lancet* 2005;366:895–906.

24. Lubsen J, et al. Effect of long-acting nifedipine on mortality and cardiovascular morbidity in patients with symptomatic stable angina and hypertension: the ACTION trial. *J Hypertens* 2005;23:641–648.

25. Pepine CJ, et al. A calcium antagonist vs a non-calcium antagonist hypertension treatment strategy for patients with coronary artery disease. The International Verapamil-Trandolapril Study (INVEST): a randomized controlled trial. *JAMA* 2003;290:2805–2816.

26. Boden WE, et al. Optimal medical therapy with or without PCI for stable coronary disease. *N Engl J Med* 2007;356:1503–1516.

27. Poole-Wilson PA, et al. Effect of long-acting nifedipine on mortality and cardiovascular morbidity in patients with stable angina requiring treatment (ACTION trial): randomised controlled trial. *Lancet* 2004; 364:849–857.

28. HOT Study, Hansson L, et al. Effects of intensive blood-pressure lowering and low-dose aspirin in patients with hypertension: principal results of the Hypertension Optimal Treatment (HOT) randomised trial. *Lancet* 1998;351:1755–1762.

29. Tuomilehto J, et al. Effects of calcium-channel blockade in older patients with diabetes and systolic hypertension. *N Engl J Med* 1999;340:677–684.

30. ALLHAT Collaborative Research Group. Major outcomes in high-risk hypertensive patients randomized to angiotensin-converting enzyme inhibitor or calcium channel blocker vs diuretic. The Antihypertensive and Lipid-Lowering Treatment to Prevent Heart Attack Trial (ALLHAT). *JAMA* 2002;288:2981–2997.

31. Joint National Council 7, Chobanian AV, et al. The seventh report of the Joint National Committee on Prevention, Detection, Evaluation and Treatment of High Blood Pressure. *JAMA* 2003;289:2560–2572.

32. Schwartz JB, et al. Prolongation of verapamil elimination kinetics during chronic oral administration. *Am Heart J* 1982;104:198–203.

33. Boyer EW, et al. Treatment of calcium-channel-blocker intoxication with insulin infusion. *N Engl J Med* 2001;344:1721–1722.

34. Freedman SB, et al. Long-term follow-up of verapamil and nitrate treatment for coronary artery spasm. *Am J Cardiol* 1982;50:711–715.

35. Holzgreve H, et al. Verapamil versus hydrochlorothiazide in the treatment of hypertension: results of long term double blind comparative trial. Verapamil versus Diuretic (VERDI) Trial Research Group. *Brit Med J* 1989;299:881–886.

36. Seiler C, et al. Long-term follow-up of medical versus surgical therapy for hypertrophic cardiomyopathy: a retrospective study. *J Am Coll Cardiol* 1991;17:634–642.

37. Bagger JP, et al. Effect of verapamil in intermittent claudication: a randomized, double-blind, placebo-controlled, cross-over study after individual dose-response assessment. *Circulation* 1997;95:411–414.

38. Multicenter Diltiazem Postinfarction Trial Research Group. The effect of diltiazem on mortality and reinfarction after myocardial infarction. *New Engl J Med* 1988;319:385–392.

39. Black HR, et al. Principal results of the Controlled Onset Verapamil Investigation of Cardiovascular End Points (CONVINCE) trial. *JAMA* 2003;289:2073–2082.

40. Materson BJ, et al. Single-drug therapy for hypertension in men: a comparison of six antihypertensive agents with placebo. The Department of Veterans Affairs Cooperative Study Group on Antihypertensive Agents. *N Engl J Med* 1993;328:914–921.

41. Gottdiener JS, et al. Effect of single-drug therapy on reduction of left ventricular size in mild to moderate hypertension. Comparison of six antihypertensive agents. The Department of Veterans Affairs Cooperative Study Group on Antihypertensive Agents. *Circulation* 1998;98:140–148.

42. Schroeder J, et al. A preliminary study of diltiazem in the prevention of coronary artery disease in heart transplant recipients. *N Engl J Med* 1993;328:164–170.

43. Muller J, et al. Nifedipine therapy for patients with threatened and acute myocardial infarction: a randomized, double-blind, placebo-controlled comparison. *Circulation* 1984;69:740–747.

44. Muller J, et al. Nifedipine and conventional therapy for unstable angina pectoris: a randomized, double-blind comparison. *Circulation* 1984;69:728–733.

45. de Champlain J, et al. Different effects of nifedipine and amlodipine on circulating catecholamine levels in essential hypertensive patients. *J Hypertens* 1998;16:1357–1369.

46. Heidenreich PA, et al. Meta-analysis of trials comparing b-blockers, calcium antagonists, and nitrates for stable angina. *JAMA* 1999;281:1927–1936.

47. Simon A, et al. Differential effects of nifedipine and co-amilozide on the progression of early carotid wall changes. *Circulation* 2001;103:2949–2954.

48. Nayler WG, et al. The unique binding properties of amlodipine: a long-acting calcium antagonist. *J Human Hypertens* 1991;5(Suppl 1):55–59.

49. Julius S, et al. Outcomes in hypertensive patients at high cardiovascular risk treated with regimens based on valsartan or amlodipine: the VALUE randomised trial. *Lancet* 2004;363:2022–2031.

50. TOMH Study, Neaton JD, et al. Treatment of Mild Hypertension study (TOMH): final results. *JAMA* 1993;270:713–724.

51. Bakris GL, et al. ACCOMPLISH trial investigators renal outcomes with different fixed-dose combination therapies in patients with hypertension at high risk for cardiovascular events (ACCOMPLISH): a prespecified secondary analysis of a randomised controlled trial. *Lancet* 2010;375:1173–1181.

52. Whelton PK, et al. Clinical outcomes in antihypertensive treatment of type 2 diabetes, impaired fasting glucose concentration, and normoglycemia: Antihypertensive and Lipid-Lowering Treatment to Prevent Heart Attack Trial (ALLHAT). *Arch Intern Med* 2005;165:1401–1409.

53. Berl T, et al. Cardiovascular outcomes in the Irbesartan diabetic nephropathy trial of patients with type 2 diabetes and overt nephropathy. *Ann Intern Med* 2003;138:542–549.

54. Brener SJ, et al. Antihypertensive therapy and regression of coronary artery disease: insights from the Comparison of Amlodipine versus Enalapril to Limit Occurrences of Thrombosis (CAMELOT) and Norvasc for Regression of Manifest Atherosclerotic Lesions by Intravascular Sonographic Evaluation (NORMALISE) trials. *Am Heart J* 2006;152:1059–1063.

55. Pitt B, et al. Effect of amlodipine on the progression of atherosclerosis and the occurrence of clinical events. *Circulation* 2000;102:1503–1510.

56. Davies RF, et al. Effect of amlodipine, atenolol and their combination on myocardial ischemia during treadmill exercise and ambulatory monitoring. *J Am Coll Cardiol* 1995;25:619–625.

57. Rinaldi CA, et al. Randomized, double-blind crossover study to investigate the effects of amlodipine and isosorbide mononitrate on the time course and severity of exercise-induced myocardial stunning. *Circulation* 1998;98:749–756.

58. Emanuelsson H, et al. For the TRAFFIC Study Group. Antianginal efficacy of the combination of felodipine-metoprolol 10/100 mg compared with each drug alone in patients with stable effort-induced angina pectoris: a multicenter parallel group study. *Am Heart J* 1999;137:854–862.

59. Cohn JN, et al. Effect of the calcium antagonist felodipine as supplementary vasodilator therapy in patients with chronic heart failure treated with enalapril (V-HeFT III Study). *Circulation* 1997;96:856–863.

60. Morimoto S, et al. Renal and vascular protective effects of cilnidipine in patients with essential hypertension. *J Hypertens* 2007;25:2178–2183.

61. Zanchetti A, et al. Prevalence and incidence of the metabolic syndrome in the European Lacidipine Study on Atherosclerosis (ELSA) and its relation with carotid intima-media thickness. *J Hypertens* 2007;25:2463–2470.

62. Liao Y, et al. Benidipine, a long-acting calcium channel blocker, inhibits cardiac remodeling in pressure-overloaded mice. *Cardiovasc Res* 2005;65:879–888.

63. Matsuzaki M, et al. Prevention of cardiovascular events with calcium channel blocker-based combination therapies in patients with hypertension: a randomized controlled trial. *J Hypertens* 2011;29:1649–1659.

64. Nakagomi A, et al. Secondary preventive effects of a calcium antagonist for ischemic heart attack: randomized parallel comparison with β-blockers. *Circ J* 2011;75:1696–1705.

65. Ruggenenti P, et al. For the DEMAND Study Investigators. Effects of manidipine and delapril in hypertensive patients with type 2 diabetes mellitus: the Delapril and Manidipine for Nephroprotection in Diabetes (DEMAND) randomized clinical trial. *Hypertension* 2011;58:776–783.

4

Diuretics

LIONEL H. OPIE · RONALD G. VICTOR
· NORMAN M. KAPLAN

*"Little benefit is to be derived from using large doses of oral diuretics to
reduce blood pressure."*

Cranston et al., 1963[1]

Diuretics alter physiologic renal mechanisms to increase the flow
of urine with greater excretion of sodium (natriuresis, Fig. 4-1). Diuretics have traditionally been used in the treatment of symptomatic
heart failure with fluid retention, added to standard therapy such
as angiotensin-converting enzyme (ACE) inhibition. In hypertension,
diuretics are recommended as first-line therapy, especially because a
network metaanalysis found low-dose diuretics the most effective first-
line treatment for prevention of cardiovascular complications.[2] However, increased awareness of diuretic-associated diabetes[3] has damp-
ened but not extinguished enthusiasm for first-line diuretics.[4] New
diabetes is an even greater risk of diuretic–β-blocker combinations for
hypertension (see Chapter 7, p. 257). Thus current emphasis is toward
diuretic combinations with ACE inhibitors or angiotensin receptor
blockers (ARBs) to allow lower diuretic doses, to reduce the blood pressure (BP) quicker, and to offset adverse renin-angiotensin activation.

Differing Effects of Diuretics in Congestive Heart Failure and Hypertension

In *heart failure with fluid retention,* diuretics are given to control
pulmonary and peripheral symptoms and signs of congestion. In non-
congested heart failure, diuretic-induced renin activation may outweigh advantages.[5] Diuretics should rarely be used as monotherapy,
but rather should be combined with ACE inhibitors and generally a
β-blocker.[6] Often the loop diuretics (Fig. 4-2) are used preferentially,
for three reasons: (1) the superior fluid clearance for the same degree
of natriuresis; (2) loop diuretics work despite renal impairment
that often accompanies severe heart failure; and (3) increasing doses
increase diuretic responses, so that they are "high ceiling" diuretics. Yet
in mild fluid retention thiazides may initially be preferred, especially
when there is a background of hypertension. In general, diuretic doses
for congestive heart failure (CHF) are higher than in hypertension.

In *hypertension,* to exert an effect, the diuretic must provide
enough natriuresis to achieve some persistent volume depletion.
Diuretics may also work as vasodilators[7] and in other ways. Therefore, once-daily furosemide is usually inadequate because the initial

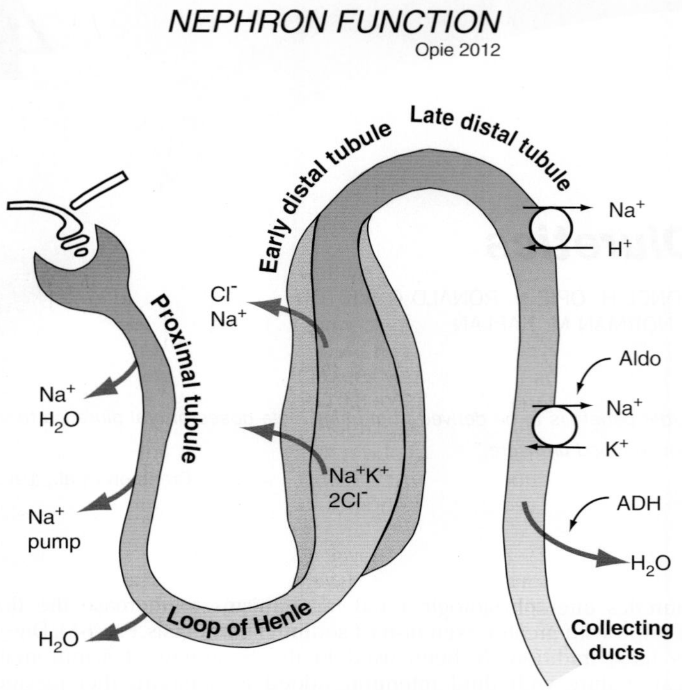

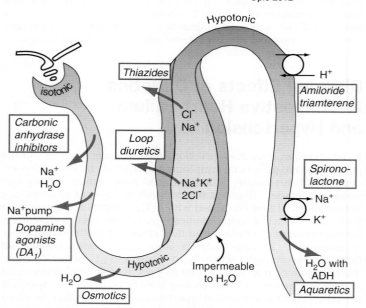

NEPHRON FUNCTION
Opie 2012

Figure 4-1   Nephron anatomy and function. *ADH,* Antidiuretic hormone; *aldo,* aldosterone. (Figure © L.H. Opie, 2012.)

DIURETIC SITES OF ACTION
Opie 2012

Figure 4-2   The multiple sites of action of diuretic agents from which follows the principle of sequential nephron block. A common maximal combination, using this principle, is a loop diuretic plus a thiazide plus a K^+-sparing agent. For aquaretics, see Figure 4-4. *ADH,* Antidiuretic hormone. (Figure © L.H. Opie, 2012.)

sodium loss is quickly reconstituted throughout the remainder of the day. Thus a longer-acting thiazide-type diuretic is usually chosen for hypertension.[8,9]

The three major groups of diuretics are the loop diuretics, the thiazides, and the potassium-sparing agents. Aquaretics constitute a recent fourth. Each type of diuretic acts at a different site of the nephron (see Fig. 4-2), leading to the concept of *sequential nephron blockade.* All but the potassium sparers must be transported to the luminal side; this process is blocked by the buildup of organic acids in renal insufficiency so that progressively larger doses are needed. Especially thiazides lose their potency as renal function falls.

Loop Diuretics

Furosemide

Furosemide *(Lasix, Dryptal, Frusetic, Frusid),* one of the standard loop diuretics for severe CHF, is a sulfonamide derivative. Furosemide is initial therapy in acute pulmonary edema and in the pulmonary congestion of left-sided failure of acute myocardial infarction (AMI). Relief of dyspnea even before diuresis results from venodilation and preload reduction.[10]

Pharmacologic effects and pharmacokinetics. Loop diuretics including furosemide inhibit the $Na^+/K^+/2Cl^-$ cotransporter concerned with the transport of chloride across the lining cells of the ascending limb of the loop of Henle (see Fig. 4-2). This site of action is reached intraluminally, after the drug has been excreted by the proximal tubule. The effect of the cotransport inhibition is that chloride, sodium, potassium, and hydrogen ions all remain intraluminally and are lost in the urine with the possible side effects of hyponatremia, hypochloremia, hypokalemia, and alkalosis. However, in comparison with thiazides, there is a relatively greater urine volume and relatively less loss of sodium. Venodilation reduces the preload in acute left ventricular (LV) failure within 5-15 min; the mechanism is not well understood. Conversely, there may follow a reactive vasoconstriction.

Dose. *Intravenous furosemide* is usually started as a slow 40-mg injection (no more than 4 mg/min to reduce ototoxicity; give 80 mg over 20 min intravenously 1 hour later if needed). When renal function is impaired, as in older adult patients, higher doses are required, with much higher doses for renal failure and severe CHF. *Oral furosemide* has a wide dose range (20 to 240 mg/day or even more; 20, 40, and 80 mg tablets in the United States; in Europe, also scored 500 mg tablets) because of absorption varying from 10% to 100%, averaging 50%.[11] In contrast, absorption of bemetanide and torsemide is nearly complete. Furosemide's short duration of action (4 to 5 hours) means that frequent doses are needed when sustained diuresis is required. Twice-daily doses should be given in the early morning and midafternoon to obviate nocturia and to protect against volume depletion. For *hypertension,* furosemide 20 mg twice daily may be the approximate equivalent of hydrochlorothiazide (HCTZ) 25 mg. Furosemide causes a greater earlier (0 to 6 hours) absolute loss of sodium than does HCTZ but, because of its short duration of action, the total 24-hour sodium loss may be insufficient to maintain the slight volume contraction needed for sustained antihypertensive action,[12] thus requiring furosemide twice daily. In *oliguria* (not induced by volume depletion), as the glomerular filtration rate (GFR) drops to less than 20 mL/min, from 240 mg up to 2000 mg of furosemide may be required because of decreasing luminal excretion. Similar arguments lead to increasing doses of furosemide in *severe refractory heart failure.*

Indications. Furosemide is frequently the diuretic of choice for *severe heart failure* and acute pulmonary edema for reasons already discussed. After initial intravenous use, oral furosemide is usually continued as standard diuretic therapy, sometimes to be replaced by thiazides as the heart failure ameliorates. In *AMI* with clinical failure, intravenous furosemide has rapid beneficial hemodynamic effects and is often combined with ACE inhibition.[13] In *hypertension*, twice-daily low-dose furosemide can be effective even as monotherapy or combined with other agents and is increasingly needed as renal function deteriorates.[14] In *hypertensive crisis*, intravenous furosemide is used if fluid overload is present. In a placebo-controlled study, high-dose furosemide given for acute renal failure increased the urine output but failed to alter the number of dialysis sessions or the time on dialysis.[15]

Contraindications. In heart failure without fluid retention, furosemide can increase aldosterone levels with deterioration of LV function.[16] Anuria, although listed as a contraindication to the use of furosemide, is sometimes treated (as is oliguria) by furosemide in the hope for diuresis; first exclude dehydration and a history of hypersensitivity to furosemide or sulfonamides.

Hypokalemia with furosemide. Clearly, much depends on the doses chosen and the degree of diuresis achieved. *Furosemide should not be used intravenously when electrolytes cannot be monitored.* The risk of hypokalemia is greatest with high-dose furosemide, especially when given intravenously, and at the start of myocardial infarction when hypokalemia with risk of arrhythmias is common even in the absence of diuretic therapy. Carefully regulated intravenous potassium supplements may be required in these circumstances. In heart failure, digitalis toxicity may be precipitated by overdiuresis and hypokalemia.

Other side effects. The chief side effects, in addition to *hypokalemia,* are *hypovolemia* and *hyperuricemia.* Hypovolemia, with risk of prerenal azotemia, can be lessened by a low starting initial dose (20 to 40 mg, monitoring blood urea). A few patients on high-dose furosemide have developed severe hyperosmolar nonketotic *hyperglycemic states. Atherogenic blood lipid changes,* similar to those found with thiazides, may also be found with loop diuretics. Occasionally diabetes may be precipitated. Minimizing hypokalemia should lessen the risk of glucose intolerance. Furosemide (like other sulfonamides) may precipitate photosensitive skin eruptions or may cause blood dyscrasias. Reversible dose-related *ototoxicity* (electrolyte disturbances of the endolymphatic system) can be avoided by infusing furosemide at rates not greater than 4 mg/min and keeping the oral dose less than 1000 mg daily. *Urinary retention* may by noted from vigorous diuresis in older adults. In pregnancy, furosemide is classified as Category C. In *nursing mothers,* furosemide is excreted in the milk.

Loss of diuretic potency. *Braking* is the phenomenon whereby after the first dose, there is a decrease in the diuretic response caused by renin-angiotensin activation and prevented by restoring the diuretic-induced loss of blood volume.[11] *Long-term tolerance* refers to increased reabsorption of sodium associated with hypertrophy of the distal nephron segments (see "Diuretic Resistance" later in this chapter). The mechanism may be increased growth of the nephron cells induced by increased aldosterone.[12]

Drug interactions with furosemide. Co-therapy with certain *aminoglycosides* can precipitate ototoxicity. *Probenecid* may interfere with the effects of thiazides or loop diuretics by blocking their secretion into the urine of the proximal tubule. *Indomethacin* and other nonsteroidal antiinflammatory drugs (*NSAIDs*) lessen the renal response to loop diuretics, presumably by interfering with formation of vasodilatory prostaglandins.[17]

High doses of furosemide may competitively inhibit the excretion of *salicylates* to predispose to salicylate poisoning with tinnitus. *Steroid* or adrenocorticotropic hormone therapy may predispose to hypokalemia. Furosemide, unlike thiazides, does not decrease renal excretion of *lithium*, so that lithium toxicity is not a risk. Loop diuretics do not alter blood digoxin levels, nor do they interact with warfarin.

Bumetanide

The site of action of bumetanide (*Bumex, Burinex*) and its effects (and side effects) are very similar to that of furosemide (Table 4-1). As with furosemide, higher doses can cause considerable electrolyte disturbances, including hypokalemia. As in the case of furosemide, a combined diuretic effect is obtained by addition of a thiazide diuretic. In contrast to furosemide, oral absorption is predictable at 80% or more.[11]

Dosage and clinical uses. In *CHF,* the usual oral dose is 0.5 to 2 mg, with 1 mg bumetanide being approximately equal to 40 mg furosemide. In acute pulmonary edema, a single intravenous dose of 1 to 3 mg over 1 to 2 minutes can be effective; repeat if needed at 2- to 3-hour intervals to a maximum of 10 mg daily. In *renal edema,* the effects of bumetanide are similar to those of furosemide. In the United States, bumetanide is not approved for hypertension.

Side effects and cautions. Side effects associated with bumetanide are similar to those of furosemide; ototoxicity may be less and renal toxicity more. The combination with other potentially nephrotoxic drugs, such as aminoglycosides, must be avoided. In patients with renal failure, high doses have caused myalgia, so that the dose should not exceed 4 mg/day when the GFR is less than 5 mL/min. Patients allergic to sulfonamides may also be hypersensitive to bumetanide. In pregnancy, the risk is similar to furosemide (Category C).

Conclusion. Most clinicians will continue to use the agent they know best (i.e., furosemide). Because furosemide is widely available in generic form, its cost is likely to be less than that of torsemide or bumetanide.

Table 4-1

Loop Diuretics: Doses and Kinetics		
Drug	**Dose**	**Pharmacokinetics**
Furosemide (Lasix)	10-40 mg oral, 2× for BP 20-80 mg 2-3× for CHF Up to 250-2000 mg oral or IV	Diuresis within 10-20 min Peak diuresis at 1.5 h Total duration of action 4-5 h Renal excretion Variable absorption 10%-100%
Bumetanide (Bumex in the US, Burinex in the UK)	0.5-2 mg oral 1-2× daily for CHF 5 mg oral or IV for oliguria (not licensed for BP)	Peak diuresis 75-90 min Total duration of action 4-5 h Renal excretion Absorption 80%-100%
Torsemide (Demadex in the US)	5-10 mg oral 1× daily for BP 10-20 mg oral 1× daily or IV for CHF (up to 200 mg daily)	Diuresis within 10 min of IV dose; peak at 60 min Oral peak effect 1-2 h Oral duration of diuresis 6-8 h Absorption 80%-100%

BP, Blood pressure control; *CHF,* congestive heart failure; *IV,* intravenous.

Torsemide

Torsemide *(Demadex)* is a loop diuretic with a longer duration of action than furosemide (see Table 4-1). A subdiuretic daily dose of 2.5 mg may be antihypertensive and free of changes in plasma potassium or glucose, yet in the United States the only doses registered for antihypertensive efficacy are 5 to 10 mg daily. It remains uncertain whether torsemide or other loop diuretics cause less metabolic disturbances than do thiazides in equipotent doses.

In *heart failure,* an intravenous dose of torsemide 10 to 20 mg initiates a diuresis within 10 minutes that peaks within the first hour. Similar oral doses (note high availability) give an onset of diuresis within 1 hour and a peak effect within 1 to 2 hours, and a total duration of action of 6 to 8 hours. Torsemide 20 mg gives approximately the same degree of natriuresis as does furosemide 80 mg but absorption is much higher and constant.[12] *In hypertension,* an oral dose of 5-10 mg once daily may take 4-6 weeks for maximal effect. There are no long-term outcome studies available for either of these indications.

In *renal failure,* as in the case of other loop diuretics, the renal excretion of the drug falls as does the renal function. Yet the plasma half-life of torsemide is unaltered, probably because hepatic clearance increases. In *edema of hepatic cirrhosis,* the dose is 5 to 10 mg daily, titrated to maximum 200 mg daily, given with aldosterone antagonist. In *pregnancy,* torsemide may be relatively safe (Category B versus Category C for furosemide).

Metabolic and other side effects, cautions, and contraindications are similar to those of furosemide.

Class Side Effects of Loop Diuretics

Sulfonamide sensitivity. Ethacrynic acid *(Edecrin)* is the only non-sulfonamide diuretic and is used only in patients allergic to other diuretics. It closely resembles furosemide in dose (25 and 50 mg tablet), duration of diuresis, and side effects (except for more ototoxicity). If ethacrynic acid is not available for a sulfonamide-sensitive patient, a gradual challenge with furosemide or, even better, torsemide may overcome sensitivity.[18]

Hypokalemia. Hypokalemia may cause vague symptoms such as fatigue and listlessness, besides electrocardiographic and rhythm abnormalities. In the doses used for mild hypertension (furosemide 20 mg twice daily, torsemide 5 to 10 mg), hypokalemia is limited and possibly less than with HCTZ 25 to 50 mg daily. In heart failure, hypokalemia is more likely; similar cautions apply.

Hyperglycemia. Diuretic-induced glucose intolerance is likely related to hypokalemia, or to total body potassium depletion.[19] An interesting proposal is that the transient postprandial fall of potassium impairs the effect of insulin at that time and hence leads to intermittent hyperglycemia.[20] Although there are no large prospective studies on the effects of loop diuretics on insulin insensitivity or glucose tolerance in hypertensive patients, it is clearly prudent to avoid hypokalemia and to monitor both serum potassium and blood glucose values.

Gout. Use of loop diuretics more than doubles the risk of gout, with a hazard ratio (HR) of 2.31. (See "Urate Excretion and Gout" later in this chapter.)

Metabolic changes with loop diuretics: recommendations. The overall evidence suggests that loop diuretics, like the thiazides, can cause dose-related metabolic disturbances. High doses used for heart failure might therefore pose problems. It makes sense to take special precautions against the hypokalemia of high-dose loop diuretics because of the link between intermittent falls in plasma potassium and hyperglycemia. A sensible start is addition of an ACE inhibitor or ARB.

Thiazide Diuretics

Thiazide diuretics (Table 4-2) remain the most widely recommended first-line therapy for hypertension,[8,9] although challenged by other agents such as ACE inhibitors, ARBs, and calcium channel blockers (CCBs). Thiazides are also standard therapy for chronic CHF, when edema is modest, either alone or in combination with loop diuretics. Recently, chlorthalidone a "thiazide-like diuretic" have been distinguished from HCTZ and other standard thiazides; chlorthalidone is preferred for hypertension, the major reason being that HCTZ has no outcome studies in hypertension when used at the presently recommended doses.[21]

Pharmacologic action and pharmacokinetics. Thiazide diuretics act to inhibit the reabsorption of sodium and chloride in the more distal part of the nephron (see Fig. 4-2). This co-transporter is insensitive to the loop diuretics. More sodium reaches the distal tubules to stimulate the exchange with potassium, particularly in the presence of an activated renin-angiotensin-aldosterone system. Thiazides may also increase the active excretion of potassium in the distal renal tubule. Thiazides are rapidly absorbed from the gastrointestinal (GI) tract to produce a diuresis within 1 to 2 hours, which lasts for 16 to 24 hours in the case of the prototype thiazide, HCTZ.[22] Some major differences from the loop diuretics are (1) the longer duration of action (Table 4-2), (2) the different site of action (see Fig. 4-2), (3) the fact that thiazides are *low ceiling diuretics* because the maximal response is reached at a relatively low dosage (Fig. 4-3), and (4) the much decreased capacity of thiazides to work in the presence of renal failure (serum creatinine >2 mg/dL or approximately 180 μmol/L; GFR below 15 to 20 mL/min).[11] The fact that thiazides, loop diuretics and potassium-sparing agents all act at different tubular sites explains their additive effects *(sequential nephron block)*.

Thiazide doses and indications. In *hypertension,* low-dose diuretics are often the initial agent of choice especially in low-renin groups such as older adults and in black patients.[23] By contrast, in younger whites (mean age 51 years) only one-third responded to escalating doses of HCTZ over 1 year.[24] The thiazide doses generally used have been too high. Lower doses with fewer biochemical alterations provide full antihypertensive as shown in several large trials. In the SHEP (Systolic Hypertension in the Elderly Program) study, chlorthalidone 12.5 mg was initially used and after 5 years 30% of the subjects were still on this lower dose.[25] Overall, documented biochemical changes were small including an 0.3 mmol/L fall in potassium, a rise in serum uric acid, and small increases in serum cholesterol and in glucose (1.7% more new diabetes than in placebo). Regarding HCTZ, exceeding 25 mg daily clearly creates metabolic problems.[26,27] Increasing the dose from 12.5 to 25 mg may precipitate hyperglycemia[28] and only induces a borderline better reduction of BP.[29] In the case of bendrofluazide, a low dose (1.25 mg daily) causes less metabolic side effects and no effects on postabsorptive hepatic insulin production when compared with the conventional 5-mg dose.[30] Even higher doses have greater risks of undesirable side-effects (Table 4-3).

The *response rate in hypertension* to thiazide monotherapy is variable and may be disappointing, depending in part on the age and race of the patient and probably also on the sodium intake. With HCTZ, the full antihypertensive effect of low dose 12.5 mg daily may take up to 6 weeks. By 24-hour ambulatory monitoring, 12.5 to 25 mg of HCTZ lowers BP less than the commonly prescribed doses of the other antihypertensive drug classes, with no difference in BP reduction between 12.5 and 25 mg doses of HCTZ.[31]

Table 4-2

Thiazide and Thiazide-Type Diuretics: Doses and Duration of Action

	Trade Name (UK-Europe)	Trade Name (US)	Dose	Duration of Action (H)
Hydrochlorothiazide	Esidrex HydroSaluric	HydroDiuril, Microzide	12.5-25 mg, 12.5 mg preferred (BP); 25-100 mg (CHF)	16-24
Hydroflumethiazide	Hydrenox	Saluron, Diucardin	12.5-25 mg, 12.5 mg preferred (BP); 25-200 mg (CHF)	12-24
Chlorthalidone	Hygroton	Thalitone	12.5-50 mg, 12.5 to 15 preferred (BP)	≈40-60
Metolazone	Metenix; Diulo	Zaroxolyn, Mykrox	2.5-5 mg (BP); 5-20 mg (CHF)	24
Bendrofluazide (bendroflumethiazide)	Aprinox; Centyl; Urizide	Naturetin	1.25-2.5 mg, 1.25 preferred (BP); 10 mg (CHF)	12-18
Benzthiazide	—	Aquatag, Exna, Diurin, Fovane, Hydrex, Proaqua, Regulon	50*-200 mg	12-18
Chlorothiazide	Saluric	Diuril, Chlotride	250*-1000 mg	6-12
Trichlormethiazide	Fluitran (not in UK)	Metahydrin, Naqua, Diurese	1*-4 mg	24
Indapamide	Natrilix	Lozol	1.25-2.5 mg, 1.25 mg preferred (BP); 2.5-5 mg (CHF)	24
Xipamide	Diurexan	—	10-20 mg, 5 mg preferred (BP)	6-12

BP, Blood pressure; *CHF,* congestive heart failure.

*Lowest effective antihypertensive dose not known; may prefer to use other agents for BP control.

Julie M Groth, MPH, Heart Institute, Cedars Sinai Medical Center, is thanked for valuable assistance.

NB: The doses given here for antihypertensive therapy are generally *lower* than those recommended by the manufacturers (exception: Lozol 1.25 mg is recommended).

LOW VS HIGH CEILING DIURETICS
Opie 2012

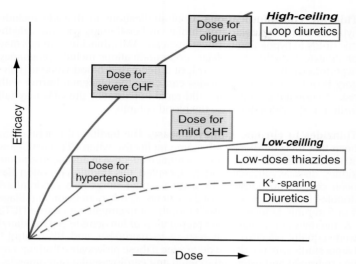

Figure 4-3 **High- and low-ceiling diuretics,** their differences, and the doses of each group used for various indications. Lowest doses are used for hypertension. *CHF,* Congestive heart failure. (Figure © L.H. Opie, 2012.)

Table 4-3

Side Effects of High-dose Diuretic Therapy for Hypertension

Causing Withdrawal of Therapy:

Impaired glucose tolerance, diabetes mellitus
Gout
Impotence, erectile dysfunction
Nausea, dizziness, or headache

Blood Biochemical Changes:

Potassium: hypokalemia
Glucose: hyperglycemia
Uric acid: hyperuricemia
Urea, creatinine: prerenal fall in glomerular filtration rate
Lipid profile: rise in serum cholesterol, triglyceride, and ratio apolipoprotein B
  to A; fall in high-density lipoprotein cholesterol level

Dose of bendrofluazide was 10 mg daily (Peart, Lancet 1981;2:539–543), but now would be 1.25-2.5 mg. All effects are minimized by appropriately lower doses such as hydrochlorothiazide 12.5 mg daily.

Combination therapy, for example, with an ACE inhibitor or ARB, becomes preferable rather than increasing the dose beyond 25 mg daily[22] or even beyond 12.5mg daily.[28,29] In *CHF,* higher doses are justified (50 to 100 mg HCTZ daily are probably ceiling doses), while watching the serum potassium. Considerable diuretic advantage in CHF can result from combining a loop diuretic with a thiazide.[11] Specifically, the thiazides block the nephron sites at which hypertrophy occurs during long term loop diuretic therapy (see "Diuretic Resistance" later in this chapter).

Which thiazide? In the United States, *HCTZ* is by far the most popular. *Bendrofluazide* is still popular in the United Kingdom, but the British Hypertension Society has come out against its prime use. The standard dose is 2.5 versus previous 5-10 mg daily with fewer serious side effects (see Table 4-3). However, a lower dose (1.25 mg once daily) reduces the

BP without metabolic side effects.[30,32] Benzthiazide is available in the United States (see Table 4-2). As with the other thiazides, there are no outcome studies with these drugs.

Thiazide contraindications. Contraindications to thiazide include hypokalemia, ventricular arrhythmias, and co-therapy with proarrhythmic drugs. In hypokalemia (including early AMI), thiazide diuretics may precipitate arrhythmias. Relative contraindications include pregnancy hypertension because of the risk of a decreased blood volume (category B or C); moreover, thiazides can cross the placental barrier with risk of neonatal jaundice. In mild renal impairment, the GFR may fall further as thiazides decrease the blood volume.

Thiazides in chronic kidney disease. The traditional teaching has been that thiazide diuretics become ineffective when GFR falls below 30 mL/min, whereas loop diuretics remain effective in advanced chronic kidney disease. Although widely accepted, this traditional notion has been called into question by a recent pilot study: in a randomized, double-blind, crossover trial of 23 patients with hypertension and Stage 4 or 5 chronic kidney disease, 3 months of treatment with either HCTZ (25 mg daily) or a long-acting preparation of furosemide (60 mg daily) were equally effective with respect to natriuresis and BP control.[33] Larger studies are needed to determine if these provocative findings can be confirmed and extended to renal and cardiovascular outcomes.

Thiazide side effects. In addition to the metabolic side effects seen with previously used high doses (see Table 4-3), thiazide diuretics rarely cause sulfonamide-type immune side effects including intrahepatic jaundice, pancreatitis, blood dyscrasias, angiitis, pneumonitis, interstitial nephritis, and photosensitive dermatitis. Erectile dysfunction is seen more commonly than with any other class of drugs in the TOMH study.[34]

Adherence (measured by medication refill data) is lower with thiazide diuretics than with the other major classes of antihypertensive drugs, including β-blockers, CCBs, ACEs, and ARBs.[35]

Thiazide drug interactions. *Steroids* may cause salt retention to antagonize the action of thiazide diuretics. *Indomethacin* and other NSAIDs blunt the response to thiazide diuretics.[17] *Antiarrhythmics* that prolong the QT-interval, such as Class IA or III agents including sotalol, may precipitate torsades de pointes in the presence of diuretic-induced hypokalemia. The *nephrotoxic effects of certain antibiotics,* such as the aminoglycosides, may be potentiated by diuretics. *Probenecid* (for the therapy of gout) and *lithium* (for mania) may block thiazide effects by interfering with thiazide transport into the tubule. Thiazide diuretics also interact with lithium by impairing renal clearance with risk of lithium toxicity.

Thiazide-Like Agents

These differ from the standard thiazides in structure and by being evidence-based.

Chlorthalidone. Chlorthalidone was chosen for the two most important trials: SHEP[25] and ALLHAT.[36] Lower doses gave approximately as much BP reduction as did the higher, suggesting that low doses should be used to avoid metabolic problems, especially in older adults.[22]

Chlorthalidone versus hydrochlorothiazide. A small comparative study set the ball rolling by finding that chlorthalidone was better than HCTZ in reducing nocturnal BP, in agreement with its longer half-life.[37] The doses were chlorthalidone 12.5 mg/day (force-titrated to 25 mg/day) and HCTZ 25 mg/day (force-titrated to 50 mg/day). In a metaanalysis of 108 trials, chlorthalidone was somewhat better in lowering systolic BP, at the cost of more hyperkalemia.[38]

Retrospective analyses of the large Multiple Risk Factor Intervention Trial (MRFIT) add to the arguments for chlorthalidone.[39,40] In this prolonged trial, lifestyle, active BP and statin therapy were given as needed with long-term follow up of men 35 to 57 years of age beginning in 1973. Chlorthalidone addition for hypertension was compared with HCTZ, both in the dose range of 50-100 mg per day, which were the standard doses used at that time. Chlorthalidone had lower systolic BP, lower total cholesterol, and lower low-density lipoprotein (LDL) cholesterol, but also lower potassium and higher uric acid (all comparisons P < 0.001). Compared with neither diuretic, cardiovascular events were lower both in those on chlorthalidone (HR: 0.51; P < 0.0001) and those on HCTZ (HR: 0.65; P < 0.0001), but chlorthalidone was better than HCTZ. Furthermore, left ventricular hypertrophy (LVH) also decreased more with chlorthalidone.[40] Importantly, however, MRFIT was not randomized but was rather a retrospective cohort study. Nonetheless, in summary, the overall data favor chlorthalidone instead of HCTZ.

Indapamide. Indapamide *(Lozol, Natrilix)* is a thiazide-like diuretic, albeit with a different indoline structure and added vasodilation.[41] Widely used in Europe, it is available but less used in the United States. Indapamide has a terminal half-life of 14 to 16 hours, and effectively lowers the BP over 24 hours. The initial dose is 1.25 mg once daily for 4 weeks, then if needed 2.5 mg daily. Indapamide appears to be more lipid-neutral than other thiazides[42] but seems equally likely to cause dose-dependent metabolic problems such as hypokalemia, hyperglycemia, or hyperuricemia. In the slow-release formula (not available in the United States), it reduced BP variability[43] and hence decreased a new risk factor for stroke.[44]

The major outcome trial is the HYVET study.[45] Patients 80 years of age or older with a sustained systolic BP of 160 mm Hg or more received indapamide (sustained release, 1.5 mg), with the ACE inhibitor perindopril (2 or 4 mg) added if necessary to achieve the target BP of 150/80 mm Hg. Benefits were a 21% reduction in death from any cause (95% confidence interval [CI], 4 to 35; P = 0.02), with 39% reduction in stroke deaths (P = 0.05), and a 64% reduction in heart failure (95% CI, 42 to 78; P < 0.001). Fewer serious adverse events occurred in the active-treatment group (P = 0.001).

Regarding side effects, with a reduced but still antihypertensive dose of only 0.625-1.25 mg of the standard preparation, combined with the ACE inhibitor perindopril 2-4 mg, the serum potassium fell by only 0.11 mmol/L over 1 year, whereas the blood glucose was unchanged from placebo.[46] This combination reduced mortality in ADVANCE, a megatrial in diabetics.[47] Regarding *regression of LVH,* indapamide was better than enalapril in the LIVE study (LVH with Indapamide Versus Enalapril).[48] In *cardiac edema,* higher doses such as 2.5 to 5 mg give a diuresis. In general, its side-effect profile resembles that of the thiazides, including the low risk of sulfonamide sensitivity reactions. In Europe, a new sustained release preparation (1.5 mg) gives equal BP reduction to 2.5 mg indapamide, yet the incidence of hypokalemia at less than 3.4 mmol/L is more than 50% lower.[49]

Metolazone. Metolazone *(Zaroxolyn, Diulo, Metenix)* is a powerful diuretic with a quinazoline structure falling within the overall thiazide family and with similar side effects. There may be an additional site of action beyond that of the standard thiazides. An important advantage of metolazone is efficacy even *despite reduced renal function.* The duration of action is up to 24 hours. The standard dose is 5 to 20 mg once daily for CHF or renal edema and 2.5 to 5 mg for hypertension. In combination with furosemide, metolazone may provoke a profound diuresis, with the risk of excessive volume and potassium depletion. Nonetheless, metolazone may be added to furosemide with care, especially in patients with renal as well as cardiac failure. Metolazone 1.25 to 10 mg once daily was given in titrated doses to 17 patients with severe CHF, almost all of whom were already on furosemide, captopril, and digoxin; most responded by a brisk diuresis within 48 to 72 hours.[50] Consequently, metolazone is often used in addition to a prior combination of a loop diuretic, a thiazide, and aldosterone inhibitor in patients with chronic heart failure and resistant peripheral edema.

Mykrox. Mykrox is a rapidly acting formulation of metolazone with high bioavailability, registered for use in hypertension only in a dose of 0.5 to 1 mg once daily. The maximum antihypertensive effect is reached within 2 weeks.

Metabolic and Other Side Effects of Thiazides

Many side effects of thiazides are similar to those of the loop diuretics and are dose dependent (see Table 4-3).

Hypokalemia. Hypokalemia is probably an over-feared complication, especially when low doses of thiazides are used.[51] Nonetheless, the frequent choice of combination of thiazides with the potassium-retaining agents including the ACE inhibitors, ARBs, or aldosterone blockers is appropriate, with the alternative, but lesser, risk of *hyperkalemia*, especially in the presence of renal impairment.

Ventricular arrhythmias. Diuretic-induced hypokalemia can contribute to torsades de pointes and hence to sudden death, especially when there is co-therapy with agents prolonging the QT-interval. Of importance, in the SOLVD study on heart failure, the baseline use of a non–potassium-retaining diuretic was associated with an increased risk of arrhythmic death compared with a potassium-retaining diuretic.[52] In hypertension, the degree of hypokalemia evoked by low-dose thiazides seldom matters.

Therapeutic strategies to avoid hypokalemia. In patients with a higher risk of arrhythmias, as in ischemic heart disease, heart failure on digoxin, or hypertension with LV hypertrophy, a potassium- and magnesium-sparing diuretic should be part of the therapy unless contraindicated by renal failure or by co-therapy with an ACE inhibitor or ARB. A potassium sparer may be better than potassium supplementation, especially because the supplements do not correct hypomagnesemia.

Hypomagnesemia. Conventional doses of diuretics rarely cause magnesium deficiency,[53] but hypomagnesemia, like hypokalemia, is blamed for arrhythmias of QT-prolongation during diuretic therapy. Hypomagnesemia may be prevented by adding a potassium-retaining component such as amiloride to the thiazide diuretic.

Hyponatremia. Thiazides and thiazide-like diuretics can cause hyponatremia especially in older patients (more so in women) in whom free water excretion is impaired. In the Systolic Hypertension in the Elderly Program (SHEP),[25] hyponatremia occurred in 4% of patients treated with chlorthalidone versus 1% in the placebo group. Occurring rapidly (within 2 weeks), mild thiazide-induced hyponatremia can cause vague symptoms of fatigue and nausea, but when severe, can cause confusion, seizures, coma, and death.

Diabetogenic effects. Diuretic therapy for hypertension increases the risk of new diabetes by approximately one-third, versus placebo.[3] The thiazides are more likely to provoke diabetes if combined with a β-blocker.[54-58] This risk presumably depends on the thiazide dose and possibly on the type of β-blocker, in that carvedilol or nebivolol are exceptions (see Chapter 1, sections on these agents). Patients with a familial tendency to diabetes or those with the metabolic syndrome are probably more prone to the diabetogenic side effects, so that thiazides should be avoided or only given in low doses, such as HCTZ 12.5 mg daily or chlorthalidone 6.25 to 15 mg daily. In addition, plasma potassium and glucose should be monitored. Common sense but no good trial data suggest that the lowest effective dose of HCTZ (12.5 mg) should be used with the expectation that a significant proportion of the antihypertensive effect should be maintained without impairing glucose tolerance, as in the case of low-dose bendrofluazide.[30] *There is no evidence that changing from a thiazide to a loop diuretic improves glucose tolerance.*

How serious is new diuretic-induced diabetes? During the 4.5 years of follow-up in the VALUE trial, new-onset diabetes posed a cardiac risk between no diabetes and prior diabetes, and in the longer follow-up, equal risks.[59]

Urate excretion and gout. Most diuretics decrease urate excretion with the risk of increasing blood uric acid, causing gout in those predisposed. In 5789 persons with hypertension, 37% were treated with a diuretic. Use of any diuretic (HR 1.48; CI 1.11-1.98), a thiazide diuretic (HR 1.44; CI 1.00-2.10), or a loop diuretic (HR 2.31; CI 1.36-3.91) increased the risk of gout.[60] Thus a personal or family history of gout further emphasizes that only low-dose diuretics should be used. Co-therapy with *losartan* lessens the rise in uric acid.[61] When *allopurinol* is given for gout, or when the blood urate is high with a family history of gout, the standard dose of 300 mg daily is only for a normal creatinine clearance. With a clearance of only 40 mL/min, the dose drops to 150 mg daily and, for 10 mL/min, down to 100 mg every 2 days. *Dose reduction is essential* to avoid serious reactions, which are dose-related and can be fatal. *Benemid,* a uricosuric agent may protect against hyperuricemia with less potential toxicity.[62]

Atherogenic changes in blood lipids. Thiazides may increase the total blood cholesterol in a dose-related fashion.[63] LDL cholesterol and triglycerides increase after 4 months with HCTZ (40-mg daily mean dose).[27] In the TOMH study, low-dose chlorthalidone (15 mg daily) increased cholesterol levels at 1 year but not at 4 years.[64] Even if total cholesterol does not change, triglycerides and the ratio of apolipoprotein B to A may rise, whereas high-density lipoprotein cholesterol may fall.[57] During prolonged thiazide therapy occasional checks on blood lipids are ideal and a lipid-lowering diet is advisable.

Hypercalcemia. Thiazide diuretics tend to retain calcium by increasing proximal tubular reabsorption (along with sodium). The benefit is a decreased risk of hip fractures in older adults.[65] Conversely, especially in hyperparathyroid patients, hypercalcemia can be precipitated.

Erectile dysfunction. In the TOMH study, low-dose chlorthalidone (15 mg daily given over 4 years) was the only one of several antihypertensive agents that doubled impotence.[34] Pragmatically, sildenafil or similar drugs should help, provided the patient is not also receiving nitrates.

Prevention of metabolic side effects. Reduction in the dose of a diuretic is the basic step. In addition, restriction of dietary sodium and additional dietary potassium will reduce the frequency of hypokalemia. Combination of a thiazide with a potassium sparer lessens hypokalemia, as does the addition of an ACE inhibitor or ARB. In the treatment of hypertension, standard doses of diuretics should not be combined, if possible, with other drugs with unfavorable effects on blood lipids, such as the β-blockers, but rather with ACE inhibitors, ARBs, or CCBs, which are lipid-neutral (see Table 10-5).

Potassium-Sparing Agents

Potassium-retaining agents lessen the incidence of serious ventricular arrhythmias in heart failure[52] and in hypertension.[66]

Amiloride and triamterene. Amiloride acts on the renal epithelial sodium channel (ENaC)[67] and triamterene inhibits the sodium-proton exchanger, so that both lessen sodium reabsorption in the distal tubules and collecting tubules. Thereby potassium loss is indirectly decreased (Table 4-4). Relatively weak diuretics on their own, they are frequently used in combination with thiazides (Table 4-5).[68] Advantages are that (1) the loss of sodium is achieved without a major loss of potassium or magnesium, and (2) there is potassium retention independent of the activity of aldosterone. Side effects are few: hyperkalemia (a contraindication) and acidosis may seldom occur, mostly in renal disease. In particular, the thiazide-related risks of diabetes mellitus and gout have not been reported with these agents. Amiloride also helps to retain magnesium and is of special benefit to the relatively small percentage of black patients with low-renin, low-aldosterone hypertension and a genetic defect in the epithelial sodium channel.[69]

Spironolactone and eplerenone. Spironolactone and eplerenone are *aldosterone blockers* that spare potassium by blocking the mineralocorticoid receptor that binds aldosterone as well as cortisol and deoxycorticosterone. Eplerenone is a more specific blocker of the mineralocorticoid receptor, thereby preventing the gynecomastia and sexual dysfunction seen in up to 10% of those given spironolactone. Eplerenone should become the preferred potassium sparer for primary hypertension, especially if costs of the generic preparation go down as expected. In patients with hypertensive heart disease, eplerenone was

Table 4-4

Potassium-sparing Agents (Generally also Magnesium Sparing)			
	Trade Names	**Dose**	**Duration of Action**
Amiloride	Midamor	2.5-20 mg	6-24 h
Triamterene	Dytac, Dyrenium	25-200 mg	8-12 h
Spironolactone	Aldactone	25-200 mg	3-5 days
Eplerenone	Inspra	50-100 mg	24 h

Table 4-5

Some Combination K⁺-Retaining Diuretics			
	Trade Name	**Combination (mg)**	**Preferred Daily Dose**
Hydrochlorothiazide + triamterene	Dyazide	25 50	½ (up to 4 in CHF)
Hydrochlorothiazide + amiloride	Moduretic	50 5	¼* (up to 2 in CHF)
Hydrochlorothiazide + triamterene	Maxzide	50 75	¼*
Hydrochlorothiazide + triamterene	Maxzide-25	25 37.5	½
Spironolactone + hydrochlorothiazide	Aldactazide	25 25	1-4/day
Furosemide + amiloride	Frumil†	40 5	1-2/day

CHF, Congestive heart failure.

    *Quarter[68] is best avoided by use of alternate combinations.

    †Not in the United States.

    For hypertension, see text; low doses generally preferred and high doses are contraindicated.

as effective as enalapril (40 mg daily) in regressing LVH and lowering BP and was equally effective in lowering BP in black and white patients with hypertension.[70] Another advantage of mineralocorticoid receptor antagonists over thiazides is that they do not cause reflex sympathetic activation.[71,72] Aldosterone receptor blockers have an obvious place in the treatment of primary aldosteronism.

In patients with *resistant hypertension* without primary aldosteronism, aldosterone receptor blockers are becoming standard add-on therapy, and are potentially more used even in the larger population of patients with primary hypertension while monitoring serum potassium.[73] Eplerenone (100-300 mg daily) was only half as effective as spironolactone (75-225 mg daily) in lowering BP in patients with primary aldosteronism.[74] The real problem is that there are no good prospective outcome studies of resistant hypertension.[75] A metaanalysis of five small randomized crossover studies[76] found that spironolactone reduced BP by 20/7 mmHg, with *daily doses of more than 50 mg not producing further BP reductions.*

ACE inhibitors and ARBs. Because ACE inhibitors and ARBs ultimately exert an antialdosterone effect, they too act as mild potassium-retaining diuretics. Combination therapy with other potassium retainers should be avoided in the presence of renal impairment, but can successfully be undertaken with care and monitoring of serum potassium, as in the RALES study.[77]

Hyperkalemia: a specific risk. Amiloride, triamterene, spironolactone and eplerenone may all cause hyperkalemia (serum potassium equal to or exceeding 5.5 mEq/L), especially in the presence of preexisting renal disease, diabetes (type IV renal tubular acidosis), in older adult patients during co-therapy with ACE inhibitors or ARBs, or in patients receiving possible nephrotoxic agents. Mechanisms causing hyperkalemia include prolonged solute-driven water loss as well as diuretic-driven renin-angiotensin aldosterone activation and negative diuretic effects on nephron function.[78]

Aquaretics

Chronic heart failure is often associated with increased vasopressin plasma concentrations, which may underlie the associated fluid retention and hyponatremia. Arginine vasopressin (AVP) acts via V1 and V2 receptors to regulate vascular tone (V1), and fluid retention (V2). *Aquaretics* are antagonists of AVP-2 receptors in the kidney to promote solute-free water clearance to correct hyponatremia. Specific examples are tolvaptan, conivaptan, satavaptan, and lixivaptan, a grouping often called the *vaptans.* Experimentally, they inhibit aquaporin-2, the AVP-sensitive water transport channel found in the apices of the renal collecting duct cells (Fig. 4-4).[79] In clinical trials, vaptans increase free water clearance and urine volume, while decreasing urine osmolality, thereby increasing serum sodium when administered to patients with hyponatremia. Hypotension and thirst are among the side effects.

Conivaptan is a combined V1/V2 receptor antagonist now approved and available in the United States for intravenous administration in treatment of euvolemic or hypervolemic hyponatremia in hospitalized patients (intravenous 20 mg loading dose over 30 min, then 20-40 mg continuously infused over 24 hours; up to 40 mg to correct hyponatremia; infuse up to 3 days thereafter, the total duration not exceeding 4 days). In 74 hyponatremic patients, oral doses (20-40 mg twice daily) increased serum sodium by 3 and 4.8 mEq/L, respectively (placebo corrected).[80]

Tolvaptan, an oral V2 antagonist (30-90 mg once daily) added to standard therapy for patients hospitalized with worsening heart failure, decreased body weight, increased urine output, and increased serum sodium by approximately 4 mEq/L from approximately 138 mEq/L.[81]

AQUARETICS
Opie 2012

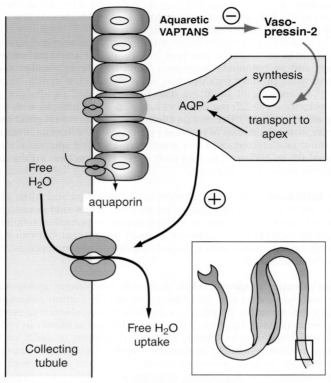

Figure 4-4 Mechanism of action of aquaretics ("vaptans"). These inhibit the vasopressin-2 receptors whose activity promotes the synthesis and transport of aquaporin (AQP) to the apex of the cells of the collecting duct. Aquaporin is the vasopressin-regulated water channel that mediates water transport across the apical cell membranes of the renal collecting duct. *AQP,* Aquaporin. (Figure © L.H. Opie, 2012.)

However, a mortality trial (EVEREST) with 30 mg daily given to selected heart failure patients for a mean of 9.9 months was negative, although early changes were loss of body weight, decreased edema, and increased serum sodium.[82]

Lixivaptan, also an oral V2 antagonist, increased solute-free urine flow in chronic heart failure without renin-angiotensin system stimulation at single doses of 30-400 mg.[83] Further studies are underway.

Combination Diuretics with K$^+$ Sparing

For *heart failure,* a standard combination daily therapy might be one to two tablets of HCTZ 50 mg, amiloride 5 mg (Moduretic); two to four tablets of HCTZ 25 mg, triamterene 50 mg (Dyazide); or one to two tablets of HCTZ 50 mg, triamterene 75 mg (Maxzide). When used for *hypertension,* special attention must be given to the thiazide dose (25 mg HCTZ in Dyazide, 50 mg in Moduretic, and both 25 mg and 50 mg in Maxzide), in which the initial aim is only 12.5 mg HCTZ. With Aldactazide (25 mg of spironolactone and 25 mg of HCTZ), the starting dose should be half a tablet. A potassium-retaining furosemide combination is available and much used in Europe (furosemide 40 mg, amiloride 5 mg *[Frumil]*). A logical combination is that of ACE inhibitor or ARB with low-dose thiazide, for example, low dose perindopril with low dose indapamide.[46] Thiazide diuretics increase renin levels and ACE inhibitors or ARBs decrease the metabolic side effects of thiazides (see Chapter 5, p. 134).

Minor Diuretics

Carbonic anhydrase inhibitors. Carbonic anhydrase inhibitors such as acetazolamide *(Diamox)* are weak diuretics. They decrease the secretion of hydrogen ions by the proximal renal tubule, with increased loss of bicarbonate and hence of sodium. These agents, seldom used as primary diuretics, have found a place in the therapy of *glaucoma* because carbonic anhydrase plays a role in the secretion of aqueous humor in the ciliary processes of the eye. They also protect from altitude illness. In *salicylate poisoning,* the alkalinizing effect of carbonic anhydrase inhibitors increases the renal excretion of lipid-soluble weak organic acids.

Calcium channel blockers. CCBs are mild direct diuretics that may contribute to the long-term antihypertensive effect.[84]

Dopamine. Dopamine has a diuretic action apart from the improvement in cardiac function and indirect diuresis that it induces. The mechanism of the diuresis, found only in conditions of fluid retention, appears to involve dopamine agonists (DA_1) receptors on the renal tubular cells where dopamine stimulation opposes the effects of antidiuretic hormone (ADH).

A_1-Adenosine receptor antagonists. A_1-adenosine receptor antagonists are another new approach to diuresis that increase urine flow and natriuresis. They may act by afferent arteriolar dilation, thereby increasing glomerular filtration. In patients with acute heart failure, they enhance the response to loop diuretics.[85]

Limited Role of Potassium Supplements

The use of potassium supplements with loop diuretics is usually unnecessary and does not appear to protect from the adverse effects of non–K-sparing diuretics. Supplements lead to extra cost and loss of compliance. Rather, addition of low-dose potassium-retaining agents is usually better (see Table 4-4) and can often be accompanied by a lower dose of the loop diuretic. Even high doses of furosemide may not automatically require potassium replacement because such doses are usually given in the presence of renal impairment or severe CHF when renal potassium handling may be abnormal. *Clearly potassium levels need periodic checking during therapy with all diuretics.* A high-potassium, low-salt diet is advised and can be simply and cheaply achieved by choosing fresh rather than processed foods and by the use of salt substitutes. If problematic hypokalemia develops, then a potassium supplement may become necessary. Persistent hypokalemia in hypertension merits investigation for primary aldosteronism.

Potassium chloride. Potassium chloride (KCl) in liquid form is theoretically best because (1) co-administration of chloride is required to fully correct potassium deficiency in hypokalemic hypochloremic alkalosis,[86] and (2) slow-release tablets may cause GI ulceration, which liquid KCl does not.[87] The dose is variable. At least 20 mEq daily are required to avoid potassium depletion and 60 to 100 mEq are required to treat potassium depletion. Absorption is rapid and bioavailability good. To help avoid the frequent GI irritation, liquid KCl needs dilution in water or another liquid and titration against the patient's acceptability. KCl may also be given in some effervescent preparations. To avoid esophageal ulceration, tablets should be taken upright or sitting, with a meal or beverage, and anticholinergic therapy should be avoided. *Microencapsulated KCl* (Micro-K, 8 mEq KCl or 10 mEq KCl) may reduce GI ulceration to only 1 per 100,000 patient years. Nonetheless, high doses of Micro-K cause GI ulcers, especially during anticholinergic therapy.

Recommendations. Diet is the simplest recommendation, with high-potassium, low-sodium intake achieved by fresh foods and salt substitutes. When K^+ supplements become essential, KCl is preferred. The best preparation is one that is well tolerated by the patient and that is inexpensive. No comprehensive adequately controlled studies of the relative efficacy of the various KCl preparations in clinical settings are available.

Special Diuretic Problems

Overdiuresis

During therapy of edematous states, overvigorous diuresis is common and may reduce intravascular volume and ventricular filling so that the cardiac output drops and tissues become underperfused. The renin-angiotensin axis and the sympathetic nervous system are further activated. Overdiuresis is most frequently seen during hospital admissions when a rigid policy of regular administration of diuretics is carried out. Symptoms include fatigue and listlessness. Overdiuresis is also seen when a thiazide diuretic is combined with a loop diuretic to produce diuretic synergy via sequential nephron blockade (see Fig. 4-3). Although this diuretic combination can overcome loop diuretic resistance in acute and chronic heart failure, this practice can also cause massive diuresis leading to hypokalemia, hyponatremia, hypovolemic hypotension, and acute renal failure.[88] These authors call for "pragmatic clinical trials for this commonly used therapy."

Clinical situations in which overdiuresis is most likely include (1) patients with mild chronic heart failure overtreated with potent diuretics; (2) patients requiring a high filling pressure, particularly those with a "restrictive" pathophysiologic condition as in restrictive cardiomyopathy, hypertrophic cardiomyopathy, or constrictive pericarditis; and (3) patients in early phase AMI, when excess diuresis by potent intravenous diuretics can cause a pressor response that attenuated by ACE inhibition.[13] It may be necessary to cautiously administer a *fluid challenge* with saline solution or a colloid preparation while checking the patient's cardiovascular status. If the resting heart rate falls, renal function improves, and BP stabilizes, the ventricular filling pressure has been reduced too much by overdiuresis.

Patients can manage their therapy well by tailoring a flexible diuretic schedule to their own needs, using a simple bathroom scale. Knowing how to recognize pedal edema and the time course of maximal effect of their diuretic often allows a patient to adjust his or her own diuretic dose and administration schedule to fit in with daily activities. A *practical approach* is to stabilize the patient on a combination of drugs, and then to allow self-modification of the furosemide dose, within specified limits, and according to body weight.

Diuretic resistance. Diuretic resistance may occur late or early, with the latter occurring even after one dose of a diuretic and resulting from intravascular fluid contraction (Table 4-6).[11] Repetitive diuretic administration leads to a leveling off of the diuretic effect, because (in the

Table 4-6

Some Causes of Apparent Resistance to Diuretics in Therapy of Cardiac Failure

Incorrect Use of Diuretic Agent

Combination of two thiazides or two loop diuretics instead of one of each type
Use of thiazides when GFR is low* (exception: metolazone)
Excessive diuretic dose
Poor compliance, especially caused by multiple tablets of oral K^+ supplements

Electrolyte Imbalance

Hyponatremia, hypokalemia
Hypomagnesemia may need correction to remedy hypokalemia

Poor Renal Perfusion: Diuretic-Induced Hypovolemia

Cardiac output too low
Hypotension (ACE inhibitors or ARBs in high renin states)

Excess Circulating Catecholamines

Frequent in severe congestive heart failure
Correct by additional therapy for CHF

Interfering Drugs

Nonsteroidal antiinflammatory agents inhibit diuresis
Probenecid and lithium inhibit tubular excretion of thiazides and loop diuretics

ACE, angiotensin-converting enzyme; *ARB,* angiotensin receptor blocker; *CHF,* congestive heart failure; *GFR,* glomerular filtration rate.
*GFR less than 15 to 20 mL/min.

face of a shrunken intravascular volume) the part of the tubular system not affected reacts by reabsorbing more sodium (see Fig. 4-4). Such decreased sodium diuresis is associated with hypertrophy of distal nephron cells,[11] thought to be the result of aldosterone-induced growth.[12] Of therapeutic interest, the thiazides block the nephron sites at which the hypertrophy occurs,[11] thereby providing another argument for combined thiazide-loop therapy.[89] Apparent resistance can also develop during incorrect use of diuretics (see Table 4-6), or when there is concomitant therapy with indomethacin, with other NSAIDs, or with probenecid. The thiazide diuretics will not work well if the GFR is less than 20 to 30 mL/min; metolazone is an exception (see Table 4-6). When potassium depletion is severe, all diuretics work poorly for complex reasons.

To achieve diuresis, an ACE inhibitor or ARB may have to be added cautiously to thiazide or loop diuretics, or metolazone (or other thiazide) may have to be combined with loop diuretics, all following the principle of sequential nephron blockade. Sometimes spironolactone is also required. Furthermore, intravenous *dopamine* may, through its action on DA_1-receptors, help induce diuresis acting in part by increasing renal blood flow. In outpatients, compliance and dietary salt restriction must be carefully checked and all unnecessary drugs eliminated. Sometimes fewer drugs work better than more (here the prime sinners are potassium supplements, requiring many daily tablets frequently not taken).

Hyponatremia. *In heart failure,* hyponatremia may occur in patients severely ill with CHF and in some older adult patients who consume large amounts of water despite an increased total body sodium in heart failure. Predominant water retention is caused by (1) the inappropriate release of AVP-ADH (see ADH in Fig. 4-1), and (2) increased activity of angiotensin-II.[90] Treatment is by combined furosemide and an ACE inhibitor (see Chapter 6, p. 193); restriction of water intake is also critical.

Aquaretics are novel agents that help to overcome hyponatremia (see p. 107). *In hypertension,* hyponatremia may occur especially in older women receiving a thiazide dose of 25 mg daily or more.[91]

Less Common Uses of Diuretics

Less common indications are:

1. Intravenous furosemide used in *malignant hypertension,* especially if there is associated CHF and fluid retention.

2. High-dose furosemide used for *acute or chronic renal failure* when it is hoped that the drug may initiate diuresis.

3. In *hypercalcemia,* high-dose loop diuretics increase urinary excretion of calcium; intravenous furosemide plus saline is used in the emergency treatment of severe hypercalcemia.

4. Thiazides used for the *nephrogenic form of diabetes insipidus*—the mechanism of action is not clear, but there is a diminution in "free water" clearance.

5. Thiazide diuretics decrease the urinary calcium output by promoting proximal reabsorption, so that they are used in *idiopathic hypercalciuria* to decrease the formation of renal stones. (In contrast, loop diuretics increase urinary excretion of calcium.)

The inhibitory effect of thiazides on urinary calcium loss may explain why these agents may increase bone mineralization and decrease the incidence of hip fractures.[92] The latter benefit is another argument for first-line low-dose diuretic therapy in older adult patients with hypertension.

Diuretics in Step-Care Therapy of CHF

In *mild to moderate heart failure with fluid retention,* diuretics are standard first-line therapy (Fig. 4-5). The choice of diuretic lies between standard thiazide, a K-retainer plus thiazide, furosemide, spironolactone, and eplerenone. The latter are known to save lives in severe CHF when added to otherwise standard therapy.[77,93] Furthermore, a retrospective analysis showed that use of non-K retaining diuretics in the SOLVD study was associated with increased arrhythmic death.[52] By contrast, a K-retainer alone or in combination with a non-K retainer, gave no such increase in risk of arrhythmic death. ACE inhibition plus a non-K retaining diuretic also did not protect from arrhythmic death. These studies, although retrospective and observational, are bound to influence clinicians toward the preferential use of spironolactone, eplerenone or combination diuretics containing K-retainers (see Tables 4-4 and 4-5).

Step-care diuretic therapy in symptomatic heart failure (see Fig. 6-9) with fluid retention is not clearly delineated by adequate trials, but four potential agents are (1) thiazide diuretics with ACE inhibitors, (2) low-dose furosemide with ACE inhibitors, (3) thiazides together with low-dose furosemide with ACE inhibitors, and (4) spironolactone or eplerenone added to the others. High-dose furosemide is now less used, chiefly for acute heart failure. The current practice is to add ACE inhibitors or ARBs whenever the patient is given a diuretic, unless there is a contraindication. ACE inhibition or ARBs should offset the deleterious renin-angiotensin activation induced by diuretics. Regarding *sodium restriction,* modest restriction is advisable throughout, starting with no added salt, then cutting out obvious sources of salt as in processed or fast foods, and then going on to salt-free bread. Downregulation of the salt-sensitive taste buds means that after approximately

DIURETIC RESISTANCE IN CHF

Opie 2012

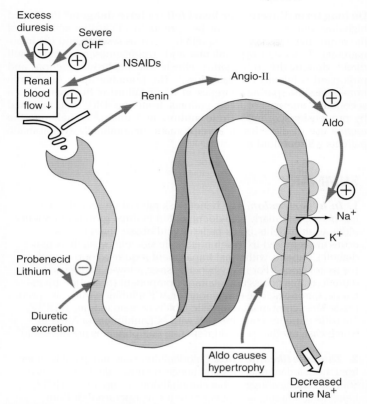

Figure 4-5 **Diuretic resistance** has several causes including reduced renal blood flow and the stimulation of the renin-angiotensin-aldosterone system. Hypothetically, increased aldosterone (aldo) may promote distal tubular hypertrophy to reabsorb greater amounts of sodium. For early "braking," not shown here, see text. *Angio II,* angiotensin II; *CHF,* congestive heart failure; *NSAID,* nonsteroidal antiinflammatory drug. (Figure © L.H. Opie, 2012.)

6 weeks of modest sodium restriction, a low-salt diet becomes the preferred norm.

For *severe CHF,* when congestion and edema are prominent symptoms, initial therapy is usually with furosemide, especially when renal perfusion may be impaired. In severely ill patients complete bed rest, although old-fashioned, may promote an early diuresis. The dose of furosemide required in resistant CHF may be very high (500 to 1500 mg daily). Alternatively, the principle of sequential nephron blockade may be used with a lower dose of furosemide, and consideration should be given to intermittent dopamine.

Sequential nephron blockade. *Sequential nephron blockade* is the principle whereby addition of a diuretic acting at a different site, such as a thiazide to a loop diuretic, is logical (see Fig. 4-3). However, beware of overdiuresis as previously warned.[88]

ACE inhibitors. ACE inhibitors are now standard agents for all stages of heart failure. In CHF, the action of diuretics may be inhibited by poor renal perfusion and vasoconstrictive formation of renin, with a low GFR lessening sodium excretion. Hence ACE inhibitors are logical additions to diuretics. They have an indirect diuretic effect ultimately by inhibiting aldosterone release. They also help to maintain cell potassium and magnesium.

Do long-term diuretics for heart failure have dangers? Prolonged high-dose diuretic therapy may be harmful by (1) further activation of the renin-angiotensin and sympathetic nervous systems, and (2) hyponatremia (less often hypokalemia and hypomagnesemia) can result direct diuretic-driven negative effects on nephron function and prolonged solute-driven water loss.[78] The potential harm of chronic non–potassium-sparing diuretics in heart failure is highlighted in a secondary analysis of 7788 patients from the DIG trial, matched by propensity scoring.[94] These authors and others[5,16] challenge the *routine* use of diuretics in asymptomatic or minimally symptomatic patients without fluid retention.

SUMMARY

1. *In hypertension.* The benefit-risk ratio of diuretic therapy has been particularly well-documented in three groups of patients: older adult patients, black patients, and obese patients. Low doses are required to lessen metabolic side effects such as new diabetes. Patients with renal impairment require a loop diuretic (or metolazone). For many hypertensives, a low-dose thiazide diuretic, with a potassium-retaining component (amiloride, triamterene, spironolactone-eplerenone or ACE inhibition–ARB) is appropriate. Most combination diuretic tablets contain too much HCTZ. Thiazide diuretics combine well with ACE inhibitors or ARBs, in which case another potassium-sparing component is not advisable.

2. *Thiazide-like diuretics.* Chlorthalidone and indapamide differ from the standard thiazides, and hence are now called *thiazide-like*. Some recent data suggest that chlorthalidone is superior to HCTZ, being longer acting and better at reducing nocturnal BP. Both chlorthalidone and indapamide slow-release are preferentially recommended for hypertension by the British NICE group as having positive outcome studies in hypertension, which the standard thiazides do not have.

3. *Amiloride, triamterene, and spironolactone.* Amiloride, triamterene, and spironolactone are "old-fashioned drugs" making a comeback, the first two for hypertension associated with renal epithelial sodium channel defects, and spironolactone for resistant hypertension and heart failure.

4. *CHF with fluid retention.* The benefit-risk ratio of diuretics is high and their use remains standard. Yet not all patients require vigorous diuresis; rather, each patient needs careful clinical evaluation with a specific cardiologic diagnosis so that surgically correctable defects are appropriately handled. First choice of therapy for mild fluid retention is a thiazide logically combined with an ACE inhibitor or ARB. With increasing severities of failure, larger doses of thiazide are used before switching to or combining with a loop diuretic such as furosemide.

5. *Non-congested heart failure.* Diuretics may be harmful by renin-aldosterone stimulation but countered by spironolactone-eplerenone.

6. *Sequential nephron block.* Sequential nephron block is an important principle calling for the progressive addition of diuretics acting at different nephron sites as the severity of heart failure increases: thiazides, loop diuretics, and then aldosterone antagonists.

With concurrent use of ACE inhibitors or ARBs, hyperkalemia is best limited by low doses of spironolactone—eplerenone.

7. *Hypokalemia*. Hypokalemia remains one of the frequent complications of diuretic therapy. In hypertension this is avoided by the use of a low-dose thiazide with a potassium-retaining component: amiloride, triamterene, spironolactone, or eplerenone. In heart failure, we stress that automatic addition of oral potassium supplements is far from ideal practice. Rather, the combination of a loop diuretic plus low-dose thiazide plus potassium-retaining agent is reasonable. Concurrent ACE inhibitor or ARB therapy also counters hypokalemia by an antialdosterone effect. For mild to moderate heart failure with fluid retention, some combination of diuretics, plus ACE inhibitors and ideally with β-blockade, is standard therapy.

8. *Hyponatremia*. Hyponatremia is a potentially serious complication of chronic heart failure, often associated with increased plasma vasopressin and prolonged use of loop diuretics. Thiazides can cause hyponatremia in older hypertensives. *Aquaretics* are a new class of diuretic that promote solute-free water clearance to correct hyponatremia by inhibiting aquaporin, the vasopressin-sensitive water transport channel found in the apices of the renal collecting duct cells. Specific examples are conivaptan, tolvaptan, and lixivaptan, a grouping often called the *vaptans*. However, an outcome study with tolvaptan was disappointing (see Chapter 6, p. 189).

References

1. Cranston W, et al. Effects of oral diuretics on raised arterial pressure. *Lancet* 1963;2:966–969.
2. Psaty BM, et al. Health outcomes associated with various antihypertensive therapies used as first-line agents. *JAMA* 2003;289:2534–2544.
3. Lam SK, et al. Incident diabetes in clinical trials of antihypertensive drugs. *Lancet* 2007;369:1513-1514; author reply 1514–1515.
4. Messerli FH, et al. Essential hypertension. *Lancet* 2007;370:591–603.
5. Gupta S, et al. Diuretic usage in heart failure: a continuing conundrum in 2005. *Eur Heart J* 2005;26:644–649.
6. Hunt SA, et al. ACC/AHA guidelines for the evaluation and management of chronic heart failure in the adult: executive summary. A report of the American College of Cardiology/American Heart Association Task Force on Practice Guidelines (Committee to Revise the 1995 Guidelines for the Evaluation and Management of Heart Failure): developed in collaboration with the International Society for Heart and Lung Transplantation; endorsed by the Heart Failure Society of America. *Circulation* 2001;104: 2996–3007.
7. Zhu Z, et al. Thiazide-like diuretics attenuate agonist-induced vasoconstriction by calcium desensitization linked to Rho kinase. *Hypertension* 2005;45:233–239.
8. Joint National Committee 7, Chobanian AV, et al. The seventh report of the Joint National Committee on Prevention, Detection, Evaluation and Treatment of High Blood Pressure. *JAMA* 2003;289:2560–2572.
9. WHO/ISH Writing Group. 2003 World Health Organisation (WHO)/International Society of Hypertension (ISH) statement on management of hypertension. *J Hypertens* 2003;21:1983–1992.
10. Gammage M. Treatment of acute pulmonary edema: diuresis or vasodilation? (commentary). *Lancet* 1998;351:382–383.
11. Brater DC. Diuretic therapy. *New Engl J Med* 1998;339:387–395.
12. Reyes AJ, et al. Diuretics in cardiovascular therapy: the new clinicopharmacological bases that matter. *Cardiovasc Drugs Ther* 1999;13:371–398.
13. Goldsmith SR, et al. Attenuation of the pressor response to intravenous furosemide by angiotensin converting enzyme inhibition in congestive heart failure. *Am J Cardiol* 1989;64:1382–1385.
14. Vlase HL, et al. Effectiveness of furosemide in uncontrolled hypertension in the elderly: role of renin profiling. *Am J Hypertens* 2003;16:187–193.
15. Cantarovich F, et al. High-dose furosemide for established ARF: a prospective, randomized, double-blind, placebo-controlled, multicenter trial. *Am J Kidney Dis* 2004;44: 402–409.
16. McCurley JM, et al. Furosemide and the progression of left ventricular dysfunction in experimental heart failure. *J Am Coll Cardiol* 2004;44:1301–1307.
17. Johnson AG. NSAIDs and blood pressure: clinical importance for older patients. *Drugs Aging* 1998;12:17–27.
18. Wall GC, et al. Ethacrynic acid and the sulfa-sensitive patient. *Arch Intern Med* 2003;163:116–117.

19. Zillich AJ, et al. Thiazide diuretics, potassium, and the development of diabetes: a quantitative review. *Hypertension* 2006;48:219–224.
20. Santoro D, et al. Effects of chronic angiotensin-converting enzyme inhibition on glucose tolerance and insulin sensitivity in essential hypertension. *Hypertension* 1992;20:181–191.
21. Krause T, et al for the Guideline Development Group. Management of hypertension: summary of NICE guidance. *Brit Med J* 2011;343:d4891.
22. Carter BL, et al. Hydrochlorothiazide versus chlorthalidone: evidence supporting their interchangeability. *Hypertension* 2004;43:4–9.
23. Wright Jr JT, et al. Outcomes in hypertensive black and nonblack patients treated with chlorthalidone, amlodipine, and lisinopril. *JAMA* 2005;293:1595–1608.
24. Materson BJ, et al. Single-drug therapy for hypertension in men: a comparison of six antihypertensive agents with placebo. The Department of Veterans Affairs Cooperative Study Group on Antihypertensive Agents. *N Engl J Med* 1993;328:914–921.
25. SHEP Cooperative Research Group. Prevention of stroke by antihypertensive drug treatment in older persons with isolated systolic hypertension: final results of the Systolic Hypertension in the Elderly Program (SHEP). *JAMA* 1991;265:3255–3264.
26. Brown MJ, et al. Morbidity and mortality in patients randomised to double-blind treatment with a long-acting calcium-channel blocker or diuretic in the International Nifedipine GITS study: intervention as a goal in hypertension treatment. *Lancet* 2000;356:366–372.
27. Pollare T, et al. A comparison of the effects of hydrochlorothiazide and captopril on glucose and lipid metabolism in patients with hypertension. *N Engl J Med* 1989;321:868–873.
28. Pepine CJ, et al. A calcium antagonist vs a non-calcium antagonist hypertension treatment strategy for patients with coronary artery disease. The International Verapamil-Trandolapril Study (INVEST): a randomized controlled trial. *JAMA* 2003;290:2805–2816.
29. Lacourciere Y, et al. Antihypertensive effects of two fixed-dose combinations of losartan and hydrochlorothiazide versus hydrochlorothiazide monotherapy in subjects with ambulatory systolic hypertension. *Am J Hypertens* 2003;16:1036–1042.
30. Harper R, et al. Effects of low dose versus conventional dose thiazide diuretic on insulin action in essential hypertension. *Brit Med J* 1994;309:226–230.
31. Messerli FH, et al. Antihypertensive efficacy of hydrochlorothiazide as evaluated by ambulatory blood pressure monitoring. *J Am Coll Cardiol* 2011;57:590–600.
32. Wiggam MI, et al. Low dose bendrofluazide (1.25 mg) effectively lowers blood pressure over 24 h: results of a randomized, double-blind, placebo-controlled crossover study. *Am J Hypertens* 1999;12:528–531.
33. Dussol B, et al. A pilot study comparing furosemide and hydrochlorothiazide in patients with hypertension and stage 4 or 5 chronic kidney disease. *J Clin Hypertens* 2012;14:32–37.
34. Grimm RH, et al. Long-term effects on sexual function of five antihypertensive drugs and nutritional hygienic treatment in hypertensive men and women. Treatment of Mild Hypertension Study (TOMHS). *Hypertension* 1997;29:8–14.
35. Kronish IM, et al. Meta-analysis: impact of drug class on adherence to antihypertensives. *Circulation* 2011;123:1611–1621.
36. ALLHAT Collaborative Research Group. Major outcomes in high-risk hypertensive patients randomized to angiotensin-converting enzyme inhibitor or calcium channel blocker vs diuretic. The Antihypertensive and Lipid-Lowering Treatment to Prevent Heart Attack Trial (ALLHAT). *JAMA* 2002;288:2981–2997.
37. Ernst ME, et al. Comparative antihypertensive effects of hydrochlorothiazide and chlorthalidone on ambulatory and office blood pressure. *Hypertension* 2006;47:352–358.
38. Ernst ME, et al. Meta-analysis of dose-response characteristics of hydrochlorothiazide and chlorthalidone: effects on systolic blood pressure and potassium. *Am J Hypertens* 2010;23:440–446.
39. Dorsch MP, et al. Chlorthalidone reduces cardiovascular events compared with hydrochlorothiazide: a retrospective cohort analysis. *Hypertension* 2011;57:689–694.
40. Ernst ME, et al. for the Multiple Risk Factor Intervention Trial Research Group. Long-Term effects of chlorthalidone versus hydrochlorothiazide on electrocardiographic left ventricular hypertrophy in the Multiple Risk Factor Intervention Trial. *Hypertension* 2011;58:1001–1007.
41. Kreeft J, et al. Comparative trial of indapamide and hydrochlorothiazide in essential hypertension with forearm plethysmography. *J Cardiovasc Pharmacol* 1984;6:622–626.
42. Ames RP. A comparison of blood lipid and blood pressure responses during the treatment of systemic hypertension with indapamide and with thiazides. *Am J Cardiol* 1996;77:12B–16B.
43. Zhang Y, et al. Effect of antihypertensive agents on blood pressure variability: the Natrilix SR versus candesartan and amlodipine in the reduction of systolic blood pressure in hypertensive patients (X-CELLENT) study. *Hypertension* 2011;58:155–160.
44. Webb AJ, et al. Effect of dose and combination of antihypertensives on interindividual blood pressure variability: a systemic review. *Stroke* 2011;42:2860–2865.
45. Beckett N, et al. for the HYVET Study Group. Treatment of hypertension in patients 80 years of age or older. *N Engl J Med* 2008;358:1887–1898.
46. Chalmers J, et al. Long-term efficacy of a new, fixed, very-low-dose angiotensin-converting enzyme inhibitor/diuretic combination as first-line therapy in elderly hypertensive patients. *J Hypertens* 2000;18:327–337.
47. ADVANCE Collaborative Group, Patel A, et al. Effects of a fixed combination of perindopril and indapamide on macrovascular and microvascular outcomes in patients with type 2 diabetes mellitus (the ADVANCE trial): a randomised controlled trial. *Lancet* 2007;370:829–840.

48. Gosse P, et al. On behalf of the LIVE investigators. Regression of left ventricular hypertrophy in hypertensive patients treated with indapamide SR 1.5 mg versus enalapril 20 mg: the LIVE study. *J Hypertens* 2000;18:1465–1475.

49. Ambrosioni E, et al. Low-dose antihypertensive therapy with 1.5 mg sustained-release indapamide: results of randomised double-blind controlled studies. *J Hypertens* 1998;16:1677–1684.

50. Sica DA, et al. Diuretic combinations in refractory edema states: pharmacokinetic-pharmacodynamic relationships. *Clin Pharmacokinet* 1996;30:229–249.

51. Franse LV, et al. Hypokalemia associated with diuretic use and cardiovascular events in the Systolic Hypertension in the Elderly Program. *Hypertension* 2000;35:1025–1030.

52. Domanski M, et al. Diuretic use, progressive heart failure, and death in patients in the Studies Of Left Ventricular Dysfunction (SOLVD). *J Am Coll Cardiol* 2003;42: 705–708.

53. Wilcox CS. Metabolic and adverse effects of diuretics. *Semin Nephrol* 1999;19:557–568.

54. Gress TW, et al. For the Atherosclerosis Risk in Communities Study. Hypertension and antihypertensives therapy as risk factors for type 2 diabetes mellitus. *N Engl J Med* 2000;342:905–912.

55. Holzgreve H, et al. Antihypertensive therapy with verapamil SR plus trandolapril versus atenolol plus chlorthalidone on glycemic control. *Am J Hypertens* 2003;16:381–386.

56. LIFE Study Group, Dahlöf B, et al. Cardiovascular morbidity and mortality in the Losartan Intervention For Endpoint reduction in hypertension study (LIFE): a randomised trial against atenolol. *Lancet* 2002;359:995–1003.

57. Lindholm LH, et al. Metabolic outcome during 1 year in newly detected hypertensives: results of the Antihypertensive Treatment and Lipid Profile in a North of Sweden Efficacy Evaluation (ALPINE study). *J Hypertens* 2003;21:1563–1574.

58. Swislocki ALM, et al. Insulin resistance, glucose intolerance and hyperinsulinemia in patients with hypertension. *Am J Hypertens* 1989;2:419–423.

59. Aksnes TA, et al. Impact of new-onset diabetes mellitus on cardiac outcomes in the Valsartan Antihypertensive Long-term Use Evaluation (VALUE) trial population. *Hypertension* 2007;50:467–473.

60. McAdams DeMarco MA, et al. Diuretic use, increased serum urate levels, and risk of incident gout in a population-based study of adults with hypertension: The Atherosclerosis Risk in Communities cohort study. *Arthritis & Rheumatism* 2012;64:121–129.

61. Owens P, et al. Comparison of antihypertensive and metabolic effects of losartan and losartan in combination with hydrochlorothiazide—a randomized controlled trial. *J Hypertens* 2000;18:339–345.

62. Rayner BL, et al. Effect of losartan versus candesartan on uric acid, renal function, and fibrinogen in patients with hypertension and hyperuricemia associated with diuretics. *Am J Hypertens* 2006;19:208–213.

63. Kasiske BL, et al. Effects of antihypertensive therapy on serum lipids. *Ann Intern Med* 1995;122:133–141.

64. TOMH Study, Neaton JD, et al. Treatment of Mild Hypertension study (TOMH). Final results. *JAMA* 1993;270:713–724.

65. LaCroix AZ, et al. Thiazide diuretic agents and the incidence of hip fracture. *New Engl J Med* 1990;322:286–290.

66. Siscovick DS, et al. Diuretic therapy for hypertension and the risk of primary cardiac arrest. *New Eng J Med* 1994;330:1852–1857.

67. Teiwes J, et al. Epithelial sodium channel inhibition in cardiovascular disease: a potential role for amiloride. *Am J Hypertens* 2007;20:109–117.

68. Krown KA, et al. Tumor necrosis factor alpha-induced apoptosis in cardiac myocytes. Involvement of the sphingolipid signaling cascade in cardiac cell death. *J Clin Invest* 1996;98:2854–2865.

69. Rayner BL, et al. A new mutation, R563Q, of the beta subunit of the epithelial sodium channel associated with low-renin, low-aldosterone hypertension. *J Hypertens* 2003;21: 921–926.

70. Pitt B, et al. Effects of eplerenone, enalapril, and eplerenone/enalapril in patients with essential hypertension and left ventricular hypertrophy: the 4E-left ventricular hypertrophy study. *Circulation* 2003;108:1831–1838.

71. Menon DV, et al. Differential effects of chlorthalidone versus spironolactone on muscle sympathetic nerve activity in hypertensive patients. *J Clin Endocrinol Metab* 2009;94: 1361–1366.

72. Wray DW, et al. Impact of aldosterone receptor blockade compared with thiazide therapy on sympathetic nervous system function in geriatric hypertension. *Hypertension* 2010;55:1217–1223.

73. Chapman N, et al. Effect of spironolactone on blood pressure in subjects with resistant hypertension. *Hypertension* 2007;49:839–845.

74. Parthasarathy HK, et al. A double-blind randomized study comparing the antihypertensive effect of eplerenone and spironolactone in primary aldosteronism. *J Hypertens* 2011;29:980–990.

75. Zannad F. Aldosterone antagonist therapy in resistant hypertension. *J Hypertens* 2007;25:747–750.

76. Batterink J, et al. *Spironolactone for hypertension (Review)*, The Cochrane Collaboration, Hoboken, NJ: John Wiley & Sons; 2010. p. 1–37.

77. RALES Study, Pitt B, et al. For the Randomized Aldactone Evaluation Study Investigators. The effect of spironolactone on morbidity and mortality in patients with severe heart failure. *New Engl J Med* 1999;341:709–717.

78. de Goma EM, et al. Emerging therapies for the management of decompensated heart failure: from bench to bedside. *J Am Coll Cardiol* 2006;48:2397–2409.

79. Martin PY, et al. Selective V2-receptor vasopressin antagonism decreases urinary aquaporin-2 excretion in patients with chronic heart failure. *J Am Soc Nephrol* 1999;10: 2165–2170.

80. Ghali JK, et al. Efficacy and safety of oral conivaptan: a V1A/V2 vasopressin receptor antagonist, assessed in a randomized, placebo-controlled trial in patients with euvolemic or hypervolemic hyponatremia. *J Clin Endocrinol Metab* 2006;91:2145–2152.

81. Gheorghiade M, et al. Effects of tolvaptan, a vasopressin antagonist, in patients hospitalized with worsening heart failure: a randomized controlled trial. *JAMA* 2004;291: 1963–1971.

82. Konstam MA, et al. Effects of oral tolvaptan in patients hospitalized for worsening heart failure: the EVEREST Outcome Trial. *JAMA* 2007;297:1319–1331.

83. Abraham WT, et al. Aquaretic effect of lixivaptan, an oral, non-peptide, selective V2 receptor vasopressin antagonist, in New York Heart Association functional class II and III chronic heart failure patients. *J Am Coll Cardiol* 2006;47:1615–1621.

84. Segal AS, et al. On the natriuretic effect of verapamil: inhibition of ENaC and transepithelial sodium transport. *Am J Physiol Renal Physiol* 2002;283:F765–770.

85. Givertz MM, et al. The effects of KW-3902, an adenosine A1-receptor antagonist, on diuresis and renal function in patients with acute decompensated heart failure and renal impairment or diuretic resistance. *J Am Coll Cardiol* 2007;50:1551–1560.

86. Stanaszek WF, et al. Current approaches to management of potassium deficiency. *Drug Intell Clin Pharm* 1985;19:176–184.

87. Patterson DJ, et al. Endoscopic comparison of solid and liquid potassium chloride supplements. *Lancet* 1983;2:1077–1078.

88. Jentzer JC, et al. Combination of loop diuretics with thiazide-type diuretics in heart failure. *J Am Coll Cardiol* 2010;56:1527–1534.

89. Dormans TPJ, et al. Combination of high-dose furosemide and hydrochlorothiazide in the treatment of refractory congestive heart failure. *Eur Heart J* 1996;17:1867–1874.

90. Opie LH, et al. Diuretic therapy. In: Opie LH, editor. *Drugs for the heart.* 2nd ed. Philadelphia: Grune and Stratton; 1987. p. 111–130.

91. Sharabi Y, et al. Diuretic induced hyponatraemia in elderly hypertensive women. *J Hum Hypertens* 2002;16:631–635.

92. LaCroix AZ, et al. Low-dose hydrochlorothiazide and preservation of bone mineral density in older adults: a randomized, double-blind, placebo-controlled trial. *Ann Intern Med* 2000;133:516–526.

93. Pitt B. Aldosterone blockade in patients with systolic left ventricular dysfunction. *Circulation* 2003;108:1790–1794.

94. Ahmed A, et al. Heart failure, chronic diuretic use, and increase in mortality and hospitalization: an observational study using propensity score methods. *Eur Heart J* 2006; 27:1431–1439.

5

Inhibitors of the Renin-Angiotensin-Aldosterone System

LIONEL H. OPIE · MARC A. PFEFFER

"Angiotensin-converting enzyme inhibitors have been shown to have the broadest impact of any drug in cardiovascular medicine."

Harvey White, 2003[1]

Since the description in 1977 of the first angiotensin-converting enzyme (ACE) inhibitor, captopril, by the Squibb group led by Ondetti and Cushman, ACE inhibitors have become the cornerstone not only of the treatment of heart failure and left ventricular (LV) dysfunction, but increasingly also play a major role in hypertension and in cardiovascular (CV) protection.[1,2] The purpose of this chapter is to survey the pharmacologic characteristics, the use, and the limitations of these agents and their new relatives, the angiotensin receptor blockers (ARBs).

Frequent reference is made to the role of the renin-angiotensin-aldosterone system (RAAS) in CV pathologic conditions, with excess activities of angiotensin II and of aldosterone contributing to major adverse maladaptive roles. ACE inhibitors act on the crucial enzyme that generates angiotensin II and mediates the breakdown of bradykinin, whereas the ARBs act directly by blocking the major angiotensin II receptor subtype 1 (AT-1 subtype) that responds to angiotensin-II stimulation. As the result of many careful long and large trials, it is now clear that ACE inhibitors give both primary and secondary protection from cardiovascular disease (CVD), thereby interrupting the vicious circle from risk factors to LV failure at many sites (Fig. 5-1).[3] The ARBs are very well tolerated, and have been shown in several but not all outcome trials to give benefits equal to those provided by the ACE inhibitors. The final step in the RAAS, aldosterone, is increased in heart failure. Aldosterone inhibitors have additive protective effects to those of ACE inhibitors in heart failure and in high-risk postmyocardial infarction (MI) patients. The newer direct renin inhibitors are antihypertensive, but clinical outcome data are currently lacking.

Mechanisms of Action of ACE Inhibitors

Logically, ACE inhibition should work by lessening the complex and widespread effects of angiotensin II (Table 5-1). This octapeptide is formed from its precursor, a decapeptide *angiotensin I,* by the activity of the ACE. ACE activity is found chiefly in the vascular endothelium of the lungs, but occurs in all vascular beds, including the coronary arteries.

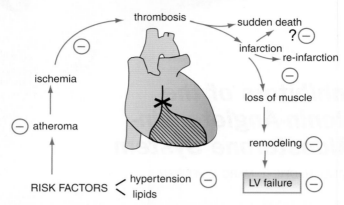

ACEi EFFECTS

Dzau and Braunwald, 1991

Figure 5-1 Dual role of angiotensin-converting enzyme (ACE) inhibitors, both preventing and treating cardiovascular disease. Note multiple sites of action in both primary and secondary prevention. ACE inhibitors (ACEi) have an indirect effect in primary prevention by lessening hypertension and by decreasing left ventricular (LV) hypertrophy. They protect the blood vessels indirectly by an antihypertensive effect, and directly inhibit carotid atherogenesis and thrombogenesis. Given at the start of myocardial infarction, they improve mortality in high-risk patients. By an antiarrhythmic effect, they may act to prevent postinfarct sudden death. By lessening wall stress, they beneficially improve postinfarct remodeling and decrease the incidence of LV failure. The concept of sequential changes leading to a chain of events from risk factors to LV failure is based on concepts of Dzau and Braunwald.[3] (Figure © L.H. Opie, 2012, and adapted from *Angiotensin-Converting Enzyme Inhibitors. The Advance Continues,* 3rd ed, Authors' Publishing House, New York & University of Cape Town Press, 1999.)

Table 5-1

Potential Pathogenic Properties of Angiotensin II
Heart
• Myocardial hypertrophy
• Interstitial fibrosis
Coronary Arteries
• Endothelial dysfunction with deceased release of nitric oxide
• Coronary constriction via release of norepinephrine
• Increased oxidative stress; oxygen-derived free radicals formed via NADH oxidase
• Promotion of inflammatory response and atheroma
• Promotion of LDL cholesterol uptake
Kidneys
• Increased intraglomerular pressure
• Increased protein leak
• Glomerular growth and fibrosis
• Increased sodium reabsorption
Adrenals
• Increased formation of aldosterone
Coagulation System
• Increased fibrinogen
• Increased PAI-1 relative to tissue plasminogen factor

LDL, Low-density lipoprotein; *NADH,* nicotine adenine dinucleotide, reduced; *PAI,* plasminogen activator inhibitor.

Angiotensin I originates in the liver from *angiotensinogen* under the influence of the enzyme *renin,* a protease that is formed in the renal juxtaglomerular cells. Classic stimuli to the release of renin include (1) impaired renal blood flow as in ischemia or hypotension, (2) salt depletion or sodium diuresis, and (3) β-adrenergic stimulation. The *ACE* is a protease that has two zinc groups, only one of which participates in the high-affinity binding site that interacts with angiotensin I or with the ACE inhibitors. ACE not only converts angiotensin I to angiotensin II, but also inactivates the breakdown of bradykinin. ACE inhibition is vasodilatory by decreased formation of angiotensin II and potentially by decreased degradation of bradykinin (Fig. 5-2).

Alternate Modes of Angiotensin II Generation

Not all angiotensin II is generated by ACE. Non-ACE pathways, involving chymaselike serine proteases, can also form angiotensin II, but their exact role is still the subject of controversy. One view is that more than 75% of the cardiac angiotensin II formed in severe human heart failure is formed by chymase activity, and that inhibition of chymase prevents cardiac fibrosis and limits experimental heart failure.[4] However, because ARBs are not more efficacious than ACE inhibitors in heart failure, this view is not supported by the clinical trial data.

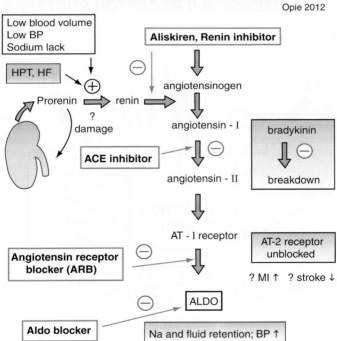

Figure 5-2 The renin-angiotensin-aldosterone system (RAAS) and where inhibitors act. Angiotensin-converting enzyme (ACE) inhibitors have dual vasodilatory actions, chiefly on the renin-angiotensin system with ancillary effects on the breakdown of vascular protective bradykinin. The angiotensin receptor blockers (ARBs) inhibit the angiotensin type 1 receptor (AT-1). The renin inhibitor aliskiren could block the whole RAAS with the theoretical downside of increased formation of prorenin. *AT-2,* Angiotensin type 2; *BP,* blood pressure; *HF,* heart failure; *HPT,* hypertension; *Na,* sodium. (Figure © L.H. Opie, 2012.)

Angiotensin II and Intracellular Messenger Systems

There are many complex steps between occupation of the angiotensin II receptor and ultimate mobilization of calcium with a vasoconstrictor effect in vascular smooth muscle. Occupation of the angiotensin II receptor stimulates the phosphodiesterase (called *phospholipase C*) that leads to a series of signals that activate a specialized enzyme, *protein kinase C,* that in turn evokes the activity growth pathways that stimulate ventricular remodelling.[5] Phospholipase C also activates the *inositol trisphosphate signaling pathway* in blood vessels to liberate calcium from the intracellular sarcoplasmic reticulum to promote vasoconstriction as well as cardiac and vascular structural alterations.

Angiotensin II Receptor Subtypes: The AT-1 and AT-2 Receptors

There are at least two angiotensin II receptor subtypes, the AT-1 and AT-2 receptors (Fig. 5-3). Note the potentially confusing nomenclature: both receptors respond to angiotensin II, but are subtypes 1 and 2. These link to separate internal signaling paths.[6] Clinically used ARBs should be considered as AT-1 blockers. The effects of angiotensin II acting via AT-1 receptors on the diseased heart and failing circulation are often regarded as adverse, such as stimulation of contraction, vasoconstriction, myocyte hypertrophy, fibrosis,[7] and antinatriuresis. In fetal life, these AT-1

ANGIOTENSION-*II* RECEPTOR SUBTYPES

Opie 2012

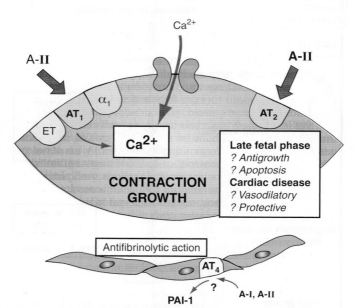

Figure 5-3 Proposed roles of angiotensin II receptor subtypes, which are called AT-1, AT-2, and (possibly) AT-4 subtypes. Most of the physiologic effects in adult vascular smooth muscle cells are conveyed by the AT-1 receptor subtype. The AT-2 receptor is of substantial importance in late fetal vascular growth, exerting an antigrowth effect. Hypothetically, these receptors may also play a beneficial role in various myocardial pathophysiologic conditions (see text). AT-4 receptors are postulated to have an antifibrinolytic effect. (Figure © L.H. Opie, 2012, and adapted from *Angiotensin-Converting Enzyme Inhibitors. The Advance Continues,* 3rd ed, Authors' Publishing House, New York & University of Cape Town Press, 1999.)

receptors act as teratogenic growth stimulators, which explains why ACE inhibitors and ARBs are prohibited therapy in pregnancy. The physiologic role of the AT-2 receptor includes the inhibition of growth in the late fetal phase (growth can't keep on forever). In adult life, the role of the AT-2 receptors is much less well understood and controversial, but could become more relevant in pathophysiologic conditions, the receptors being upregulated in hypertrophy and in heart failure and having a postulated protective function. Again, the comparable clinical results of ACE inhibitors and ARBs (see p. 145) raise questions about the importance of unopposed AT-2 stimulation with ARBs.

Renin-Angiotensin-Aldosterone System

The major factors stimulating *renin release* from the juxtaglomerular cells of the kidney and, hence, angiotensin activation are (Fig. 5-4): (1) a low arterial blood pressure (BP); (2) decreased sodium reabsorption in the distal tubule, as when dietary sodium is low or during diuretic therapy; (3) decreased blood volume; and (4) increased beta$_1$-sympathetic activity. *Stimulation of aldosterone by angiotensin II* means that the latter stimulus releases the sodium-retaining hormone aldosterone from the adrenal cortex. Hence ACE inhibition is associated with aldosterone reduction and has potential indirect natriuretic and potassium-retaining effects. Aldosterone formation does not, however, stay fully blocked during prolonged ACE-inhibitor therapy. This late "escape" does not appear to compromise the antihypertensive effects achieved by ACE inhibitors; nonetheless, it might detract from the prolonged benefit of these agents in heart failure. In the RALES study, *added low-dose spironolactone on top of diuretics and ACE inhibition reduced mortality* (see p. 159).

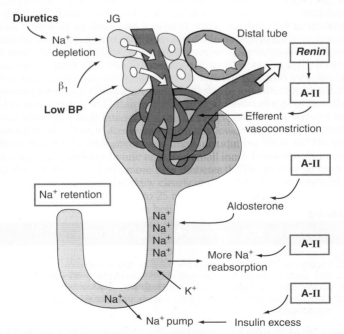

A-II AND Na$^+$ BALANCE

Opie 2012

Figure 5-4   Renal mechanisms whereby renin-angiotensin-aldosterone system promotes sodium retention. *A-II,* angiotensin II; *JG,* juxtaglomerular cells. (Figure © L.H. Opie, 2012.)

Adverse Effects of Excess Aldosterone

Aldosterone, released either in response to angiotensin II or to stimulation by adrenocorticotropic hormone (ACTH) or increased potassium, has major effects on electrolyte balance. Aldosterone acts on the distal tubule to retain sodium and excrete potassium by inhibition of sodium-potassium exchange (see Fig. 5-4). Water is retained with sodium. In heart failure, plasma aldosterone rises up to 20 times normal, in response to increased angiotensin II, coupled with decreased hepatic clearance.[8] Aldosterone, some of it locally produced, may adversely alter the structure of the myocardium by promotion of cardiac fibrosis.[8] Aldosterone also promotes endothelial dysfunction.[9]

Autonomic Interactions of Angiotensin II

ACE inhibitors have indirect permissive antiadrenergic effects. Angiotensin II promotes the release of norepinephrine from adrenergic terminal neurons, and also enhances adrenergic tone by central activation and by facilitation of ganglionic transmission. Furthermore, angiotensin II amplifies the vasoconstriction achieved by alpha$_1$-receptor stimulation. Thus angiotensin II has facilitatory adrenergic actions leading to increased activity of vasoconstrictor norepinephrine. Vagomimetic effects could explain why tachycardia is absent despite peripheral vasodilation. The combined antiadrenergic and vagomimetic mechanisms could contribute to the *antiarrhythmic effects* of ACE inhibitors and the reduction of sudden death in several trials in congestive heart failure (CHF), especially post-MI.[10] An additional factor is probably better potassium retention (as a result of aldosterone inhibition).

Kallikrein-Kinin System and Bradykinin

Besides decreased formation of angiotensin II, increased bradykinin is another alternate site of action of ACE inhibitors (see Fig. 5-2; Table 5-2). This nonapeptide, originally described as causing slow contractions in the gut (hence the *brady* in the name) is of potential CV importance. Bradykinin is inactivated by two kininases, kininase I and II. The latter is identical to ACE. ACE inhibition therefore also leads to increased local formation of bradykinin, as well as a reduction in angiotensin II production. Bradykinin acts on its receptors in the vascular endothelium to promote the release of two vasodilators (Table 5-2), nitric oxide and vasodilatory prostaglandins, such as prostacyclin and prostaglandin E$_2$ (PGE$_2$). Indomethacin, which inhibits prostaglandin synthesis, partially reduces the hypotensive effect of ACE inhibitors. The current concept is that bradykinin formation, occurring locally and thus not easily measured, can participate in the hypotensive effect of ACE inhibitors and may act via nitric oxide to protect the endothelium. These potentially favorable actions of an ACE inhibitor, mediated via bradykinin, would not occur with an ARB (but there would also be fewer adverse effects of bradykinin such as cough and angioedema).

Table 5-2

Indications for ACE Inhibitors Based on Trial Data

1. Heart failure, all stages
2. Hypertension especially in high-risk patients and in diabetics
3. AMI, acute phase for high-risk patients, postinfarct LV dysfunction
4. Nephropathy, nondiabetic and diabetic type 1
5. Cardiovascular protection in specified doses (ramipril, perindopril, trandolapril)

Caution: Not all the above are licensed indications and the license for a specific ACE inhibitor may vary. Check the package insert.

ACE, Angiotensin-converting enzyme; *AMI,* acute myocardial infarction; *LV,* left ventricular.

ACE 2

A newly described enzyme, ACE 2, generates angiotensin-(1-7) (Ang-[1-7]) from angiotensin II. Ang-(1-7) acts on its vascular receptor to inhibit vasoconstriction and sodium retention[11] and metabolize angiotensin II to Ang-(1-7). Ang-(1-7) antagonizes angiotensin II actions via the G-coupled Mas receptor.[12] Genetic ablation of ACE 2 leads to heart failure in mice.[13] ACE 2 also acts on angiotensin I to form Ang-(1-9).[14] Ang-(1-9) blocks cardiomyocyte hypertrophy via the angiotensin type 2 receptor. Ang-(1-9) infusion acted on the AT-2 receptor to lessen cardiac fibrosis in stroke-prone rats, thereby supporting a direct role for Ang-(1-9) in the renin-angiotensin system (RAS).[14] Furthermore, Ang-(1-9) can be hydrolyzed to form Ang-(1-7).[12] ACE 2 agonists may soon have clinical testing because similar paths exist in human heart tissue.[15]

Tissue Renin-Angiotensin Systems

Although the acute hypotensive effects of ACE inhibition can clearly be linked to decreased circulating levels of angiotensin II, during chronic ACE inhibition there is a reactive hyperreninemia linked to reemergence of circulating angiotensin II and aldosterone. Hence, the present proposal is that ACE inhibitors exert their sustained antihypertensive, favorable structural effects, and antiheart failure effects at least in part by acting on the tissue RASs, lessening formation of angiotensin II within the target organ. Likewise, this is the proposed site of action, in addition to BP reduction, in the regression of left ventricular hypertrophy (LVH) and vascular remodeling (Fig. 5-5).

Cerebral Effects and Renin-Angiotensin Inhibitors

In patients with heart failure, central mechanisms play an important role in postinfarct remodelling.[5] Do brain-penetrant renin-angiotensin inhibitors improve cognition?[16,17] If so, such agents could preferentially be used in the therapy of hypertension in older adults. However, in ONTARGET and TRANSCEND, large double-blind studies with telmisartan, ramipril, and their combination, different approaches to blocking the RAS had no clear effects on cognitive outcomes.[18] More specific prospective studies due to be presented soon are awaited.[17]

Genotypes and Response to ACE Inhibitors

There is no direct relevance to clinical practice at present as the phenotype does influence clinical response to pharmacologic therapy.

Pharmacologic Characteristics of ACE Inhibitors

Major Indications and Classes

Major indications are heart failure, hypertension, acute and chronic MI, renoprotection, diabetic nephropathy and hypertension, and CV protection. ACE inhibitors play a major role in secondary CVD prevention (Table 5-3 and Fig. 5-6).

Side Effects of ACE Inhibitors

Cough remains as one of the most troublesome and common of the various side-effects (Fig. 5-7; see later, Table 5-6), some serious and some not. Patients with heart failure often cough as a result of pulmonary congestion (which may need more rather than less ACE inhibitor), and

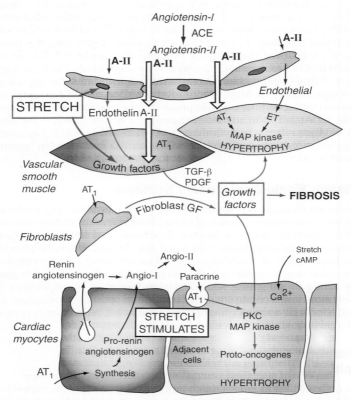

Figure 5-5   Role of cardiac tissue renin-angiotensin system, hypothetically as in left ventricular hypertrophy (hypertrophy), involving myocytes, fibroblasts, vascular smooth muscle and endothelium. *ACE,* Angiotensin-converting enzyme; *AT-1,* angiotensin II receptor, subtype 1; *cAMP,* cyclic adenosine monophosphate; *ET,* endothelin; *GF,* growth factor; *MAP kinase,* mitogen activated protein kinase; *PDGF,* platelet-derived growth factor; *PKC,* protein kinase C; *TGF,* transforming growth factor. Other abbreviations as in Fig. 5-2. (Figure © L.H. Opie, 2012, and adapted from *Angiotensin-Converting Enzyme Inhibitors. The Advance Continues,* 3rd ed, Authors' Publishing House, New York & University of Cape Town Press, 1999.)

in patients with hypertension such side effects are generally discovered only if volunteered. In some centers, the incidence of cough is thought to be as high as 10% to 15%, whereas others report a much lower incidence such as 5.5% in HOPE.[19] The cough is due to an increased sensitivity of the cough reflex resulting in a dry, irritating, nonproductive cough, quite different from bronchospasm. Increased formation of bradykinin and prostaglandins may play a role because ARBs have a much lower incidence of cough. Several studies suggest relief of the cough by added nonsteroidal antiinflammatory drugs (NSAIDs),[20] with the downside of diminished antihypertensive effects. Logically, and most often tried with success, a change to an angiotensin II receptor blocker consistently lessens the cough.[21]

Hypotension

Particularly in CHF, orthostatic symptoms caused by excess hypotension are common and may necessitate dose reduction or even cessation of ACE-inhibitor therapy. In general, so long as orthostatic

Table 5-3

ACE Inhibitors and Other RAAS Inhibitors for Secondary Prevention in CHD and Other Atherosclerotic Diseases (AHA/ACC Foundation Recommendations)

1. ACE inhibitors should be started and continued indefinitely in all patients with LV EF ≤40% and in those with hypertension, diabetes, or chronic kidney disease, unless contraindicated. (Class I, *Level of Evidence: A)* It is reasonable to use ACE inhibitors in all other patients. *(Class IIa, Level: B)*
2. ARBs are recommended for ACE-intolerant patients with HF or post-MI with EF ≤40%. (Class I, *Level: A)* It is reasonable to use ARBs in other ACE-intolerant patients. (Class IIa, *Level: B)*
3. ARB use combined with an ACE inhibitor is not well established in those with systolic HF. *(Class IIb, Level: A)*
4. Aldosterone blockade is recommended in post-MI patients without significant renal dysfunction or hyperkalemia and already receiving an ACE inhibitor and β-blocker with LV EF ≤40% plus either with diabetes or HF. *(Class I, Level: A)*

ACC, American College of Cardiology; *ACE,* angiotensin-converting enzyme; *AHA,* American Heart Association; *ARB,* angiotensin receptor blocker; *CHD,* coronary heart disease; *EF,* ejection fraction; *HF,* heart failure; *LV,* left ventricular; *MI,* myocardial infarction.

From Smith Jr SC. Secondary prevention and risk reduction therapy for patients with coronary and other atherosclerotic vascular disease: 2011 update: a guideline from the AHA and ACC Foundation. *Circulation* 2011;124:2458–2473.

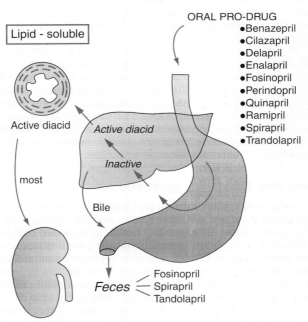

KINETIC GROUP: PRO-DRUGS
Opie 2012

Figure 5-6 Pharmacokinetic patterns of prodrugs that are converted to active diacids and then excreted (Class II). The predominant pattern for most is renal excretion but with some drugs, especially fosinopril, biliary and fecal excretion may be as important. (Figure © L.H. Opie, 2012 and adapted from *Angiotensin-Converting Enzyme Inhibitors. The Advance Continues,* 3rd ed, Authors' Publishing House, New York & University of Cape Town Press, 1999.)

ACE INHIBITORS: POTENTIAL SIDE EFFECTS

Opie 2012

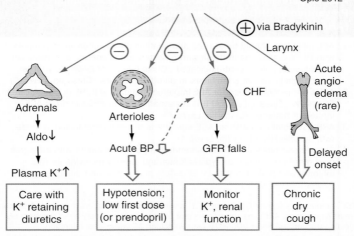

Figure 5-7   Potential side effects of angiotensin-converting enzyme (ACE) inhibitors include cough, hypotension, and renal impairment. Angioedema is rare but potentially fatal. To avoid hypotension in heart failure patients, a low first test dose is usually given. *Aldo,* Aldosterone; *BP,* blood pressure; *CHF,* congestive heart failure; *GFR,* glomerular filtration rate; *K,* potassium. (Figure © L.H. Opie, 2012.)

symptoms do not occur, the absolute BP is not crucial and some heart failure patients do well with systolic pressures of 80 to 90 mm Hg. *Hyponatremia* can be an indicator of heightened RAAS activity, and when present, there is an increased risk of hypotension (see later in this chapter).

Hyperkalemia is a risk, especially when ACE inhibitors are given with aldosterone antagonists, ARBs, or potassium-sparing diuretics, or in the presence of renal failure. A rough rule is that increasing RAAS block may improve the heart failure at the risk of increasing hyperkalemia. The RALES study showed the safety and efficacy of low doses of spironolactone when carefully added to β-blockers, ACE inhibitors, and diuretics in the therapy of severe systolic heart failure.[22] Careful monitoring of serum potassium is essential because hyperkalemia is potentially lethal.

Renal Side Effects and Hyponatremia

Reversible renal failure can be precipitated by hypotension, and hyponatremia is the most reliable sign of trouble. Predisposing characteristics are a fixed low renal blood flow as in severe CHF or severe sodium and volume depletion, or underlying renal disease, including renal artery stenosis. In these conditions, efferent glomerular arterial constriction resulting from angiotensin II may be crucial in retaining the glomerular filtration rate (GFR). Rarely, irreversible renal failure has occurred in patients with bilateral renal artery stenosis, a contraindication to ACE inhibitors. In unilateral renal artery disease, with high circulating renin values, ACE inhibitors may also cause excessive hypotensive responses with oliguria or azotemia. To obviate such problems, and especially when there is unilateral renal artery stenosis or a low sodium state, a low first test dose of the ACE inhibitor should be given, although this is seldom done. An arbitrary high value of serum creatinine is often taken as a contraindication (see later in chapter). A slight stable increase in serum creatinine after the introduction of an ACE inhibitor should not limit use. A 20% rise in creatinine should make one consider renal artery stenosis.

Angioedema

Although uncommon (approximately 0.3% in ALLHAT, rising to 0.6%-1.6% in black individuals),[23,24] this condition can very rarely be fatal, the incidence of death increasing from 0 in a large study on 12,634 patients given enalapril for 24 weeks[24] to approximately 1 in 5-10,000 patients.[23,25] The mechanism depends on bradykinin,[26] with a further contribution from impaired breakdown of substance P.[27] The enzyme breaking down both peptides is dipeptidyl peptidase IV, which is inhibited by a group of antidiabetic drugs (see Chapter 11, page 451). Indirect evidence suggests increased angioedema in patients taking antidiabetics such as sitagliptin.[27] For urgent therapy, prompt subcutaneous epinephrine and rarely even intubation may be needed.[28] The ACE inhibitor must be stopped. Switching to an ARB may be considered,[21] yet there are isolated instances of ARB-associated angioedema.

Pregnancy Risks

All ACE inhibitors (also ARBs and renin inhibitors) are embryopathic and contraindicated in pregnancy in all trimesters.[29] The Food and Drug Administration (FDA) requires a boxed warning in the package insert. *Avoid giving these drugs to women of childbearing age unless pregnancy is avoided.*

Neutropenia

Once the bane of captopril therapy, neutropenia now seems to be rare. The association with high-dose captopril, usually occurring in patients with renal failure and especially those with a collagen vascular disorder, is undoubted. In the case of all other ACE inhibitors, the American package inserts all warn that available data for all other ACE inhibitors are not sufficient to exclude agranulocytosis at similar rates to those found with captopril.

ACE Inhibitors: Contraindications

Contraindications include bilateral renal artery stenosis, pregnancy, known allergy or hypersensitivity, and hyperkalemia. Often a high serum creatinine of more than 2.5-3 mg/dL (220-265 μmol/L) is taken as an arbitrary cut-off point for the use of ACE inhibitors and for ARBs, especially in heart failure. However, patients with higher creatinine values might be evaluated in the context of the renoprotection that may be achieved and nephrologists might elect to start ACE inhibition with caution. Overall benefits can be attained with lesser degrees of renal insufficiency.[30]

ACE Inhibitors for Heart Failure

Neurohumoral Effects of Overt Heart Failure

A crucial problem in CHF is *the inability of the left ventricle to maintain a normal BP and organ perfusion. Enhanced activity of the RAS* (Fig. 5-8) follows from (1) hypotension, which evokes baroreflexes to increase sympathetic adrenergic discharge, thereby stimulating the beta$_1$ renal receptors involved in renin release; (2) activation of chemoreflexes and ergoreflexes; (3) decreased renal perfusion resulting in renal ischemia, which enhances renin release; and (4) β-adrenergic simulation. However, even in compensated CHF, plasma renin may not be persistently elevated[31] without simultaneous diuretic therapy. Angiotensin II promotes secretion of aldosterone and the release of vasopressin. Both contribute to abnormal fluid retention and volume regulation in severe CHF. Generally, such changes are thought to be

NEUROHUMORAL EFFECTS OF HEART FAILURE

Opie 2012

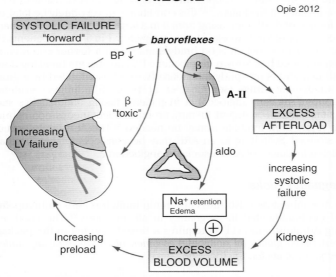

Figure 5-8 Neurohumoral adaptation in heart failure. The crucial consequence of left ventricular (LV) failure is the inability to maintain a normal blood
pressure and normal organ perfusion. As a result of reflex baroreflex activation and excess adrenergic stimulation, there is alpha (α)–mediated peripheral vasoconstriction that increases the afterload and leads to increased LV
failure. Excess alpha (α) adrenergic stimulation leads to peripheral vasoconstriction. Furthermore, excess beta (β)–adrenergic stimulation promotes renin
release with increased vasoconstrictive angiotensin-II (A-II) and release of
aldosterone. Increasing preload and afterload leads to increasing LV failure.
A-II, Angiotensin II; *aldo,* aldosterone; *BP,* blood pressure; *Na,* sodium. (Figure
© L.H. Opie, 2012, and adapted from *Angiotensin-Converting Enzyme Inhibitors. The Advance Continues,* 3rd ed, Authors' Publishing House, New York &
University of Cape Town Press, 1999.)

adverse because of the resultant increased vasoconstriction, fluid
and sodium retention, and dilutional hyponatremia.

The peripheral vascular resistance is greatly increased. Thus the
greater afterload against which the failing heart must work is explained by (1) increased formation of angiotensin II, (2) reflex release
of norepinephrine, (3) release of vasoconstrictor *endothelin* from
the dysfunctional vascular *endothelium,* (4) reduced muscle mass,
(5) thickened capillary membranes, and (6) altered endothelial cell
response to muscle metabolites. Systemic and renal vascular vasoconstriction reduces renal plasma flow, which detrimentally affects salt
excretion and further promotes renin formation. Vasodilator hormones
of cardiac origin such as atrial and brain natriuretic peptides (BNPs),
and prostaglandins of vascular origin, are also activated, but fail to
achieve compensatory vasodilation for complex reasons including
receptor downgrading.

The LV wall stress increases. Especially during exertion, both systolic
and diastolic wall stresses become too high for the depressed contractility of the failing myocardium. The inability of the left ventricle to empty
itself during systole increases the preload. The combination of increased
pre- and afterload, so common in CHF, leads to progressive ventricular
dilation with wall remodeling (myocyte hypertrophy and slippage with
matrix changes) so that the ejection fraction progressively declines with
time. Load reduction and in particular angiotensin II inhibition retards
this detrimental remodeling process.[32] According to *Laplace's law,* the

stress on the wall of a thin-walled sphere is proportional to the product of the intraluminal pressure and the radius, and inversely related to the wall thickness. Wall stress is one of the major determinants of myocardial oxygen uptake. Afterload and preload reduction, by decreasing the radius of the left ventricle, decreases the myocardial oxygen demand. ACE inhibition, by reducing the preload and the afterload, lessens excessive LV wall stress, limits remodeling, and enhances ventricular emptying.[33] Inhibiting these factors improves the myocardial oxygen balance and attenuates further LV chamber enlargement.

Beneficial neurohumoral effects of ACE-inhibitors are as follows: ACE inhibitors have a consistent effect in increasing plasma renin and decreasing angiotensin II and aldosterone, with a fall in norepinephrine, epinephrine, and in vasopressin. Angiotensin II production falls. Parasympathetic activity, reduced in heart failure, is improved by ACE inhibition. Although there are some exceptions to the patterns noted, most of the results are reasonably consistent. From these data it can be concluded that chronic ACE inhibition ameliorates the neurohumoral changes found in CHF.

ACE Inhibitors as Preventative Therapy in Early LV Dysfunction

ACE inhibitors have earned their place as preventative therapy in early LV dysfunction, as shown for captopril in SAVE[34] and enalapril in SOLVD.[35] Longer-term 12-year follow up of such asymptomatic patients has revealed a mortality benefit of early ACE-inhibitor use.[36] This mortality benefit of ACE inhibitors can be found even in the absence of initial diuretic therapy.[37] Note the challenge posed by β-blockers to ACE inhibitors as first-line therapy in early chronic heart failure (see Chapter 6, p. 195).

How Do Diuretics Compare with ACE Inhibitors?

In postinfarct patients without clinical heart failure but with modestly depressed LV function, the ACE inhibitor captopril was better able to maintain LV function and size than the diuretic furosemide.[38] There could be many adverse effects of diuretics, including activation of the renin-angiotensin axis. Yet in overt LV failure and in CHF, diuretic therapy is still universally accepted as first-step therapy to reduce symptoms because diuretics are superior to ACE in diminishing sodium and water retention. There is no evidence that chronic diuretic therapy prolongs life, although it is clinically evident that an intravenous loop diuretic is life-saving when given to a patient with severe LV failure and pulmonary edema. Long term, it is now clear that ACE inhibitors prolong life, whereas digoxin does not, so that the automatic choice of agent to combine with a diuretic in CHF is an ACE inhibitor.

ACE Inhibitors Plus β-blockers for Heart Failure

Historically, ACE inhibitors came first in the therapy of heart failure, before β-blockers, which were better at reducing mortality. The consistently positive survival-prolonging results with bisoprolol,[39] the MERIT study with metoprolol, and several carvedilol studies[40] given in addition to ACE inhibitors were such that β-blockers are now viewed as an integral part of the standard therapy of heart failure. *Thus the combination we should strive for is that of ACE inhibitors plus β-blockers.* The β-blocker should be carefully introduced when the patient is stable, not when there is hemodynamic deterioration (see Table 1-2). Mortality reductions with β-blockers (relative risk of 0.68) was demonstrated with and without an ACE inhibitor and the combination was optimal (relative risk of 0.83).[37] *The β-blocker can be given first.*[39]

Potential Problems with Drug Combinations in CHF

1. *Diuretics plus ACE inhibitors.* Additive effects on the preload may lead to syncope or hypotension; thus the diuretic dose is usually halved before starting ACE inhibitors. The result may be a true diuretic-sparing effect in approximately half of patients with mild CHF following the addition of the ACE-inhibitor, whereas in others the full diuretic dose must be reinstituted.

2. *ACE inhibitors plus spironolactone or eplerenone.* The major danger is hyperkalemia and the lesser is an increasing serum creatinine,[22,41] so frequent checks are needed. Some safety guidelines to evaluate before using this combination are the prior use of potassium-retaining diuretics, a serum creatinine exceeding 2.5 mg/dL (220 μmol/L) or an estimated glomerular filtration rate (eGFR) of less than 30 (mL/min/1.73 m^2 of body-surface area) and a serum potassium exceeding 5 mm/L. Sometimes the dose of the ACE inhibitor must be adjusted downward.

3. *ACE inhibitors and aspirin or NSAIDs.* Formation of bradykinin and thereby prostaglandins may play an important role in peripheral and renal vasodilation. Hence, NSAIDs, especially indomethacin, lessen the effectiveness of ACE inhibitors in hypertension.[42] Sulindac may have less effect and ARBs seem to interact less.[42] In CHF the interaction with NSAIDs is less studied. Restrictions on renal blood flow invoked by NSAIDs are most likely to be serious in those with major renin-angiotensin inhibition receiving high-dose diuretics and with hyponatremia. If an NSAID has to be used in heart failure, frequent checks of renal function are required. In practice, low-dose (approximately 80 mg daily) aspirin is often combined with an ACE inhibitor in the therapy of ischemic heart failure.

How to Start an ACE Inhibitor in Severe Heart Failure

First the patient must be fully assessed clinically, including measurements of serum creatinine, eGFR, and electrolytes. It is important to avoid first-dose hypotension and thereby lessen the risk of temporary renal failure. Patients at high *risk of hypotension* include those with serum sodium levels less than 130 mmol/L, a increased serum creatinine in the range of 1.5 to 3 mg/dL or 135 to 265 μmol/L. Hyponatremia is serious. Patients with creatinine values exceeding 3 mg/dL should be considered separately (see later in this chapter). All these patients need to have diuretic therapy stopped for 1 to 2 days and are then ideally given a test dose under supervision. Alternatively, a low initial dose of enalapril (1.25 mg) or 2 mg of perindopril (with its slow onset of action) is given. If there is no symptomatic hypotension, the chosen drug is continued, renal function is monitored, and the dose gradually is increased. Absence of first-dose hypotension suggests but does not securely establish that the subsequent course will be smooth. If the patient is fluid overloaded with an elevated jugular venous pressure, then the test dose of the ACE inhibitor can be given without first having to stop diuretic therapy.

Preexisting Renal Failure

In general, the serum creatinine can be expected to rise modestly and then to stabilize. In severe CHF, in which renal function is already limited by hypotension and by poor renal blood flow, it may be difficult to decide whether to introduce ACE-inhibitor therapy. For example, the serum creatinine may exceed 2.5-3 mg/dL or 220-265 μmol/L. The danger of exaggeration of renal failure must be balanced against the possible benefit from an improved cardiac output and decreased renal afferent arteriolar vasoconstriction resulting from ACE-inhibitor therapy. Problems can be expected, especially when the eGFR is low and the renin-angiotensin axis is highly stimulated. The best policy may be to improve the hemodynamic status as far as possible by the combined use of optimal doses of diuretics and other agents. Then the diuretic dose could be briefly reduced or stopped, and a very low dose of an ACE inhibitor introduced.

Hyponatremia and Salt and Water Limitation

Patients with severe hyponatremia are 30 times more likely to develop hypotension in response to ACE-inhibitor therapy and require special care. The cause of the hyponatremia is, at least in part, release of vasopressin (antidiuretic hormone) as can result from renin-angiotensin activation following intense diuretic therapy. Vasopressin antagonists (see Fig. 4-4) may be tried to combat hyponatremia. Modest, tolerable *salt restriction* is standard practice. Patients already on strict low-sodium diets are at increased risk of first-dose hypotension. In patients who are not volume depleted, restriction of water intake is advisable because delayed water diuresis may contribute to hyponatremia in severe CHF.

Outstanding Clinical Problems in the Therapy of Heart Failure

1. *Drug dose.* Whereas in hypertension the dose-response curve is flat and can be monitored from the BP response, in CHF the problem of the optimal dose does arise. Is the dose large enough to give as complete renin-angiotensin inhibition as possible? Standard medium doses were not tested. In the case of enalapril, the standard target dose is 10 mg twice daily. Increasing this to 60 mg/day did not alter death rate nor hemodynamic parameters.[43] In clinical practice lower doses than in the trials are commonly used. Although the optimal doses of ACE inhibitors in CHF have not been established by clinical studies, our opinion is that the dose should be titrated upward to the effective trial doses without going higher.

2. *Diastolic dysfunction.* Most heart failure studies have concentrated on the role of ACE inhibition in systolic failure. Diastolic failure is an early event, particularly in LVH in response to hypertension or aortic stenosis, as well as in older adults. Therapy remains challenging (see Chapter 6, p. 207).

3. *Myopathies.* The skeletal muscle myopathy found in heart failure is associated with increased proton production that stimulates the ergoreflexes that worsen the symptoms of exertional intolerance.[44] The causes of the myopathy are not clear. Increased circulating angiotensin II may play a role. Clinical studies with ACE inhibitors or ARBs geared to this problem are still lacking, yet may be very difficult to interpret because deconditioning may play a prominent role in the skeletal weakness in heart failure,[45] making exercise a more logical choice of therapy. In some patients there is a genetic link between heart failure and myopathy.[46] In a small study on Duchenne muscular dystrophy, perindopril decreased mortality at 10 years.[47]

4. *Anemia.* A low hemoglobin is a poorly understood risk factor for CVD.[48] A small decrease in hemoglobin to the order of 0.3 g/dL may occur and ACE inhibitors may be used therapeutically to treat the erythrocytosis that follows renal transplantation.[49] Attention should be paid to the possible development of anemia during ACE inhibitor therapy, especially because anemia is now recognized as an adverse risk factor in heart failure.[50] However, the development of anemia should generally not be attributed to an ACE inhibitor and other investigations should be pursued.

ACE Inhibitors for Hypertension

The RAAS is one of several major mechanisms that help to maintain the BP both in normal persons and in persons with essential hypertension, especially when sodium is restricted or diuretics are in use. In malignant hypertension or in renal artery stenosis, renal ischemia stimulates the release of renin from the juxtaglomerular apparatus to increase the BP. Although ACE inhibition leads to the most dramatic falls of BP in the presence of such an underlying renal mechanism, ACE inhibition is also effectively antihypertensive in mild to moderate hypertension even when plasma renin is not high. ACE inhibitors lower BP by multiple mechanisms (see Fig. 7-9). In general, ACE inhibitors are more effective in white patients who also respond to β-blockers.[51] Lesser BP efficacy in black patients, especially in older adults, can be overcome by addition of low-dose diuretics or higher doses of the ACE inhibitor. In the ALLHAT trial, the somewhat lesser efficacy of an ACE inhibitor than the diuretic[23] may be ascribed to (1) the trial design, which did not allow addition of a diuretic; and (2) the relatively high proportion of black patients, approximately one third of the study population, in whom the lack of diuretic was more serious. In the Australian study on older white subjects, enalapril gave overall better results than did the diuretic at equal BP control.[52] Because ACE inhibitors do not alter glucose tolerance, blood uric acid, or cholesterol levels with few side effects apart from cough, their use in hypertension has rapidly increased. Their ideal combination may well not be with a diuretic, as often thought, but with a calcium channel blocker (CCB), as in the ACCOMPLISH study.[53]

Less New Diabetes

Rather than precipitating diabetes, as may occur with diuretic or β-blocker therapy, ACE inhibitors may lessen the development of new diabetes in hypertensives,[50,54-57] in heart failure,[58] and in those at risk of CVD.[19] Because similar protection is found with ARBs (see Fig. 7-7), the mechanism is likely to involve AT-1 receptor blockade. Note, however, in the DREAM study, ramipril decreased fasting blood glucose but not diabetes, perhaps because the study was only 3 years in duration.[59]

ACE Inhibitors for Early-Phase Acute Myocardial Infarction or Postinfarct Left Ventricular Dysfunction or Failure

ACE Inhibition within 24 Hours of Onset of Acute Myocardial Infarction

ACE inhibitors are given for overt LV failure or LV dysfunction[60-62] starting slowly on the first day.[63] The selective policy, favored by the authors, is to give ACE inhibitors to all high-risk patients: diabetics, those with anterior infarcts,[64] or tachycardia or overt LV failure. Logically, the sicker the patients, the greater the activation of the RAAS, and the better the expected result with the use of an ACE inhibitor. The selective policy receives a class 1A (highest) recommendation from the American Heart Association and American College of Cardiology, and is based on results from several major trials. For example, in nearly 19,000 patients in GISSI-3,[65] lisinopril reduced mortality at 6 weeks from the already low value of 7.1% in controls to 6.3%. Nondiabetics can also benefit, as found in an overview of nearly 100,000 high-risk patients with acute myocardial infarction (AMI).[66] Of note, the benefit of early ACE inhibition is not annulled by early administration of aspirin.[61] Nor is the

POST-INFARCT REMODELING

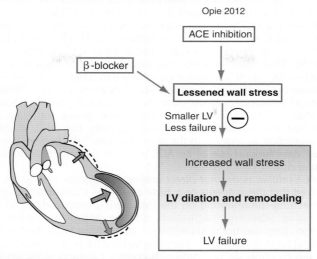

Opie 2012

Figure 5-9   Postinfarction remodeling. Increased wall stress promotes adverse remodeling and left ventricular (LV) failure by Laplace's law (see equation). The proposal, based on substantial animal data and human studies, is that angiotensin-converting enzyme (ACE) inhibition will attenuate postinfarct LV enlargement and promote beneficial remodeling with better LV mechanical function. (Figure © L.H. Opie, 2012.)

benefit explained by reduction of infarct size, which is better accomplished by β-blockade.[67]

ACE Inhibitors in Postinfarct Left Ventricular Dysfunction or Clinical Failure

ACE-inhibitors attenuate LV remodeling and reduce the risk of subsequent MI (Fig. 5-9). If ACE inhibitors have not been started within 24 hours of the onset of AMI, then the next opportunity is a few days later. Three major trials used rather different entry criteria, one being clinical[60] and two based on LV functional measurements.[34,62] All three showed major mortality reduction. Long-term follow-up in AIRE found that all-cause mortality was reduced by 36% with an absolute reduction of 11.4%.[68] In a 6-year follow up to the TRACE study,[69] the mean prolongation of life was 15.3 months. These impressive data strongly argue for the prolonged use of ACE inhibitors in postinfarct patients with clinical or echocardiographic LV failure, noting that the survival benefit observed was similar in those with or without pulmonary congestion, including those with asymptomatic LV dysfunction.[34,60,62]

ACE Inhibitors: Long-Term Cardiovascular Protection

Do ACE inhibitors as a group protect against coronary heart disease? One argument is that high-risk patients are better protected.[70] Dagenais and colleagues argue that the protection extends even to low-risk groups.[71] The background to this controversy is as follows. The meta-analysis of three major ACE-inhibitor prevention trials, HOPE, EUROPA, and Prevention of Events with Angiotensin-Converting Enzyme Inhibition (PEACE), found an 18% reduction in the odds ratio for the combined outcomes of CV death, nonfatal MI, or stroke (P < 0.0001). The issue relates to the PEACE trial in which 8290 patients with stable coronary artery disease and normal or near-normal LV function were randomly assigned to 4 mg of trandolapril daily or to placebo.[72] There was a non-significant fall of 7% in the composite CV primary end-point, which, when merged with the larger reductions in HOPE and EUROPA, resulted in an overall decrease (odds ratio 0.82, cardiac index 0.76-0.88). These authors argue that all patients with vascular disease should receive an ACE inhibitor (in addition to other proven preventative measures such as other antihypertensives to control BP, antiplatelet agents, β-blockers, and statins). Note that in the PEACE trial trandolapril did reduce total mortality in a higher risk group with impaired renal function, supporting the alternate theory that ACE inhibitors give protection in relation to the degree of risk.[73] We believe that the overall data support use of an ACE inhibitor incrementally to lower vascular risk.

ACE-inhibitors are not direct antianginal agents. It must be emphasized that these agents only have an indirect antiischemic effect by lessening the afterload on the myocardial oxygen demand[74] by decreasing adrenergic activation, and by improving endothelial function. They are not antianginals.[75] In the long term, they reduce the need for coronary bypass grafting but not for percutaneous coronary intervention (PCI).[71] Although coronary surgery activates neurohumoral mechanisms that could be improved by ACE inhibition, when added early after surgery, quinapril unexpectedly increased rather than decreased CV events within the first 3 months.[76] However, this finding with a lesser used ACE inhibitor has never been confirmed.

Diabetes: Complications and Renoprotection

In patients with diabetes, the BP goals are lower than in nondiabetics. The Seventh Report of the Joint National Committee on Prevention, Detection, Evaluation, and Treatment of High Blood Pressure (JNC 7) recommends a goal BP of 130/80 mm Hg. Both diabetes (type 2, maturity onset, noninsulin-dependent) and hypertension are associated with insulin resistance. Both high-dose thiazides and β-blockers can impair insulin sensitivity in nondiabetic hypertensives. Therefore there are arguments for the use of ACE inhibition or an ARB,[77] often with a CCB and diuretic.

The ACCORD Studies

The ACCORD trials examined whether ultra-intense CV risk factor reduction could improve clinical outcomes. To improve on the impressive baseline control of risk factors in the patients assigned to standard therapy in ACCORD was a formidable task, illustrating the synergistic effects of the multifactorial risk-reduction regimen. The respective intense arms achieved a more than 1% absolute difference in hemoglobin A_{1C}, a 14.2-mm Hg lower systolic pressure, and plasma triglycerides of approximately 145 mg/dL. For each of the three separate questions—further reduction of BP, glycemia, or triglycerides—the primary clinical composite was not significantly reduced despite the more intense therapies, as assessed in a Circulation editorial.[78]

Diabetes and Steatosis

Impaired glucose tolerance is accompanied by cardiac lipid loading (steatosis) preceding the onset of type 2 diabetes mellitus and LV systolic dysfunction as shown in human cardiac myocytes.[79] There have been no studies with ACE inhibitors or ARBs in such patients.

Diabetics with Nephropathy

In type 1 diabetic nephropathy, ACE inhibitors have repeatedly been shown to reduce proteinuria and protect against progressive glomerular sclerosis and loss of renal function.[77] In type 2 diabetic nephropathy, four trials with ARBs have shown similar renal protection.[77] Evidence-based guidelines therefore suggest ACE inhibitors for type I and ARBs for type 2 diabetic renal disease.[80] The strong likelihood is that ACE inhibitors would be as effective in type 2 patients if they had been tested, so in practice ACE inhibitors are used whenever ARBs cannot be afforded. They often have to be combined with other drugs, including diuretics, β-blockers, and CCBs to reduce the BP to less than 130/80 mm Hg.

Diabetic Microalbuminuria

Microalbuminuria is one of the strongest predictors of both adverse renal and CVD outcomes in patients with type 2 diabetes mellitus. Current guideline recommendations are to screen for urinary albumin excretion (UAE) in all patients with type 2 diabetes, even in the absence of nephropathy. In a 10-year follow study, serial UAE measurements even after the initiation of antihypertensive therapy were found to have prognostic value independent of traditional CV risk factors.[81] ACE inhibition delays the onset of microalbuminuria, which is the initial step from normoalbuminuria toward potentially lethal nephropathy.[82] In MICRO-HOPE, in which ramipril reduced the development of overt nephropathy and all-cause mortality both by 24%, one entry criterion was diabetes with microalbuminuria, yet without macroalbuminuria.[83]

Diabetic Albuminuria

VA NEPHRON-D is a randomized, double-blind, multicenter clinical trial in progress to evaluate whether combined ARB-ACE inhibitor therapy might benefit patients with diabetes and overt albuminuria (more than 300 mg/g creatinine). The study is assessing losartan 100 mg plus lisinopril 10-40 mg, versus losartan alone, on the progression of kidney disease in patients with diabetes and overt proteinuria.[84]

ACE Inhibition for Nondiabetic Renal Failure

In progressive renal failure, from whatever cause, there is a steady rise in serum creatinine, a fall in glomerular function, and increasing proteinuria. Angiotensin II may play a crucial role in the progression of glomerular injury and the growth and destruction of the glomeruli (Fig. 5-10). Using the combined data of the RENAAL and IDNT trials, across all systolic blood pressure (SBP) ranges, a progressively lower CV risk was observed with a lower albuminuria level.[85] This was particularly evident in patients who reached the guideline recommended SBP target of 130 mm Hg or less. Therapies intervening in the RAAS with the aim of improving CV outcomes may therefore require a dual approach separately targeting both BP and albuminuria.

Ramipril in Overt Proteinuria

To the RENAAL and IDNT trials must be added the very impressive Ramipril Efficacy in Nephropathy (REIN) study and its long-term follow up.[86] In the initial core study, patients with proteinuria of more than 3 g per 24 hr were selected. Ramipril reduced the rate of GFR decline more than expected from the BP drop. In the follow-up study,

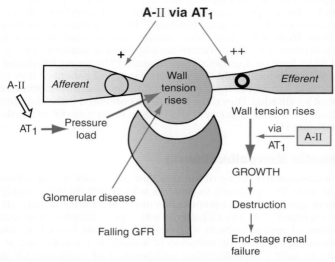

Figure 5-10 Role of angiotensin II and AT-1 receptor in glomerular injury and progressive renal failure. An increased intraglomerular pressure as from a pressure load in hypertension or primary renal disease or diabetes can evoke mesangial growth with threat of complete glomerular closure. Angiotensin II may be an important growth signal accelerating the disease process. (Figure © L.H. Opie, 2012, and adapted from *Angiotensin-Converting Enzyme Inhibitors. The Advance Continues,* 3rd ed, Authors' Publishing House, New York & University of Cape Town Press, 1999.)

those who were originally allocated to nonramipril therapy and then switched to ramipril at the end of the initial core study never caught up with those kept on ramipril from the start. This occurred even though the BP reduction in the switched group was greater than in those who stayed on ramipril throughout.

Studies of Kidney Disease and Hypertension in Black Patients

Despite a lack of compelling evidence, numerous guidelines recommend a reduced BP target in patients with chronic kidney disease. In observational studies, the relationship between BP and end-stage renal disease (ESRD) is direct and progressive. The burden of hypertension-related chronic kidney disease and ESRD is especially high among black patients. Does intensive BP control retard the progression of chronic kidney disease among black patients? In 1094 black patients with hypertensive chronic kidney disease receiving either intensive or standard BP control, follow-up ranged from 8.8 to 12.2 years. Intensive BP control had no effect on kidney disease progression.[87] Intensive BP control had no effect on kidney disease progression. However, there was a potential benefit in patients with a protein/creatinine ratio of more than 0.22 (hazard ratio, 0.73; $P = 0.01$). Some earlier studies at earlier stages of renal disease were more promising. With the entry point as established hypertension with a low GFR, rather than end-stage renal failure,[88] ramipril-based therapy was more effective than amlodipine at equal BP levels in reducing the clinical endpoints, including dialysis and proteinuria. The greater renoprotection with the ACE inhibitor was independent of the BP reduction and despite the high serum creatinine. Importantly, fewer ACE inhibitor–treated black patients ended up on dialysis.[89]

Properties of Specific ACE Inhibitors

Captopril, The Grand Daddy

Captopril (Capoten, Lopril in France, Lopirin in Germany, and Captopril in Japan), the first widely available ACE inhibitor and available as a generic, was originally seen to be an agent with significant and serious side effects such as loss of taste, renal impairment, and neutropenia. Now it is recognized that these are rather rare side effects that can be avoided largely by reducing the daily dose and practicing appropriate monitoring. Captopril is widely licensed in the United States for hypertension, heart failure, postinfarct LV dysfunction, and type 1 diabetic nephropathy. It is the best-studied ACE inhibitor and has the widest range of approved indications. In the United Kingdom, it is also licensed for prevention of reinfarction and for diabetic microproteinuria. Pharmacokinetically, it belongs to a specific pattern, namely a molecule that is active as it is, but is further metabolized in the liver to active metabolites. After absorption from the stomach, captopril is largely excreted by the kidneys, approximately half as is and half as active metabolites formed in the liver and kidney. The elimination half-life is approximately 4 to 6 hours (Table 5-4). In hypertension, its biologic half-life is long enough to allow twice-daily dosage. *Of note, captopril, when optimally dosed, has never been bettered by other RAS blockers.*

Dose and Indications

In *hypertension,* captopril has an average daily dose of 25 to 50 mg orally given twice or three times daily (instead of much higher previous doses). The risk of excess hypotension is highest in patients with high renin states (renal artery stenosis, preexisting vigorous diuretic therapy, severe sodium restriction, or hyponatremia) when the initial dose should be low (6.25 to 12.5 mg). In *CHF,* during initiation captopril may cause excessive hypotension, especially in vigorously diuresed patients so that a *test dose* of 6.25 mg may be required, followed by 12.5 mg three times daily, and working up to 50 mg three times daily as tolerated. The diuretic may have to be stopped prior to captopril to avoid an excess renin state. In *postinfarct patients with LV dysfunction* (ejection fraction 40% or less), captopril is licensed to improve survival and prevent overt heart failure and, in the United Kingdom, to reduce recurrent MI and coronary revascularization procedures. In VALIANT, valsartan was noninferior to captopril.[90] In *diabetic nephropathy,* captopril improves proteinuria and decreases hard end-points, such as death, transplantation, or dialysis. However, captopril is largely renal excreted, so doses should be reduced as in *renal disease.*

Contraindications

Contraindications include bilateral renal artery stenosis; renal artery stenosis in a single kidney; immune-based renal disease, especially collagen vascular disease; severe renal failure (serum creatinine >3 mg/dL or >265 μmol/L [see p.128 for renal side-effects of ACE-inhibitors]); preexisting neutropenia; and systemic hypotension. Pregnancy is an absolute contraindication for all ACE inhibitors for all trimesters.[29]

Side Effects

In general, the serious side effects initially described are seldom found today when the total daily dose is 150 mg daily or less. Cough is the most common side effect with all ACE inhibitors. Other class side effects include transient renal failure, angioedema, and hyperkalemia.

Table 5-4

Summary of Pharmacologic Properties, Clinical Indications, and Doses of ACE-Inhibitors

Drug	Zinc Ligand	Active Drug	Elim $T_{1/2}$ (hours)	T/P Ratio % (FDA)	Hypertension (usual daily dose)	Heart Failure or Postinfarct, Target Doses Used in Large Trials
Class I: Captopril-like						
Captopril	SH	Captopril	4-6 (total captopril)	—	25-50 mg 2× or 3×	50 mg 3×
Class II: Prodrugs						
Alacepril	Carboxyl	Captopril	8 (total captopril)	—	12.5-25 mg 2×	Not established
Benazepril	Carboxyl	Benazeprilat	11	—	10-80 mg in 1-2 doses	Not established
Cilazapril	Carboxyl	Cilazaprilat	9	—	2.5-5 mg 1×	Not established
Delapril	Carboxyl	Delaprilat 5-OH-delaprilat	1.2-1.4	—	7.5-30 mg in 1-2 doses	Not established
Enalapril	Carboxyl	Enalaprilat	6; 11 (accum)	—	5-20 mg in 1-2 doses	10 mg 2×
Fosinopril	Phosphoryl	Fosinoprilat	12	50-80	10-40 mg 1× (or 2×	Not established
Perindopril	Carboxyl	Perindoprilat	3-10	75-100	4-8 mg 1×	Not established
Quinapril	Carboxyl	Quinaprilat	1.8	50	10-40 mg in 1-2 doses	Not established
Ramipril	Carboxyl	Ramiprilat	13-17	50-60	2.5-10 mg in 1-2 doses	5 mg 2×
Spirapril	Carboxyl	Spiraprilat	<2	—	3-6 mg 1 dose*	Not established
Trandolapril	Carboxyl	Trandoprilat	10	50-90	0.5-4 mg 1× then 4 mg 2×	4 mg 1×
Class III: Water-soluble						
Lisinopril	Carboxyl	Lisinopril	7; 12 (accum)	—	10-40 mg 1× (may need high dose if given 1×)	10-35 mg 1×

Thurman PA, *Hypertension,* 1996;28:450.

accum, Accumulation half-life; *Elim $T_{1/2}$,* elimination half-life; *FDA,* Food and Drug Administration; *T/P ratio,* trough/peak ratios, FDA-approved values. Data based on FDA-approved information if available.

Immune-based side effects are probably specific to captopril and found especially with high doses. These are taste disturbances, immune-based skin rashes, and neutropenia ($<1000/mm^3$). The latter is extremely rare in hypertensive patients with normal renal function (1/8600 according to the package insert), more common (1/500) with preexisting impaired renal function with a serum creatinine of 1.6 mg/dL or more, and is a grave risk (1/25) in patients with both collagen vascular disease and renal impairment. When captopril is discontinued, recovery from neutropenia is usual except when there is associated serious disease, such as severe renal or heart failure or collagen vascular disease. *Proteinuria* occurs in approximately 1% of patients receiving captopril, especially in the presence of preexisting renal disease or with high doses of captopril (>150 mg/day). Paradoxically, captopril is used in the therapy of diabetic type 1 nephropathy with proteinuria. *Other side-effects* include hypotension (frequent in the treatment of CHF), impaired taste (2% to 7%), skin rashes (4% to 10%) sometimes with eosinophilia, and rarely, as with all ACE inhibitors, serious angioedema (1/100 to 1/1000).

Pretreatment Precautions

Bilateral renal artery stenosis and pregnancy must be excluded as far as possible. Patients with renal impairment caused by collagen disease, or patients receiving immunosuppressives or immune system modifiers such as steroids. Pretreatment hypotension excludes therapy.

Precautions during Treatment

Regular monitoring of neutrophil counts is required in patients with preexisting serious renal impairment, especially on the basis of collagen vascular disease (pretreatment count, then twice-weekly counts for 3 months). The risk of renal damage from captopril is much reduced by limiting total daily doses to 150 mg/day, as is now standard practice.

Enalapril

Enalapril (Vasotec in the United States; Innovace in the United Kingdom; Xanef, Renitec, or Pres in Europe; Renivace in Japan) is the standard prodrug, and is also available as a generic. The major trials showing clinical benefit have been in heart failure and in hypertension for which it was at least as good as and in some ways better than, a diuretic.[52] The chief differences from captopril are (1) a longer half-life; (2) a slower onset of effect because of the requirement of hydrolysis in the liver of the pro-drug to the active form, enalaprilat, so that the therapeutic effect depends on hepatic metabolism (see Table 5-4); and (3) the absence of the sulfhydryl (SH) group from the structure, thus theoretically lessening or removing the risk of immune-based side effects. Enalapril is approved for hypertension, heart failure, and to decrease the development of overt heart failure in asymptomatic patients with LV dysfunction (ejection fraction equal to or less than 35%). In the latter group of patients, enalapril is also licensed in the United Kingdom to prevent coronary ischemic events.

Pharmacokinetics

Approximately 60% of the oral dose is absorbed with no influence by meals. Enalapril is deesterified in the liver and kidney to the active form, enalaprilat (see Table 5-4). Time to peak serum concentration is approximately 2 hours for enalapril, and approximately 5 hours for enalaprilat, with some delay in CHF. Excretion is 95% renal as enalapril or enalaprilat (hence the lower doses in renal failure). The elimination half-life of enalaprilat is approximately 4 to 5 hours in hypertension and 7 to 8 hours in CHF. Following multiple doses, the effective elimination half-life of enalaprilat is 11 hours (package insert). One oral 10-mg dose of enalapril yields sufficient enalaprilat to cause significant ACE inhibition for 19 hours. In hypertension and in CHF, the peak hypotensive response to enalapril occurs approximately 4 to 6 hours after the oral dose.

Dose and Indications

In hypertension, the dose is 2.5 to 20 mg as one or two daily doses. In some patients the effect wanes over 24 hours so that twice-daily dosing may be better. Doses higher than 10 to 20 mg daily give little added benefit. A low initial dose (2.5 mg) is a wise precaution, especially when enalapril is added to a diuretic or the patient is salt-depleted, in older adults, or when high-renin hypertension is suspected. *In asymptomatic LV dysfunction and in CHF,* in the SOLVD trials,[35,50,91] enalapril was started with an initial dose of 2.5 mg twice daily and worked up to 10 mg twice daily (mean daily dose 17 mg). *In renal failure* (GFR less than 30 mL/min), the dose of enalapril must be reduced. In severe liver disease, the dose may have to be increased (impaired conversion of enalapril to enalaprilat). In early-phase AMI, within 24 hours of symptoms, an initial dose of only 1.25 mg at 2-hour intervals for three doses was followed by 5 mg three times daily with long-term benefits.

Contraindications, Precautions, and Side Effects

Pregnancy is a clear contraindication to all ACE inhibitors (and ARBs) (see previous discussion of captopril). In hypertensives, bilateral renal artery stenosis or stenosis in a single kidney must be excluded.

Precautions

To avoid the major risks of excess hypotension, use a low initial dose and evaluate pretreatment renal function and drug co-therapy, including diuretic dose. It is presumed that enalapril, without the SH group found in captopril, does not produce the same immune-based toxic effects. Thus monitoring of the neutrophil count is not essential.

Side Effects

Cough is most common, as for all ACE inhibitors. Enalapril may be safer when captopril has induced a skin rash. As for all ACE inhibitors, angioedema is a rare but serious risk,[24] as highlighted in the package insert.

Other Prodrugs

Benazepril (*Lotensin* in the United States) is rapidly converted to an active metabolite, benazeprilat, with an elimination half-life of 22 hours (see Table 5-4). However, the trough/peak ratio is only 0.4, less than the ideal ratio of 0.5 that the FDA recommends for once-daily antihypertensive agents. The optimal dose in hypertension is 10 mg twice daily. In the influential ACCOMPLISH trial in hypertension, benazepril once daily combined with the long acting CCB amlodipine gave better CV protection than when combined with a diuretic (see Chapter 7, p. 244).

Fosinopril (*Monopril* in the United States, *Staril* in the United Kingdom) differs from other ACE inhibitors in that it uses phosphinic acid as the zinc ligand. In common with most ACE inhibitors, it is a prodrug (see Table 5-4), yet has unique pharmacokinetic features in that there are dual routes of excretion, hepatic and renal. In chronic renal failure the active fosinoprilat form accumulates less in the blood than would enalaprilat or lisinopril. In older adults, the major reason for decreasing doses of other ACE inhibitors is renal impairment. In the case of fosinopril, no dosage adjustment is required. It has not been widely tested. In one large clinical trial, 40 to 80 mg fosinopril once daily was antihypertensive, and an additional diuretic was required in approximately half the patients. Compared with amlodipine, it was less antihypertensive but reduced plasminogen activator inhibitor-1 antigen, which amlodipine did not.[92]

Perindopril (*Coversyl* in the United Kingdom, *Aceon* in the United States; 4 to 8 mg once daily for hypertension) is converted to perindoprilat, which is moderately long acting (see Table 5-4) with a good peak/trough ratio. Anglo-Scandinavian Cardiac Outcomes Trial—Blood Pressure Lowering Arm (ASCOT-BPLA) compared the effects on major hypertension outcomes of amlodipine versus atenolol.[93] The trial was prematurely stopped because of an 11% reduction in all-cause mortality in the amlodipine-perindopril arm compared with the atenolol-diuretic arm. (For overall benefits, see Chapter 7, p. 243.) In CHF, the effect of a first dose of 2 mg is well documented and appears to cause little or no hypotension, in contrast to low-dose enalapril or captopril.[94] This interesting property warrants further study. Perindopril was used in PROGRESS, a large trial aimed at prevention of repeat stroke. Unexpectedly, despite BP reduction the ACE inhibitor did not reduce stroke unless combined with a diuretic.[95] In EUROPA, a large prophylactic trial in those with stable coronary artery disease, perindopril 8 mg daily resulted in a 20% lowering of major CV effects. In the HYVET trial on older persons with hypertension (see Chapter 4, p. 103 and Chapter 7, p. 241) the initial mean BP was 173/91 mm Hg. The addition of perindopril 2 mg to the diuretic indapamide roughly doubled the percentage with a controlled BP (SBP <150 mm Hg) with a further doubling by increasing the perindopril dose from 2 to 4 mg daily.[96] In the large ADVANCE trial on more than 11,000 persons, combined BP lowering based on perindopril-indapamide plus intensive glucose control reduced macrovascular and microvascular outcomes and mortality in patients with type 2 diabetes.[97] Perindopril is licensed by the FDA "to reduce the risk of cardiovascular mortality or nonfatal MI in patients with stable coronary heart disease."

Quinapril (*Accupril* in the United States; *Accupro* in the United Kingdom) works through conversion to active but short-acting quinaprilat, which activates the parent molecule (see Table 5-4). In *hypertension*, the dose recommended in the package insert is initially 10 mg/day given once or twice daily up to a maximum of 80 mg/day. Dosage should be adjusted by measuring both the peak response (2-6 hr after the dose) and the trough (before the next dose). When combined with a diuretic, the initial dose may be reduced to 5 mg/day (package insert). In *CHF*, the initial dose of 5 mg twice daily is titrated upward to the usual maintenance dose of 10 to 20 mg twice daily (package insert). Mortality data are not available. *Impaired endothelial function* in normotensive patients with coronary artery disease could be reversed by 6 months of therapy with quinapril, 40 mg once daily.[98] However, the study was not large enough to provide clinical outcome data.

Ramipril (*Altace* in the United States, *Ramace, Tritace* elsewhere) is a very well-studied agent, active via transformation to ramiprilat, is a long-acting (see Table 5-4) antihypertensive in a dose of 2.5 to 20 mg in one or two daily doses. It is also licensed for post-MI heart failure (dose 12.5 to 5 mg twice daily) and for CV protection (see later in this chapter). It is proposed as a relatively tissue-specific ACE inhibitor. *In anterior AMI*, the ramipril dose in the HEART study was 1.25 mg on the first day, then 2.5 mg at 12 hr, then uptitrated at 24-hr intervals to a full dose of 10 mg/day.[63] In early postinfarct heart failure in the AIRE study,[60] ramipril 2.5 mg twice daily and then 5 mg twice daily, as tolerated, was used to show a major reduction (27%) in mortality of patients with diagnosed clinically. The mortality benefit was maintained over a 5-year follow-up.[68] It is also the drug used in the REIN nephropathy study to show an excellent long-term benefit (see previous section on renal failure). In the landmark prophylactic HOPE trial,[19] ramipril given to high-risk patients, starting with 2.5 mg daily and working up to 10 mg once daily at night, gave markedly positive results, including reduction in all-cause mortality. As a result of this study, the extensive cardioprotective license given to ramipril in the United States is to reduce the risk of MI, stroke and death from CV causes in those at high risk, which is defined as age 55 years or older with a history of coronary artery disease, stroke, peripheral vascular disease, or diabetes that is accompanied by at least one other risk factor (hypertension, high total cholesterol or low high-density lipoprotein cholesterol, cigarette smoking, or microalbuminuria). The dose is 2.5 mg, 5 mg, and then 10 mg once daily (for prophylaxis, given at night).

In the ONTARGET studies, which included more than 25,000 persons, the ARB telmisartan was not palpably superior to this proven dose of ramipril and had equivalent effects on major CV outcomes in patients judged to be at high CV risk.[99,100]

Trandolapril (Mavik), after conversion to trandolaprilat, has one of the longer durations of action (see Table 5-4). It has been studied in one positive postinfarct trial[62] and in a large prophylactic trial (PEACE) in those with stable coronary artery disease in which it did not reduce the primary mortality end-point.[101] These patients had predominantly preserved ejection fractions (pEFs) (mean 58%) and trandolapril decreased the risk of new heart failure.[102]

In hypertension, the initial dose is 1 mg daily in nonblack patients and 2 mg daily in black patients (packet insert). Most patients require 2-4 mg once daily. If once-daily dosing at 4 mg is inadequate, twice-daily divided dosing may be tried, or the agent combined with a diuretic (trandolapril-verapamil [Tarka]). *In postinfarct heart failure or LV dysfunction* (US license) the package insert recommends an initial dose of 1 mg going up to 4 mg. *In older adults* with normal renal function, dose adjustment is not needed. *In chronic renal failure,* despite the predominant biliary excretion, there is some accumulation of trandolaprilat. The initial dose should be reduced to 0.5 mg daily when the creatinine clearance falls to less than 30 mL/min or in hepatic cirrhosis (US package insert). In *type 2 diabetes* with hypertension and normoalbuminuria, trandolapril decreased the rate of development of new microalbuminuria in the BENEDICT study.[82]

Zofenopril contains an SH group and is metabolized to zofenoprilat, a powerful antioxidant.[103] The dose in the SMILE study on severe AMI was 7.5 mg initially, repeated after 12 hours, then doubled to a target of 30 mg twice daily.[64] During 48 weeks of follow up there was a 29% reduction in the risk of mortality.

Lisinopril: Not Metabolized

Lisinopril *(Zestril, Prinivil)* is approved for hypertension, CHF, and AMI in the United States and United Kingdom, and also for diabetic nephropathy in the United Kingdom. It differs from all the others in its unusual pharmacokinetic properties (see Table 5-4). It is not a prodrug, it is not metabolized by the liver, it is water-soluble, and it is excreted unchanged by the kidneys (reminiscent of the kinetic patterns of water-soluble β-blockers). Therefore it can be given a class of its own, Class III. The half-life is sufficiently long to give a duration of action exceeding 24 hours. Once-daily dosing for *CHF* is licensed in the United States. The initial dose is 2.5 to 5 mg in heart failure, and the maintenance dose is 5 to 20 mg per day. *In hypertension,* the initial dose is 10 mg once daily and the usual dose range is 20 to 40 mg per day. In *renal impairment* and in *older adults*, the dose should be reduced. Lisinopril was the drug used in the GISSI-3 mega-study in acute-phase AMI[65] and in the Assessment of Treatment with Lisinopril and Survival (ATLAS) study. The latter study in CHF showed modest benefits for even higher doses of lisinopril (35 mg daily or more) than those usually used.[104] In the ALLHAT antihypertensive study, lisinopril was compared with a diuretic and a CCB and, unexpectedly, failed to reduce the development of heart failure when compared with the diuretic[23] (for reasons, see this chapter, p.134).

Choice of ACE Inhibitor

In general, we see little advantage for any one agent compared with others. But when a specific ACE inhibitor is very well tested in a major outcome trial, we are more sure of the dosage of that drug for that indication. All those tested work in hypertension and heart failure. However, some drugs are much better for specific situations than others. *Captopril*, the first agent available, is now much less used than before despite its wide range of approved indications, probably in part because it requires three daily doses. In postinfarct heart failure or LV dysfunction, it gave protection from death equal to the ARB valsartan,[90] and is much cheaper. Not being a prodrug, it has a rapid onset of action, thus creating the risk of hypotension especially in heart failure. Note that captopril in high doses may incur the risk of certain side effects specific to the SH group, including ageusia and neutropenia. *Enalapril* is very well tested for all stages of heart failure in several landmark studies including the CONSENSUS study, V-HeFT II, and the SOLVD studies (prevention and treatment arms), including the remarkable 12-year follow-up.[36] It is the drug with the best data on reduction of mortality in CHF. Yet (and this point is often forgotten) it is clearly not a once-a-day drug and was used twice daily (total dose 20 mg) in all these studies. *Ramipril* is especially well tested in (1) early postinfarct clinical heart failure, in which it reduced mortality substantially; (2) renoprotection; and (3) CV prophylaxis, for which it gave such striking results in the HOPE trial at a dose of 10 mg daily given in the evening. However, its BP reduction is not sustained over 24 hr.[105] *Perindopril* was the agent used in another important prophylactic study, EUROPA, on stable coronary artery disease, at a dose of 8 mg, higher than usual. Perindopril was also the partner to amlodipine in the highly successful hypertension trial, ASCOT (see Chapter 7, p. 243) and the partner to indapamide in the mortality-saving HYVET study. *Lisinopril* has simple pharmacokinetics, being water soluble with no liver transformation and renal excretion, making it an easy drug to use and understand. It is very widely used, especially in the Veteran's Administration system. There is no risk of hepatic pharmacokinetic interactions. Lisinopril has also been studied in several major postinfarct and heart failure trials.

ACE Inhibitors versus ARBs

Before we delve into ARBs, we may pause to reflect on the outstanding common mechanisms and benefits, with some differences in side-effects, of these two major groups of CV agents that both act on the RAS. They both inhibit the adverse pathogenic properties of angiotensin II (see Table 5-1). They both have a clear role in secondary prevention (see Table 5-3). They both have an impressive series of major outcome trials (Table 5-5). Furthermore, they have similar contraindications, with the major side-effect differences being the lower rate of cough and the virtual absence of angioedema with ARBs (Table 5-6). They both have impressive studies to their credit, many in the *New England Journal of Medicine* or *The Lancet,* the doyens of clinical journals (Tables 5-7 and 5-8). Their comparative properties are summarized in table format in Table 5-9. Between them, they have considerably expanded our

Table 5-5

Major Outcome Trials with Renin-Angiotensin-Aldosterone Inhibitors

Renin-Angiotensin-Aldosterone Blocker	Risk Prevention	HPT (Stroke*)	Chronic Heart Failure	Heart Failure, Post-MI	AMI, Early Phase	Diabetic Nephropathy	Chronic Renal Disease
ACE Inhibitor							
Captopril		✓✓ CAPP	✓✓ SOLVD, V-HeFT, CONSEN-SUS	✓✓ SAVE		✓✓ Type 1	✓
Enalapril		✓✓ ANBP2					✓
Lisinopril		✓ ALLHAT	✓ ATLAS		✓✓ GISSI		
Perindopril	✓✓ EUROPA	✓ ASCOT					
Ramipril	✓✓ HOPE			✓✓ AIRE		✓✓ MICRO-HOPE	✓✓ REIN, AASK
Trandolapril	✓ PEACE	✓ INVEST		✓✓ TRACE			
ARBs							
Candesartan			✓✓ CHARM				
Eprosartan		✓✓ MOSES*					
Irbesartan						✓✓ IDNT, IRMA	
Losartan		✓✓ with LVH, LIFE	?No ? ✓ ELITE 1 & 2 (?dose too low)	No, OPTI-MAAL (?dose too low)		✓✓ RENAAL	
Valsartan		✓✓ VALUE ✓✓ JIKEI-heart	✓✓ VAL-HeFT	✓✓ VALIANT			
Aldosterone Antagonist							
Spironolactone			✓✓ RALES				
Eplerenone				✓✓ EPHE-SUS			

✓✓ = Strongly indicated in opinion of authors; ✓ = indicated; No = not indicated.
*Recurrent stroke.
ACE, Angiotensin-converting enzyme; AMI, acute myocardial infarction; ARB, angiotensin receptor blocker; HPT, hypertension; MI, myocardial infarction.

Table 5-6

ACE Inhibitors and ARBs: Side Effects and Contraindications

ACE Inhibitors: Side Effects, Class

- Cough—common
- Hypotension—variable (care with renal artery stenosis; severe heart failure)
- Deterioration of renal function (related in part to hypotension)
- Angioedema (rare, but potentially fatal)
- Renal failure (rare, risk with bilateral renal artery stenosis)
- Hyperkalemia (in renal failure, especially with K-retaining diuretics)
- Skin reactions (especially with captopril)

ACE Inhibitors: Side Effects First Described for High-Dose Captopril

- Loss of taste
- Neutropenia especially with collagen vascular renal disease
- Proteinuria
- Oral lesions; scalded-mouth syndrome (rare)

ACE Inhibitors and ARBs: Shared Contraindications and Cautions

- Pregnancy all trimesters (NB: prominent FDA warning)
- Severe renal failure (caution if creatinine > 2.5-3 mg/dL, 220-265 μmol/L)
- Hyperkalemia requires caution or cessation
- Bilateral renal artery stenosis or equivalent lesions
- Preexisting hypotension
- Severe aortic stenosis or obstructive cardiomyopathy
- Often less effective in black subjects without added diuretic

ACE, Angiotensin-converting enzyme; *ARB,* angiotensin receptor blocker; *FDA,* Food and Drug Administration; *K,* potassium.

vistas in cardiology, moving from therapy of established disease to prevention of disease development to management of CV risk factors (see Table 5-9). At the beginning of this chapter, we quoted Harvey White. That quotation can now be modified: *"Angiotensin-converting enzyme inhibitors and angiotensin receptor blockers have been shown to have the broadest impact of any drug in cardiovascular medicine."*[1]

The story does not end there. The rapid expansion of interest in aldosterone blockers and now in the renin-blocker, aliskiren, means that the concept of RAS blockers has now turned to RAAS blockade, thereby providing an even more rigorous control of the RAAS system, which is essential for life, but far too often overactive.

ARBs

Because ACE inhibitors exert their major effects by inhibiting the formation of angiotensin II, it follows that direct antagonism of the receptors for angiotensin II should duplicate many or most of the effects of ACE inhibition. ARBs should largely avoid the bradykinin-related side effects of ACE inhibitors such as cough and angioedema. Hence the ARBs, the prototype of which is losartan, are being evaluated and used more and more in hypertension, heart failure, stroke prevention, and proteinuric renal disease, including diabetic nephropathy (Tables 5-8 and 5-9).

Use in Hypertension

ARBs have the capacity to reduce BP with "an astonishing lack" of side effects, and in particular the absence or much lower incidence of cough and angioedema. In recent trials with hard end points such as end-stage renal failure in diabetic nephropathy and stroke in LVH, they have been better than comparators,[106,107] with better reduction of stroke and heart failure (Table 5-8). They are already regarded

Table 5-7

Cardiovascular Trials with ACE Inhibitors

Category	Acronym	Reference	Major Benefit
Hypertension	CAPPP	*Lancet* 1999;353:611–616[54]	Captopril vs usual BP drugs result in similar CV outcomes.
	ALLHAT	*JAMA* 2002;288:2981-2997[23]	Lisinopril vs diuretic vs amlodipine result in same primary CV outcomes and all-cause mortality.
	ANBP2	*N Engl J Med* 2003;348:583-592.[52]	ACE inhibitors in older hypertensive men result in better outcomes than diuretics.
Coronary Artery Disease and Vascular	HOPE	*N Engl J Med* 2000;342:145-153.[19]	
	EUROPA	*Lancet* 2003;362: 782-788.	Perindopril 8 mg daily reduced CV death, MI.
	PEACE	*N Engl J Med* 2004;351:2058-2068.[72]	Trandolapril did not alter major outcomes in stable CHD and preserved LV function with low rates of CV events.
	IMAGINE	*Circulation* 2008;117:24-31.[76]	In low-risk patients after CABG, early quinapril increased adverse events.
	SAVE	*N Engl J Med* 1992;327:669-677.[34]	In asymptomatic LV dysfunction post-MI, captopril improved survival and reduced CV morbidity and mortality.
Myocardial Infarction	CONSENSUS II	*N Engl J Med* 1992;327:678-684.	Enalapril within 24 hours of onset of AMI does not improve survival over 180 days.
	AIRE	*Lancet* 1993;342:821-828.[60]	Ramipril started 2nd-9th day in post-AMI patients with HF reduced all-cause premature deaths.
	GISSI-3	*Lancet* 1994;343:1115-1122.[65]	Lisinopril 5 mg initially, then 10 mg daily started within 24 hr from AMI symptoms, reduced mortality.
	SMILE	*N Engl J Med* 1995;332:80-85.[64]	Zofenopril for severe AMI initially 7.5 mg up to 30 mg twice daily reduced mortality risk by 29%.
	ISIS-4	*Lancet* 1995;345:669-685.	Captopril 6.25 mg initially titrated to 50 mg twice daily within 24 hr of the onset of suspected AMI reduced mortality by 7% in large study.
	TRACE	*N Engl J Med* 1995;333:1670-1676.[62]	Trandolapril long-term for systolic dysfunction after AMI reduced mortality by 22% and severe HF by 29%.

Heart Failure	CONSENSUS	N Engl J Med 1987;316:1429-1435.[182]	Enalapril added to conventional therapy for severe CHF reduced mortality by 31%.
	V-HeFT II	N Engl J Med 1991;325:303-310.[183]	Enalapril in HF vs hydralazine-isosorbide dinitrate resulted in 25% lower 2-year mortality.
	SOLVD	N Engl J Med 1992;327:685-691.[35]	Enalapril for asymptomatic LV dysfunction reduced heart failure and hospitalizations.
	PEP-CHF	Eur Heart J 2006;27:2338-2345.	Perindopril in older adults with HF improved symptoms and exercise capacity. Decreased HF hospitalizations. Study underpowered.
Cerebrovascular	PROGRESS	Lancet 2001;358:1033-1041[95]	In recurrent stroke study, perindopril plus indapamide reduced BP by 12.5 mm Hg and stroke risk by 43%.
Diabetes Prevention	DREAM	N Engl J Med 2006;355:1551-1562.[59]	Ramipril for 3 years given to persons with impaired fasting glucose levels or impaired glucose tolerance did not reduce the incidence of diabetes or death but increased regression to normoglycemia.
Diabetic Nephropathy	Collaborative Study Group	N Engl J Med 1993;329:1456-1462.[110]	Captopril protects against deterioration in renal function in insulin-dependent diabetic nephropathy and is more effective than BP control alone.
	REIN	Lancet 1997;349:1857-1863.	Ramipril safely reduces proteinuria and the rate of GFR decline in chronic nephropathies with proteinuria of 3 g or more per 24 hr.
	ABCD	N Engl J Med 1998;338:645-652.	Enalapril for diabetes with hypertension gave a lower incidence of MI than nisoldipine over 5 years of follow-up, a secondary end point needing confirmation.
	AASK	JAMA 2001;285:2719-2728.[88]	Ramipril, compared with amlodipine in African Americans with hypertensive renal disease, retards progression of renal disease and proteinuria.

Created by Deepak K. Gupta and Marc Pfeffer.

ACE, Angiotensin-converting enzyme; AMI, acute myocardial infarction; BP, blood pressure; CABG, coronary artery bypass surgery; CHD, coronary heart disease; CHF, congestive heart failure; CV, cardiovascular; GFR, glomerular filtration rate; HF, heart failure; LV, left ventricular; MI, myocardial infarction.

Table 5-8

Cardiovascular Trials with ARBs

Category	Acronym	Reference	Major Benefit
Hypertension	SCOPE	J Am Coll Cardiol 2004 15;44:1175-1180.	Candesartan, 42% RR reduction in stroke in older adults.
	VALUE	Lancet 2004;363:2022-2031.[57]	Valsartan = amlodipine on composite cardiac mortality and morbidity.
Vascular	JIKEI	Lancet 2007;369:1431-1439.[184]	Valsartan added to conventional therapy reduced CV events.
	ONTARGET	N Engl J Med 2008;358:1547-1559.[100]	Telmisartan = ramipril for vascular events.
	TRANSCEND	Lancet 2008;372:1174-1183.	Telmisartan: less hospitalization for CV events.
	HIJ-CREATE	Eur Heart J 2009;30:1203-1212.	Although candesartan = non-ARBs, also less new-onset diabetes.
Myocardial Infarction	OPTIMAAL	Lancet 2002;360:752-760.	Losartan (50 mg daily) = captopril (50 mg thrice daily).
	VALIANT	N Engl J Med 2003;349:1893-1906.[90]	Valsartan = captopril in high risk for CV post-MI.
Heart Failure	ELITE-II	Lancet 2000;355:1582-1587.	Survival in hypertensive older adults with HF. Losartan (50 mg daily) = captopril (50 mg thrice daily).
	Val-HeFT	N Engl J Med 2001;345:1667-1675.[116]	Valsartan added. Fewer hospitalized for HF.
	CHARM	Lancet 2003;362:759-766.	Chronic HF. Candesartan 32 mg daily: less CV deaths
	I-PRESERVE	N Engl J Med 2008;359:2456-2467.	HF preserved ejection fraction. Irbesartan 300 mg shows no benefit.
Cerebrovascular	ProFESS	N Engl J Med 2008;359:1225-1237.	Telmisartan after ischemic stroke, no benefit.
Prediabetes	NAVIGATOR	N Engl J Med 2010;362:1477-1490.	Prediabetes with CV disease or risk factors. Valsartan: less new diabetes, unchanged CV events.
Diabetic Retinopathy	DIRECT	Lancet 2008;372:1394-1402.	Type 1 diabetes. Candesartan 16 mg daily: retinopathy incidence lower but progression not delayed.
Diabetic Nephropathy	RENAAL	N Engl J Med 2001;345:861-869.[147]	Losartan 50-100 daily. Reduced end-stage renal disease. Mortality unchanged.
	IDNT	N Engl J Med 2001;345:870-878.[141]	Irbesartan 300 mg daily reduced onset of diabetic nephropathy.
	ROADMAP	N Engl J Med 2011;364:907-917.	Olmesartan 40 mg daily delayed onset of microalbuminuria. Subgroup with preexisting coronary heart disease, higher CV deaths.
	VA-NEPHRON-D	Clin J Am Soc Nephrol 2009;4:361-368.[84]	Ongoing—results not yet reported.
Atrial Fibrillation	GISSI-AF	N Engl J Med 2009;360:1606-1617.	Valsartan did not reduce incidence of recurrent atrial fibrillation.
	ACTIVE-I	N Engl J Med 2011;364:928-938.	Irbesartan did not reduce CV events in patients with atrial fibrillation.

Created by Deepak K. Gupta and Marc Pfeffer.

ARB, Angiotensin receptor blocker; CV, cardiovascular; HF, heart failure; MI, myocardial infarction; RR, relative risk.

Table 5-9

Comparison of Some Properties of ARBs Versus ACE Inhibitors Relevant to Use in Hypertension		
Property	**ARB**	**ACE Inhibitor**
Major site of block	AT-1 receptor	Converting enzyme
Major claims, basic science	More complete AT-1 block, AT-2 activity increased; latter may be beneficial (not certain)	Block of two receptors: AT-1, AT-2. Inhibition of breakdown of protective bradykinin
Side effects	Generally similar to placebo; cough unusual; angioedema very rare but reported (CHARM)[21]	Dry cough; angioedema higher in black (1.6%) than nonblack patients (0.6%), enalapril data from OCTAVE[24]
Licensed for hypertension?	Yes	Yes
Compelling indications, modified from JNC 7[185]	Heart failure, diabetes, chronic renal disease, recurrent stroke (eprosartan)	As for ARB plus post-MI, high coronary risk, recurrent stroke (with diuretic)
Favored therapy in hypertension, European Guidelines[80]	ACE inhibitor—cough, HF, LVH, diabetes, renal disease or microalbuminuria, post-MI, metabolic syndrome	HF, LVH, diabetes, renal disease or microalbuminuria, post-MI, metabolic syndrome, asymptomatic atherosclerosis
Major clinical claims in hypertension	Equal BP reduction to ACE-inhibitors, little or no cough, excellent tolerability, well tested in LVH and in diabetic nephropathy	Well tolerated, years of experience especially in CHF, good quality of life; used in coronary prevention trials (HOPE, EUROPA, PEACE)
Effect on LVH vs β-blockers	Better (losartan, valsartan) Major outcome trial, LIFE[106]	Better (lisinopril, ramipril)
Effect on sex life vs β-blockers	Better	Better
Less new diabetes	Losartan, candesartan, valsartan	CAPPP[54] STOP-2[56]
Outcome trials (death, stroke, coronary events, etc.)	LIFE (losartan better than atenolol, stroke less, deaths less in diabetics)[106]; VALUE (valsartan vs amlodipine; about equal); JIKEI-heart (valsartan)[185]	Enalapril > diuretic,[52] Diuretic > lisinopril in ALLHAT[23]

>, better than; *ACE*, angiotensin-converting enzyme; *ARB*, angiotensin receptor blocker; *AT-1*, angiotensin II receptor, subtype 1; *BP*, blood pressure; *CHF*, congestive heart failure; *HF*, heart failure; *JNC*, Joint National Committee on the Prevention, Detection, Evaluation, and Treatment of High Blood Pressure; *LVH*, left ventricular hypertrophy; *MI*, myocardial infarction.

as possible first-line therapy by the European guidelines, but not by the American JNC 7 committee, which nonetheless recognizes the following compelling indications for ARBs: heart failure, diabetes, and chronic kidney disease (see Chapter 7, p. 235). These are also recognized as compelling indications for ACE inhibitors, so that patient tolerability and price (higher for the ARBs than generic ACE inhibitors) are likely to be the deciding factors. Furthermore, systemic review of 50 studies comparing ACE inhibitors with ARBs revealed similar BP control and outcomes, yet with less cough and angioedema.[108] However, despite several comparisons, ARBs have not been superior to ACE inhibitors. Note that the established contraindications to ACE inhibitor therapy such as pregnancy and bilateral renal artery stenosis are the same for the ARBs.

Use in Chronic Renal Disease, Including Diabetic Nephropathy

ARBs have better supporting documentation for benefits in type 2 diabetes.[109] On the other hand, in type 1 diabetes, the ACE inhibitors have better evidence of benefit.[110] In neither situation are there direct comparisons between ARBs and ACE inhibitors. In proteinuric renal disease, with or without diabetes, ARBs and ACE inhibitors similarly reduced proteinuria.[111] A dual approach, targeting both BP and albuminuria, is required.[85]

Fewer Cases of New Diabetes

In hypertension, losartan was associated with fewer cases of new diabetes than atenolol,[112] candesartan was associated with fewer cases than hydrochlorothiazide (HCTZ),[113] and valsartan was associated with fewer cases than amlodipine.[57] In heart failure, there were fewer cases of new diabetes with candesartan than with placebo.[114] However, it must be cautioned that all these observations were secondary analyses. In the NAVIGATOR study of patients with impaired glucose tolerance and CVD or risk factors, administration of valsartan up to 160 mg daily for 5 years, plus lifestyle modification, reduced the incidence of diabetes by 14% without reducing the rate of CV events.[115]

Use in Heart Failure

Both ACE inhibitors and ARBs inhibit the RAAS and are now well tested in heart failure (see Table 5-9). The overall data from two major trials, Val-HeFT[116] and VALIANT,[114] show that ARBs give outcome results as good as ACE inhibitors (see Table 5-9). Therefore ARBs become a reasonable alternative for use in heart failure, not only in ACE inhibitor–intolerant patients for which the case for their use is very strong.[21] Major mechanistic arguments for using ARBs are the following: (1) Benefits of ARBs are bought almost without any costly side–effects, in particular a consistently lower incidence of cough and angioedema; (2) The adverse effects of major renin-angiotensin activation in heart failure are mediated by the stimulation by angiotensin II of the receptor subtype, AT-1, which the ARBs specifically block (Fig. 5-11); (3) Non-ACE paths may be of substantial importance in the generation of pathogenic angiotensin II;[4] (4) The AT-2 receptor is not blocked and can still respond to the increased concentrations of angiotensin II as result of the AT-1 receptor block. Unopposed AT-2 receptor activity may have benefits[117,118] and harm.[119] However, the lack of clinical superiority of ARBs places in doubt the relevance of the experimental observations.

Thus although ACE inhibitors remain the logical first-line therapy because of the vast experience with these agents in heart failure, including postinfarction LV dysfunction, this prime position is gradually being eroded by the better-tolerated ARBs.

Use in Stroke

More than 25 years ago Brown hypothesized that angiotensin II could protect against strokes to explain the early trial observations that a diuretic better protected against stroke than a β-blocker.[120] Three recent trials support the Brown hypothesis. First, in PROGRESS an ACE inhibitor reduced BP but not repeat stroke unless combined with a diuretic.[95] Second, an ARB, eprosartan, reduced repeat stroke better than a CCB,[121] although CCBs are among the best medications for stroke prevention.[122] Third, losartan gave better protection from stroke in patients with LVH than did atenolol in the LIFE study.[106] Nonetheless, in an overview of 12 trials on 94,338 patients, amlodipine was better at reduction of stroke and MI by 16% to 17% versus ARBs, possibly in part because of small differences in SBP or in aortic pressure.[122]

ACE, A-II EFFECTS and ARBs

Opie 2012

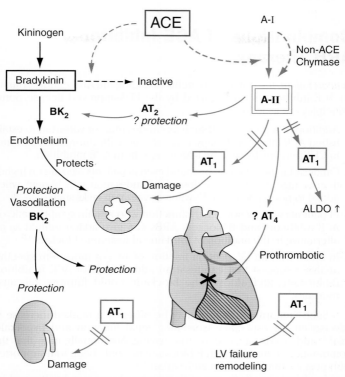

Figure 5-11   Mechanisms whereby angiotensin II (A-II) exerts adverse effects on the cardiovascular system. Most of the damaging effects are via the AT-1 receptor, with possible protection via the unopposed AT-2 receptor (see Fig. 5-3) that may unexpectedly lead to relatively small amounts of bradykinin (BK) formation. The putative AT-4 receptor may mediate prothrombotic effects. BK, formed especially during inhibition of angiotensin-converting enzyme (ACE) mediates protection by activation of the BK-2 receptor. *Double-slashed red lines* indicate effects of AT-1 receptor blockade. *Aldo,* Aldosterone. (Figure © L.H. Opie, 2012, and adapted from *Angiotensin-Converting Enzyme Inhibitors. The Advance Continues,* 3rd ed, Authors' Publishing House, New York & University of Cape Town Press, 1999.)

Nonissues with ARBs: Myocardial Infarction and Cancer

The *ARB-MI paradox* refers to the theoretical and unexpected proposal that ARBs may increase the risk of MI.[119] Because angiotensin II can be produced by non-ACE pathways (see Fig. 5-2), blocking at the receptor level by ARBs might be supposed to result in even greater reductions in the adverse actions of angiotensin II. Nonetheless, there was controversy about the effects on MI of ARBs versus ACE inhibitors, which was the subject of two articles with opposing views in *Circulation.*[119,123,124]

The controversy has been settled by the large and comprehensive analysis based on 37 randomized clinical trials including 147,020 participants with a total follow-up of 485,166 patient years.[125] This study firmly refutes the claim that ARBs increase the risk of MI (ruling out even a 0.3% absolute increase). ARBs reduce the risk of stroke, heart failure, and new-onset diabetes.

Another nonissue is the proposal that ARBs are associated with an increased incidence of cancer. Again, this stems from an inadequate assessment of all the data, and can be fully dismissed.[126]

Combinations of ACE Inhibitor–ARB Therapy

In heart failure, the outcome benefits of adding the ARB candesartan to an ACE inhibitor are recognized by the FDA-approved license. Some principles are as follows:[127]

1. Addition of a proven ARB such as candesartan or valsartan to established ACE-inhibitor therapy is associated with improved outcomes in CHF, perhaps by treating RAS escape from ACE inhibition.
2. Candesartan benefits can be found even in patients who are on higher-than-average ACE-inhibitor doses.[128] Candesartan can benefit when added to prior β-blockade,[127] whereas valsartan lacks such data.[116]
3. In patients with LV systolic dysfunction who remain symptomatic on ACE inhibitors and β-blockers, ARBs can give added benefit as an alternative to the addition of third-line aldosterone blockers.[127]
4. In those with an LV ejection fraction of 40% or more, retrospective analyses suggest that candesartan added to prior ACE inhibition, β-blockade, and aldosterone blockade could improve all-cause mortality.[129]

Such "quadruple therapy" may be offset by a marked increase in adverse effects, especially worsening renal function and hyperkalemia[130] and needs prospective trial testing. Additionally, note that the combination of an ARB with β-blockade has only been trial-supported with positive outcomes for candesartan.[114]

In chronic renal disease with proteinuria, the combination of an ARB with an ACE inhibitor reduces progression of proteinuria better than either drug alone according to an exhaustive review.[111] The accompanying editorial proposes that monotherapy with either an ACE inhibitor or an ARB is appropriate for early-stage renal disease, reserving the combination for use when monotherapy fails to decrease proteinuria to less than 0.5 g.[131] However, safety concerns remain, with hyperkalemia the major danger.[131] A more recent large observational analysis shows that the ACE inhibitor with ARB combination can be disappointing even for renal disease,[132] although the study confirms that, in addition to BP, an effect on albuminuria is a good marker for renal protection.[133] Overall, the arguments for dual therapy are much weakened by the ONTARGET and TRANSCEND investigators,[132] despite the criticisms of the study.[133]

Combined ACE inhibitor–ARB therapy provides **CV protection in high-risk persons.** The ONTARGET study tested the effects on high-risk persons of ramipril 10 mg daily compared with telmisartan 80 mg daily and with the combination.[100,134] Telmisartan was not superior to ramipril, despite telmisartan 80 mg reducing BP better over 24 hr than ramipril 10 mg.[105] The combination produced unchanged CV outcomes, although it resulted in increased hypotension, syncope, and renal dysfunction. Thus this combination is not the gold standard for RAS inhibition, whereas renin blockade needs consideration.[135]

Specific ARBs

Candesartan (Atacand)

Pharmacologically, candesartan differs from other ARBs in that active candesartan is formed during the process of gastrointestinal absorption, with a somewhat longer half-life than losartan (Table 5-10). In *hypertension,* the usual starting dose is 16 mg once daily, lower in volume depletion, with a top dose of 32 mg daily, given in one or two doses according to the package insert. However, when given once daily (dose 16 mg) there is still at 48 hr about two thirds of the effect seen at 24 hr.[136] Note that full hypotensive effect may take several weeks.

Candesartan was chosen in three large *heart failure* trials, the CHARM studies, at a target dose of 32 mg. In the CHARM-alternative trial, in patients with ACE inhibitor intolerance, candesartan significantly reduced the combined endpoint of CV death or hospitalization for CHF by 23%, with less cough and angioedema than anticipated.[21] In CHARM-added,[137] candesartan added to prior ACE inhibitor therapy reduced CV death at the cost of an increase in creatinine (3.7% more than placebo) and hyperkalemia (2.7% more than placebo). Of note, the effects of candesartan were as effective in those receiving both an ACE inhibitor and a β-blocker. Thus in these studies, the triple neurohumoral inhibitor therapy (ARB plus ACE inhibitor plus β-blocker) was successful. This hypothesis was also supported by CandHeart, a much smaller study on 514 patients

Table 5-10

Comparison of ARBs and ACE Inhibitors in Heart Failure, CV Prevention, and Stroke		
Property	**ARB**	**ACE Inhibitor**
HF: Licensed in United States	Valsartan for HF to reduce hospitalization; candesartan for class 2-4 HF with LV EF ≤40% to reduce CV deaths and hospitalization; may be added to ACEi.	Yes, several but not all.
Major clinical claims in heart failure	Use in ACEi-intolerant patients (CHARM-alternative); also when added to ACEi (CHARM-added).	Many studies with large database, at least 12,000 patients, definite mortality reduction of 20%, prevents reinfarction.
Post-MI: Major studies	VALIANT, valsartan noninferior to captopril in postinfarct heart failure.[90]	Several large studies, definite protection including LV dysfunction.
Diabetic nephropathy: Major claims	Renoprotective in type 2 diabetes independently of hypertension;[142,147] slows progress of microalbuminuria.[141]	Renoprotective in type 1 diabetes independently of hypertension; slows development of microalbuminuria in diabetics.
Nondiabetic renal disease	Decreases proteinuria.	Better outcome, REIN, AASK.
Prevention of CV complications (MI, heart failure, stroke, or CV death)	ONTARGET evaluates telmisartan vs ramipril vs combination in HOPE-like study. TRANSCEND compares telmisartan with placebo.	HOPE, reduction of this primary end-point by 22%; EUROPA, reduction of MI and combined endpoints.
Prevention of stroke	LIFE, less stroke in LVH treated by losartan usually with diuretic versus atenolol; less repeat stroke with eprosartan in MOSES.	PROGRESS, less repeat stroke with perindopril only if with diuretic.
Major warnings	Pregnancy, all trimesters.	Pregnancy, all trimesters.
Additional warnings	Hypotension, hyperkalemia, renal function.	Angioedema, hypotension, hyperkalemia, renal function.

ACE, Angiotensin converting enzyme; *ACEi,* ACE inhibitor; *ARB,* angiotensin receptor blocker; *CV,* cardiovascular; *EF,* ejection fraction; *HF,* heart failure; *LV,* left ventricular; *LVH,* left ventricular hypertrophy; *MI,* myocardial infarction.

(73% New York Heart Association [NYHA] II).[138] Candesartan (aim 32 mg daily) added to ACE inhibitors (92%) and β-blockers (85%) did not reduce circulating BNP but improved LV function and decreased aldosterone levels.

Compared with losartan in the therapy of heart failure, high doses (candesartan 16-32 mg; losartan 100 mg daily) were equal,[139] as found in the nationwide Danish National Patient Registry cohort. Note that in the CHARM studies candesartan 32 mg was the target dose.

In *acute stroke* candesartan was not successful, and was possibly harmful.[140]

Candesartan is registered in the United States for both hypertension and heart failure, class 2-4, with an LV ejection fraction of 40% or less, to reduce CV deaths and heart failure hospitalization. It is also licensed for added benefit if combined with an ACE inhibitor. It may also be added to prior therapy by β- and aldosterone-blockade, as in the CHARM studies,[129] but these combinations are not part of the licensed indications.[127] The starting dose is 4 mg daily, working up to 32 mg daily depending on the tolerance of the patient. BP, serum creatinine, and potassium must be monitored. Potassium level monitoring is especially important if combined with an ACE inhibitor or aldosterone blocker.

Irbesartan (Avapro)

Irbesartan has no active metabolite, a terminal half-life of 11-15 hr, and for hypertension there is a single daily dose of 150-300 mg (see Table 5-10). There are the usual caveats: use a lower dose for volume depletion; beware of the initial rapid hypotensive effect, then a full effect in weeks; and a better response is obtained to added diuretic than to an increased dose. The diuretic combination, Avalide, contains irbesartan 150 or 300 mg combined with 12.5 mg HCTZ. In important studies on type 2 diabetic nephropathy, IRMA2 and others, irbesartan reduced the rate of progression of microalbuminuria to overt proteinuria.[141] In established diabetic nephropathy, it lessened the primary renal endpoint, which included the rate of rise of serum creatinine and ESRD.[142] These benefits were found both in comparison with placebo and with amlodipine therapy, and were not explained by BP changes. Irbesartan is licensed in the United States for hypertension and for nephropathy in patients with type 2 diabetes with hypertension. In the ACTIVE I study on 9000 high-risk patients with atrial fibrillation, irbesartan was added to prior therapy, including an ACE inhibitor in 60%. Irbesartan did not reduce CV events, yet hospitalization was reduced (first hospitalization for heart failure, P < 0.003; fewer total hospital stays for CV events, P < 0.001).[143]

In diastolic heart failure with pEF, irbesartan had no effect on the primary outcome, yet showed unexpected benefit in lower-risk patients.[144] Irbesartan was started at 75 mg and up titrated to 300 mg daily. These patients were in the lower range of plasma natriuretic peptides, suggesting benefits early on, but not later, high-risk stages of diastolic heart failure. As this was a post-hoc analysis, prospective studies are now required.

Losartan (Cozaar)

This is the prototype ARB, historically the first, with numerous clinical studies to support its efficacy in BP reduction, and now in diabetic nephropathy and LVH (see Table 5-10). For hypertension, the standard start-up dose is 50 mg once daily, with an increase to 100 mg if needed. The package insert allows for twice daily dosing, the half-life being 6-9 hr. As with all the ARBs, a dose increase is usually less effective than the addition of a low-dose diuretic in achieving greater BP control.[145] When there is volume depletion or liver disease (risk of decreased plasma clearance), the starting dose should be only 25 mg. The combination with

HCTZ is Hyzaar (losartan 50, thiazide 12.5 mg; or losartan 100, thiazide 25 mg). As for all the ARBs, the major antihypertensive effect is present within 1 week. The full effect may take up to 3-6 weeks, and is potentiated by diuretic action or low-salt diet more than by dose increase. In *hypertensive patients with LVH,* in the LIFE study, losartan (mean dose 82 mg daily) protected from stroke when compared with equivalent BP reduction by atenolol, both agents mostly with a diuretic.[106] In addition, in LIFE substudies, mortality was reduced in diabetics[112] and in older adults with isolated systolic hypertension.[146] In *diabetic nephropathy,* in the RENAAL study, losartan (50-100 mg daily) reduced ESRD and proteinuria.[147] In *heart failure,* losartan 50 mg daily was disappointing, whereas a higher dose (150 mg daily) gave positive results.[148] The higher dose reduced the rate of death or admission for heart failure, reduced LV ejection fraction, and intolerance to ACE inhibitors compared with losartan 50 mg daily.[149] Observational data support the view that losartan 50 mg is ineffective although suggesting that 100 mg could be effective in lessening mortality in heart failure.[139] In the United States losartan is registered for hypertension, including the subgroup with LVH, in the latter only for stroke reduction, and for diabetic nephropathy with a history of hypertension.

Telmisartan (Micardis)

With no active metabolite, and a very long half life of 24 hr, this drug is attractive at 40 to 80 mg once daily (see Table 5-10). However, the formulation is such that the dose cannot be reduced to less than 40 mg even when there is hypovolemia. There is a small increase in hypotensive effect going from 40 to 80 mg daily, with the expected response to added thiazide (Micardis HCT tablets 40/12.5 mg, 80/12.5 mg). Other caveats are much the same as for all the ARBs. The US license is for hypertension, with the proviso that the fixed dose combination is not indicated for initial therapy.

In the main ONTARGET study, 25,620 participants were randomly assigned to ramipril 10 mg a day (n = 8576), telmisartan 80 mg a day (n = 8542), or the combination of both drugs. Telmisartan and ramipril had equal outcomes in patients judged to be at high CV risk.[100] In the ONTARGET renal study, telmisartan gave equal renoprotection to ramipril, but the combination of these two agents increased major adverse renal outcomes despite decreasing proteinuria.[99] In the combined TRANSCEND and ONTARGET populations, in patients at high vascular risk, telmisartan reduced new-onset electrocardiographic LVH by 37%.[150] The combination with ramipril gave no additional benefit. However, these results with telmisartan must be cautiously extrapolated to other ARBs because telmisartan has dual AT-1 blocker/PPARγ-agonist activity; the latter might account for superior reduction of microalbuminuria versus valsartan at equivalent BP levels.[151]

Valsartan (Diovan)

Valsartan also has no active metabolite (see Table 5-10). Despite the food effect of up to 50%, the package insert indicates that the drug may be given with or without food. The half-life is shorter than that of irbesartan, yet the dose is also only once daily (80-320 mg). Like the others, added diuretic is more effective in lowering BP. *Diovan HCT* has a fixed dose of 12.5 mg HCTZ with valsartan 80 or 160 mg. There are the usual caveats about volume depletion and the length of time for a full response. In the VALIANT trial, valsartan up to 160 mg twice daily was as effective as captopril up to 50 mg thrice daily in patients at high risk for fatal and nonfatal CV events after MI.[90] Combining valsartan with captopril increased the rate of adverse events without improving survival.

Besides the standard license for hypertension, FDA approval is for heart failure (NYHA class II-IV) to reduce hospitalization, with the caveat that there is no evidence that valsartan confers benefits if used with an adequate dose of an ACE inhibitor. Thus it is not approved as an add-on to ACE inhibition. It is, however, now also approved for reduction of CV mortality in clinically stable patients with LV failure or LV dysfunction.

VALUE is the largest ARB trial on 15,254 high-risk hypertensives.[57] VALUE compared valsartan 160 mg daily with the CCB, amlodipine 10 mg daily, both arms with added thiazide if needed. Despite the theoretical advantages of RAS blockade, final outcomes were similar after an initial period of accelerated BP drop with amlodipine, reflected in early decreases in all-cause mortality and in primary CV endpoints. This result supports those who argue that BP reduction by any means is what matters most, not the agent used to get it down. These conclusions are fortified by the retrospective head-to-head comparison of patients given monotherapy in whom the BP reduction patterns were virtually identical.[152] The advantage of the ARB over the CCB were less new heart failure[152] and less new diabetes.[57,152]

Unexpectedly, in the NAVIGATOR study, valsartan (up to 160 mg daily) given prophylactically to persons with impaired glucose tolerance and established CVD or CV risk factors in addition to lifestyle modification did not prevent new CVD.[115] In the accompanying editorial, the following are noted: the high rates of loss to follow-up (13%), the use of off-study ACE inhibitors or ARBs among participants assigned to placebo (24%), and nonadherence to valsartan (34% by study end), besides poor lifestyle adherence.[153]

Regarding heart failure, valsartan was compared with amlodipine in Japanese hypertensive persons with type 2 diabetes or impaired glucose tolerance. All major CV outcomes were similar with these two drugs except that new heart failure (in only 18 of a total of 1150 patients) was less common in the valsartan group.[154]

Other Agents

Eprosartan *(Teveten)* is registered for hypertension, the usual dose being 600 mg once daily, but varying from 400 to 800 mg and given once or twice daily. In the MOSES trial it was superior to the CCB nitrendipine in secondary prevention of stroke.[121]

Olmesartan *(Benicar)* is likewise licensed for hypertension, with a half-life of 13 hr, the dose being 20-40 mg once daily. This dose range decreases BP as much as equal doses of nitrendipine in isolated systolic hypertension of older adults.[155] It improves endothelial-dependent coronary dilation in hypertensives.[156] In a review of 36 studies in which the effect of various ARBs on BP was measured over 24 hr, olmesartan was one of the best taking into account a variety of modes of judging the 24-hr response, including the last 4 hr of the interdose period.[157] Olmesartan (40 mg daily) delayed the onset of microalbuminuria in patients with type 2 diabetes and normoalbuminuria. It acted beyond BP control, which was excellent.[158] Haller and colleagues state, "The higher rate of fatal cardiovascular events with olmesartan among patients with preexisting coronary heart disease is of concern."[158]

Caveats for Use of ARBs in Hypertension

There are a number of caveats common to ACE inhibitors and ARBs: reduce the dose in volume depletion, watch out for renal complications, check for hyperkalemia, and don't use in pregnancy or bilateral renal artery stenosis. In general, care is required in liver or renal disease (most ARBs are either metabolized by the liver or directly excreted by the bile or the kidneys). A good antihypertensive effect can be expected in 1 week with a full effect over 3-6 weeks, and if needed a diuretic is added rather than increasing the ARB dose. As in the case of ACE inhibitors, and in the absence of diuretic cotherapy, there is relative resistance to the antihypertensive effects of ARBs in black patients.[159]

ARBS: The Future

In view of the large number of careful trials now completed with various ARBs (see Table 5-10), the true place of these more specific inhibitors of the RAAS has emerged as follows. In hypertension, there is no question of the excellent tolerability of the ARBs, which makes them an especially attractive early option for hypertension therapy. ARBs have outcome benefit versus several other different modes of BP reduction in specialized situations such as diabetic type 2 nephropathy or LVH. In high-risk vascular patients, the ONTARGET studies showed the equivalence of telmisartan and ramipril. In heart failure, they are excellent in ACE-intolerant patients, yet also increasingly used instead of ACE inhibitors on the grounds of better tolerance and extrapolation of the benefit of candesartan in ACE-intolerant patients to the overall population of those with heart failure.

Aldosterone, Spironolactone, and Eplerenone

The RALES and EPHESUS studies have focused on the fact that aldosterone is the final link in the overactive RAAS, which underlies the lethality of heart failure.[22,160] Aldosterone production increases in response to increased stimulation by angiotensin II, and hepatic clearance decreases. Initially increased aldosterone values fall with ACE-inhibitor therapy, but later may "escape" during prolonged therapy. Because there is a correlation between aldosterone production and mortality in heart failure, the addition of the aldosterone antagonists spironolactone or eplerenone is logical (see Table 5-5).

Mechanism of Benefit: Diuresis or Tissue Effects?

Aldosterone, by sodium and water retention, tends to worsen edema (Fig. 5-12). Nonetheless, the benefits of spironolactone-eplerenone are not only the result of diuresis. Rather, there are several other beneficial mechanisms that oppose the harmful effects of aldosterone excess, including increased myocardial fibrosis, more severe heart failure, and some fatal arrhythmias.[161] Aldosterone levels are associated with adverse clinical outcomes, including mortality in ST-elevation MI.[162] Specifically, aldosterone has adverse vascular effects, including inhibition of release of nitric oxide and an increased response to vasoconstrictor doses of angiotensin I in human heart failure.[9] Aldosterone is the critical mediator of early A II–induced experimental myocardial injury.[163] Spironolactone therapy can decrease extracellular markers of fibrosis in heart failure patients.[164] Additionally, spironolactone decreases the release of cardiac norepinephrine, which should reduce ventricular arrhythmias and sudden death. Furthermore, spironolactone also has vasodilator properties.[9]

All these effects together may explain the therapeutic benefit of even the low dose of spironolactone used in the treatment of severe heart failure in RALES and why sudden cardiac death was less. It should be stressed that the patients selected did not have renal impairment, a risk factor for serious hyperkalemia. Serum potassium was carefully monitored, and there was provision for reduction of the dose of the ACE inhibitor or the aldosterone-blocker in case of hyperkalemia.

Eplerenone (Inspra)

Eplerenone is a derivative mineralocorticoid blocker with less antiandrogenic (gynecomastia, impotence) and antiprogestational (oligomenorrhea) side-effects than with spironolactone. *In hypertension*, the

ALDOSTERONE EFFECTS

Opie 2012

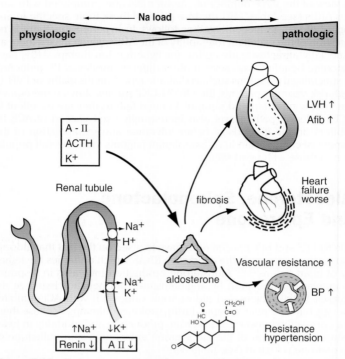

Figure 5-12 Factors promoting release of aldosterone from the adrenal cortex. During a physiologic body sodium load (left side) aldosterone exerts beneficial effects such as maintaining sodium and potassium balance and countering excess renin-angiotensin system (RAS) activation by decreasing plasma renin and thus angiotensin II. During pathologic sodium loading as in heart failure, aldosterone exerts negative effects such as increased left ventricular hypertrophy (LVH) and atrial fibrillation (Afib), worsening heart failure, and greater peripheral vascular resistance. For concepts see Dluhy R, et al. *N Engl J Med* 2004;351:8-10. *ACTH,* Adrenocorticotropic hormone; *BP,* blood pressure; *H,* hydrogen; *K,* potassium; *Na,* sodium. (Figure © L.H. Opie, 2012.)

dose is 50-100 mg once daily, and it is equally effective in white and black patients.[165] LVH is reduced and better achieved by combination with an ACE inhibitor (enalapril) in the 4E-study.[160]

In post-infarct heart failure, in EPHESUS,[160] eplerenone was added to optimal medical treatment, usually including an ACE inhibitor (86%), a β-blocker (75%), and a diuretic (60%). Morbidity and mortality were reduced. The US license is for (1) hypertension, and (2) to improve survival of stable patients with LV systolic dysfunction (ejection fraction ≤40%) and clinical evidence of CHF after an AMI. The major danger is hyperkalemia, so that in heart failure the dose is based on the serum potassium level. The starting dose of 25 mg daily is increased to 50 mg if the potassium level is less than 5 mEq/L, aiming for 5 to 5.4 mEq/L. If the serum potassium level is more than 5.5 mEq/L, the dose must be decreased or discontinued (package insert). However, one opinion is that the reduced risk of hypokalemia "more than offsets" the lesser associated risk of serious hyperkalemia. Nonetheless, there is a specific warning in the package insert against the use of eplerenone in type 2 diabetes with hypertension and microalbuminuria, because of the risk of hyperkalemia.

In the EMPHASIS-HF trial, eplerenone was compared with placebo in patients with post-MI systolic heart failure (mean ejection fraction 26%) and mild symptoms.[166] Base-line therapy included diuretics in 85%; ACE inhibitor, ARB, or both in 94%; and β-blocker in 87%. Eplerenone reduced both the risk of all-cause death (HR 0.76, CI 0.62-0.93; P = 0.008) and the risk of hospitalization (HR 0.77; CI 0.76-0.88; P < 0.001). Eplerenone was started at 25 mg once daily and increased after 4 weeks to 50 mg once daily, provided the serum potassium level was no more than 5 mmol/L. If the eGFR was 30 to 49 mL/min /1.73 sq m, the starting dose was 25 mg on alternate days, and cautiously increased to 25 mg daily. Doses were decreased if the serum potassium was 5.5-5.9 mmol/L and withheld if the serum potassium level was 6 mmol/L or more. As might be expected, hypokalemia was less common in the eplerenone group (38.8%) versus 48.4% in the placebo group (P < 0.001).

Recent Studies in Heart Failure

In EMPHASIS-HF, presented at the European Society of Cardiology in 2011 and not yet published, eplerenone was given to patients with mild systolic heart failure (NYHA class II) on top of traditional heart failure therapy, including ACE inhibitors, β-blockers, and diuretics.[167] The study was stopped prematurely after 21 months. All-cause death was reduced by 24% (p = 0.008) and hospitalization by 23%. The reviewers suggested that all systolic heart failure patients should be treated with an aldosterone antagonist irrespective of the disease severity.[167]

Does eplerenone impair renal function in HF? An early decline in eGFR by more than 20% in EPHESUS should have been associated with worse CV outcomes independent of baseline eGFR. Nonetheless, eplerenone retained its prognostic benefits even under these circumstances.[168] The benefits exceeded the harm of the decrease in GFR. The proposed postulated mechanisms are pleiotropic actions on nonepithelial tissues, thereby preventing CV remodeling.

Heart Failure: Role of Aldosterone Blockade

Does aldosterone inhibition by spironolactone or eplerenone become a new imperative for heart failure therapy? As already outlined in both RALES and EPHESUS, both aldosterone blockers reduced mortality in heart failure.[22,169] In EPHESUS eplerenone reduced death even in the subgroup already receiving both ACE inhibitors and β-blockers for postinfarct heart failure.[169] In both studies the rise in serum potassium was limited and the outcome positive. However, serum potassium *must be* carefully monitored, with reduction of the dose of the ACE inhibitor or the aldosterone blocker in case of hyperkalemia. Note that an initial serum potassium value exceeding 5 mmol/L was an exclusion criterion in both RALES and EPHESUS. Note the new analyses listed previously suggesting that aldosterone blockade should be more widely used in heart failure of all severities, including early-stage systolic heart failure.[167] Most recent studies have been with eplerenone. Extrapolation to spironolactone (much cheaper) may be justified if costs are a dominant consideration.

Is addition of an ARB an alternate third-line therapy to aldosterone blockade? Increasingly, the optimal therapy of advanced heart failure is seen as a combination of the three neurohumoral blockers. Besides ACE inhibitors and β-blockers, third line includes aldosterone blockade.[169] The CHARM studies raise the issue of adding a proven ARB, candesartan, as third-line therapy,[129] thus being an alternate to an aldosterone blocker.[127] However, there are no such studies with other ARBs, and the general lesson from ONTARGET is to avoid double blockade of the RAAS system in patients with renal problems. Thus the standard triple therapy is ACE inhibition, β-blockade, and aldosterone blockade. For choice between the two proven third-line therapies, there are no head-to-head comparisons between a proven ARB and an aldosterone blocker.

Regarding trials in progress, TOPCAT, supported by the National Heart and Lung Institute, is designed to evaluate the effect of spironolactone on morbidity, mortality, and quality of life in patients with heart failure with pEF.[170] The trial is fully recruited and underway.

The Aldo-DHF trial tests whether spironolactone 25 mg daily added to prior therapy will improve exercise capacity and diastolic function in patients with preserved LV ejection fraction (> or = 50%), and echocardiographic diastolic dysfunction.[171]

Renin Inhibition by Aliskiren

Aliskiren is the first in the class of renin blockers, which should be a one-stop shop to equal ACE inhibition or ARB, or, if there is known benefit to combining an ACE inhibitor and an ARB, as may be the case in renal disease, then aliskiren potentially could be better than either of the agents singly. Furthermore, renin inhibition decreases all the downstream messengers leading to the receptors. By contrast, as outlined by O'Brien and colleagues,[123] ACE inhibitors, ARBs, and diuretics all increase renin and plasma renin activity (PRA). Renin and its precursor, prorenin, both bind to the same newly discovered receptor to stimulate a novel path that may have adverse renal effects independently of generation of angiotensin II.[172] Furthermore, in human renin receptor transgenic rats, plasma aldosterone and BP increase.[173] ACE inhibitors increase PRA and angiotensin I, which can form angiotensin II both by ACE that is not fully blocked and by chymase, whereas ARBs and diuretics increase PRA, angiotensin I, and angiotensin II. By contrast, aliskiren neutralizes any compensatory increase in PRA even during combined therapy with a thiazide diuretic, an ACE inhibitor, or ARB and prevents the formation of both angiotensin I and angiotensin II.[123]

Despite this attractive theoretical framework, others are more skeptical because of the potentially adverse effects of excess renin secretion from the kidneys.[174] Evidence favoring the view that renin inhibition blocks RAS better than an ARB is that aliskiren 300 mg daily added to maximal antihypertensive doses of the ARB valsartan (320 mg daily) reduced PRA and further decreased BP.[175] Dual inhibition of the renin system limits the escape from chronic inhibition at any single step. Of direct relevance to aliskiren, renin inhibitors on top of ACE inhibitors or ARBs inhibit PRA despite any reactive rise in renin. In line with this concept, Oparil and colleagues found that the combination of aliskiren with valsartan reduced PRA by 44%, despite a ninefold increase in the plasma renin concentration. Dangerous hyperkalemia (≥6.0 mmL/L) was no more common than with placebo.[175] Moderate hyperkalemia (5.5-6 mmL/L) is relatively common and should warn of more serious potassium rises.[176] These studies have set the stage for the ALTITUDE, ATMOSPHERE, and ACCLERATE studies.

ALTITUDE was a large outcome study in which aliskiren was given on top of ACE inhibitor or ARB therapy in patients with type 2 diabetes and renal impairment. The study was prematurely stopped because the active treatment group experienced an increased incidence of nonfatal stroke, renal complications, hyperkalemia, and hypotension over 18 to 24 months of follow-up. In December 2011 Novartis announced termination of the ALTITUDE study with Rasilez and Tekturna. Thereafter, the European Medicines Agency declared that aliskiren-containing drugs are contraindicated in patients with diabetes or moderate to severe renal impairment who are taking ACE inhibitors or ARBs. The Agency stated, "For all other patients receiving aliskiren-containing medicines in combination with an ACE inhibitor or an ARB, the balance of benefits and risks of continuing treatment should be considered carefully." Despite this abrupt stop, final events must still be evaluated. This adverse experience with aliskiren on top of one other RAAS inhibitor is in keeping with the principle uncovered by ONTARGET, in which dual ACE inhibitor plus ARB therapy given to patients at high CV risk, including diabetics, increased serious renal outcomes when compared with monotherapy with either agent.[177]

The Aliskiren Trial of Minimizing Outcomes for Patients with Heart Failure (ATMOSPHERE) is an ongoing study of patients with systolic heart failure and an elevated BNP or N-terminal pro BNP concentration in which patients are randomized in equal proportions to receive either enalapril 10 mg twice daily, aliskiren 300 mg once daily, or the combination of both drugs.[178] The aim is to improve systolic heart failure, testing a different population from that in ALTITUDE. Furthermore, there will be an open-label run in and postrandomization checks by the Data Monitoring and Safety Committee.

ACCELERATE was a small study in which hypertensive persons were given either aliskiren (150-300 mg) or amlodipine (5-10 mg) or the combination; the BP drop, not surprisingly, was greater in the combination-therapy group. The major point of this study is that it opens the way to the further testing of the potential use of aliskiren as the theoretically ideal partner to amlodipine.[179]

Aliskiren has been tested as part of a dual or triple fixed dose combination. High-risk US minority patients with stage 2 hypertension were given aliskiren and amlodipine (300 and 10 mg) or aliskiren, amlodipine, and HCTZ (300, 10, and 25 mg). The SBP, initially at 167 mm Hg, dropped over 8 weeks to 138 mm Hg and 131 mm Hg, respectively.[180] Adverse events were experienced by 34% and 40%, but there was no placebo comparator. The concept under test is that aliskiren could become one component of a two- or three-drug combination tablet with amlodipine.

ASTRONAUT is an outcome study that will test Aliskiren on patients with chronic heart failure and acute deterioration (acute heart failure), a LV ejection fraction of 40% or less, and an eGFR of 40 mL/min/1.73 m^2 or more. Concurrent therapy with an ACE inhibitor or ARB is a contraindication.[181]

SUMMARY

1. *Inhibition of the RAAS* is established for the treatment and prevention of a wide range of CVDs. The basic concept hinges on the adverse effects of excess angiotensin II and aldosterone. ACE inhibitors both decrease the formation of angiotensin II and increase protective bradykinin. ARBs directly block the AT-1 receptor, thereby largely avoiding the side effects of excess bradykinin such as cough and angioedema. Aldosterone blockers oppose the cellular effects of aldosterone, including sodium retention and myocardial fibrosis.

2. *In CHF,* thousands of patients have been studied in many large trials that have focused attention on the important therapeutic and potential prophylactic role of the ACE inhibitors. Reduction of "hard" end-points, such as mortality, hospitalization, and prevention of disease progression, can be achieved in certain patient populations. In a minority of patients, ACE inhibitors fail to benefit. Careful use is needed to avoid potential harm (hypotension, renal dysfunction, hyperkalemia). The strong argument is to start therapy with ACE inhibition as early as possible in the course of heart failure, even when only mild to moderate, and whether symptomatic or asymptomatic. Whenever possible, ACE inhibitors are used with β-blockers, which are also life conserving (death delaying). The next step is either the addition of aldosterone blockers (spironolactone or eplerenone) or a trial-supported ARB (candesartan). Although first-line experience with ACE inhibitors is very robust, ARBs are increasingly selected because of greater tolerability. The greater the degree of RAAS inhibition by multiple inhibitors, the greater the care necessary to avoid the risk of potentially fatal hyperkalemia.

3. *In hypertension,* ACE inhibitors are effective as monotherapy in BP reduction in most patient groups except blacks, in whom higher doses may be needed. There are few side effects and contraindications. A particularly attractive combination is with diuretics because diuretics increase circulating renin activity and angiotensin II levels, which ACE inhibitors counterregulate by inhibiting the conversion of angiotensin I to angiotensin II. Another attractive combination is with a CCB, as in ACCOMPLISH (see Chapter 7, p. 244).

4. *In early-phase AMI,* ACE inhibitors achieve a modest but statistically significant reduction in mortality (6% to 11%). Best results are obtained in higher-risk patients treated long term, such as those with large infarcts or with diabetes in whom ACE inhibitors give a striking reduction of 26% in mortality.[90]

5. *In asymptomatic LV dysfunction,* whether postinfarct or otherwise, ACE inhibitors can prevent the development of overt CHF, as shown by two large trials, SAVE and SOLVD, the latter having a 12-year follow-up.

6. *In juvenile diabetic nephropathy,* ACE inhibition added to other antihypertensives has achieved reduction of hard endpoints, such as death, dialysis, and renal transplantation. Indirect evidence suggests similar protection in type 2 diabetics; RAS blockade delays the onset of microalbuminuria and the increases of proteinuria, as well as improving outcomes in advanced renal failure. Specific evidence is for ACE inhibitors for the former and for ARBs for the latter.

7. *In non-diabetic nephropathy,* renoprotection occurred independently of any BP reduction with ramipril in the REIN and AASK studies.

8. *CV prophylaxis in high- and moderate-risk patients* was studied in two large-scale preventative trials on patients at high risk of CV events, HOPE and EUROPA. The studies found reduced hard end-points, including myocardial infarction, stroke, and all-cause mortality.

9. *ARBs act at a different site from ACE-inhibitors to block the effects of angiotensin II at the AT-1 receptor.* Substantial experimental evidence shows that angiotensin II promotes vascular and myocardial hypertrophy. Theoretically, AT-1 receptor blockade gives all the benefits of ACE inhibition, except for formation of protective bradykinin. Hence, ARBs are virtually without bradykinin-attributed adverse side effects such as cough and angioedema; the latter is rare but potentially fatal. The ARBs are increasingly seen as having similar efficacy with fewer side effects. They are now used not only for ACE-intolerant patients, but when avoidance of symptomatic side effects is crucial and when these drugs can be afforded. They have the same contraindications as the ACE inhibitors, and there is also relative resistance to their BP-lowering effects in blacks.

10. *ARBs have been successful in treating heart failure.* ARBs have been tested in an era when ACE inhibitors were already the established therapy of choice for heart failure. Had the ARBs come earlier, they would probably have been the first choice. Candesartan is exceptionally well tested in heart failure in the CHARM studies. Losartan has been underdosed. Taking together the results of several large trials such as Val-HeFT, CHARM, and VALIANT, the ARBs in the specific doses used are not inferior to ACE inhibitors, whether the basic problem is heart failure or postinfarct protection.

11. *In studies of ARBs and post-MI heart failure,* valsartan was equivalent to captopril in reducing death and adverse CV outcomes, with decreased cough, rash, and taste disturbances (VALIANT trial). The downside was increased hypotension and renal problems.

12. *Combination therapy of systolic heart failure with ACE inhibitors,* *β-blockers, and aldosterone blockade is favored.* The benefits of three separate modes of RAAS blockade appear to be additive. Eplerenone was given to patients with mild systolic HF (NYHA class II) on top of standard current heart failure therapy, including diuretics.

13. *ARBs have been well-studied in those with LVH and type 2 diabetic nephropathy,* with outcome benefits. When compared with control antihypertensive regimens, ARBs were better at reducing stroke and heart failure, but not coronary heart disease.[107]

14. *ARBs and reduction of CV risk* needs to be studied. CV protection, achieved by ramipril in the HOPE trial and perindopril in EUROPA, needs to be repeated with an ARB. In 2008 the results of a large prevention trial, ONTARGET, have remedied this defect by comparing telmisartan with ramipril and with the combination. The results of this huge landmark trial set new standards for CV risk prevention.

15. *Fewer cases of new diabetes occur.* An important finding with ACE inhibitors and ARBs, especially when compared with β-blockers or diuretics, is the decreased development of new diabetes.

16. *Cautions must be taken in treatment of black patients.* Monotherapy for hypertension often requires either the addition of a diuretic or a higher dose of the ACE inhibitor or ARBs. Angioedema with ACE inhibitors occurs more commonly in black patients. In heart failure, diuretic co-therapy may explain why ACE inhibitors seem to be as effective in black patients as in others.

17. *Contraindications to ACE inhibitors and to the ARBs are few.* Bilateral renal artery stenosis and pregnancy (a boxed warning for both groups of agents) preclude use. Hypotension and a substantially increased serum creatinine require thorough evaluation before use and careful monitoring after starting the drug. Hyperkalemia is also a risk with both ACE inhibitors and the ARBs and increases with their combination.

18. *Combination ACE inhibitor–ARB therapy* can have adverse renal outcomes in patients at high CV risk, as shown in

ONTARGET and ALTITUDE. In severe heart failure, however, the candesartan–ACE inhibitor combination is approved for use. Current trials are evaluating combined ACE inhibitor–ARB therapy in overt diabetic proteinuria.

19. Aldosterone, the final effector of the RAAS, is increased in heart failure, both systemically and locally in the heart, with adverse effects including sodium retention. Inhibition by *spironolactone or eplerenone* improves the outcome beyond that of prior standard proven therapy for heart failure, usually an ACE inhibitor or ARB, β-blocker, and diuretic. The downside is the increased risk of hyperkalemia. Trials with added spironolactone or eplerenone are in progress.

20. Aliskiren is the newly developed renin blocker, still under full evaluation, with promising early results in hypertension. Currently a major trial focuses on the therapy of heart failure with due consideration of relevant safety issues.

References*

*The complete reference list is available online at www.expertconsult.com.

12. Ocaranza MP, et al. Protective role of the ACE2/Ang-(1-9) axis in cardiovascular remodeling. *Int J Hypertens* 2012;2012:594 361. Epub Jan 19, 2012.

14. Flores-Munoz M, et al. Angiotensin-(1-9) Attenuates cardiac fibrosis in the stroke-prone spontaneously hypertensive rat via the angiotensin type 2 receptor. *Hypertension* 2012; 59:300–307.

16. Opie LH. Inhibition of the cerebral renin-angiotensin system to limit cognitive decline in elderly hypertensive persons. *Cardiovasc Drugs Ther* 2011;25:277–279.

17. Sink KM, et al. Angiotensin-converting enzyme inhibitors and cognitive decline in older adults with hypertension: results from the Cardiovascular Health Study. *Arch Intern Med* 2009;169:1195–1202.

18. Anderson C, et al. For the ONTARGET and TRANSCEND Investigators. Renin-angiotensin system blockade and cognitive function in patients at high risk of cardiovascular disease: analysis of data from the ONTARGET and TRANSCEND studies. *Lancet Neurol* 2011; 10:43–53.

27. Byrd JB, et al. Dipeptidyl peptidase IV in angiotensin-converting enzyme inhibitor associated angioedema. *Hypertension* 2008;51:141–147.

45. Rehn TA, et al. Intrinsic skeletal muscle alterations in chronic heart failure patients: a disease-specific myopathy or a result of deconditioning? *Heart Fail Rev* Oct 14, 2011 [Epub ahead of print].

46. McNally EM, et al. Interplay between heart and skeletal muscle disease in heart failure: the 2011 George E. Brown memorial lecture. *Circ Res* 2012;110:749–754.

53. Jamerson KA, et al. Efficacy and duration of benazepril plus amlodipine or hydrochlorothiazide on 24-hour ambulatory systolic blood pressure control. *Hypertension* 2011; 57:174–179.

76. Rouleau JL, et al. Effects of angiotensin-converting enzyme inhibition in low-risk patients early after coronary artery bypass surgery. *Circulation* 2008;117:24–31.

78. Pfeffer MA, ACCORD(ing) to a trialist. *Circulation 2010*;122:841–843.

81. Estacio RO, et al. Relation of reduction in urinary albumin excretion to ten-year cardiovascular mortality in patients with type 2 diabetes and systemic hypertension. *Am J Cardiol* 2012;109:1743–1748.

84. Fried LF, et al. Design of combination angiotensin receptor blocker and angiotensin-converting enzyme inhibitor for treatment of diabetic nephropathy (VA NEPHRON-D). *Clin J Am Soc Nephrol* 2009;4:361–368.

85. Holtkamp FA, et al. Albuminuria and blood pressure, independent targets for cardioprotective therapy in patients with diabetes and nephropathy: a post hoc analysis of the combined RENAAL and IDNT trials. *Eur Heart J* 2011;32:1493–1499.

87. Appel LJ, et al. For the AASK Collaborative Research Group. Intensive blood-pressure control in hypertensive chronic kidney disease. *N Engl J Med* 2010;363:918–929.

96. Bulpitt CJ, et al. Blood pressure control in the Hypertension in the Very Elderly trial (HYVET). *J Hum Hypertens* 2012;26:157–163.

97. Zoungas S, et al. Combined effects of routine blood pressure lowering and intensive glucose control on macrovascular and microvascular outcomes in patients with type 2 diabetes: new results from the ADVANCE trial. *Diabetes Care* 2009;32: 2068–2074.

99. Mann JF, et al. ONTARGET investigators. Renal outcomes with telmisartan, ramipril, or both, in people at high vascular risk (the ONTARGET study): a multicentre, randomised, double-blind, controlled trial. *Lancet* 2008;372:547–553.

100. ONTARGET Investigators, Yusuf S, et al. Telmisartan, ramipril, or both in patients at high risk for vascular events. *N Engl J Med* 2008;358:1547–1559.

102. Lewis EF, et al. PEACE Investigators predictors of heart failure in patients with stable coronary artery disease: a PEACE study. *Circ Heart Fail* 2009;2:209–216.

103. Donnini S, et al. Sulfhydryl angiotensin-converting enzyme inhibitor promotes endothelial cell survival through nitric-oxide synthase, fibroblast growth factor-2, and telomerase cross-talk. *J Pharmacol Exp Ther* 2010;332:776–784.

108. Matchar DB, et al. Systematic review: comparative effectiveness of angiotensin-converting enzyme inhibitors and angiotensin II receptor blockers for treating essential hypertension. *Ann Intern Med* 2008;148:16–29.

111. Kunz R, et al. Meta-analysis: effect of monotherapy and combination therapy with inhibitors of the renin angiotensin system on proteinuria in renal disease. *Ann Intern Med* 2008;148:30–48.

115. NAVIGATOR Study Group, McMurray JJ, et al. Effect of valsartan on the incidence of diabetes and cardiovascular events. *N Engl J Med* 2010;362:1477–1490. Erratum in *N Engl J Med* 2010;362:1748.

125. Bangalore S, et al. Angiotensin receptor blockers and risk of myocardial infarction: meta-analyses and trial sequential analyses of 147,020 patients from randomised trials. *BMJ* 2011;342:d22–d34.

126. Pfeffer MA. Cancer in cardiovascular drug trials and vice versa: a personal perspective. *Eur Heart J* 2012 [in press].

131. Parfrey PS. Inhibitors of the renin angiotensin system: proven benefits, unproven safety. *Ann Intern Med* 2008;148:76–77.

132. Tobe SW, et al. ONTARGET and TRANSCEND Investigators. Cardiovascular and renal outcomes with telmisartan, ramipril, or both in people at high renal risk: results from the ONTARGET and TRANSCEND studies. *Circulation* 2011;123:1098–1107.

133. Lambers Heerspink HJ, et al. ONTARGET still OFF-TARGET? *Circulation* 2011;123:1049–1051.

138. Aleksova A, et al. Effects of candesartan on left ventricular function, aldosterone and BNP in chronic heart failure. *Cardiovasc Drugs Ther* Feb 3, 2012.

139. Svanström H, et al. Association of treatment with losartan vs candesartan and mortality among patients with heart failure. *JAMA* 2012;307:1506–1512.

140. Sandset EC, et al. The angiotensin-receptor blocker candesartan for treatment of acute stroke (SCAST): a randomised, placebo-controlled, double-blind trial. *Lancet* 2011; 377:741–750.

143. ACTIVE I Investigators, Yusuf S, et al. Irbesartan in patients with atrial fibrillation. *N Engl J Med* 2011;364:928–938.

144. Rector TS, et al. Assessment of long-term effects of irbesartan on heart failure with preserved ejection fraction as measured by the Minnesota Living with Heart Failure Questionnaire in the I-PRESERVE trial. *Circ Heart Fail* Jan 20, 2012;5:217–225.

148. Konstam MA, HEAAL Investigators. Effects of high-dose versus low-dose losartan on clinical outcomes in patients with heart failure (HEAAL study): a randomised, double-blind trial. *Lancet* 2009;374:1840–1848.

149. Eklind-Cervenka M, et al. Association of candesartan vs losartan with all-cause mortality in patients with heart failure. *JAMA* 2011;305:175–182.

150. Verdecchia P, et al. ONTARGET/TRANSCEND Investigators. Effects of telmisartan, ramipril, and their combination on left ventricular hypertrophy in individuals at high vascular risk in the Ongoing Telmisartan Alone and in Combination With Ramipril Global End Point Trial and the Telmisartan Randomized Assessment Study in ACE Intolerant Subjects With Cardiovascular Disease. *Circulation* 2009;120:1380–1389.

153. Nathan DM. Navigating the choices for diabetes prevention. *N Engl J Med* 2010;362: 1533–1535.

154. Muramatsu T, et al. Comparison between valsartan and amlodipine regarding cardiovascular morbidity and mortality in hypertensive patients with glucose intolerance: NAGOYA HEART Study. *Hypertension* 2012;59:580–586.

158. Haller H, et al. For the ROADMAP Trial Investigators. Olmesartan for the delay or prevention of microalbuminuria in type 2 diabetes. *N Engl J Med* 2011;364:907–917.

166. Zannad F, et al for the EMPHASIS-HF Study Group. Eplerenone in patients with systolic heart failure and mild symptoms. *N Engl J Med* 2011;364:11–21.

167. Rosenson R, et al. Clinical trials update ESC Congress 2011. *Cardiovasc Drugs Ther* 2012; 26:77–84.

168. Rossignol P, et al. Determinants and consequences of renal function variations with aldosterone blocker therapy in heart failure patients after myocardial infarction: insights from the Eplerenone Post-Acute Myocardial Infarction Heart Failure Efficacy and Survival Study. *Circulation* 2012;125:271–279.

170. Desai AS, et al. The TOPCAT study. Rationale and design of the treatment of preserved cardiac function heart failure with an aldosterone antagonist trial: a randomized, controlled study of spironolactone in patients with symptomatic heart failure and preserved ejection fraction. *Am Heart J* 2011;162:966–972.

171. Edelmann F, et al. Rationale and design of the aldosterone receptor blockade in diastolic heart failure trial: a double-blind, randomized, placebo-controlled, parallel group study to determine the effects of spironolactone on exercise capacity and diastolic function in patients with symptomatic diastolic heart failure (Aldo-DHF). *Eur J Heart Fail* 2010;12:874–882.

176. Harel Z, et al. The effect of combination treatment with aliskiren and blockers of the renin-angiotensin system on hyperkalaemia and acute kidney injury: systematic review and meta-analysis. *BMJ* 2012;344:e42.

177. Mann JF, et al. ONTARGET investigators. Renal outcomes with telmisartan, ramipril, or both, in people at high vascular risk (the ONTARGET study): a multicentre, randomised, double-blind, controlled trial. *Lancet* 2008;372:547–553.

178. McMurray JJ, et al. Aliskiren, ALTITUDE, and the implications for ATMOSPHERE. *Eur J Heart Fail* 2012;14:341–343.
179. Brown MJ, et al. Aliskiren and the calcium channel blocker amlodipine combination as an initial treatment strategy for hypertension control (ACCELERATE): a randomised, parallel-group trial. *Lancet* 2011;377:312–320.
180. Ferdinand KC, et al. Aliskiren-based dual- and triple-combination therapies in high-risk US minority patients with stage 2 hypertension. *J Am Soc Hypertens* 2012;6:219–227.
181. Gheorghiade M, et al. Rationale and design of the multicentre, randomized, double-blind, placebo-controlled Aliskiren Trial on Acute Heart Failure Outcomes (ASTRONAUT). *Eur J Heart Fail* 2011;13:100–106.

6

Heart Failure

JOHN R. TEERLINK · KAREN SLIWA · LIONEL H. OPIE

"There is but one meaning for the term cardiac failure—*it signifies inability of the heart to discharge its contents adequately."*

Sir Thomas Lewis, 1933[1]

"Management of [heart failure] can only grow as a concern for patients, doctors and health-system architects worldwide."

Editorial, *Lancet,* 2011[2]

"No single end point can capture all elements of the clinical course of acute heart failure syndromes, and therefore, no single end point will be appropriate for all interventions or patient populations."

Felker GM, et al., 2010[3]

Acute versus Chronic Heart Failure

Heart failure is a clinical condition in which a functional or structural abnormality of the heart results in the common symptoms of exertional shortness of breath and tiredness. Despite this simple definition, establishing the presence and cause of heart failure is often challenging. Chronic heart failure is common (prevalence 1%-3% in populations, increasing with age to 10%), debilitating, detectable, treatable, and has a major economic effect on public health systems. The prognosis is poor depending on severity at the time of presentation; in the past up to 50% of treated patients were dead within 4 years. Current comprehensive therapy is improving the outlook. The two major causes in Western countries are hypertension and coronary artery disease (Fig. 6-1), with cardiomyopathy as another common cause in Africa. Lesser causes include genetic and familial abnormalities, and peripartum cardiomyopathy (PPCM) of hormonal-molecular causation has been recently recognized.

Heart failure has been recognized and described for many centuries. As a consequence numerous words or phrases have become established in clinical practice. These include older terms such as *forward* and *backward failure, high* and *low output failure,* and *right* and *left heart failure.* More useful and current terminology includes *acute* and *chronic heart failure, systolic* (heart failure with reduced ejection fraction [HFrEF]; enlarged heart and reduced ejection fraction) and *diastolic* (heart failure with preserved ejection fraction [HFpEF]; near normal size heart or ejection fraction) *heart failure,* and adjectives such as *overt, treated, compensated, relapsing, congestive,* or *undulating.*

Two recognizable clinical categories are practically useful. (1) *Acute versus chronic heart failure:* Acute heart failure is characterized by the onset of severe symptoms, usually shortness of breath, requiring urgent or emergent treatment, and therapy is directed to the rapid improvement in these symptoms. Chronic heart failure may also be characterized by persistent but usually stable symptoms, and therapy has also been

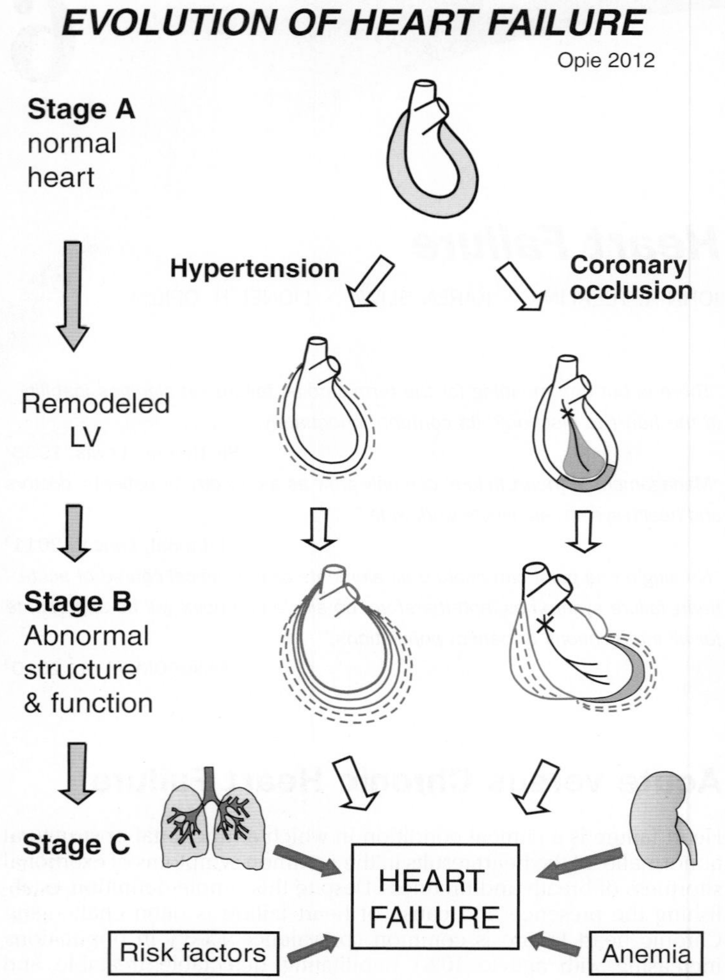

EVOLUTION OF HEART FAILURE

Opie 2012

Stage A
normal
heart

Hypertension

**Coronary
occlusion**

**Remodeled
LV**

Stage B
Abnormal
structure
& function

Stage C

HEART
FAILURE

Risk factors

Anemia

Figure 6-1 Evolution of heart failure. The two major routes to heart failure are, first, chronic hypertension and, second, coronary artery disease. Renal disease is one of the predisposing diseases, which include diabetes. Cardiomyopathy is more common in Africa. *LV,* Left ventricular. (Figure © L.H. Opie, 2012.)

demonstrated to improve mortality and morbidity. Although there are cases of de novo acute heart failure, most cases of acute heart failure are decompensations of chronic heart failure. Whether acute and chronic heart failure represent distinct pathophysiologic entities or are merely expressions of different severity is still debated, and beyond the scope of this chapter. (2) *Hypervolemic versus low output:* Most patients with heart failure present with signs and symptoms of volume overload, often including peripheral edema, rales, elevated central venous pressures, and dyspnea. Low-output heart failure, the extreme manifestation of which is cardiogenic shock, is recognized by peripheral constriction (cold peripheries, confusion, sweating), decreased end organ function (usually renal insufficiency with either anuria or oliguria), and a low systolic blood pressure (BP; less than 90 mm Hg). However, renal dysfunction may also be present in hypervolemic heart failure and should not be considered solely indicative of low output failure. Hypervolemic and low output heart failure are not mutually exclusive and may be present simultaneously, as well.

Table 6-1

Classification of Shock			
		Congestion	
		—	+
Adequate Perfusion	+	Dry-warm	Wet-warm
	—	Dry-cold	Wet-cold

Based on Nohria A, et al. *J Am Coll Cardiol* 2003;41(10):1797–1804.

Acute Heart Failure

In *acute heart failure* the symptom of shortness of breath is often related to high left atrial pressure. Treatment is aimed at immediate reduction of left atrial pressure (preload). Diuretics, nitrates, and possibly morphine (antianxiolytic) are used expeditiously. Intravenous natriuretic peptides (NPs; nesiritide) are now available, but their added benefit is questionable. Vasopressin is used in some acute situations for BP support and vasopressin antagonists, which reduce vasoconstriction and may aid diuresis, have been recently investigated.

Therapy of Acute Heart Failure

A *new classification* of acute heart failure is (1) acute decompensated heart failure, dominated by fluid retention; and (2) acute vascular failure often caused by acute hypertension or other hemodynamic causes of acute pulmonary edema.[4] Clinically, however, it is acute pulmonary edema and cardiogenic shock that must be urgently managed. Here the classification into dry-warm, wet-warm, dry-cold, and wet-cold (Table 6-1) provides prognostic information. "Wet" shock increases the risk of death by about twofold.[5] Urgent clinical examination decides whether the dominant problem is a shocklike state with hypotension (dry shock), or acute pulmonary edema with acute dyspnea (wet shock), or both, the most serious. This complex situation often requires multiple drugs acting at various sites, depending on the overall hemodynamic status (Fig. 6-2). The major drug choices are shown in Table 6-2. The immediate treatment is upright sitting posture, oxygen, intravenous loop diuretics, and perhaps morphine with or without an antiemetic. However, the use of morphine has been questioned in the setting of acute coronary syndromes[6] and acute heart failure,[7] in which morphine was associated with worse clinical outcomes, even after adjustments for clinical and prognostic variables.

Diuretics. Given that the great majority of patients present with hypervolemia, intravenous diuretics are the most commonly administered therapy for acute heart failure. A small study of 304 patients used a factorial design to compare low versus high dose and bolus versus continuous furosemide infusion strategies, and suggested that patients treated with high-dose strategies (2.5× the previous oral dose) had a trend toward greater diuresis, improved symptoms, and transient worsening of renal function.[8] Although there was no apparent short-term difference between the bolus compared with continuous infusion strategies, the attention of the clinical trial personnel and the regular frequency of the bolus dose administration may not be representative of a "real-world" clinical setting.

Diuretic dose and mortality. There are no good randomized trials. Two studies using propensity matching with mortality as an outcome came to different conclusions. The ALARM-HF study recorded in-hospital heart failure therapy in 4953 patients receiving high- or low-dose intravenous furosemide if their total initial 24-hour dose was more than or less than 1 mg/kg.[9] No association was found between diuretic dosing and

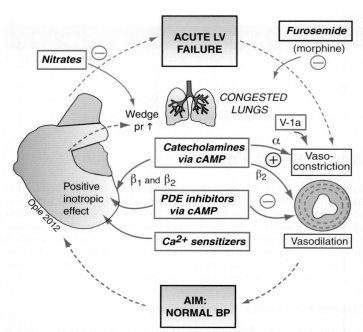

Figure 6-2   Sites of action of drugs used for acute left ventricular (LV) failure. Note opposing effects of (1) vasoconstriction resulting from α-adrenergic effects (norepinephrine, high doses of epinephrine or dopamine), and (2) vasodilation resulting from vascular cyclic adenosine monophosphate (cAMP) elevation from β$_2$-effects or phosphodiesterase (PDE) inhibition (see Fig. 6-5). *alpha,* α-adrenergic; *BP,* blood pressure; *pr,* pressure; *V-1a,* vasopressin agonist acting on receptor subtype 1a. (Figure © L.H. Opie, 2012.)

Table 6-2

Drugs Used for Acute Heart Failure

1. **Vasodilators**—if signs of congestion and BP maintained, nitrates, sodium nitroprusside, nesiritide
2. **Diuretics**—for fluid retention, with strategies against diuretic resistance (check electrolytes; combinations of diuretics; added dopamine; reduced ACE inhibitor dose); vasopressin-2 antagonist aquaretics for hyponatremia
3. **Inotropes**—if peripheral hypoperfusion, dopamine, dobutamine, epinephrine, norepinephrine, levosimendan, phosphodiesterase inhibitors
4. **Vasopressin** (AVP) for septic shock, CPR, intraoperative hypotension

Role of BP in drug choice:

1. Severe hypotension and shock: dopamine 5-20 mcg/kg/min or NE 0.5-30 mcg/min
2. Modest hypotension: Vasodilator or inotrope (dobutamine or phosphodiesterase inhibitor or levosimendan)
3. BP above 100 mm Hg: Nitroglycerin or nesiritide or BNP or nitroprusside

Role of sympathetic tone in acute heart failure:[*]

1. **Tachycardia and atrial fibrillation.** Paradoxical use of β-blockade when AHF is related to AF with rapid ventricular response: IV esmolol (see Table 8-2)
2. **Acute hypertension.** IV esmolol may be used at higher dose than above (80 mg over 30 sec, then 150-300 mcg/min; see Chapter 1, p. 30)

ACE, Angiotensin-converting enzyme; *AF,* atrial fibrillation; *AHF,* acute heart failure; *AVP,* arginine vasopressin; *BNP,* B-type natriuretic peptide; *BP,* blood pressure; *CPR,* cardiopulmonary resuscitation; *IV,* intravenous; *NE,* norepinephrine.

[*]Data from Pang PS, et al. The current and future management of acute heart failure syndromes. *Eur Heart J* 2010;31:784–793.

death in any of the subgroups. In the second study, on 1354 patients with advanced systolic heart failure, patients were divided into quartiles of equivalent total daily loop diuretic dose. Even after extensive co-variate adjustment, there was a decrease in survival with increasing diuretic dose, 0-40 mg , 41-80 mg, 81-160 mg, and more than 160 mg (83%, 81%, 68%, and 53% for quartiles 1, 2, 3, and 4, respectively).[10] Thus there are indirect arguments for both points of view; maybe a randomized trial will yet be done.

Worsening renal function. In patients with acute heart failure, the high central venous pressure impairs renal function.[11,12] Urine output must be closely monitored. Diuretics, by relieving elevated central venous pressure, help preserve renal function.

Vasodilator therapy. Vasodilator therapy is often coupled with diuretics in the treatment of choice for acute pulmonary edema. Sometimes the dyspnea is so severe that assisted ventilation is required. Abnormal vasoconstriction can be viewed as the central defect in many acute heart failure episodes.[13,14] Vasodilator treatment frequently achieves dramatic short-term benefits to save the patient from drowning in his or her own secretions, but is also useful in patients with less severe pulmonary congestion. It is likely that vasodilator therapy is underused, particularly in the United States. A small randomized trial of primarily nitrate therapy compared to a predominant diuretic approach in 110 patients with acute pulmonary edema and congestive heart failure (CHF) suggested clinical superiority of the vasodilator approach. Patients treated with *intravenous isosorbide dinitrate* had less need for mechanical ventilation and reduced frequency of myocardial infarction (MI).[15] Interestingly, an analysis from the ALARM-HF registry suggested that patients treated with a combination of intravenous diuretics and vasodilators had lower in-hospital mortality than those patients treated solely with diuretics.[16]

Sympathomimetic inotropes and inotropic dilators. Sympathomimetic inotropes and inotropic dilators may provide some limited additional benefit in some patients with hypervolemic presentations, but are typically used for low cardiac output. There is little or no evidence that they provide long-term benefit, but rather, mortality may be increased (see "Milrinone" later in this chapter). Such drugs are best used as a means of temporarily supporting the failing heart, or as a bridge to a left ventricular (LV) assist device or transplantation. Inotropes or inodilators are indicated when the BP is low and renal perfusion is reduced. An important choice, largely depending on the BP and the peripheral perfusion, is whether to give an agent increasing or decreasing the peripheral vascular resistance by increasing or decreasing vasoconstriction, and whether to choose an inotropic agent or a vasodilator. Helpful algorithms are given in the European guidelines on the diagnosis and treatment of acute heart failure.[17] Once acute intervention has stabilized the patient, the cause of the acute shocklike condition or the acute deterioration must be established. Thereafter the management is that of chronic heart failure.

Inotropic versus vasodilator therapy. There are few outcome studies comparing inotropic versus vasodilator therapy in acute heart failure. In the ADHERE registry, a retrospective review of more than 65,000 patients suggested that mortality was lower with the vasodilators nitroglycerin or nesiritide than with dobutamine or milrinone.[18] However, those treated by vasodilators had higher initial systolic BPs than those treated by inotropes, as might be expected. Corrections were made but this remains a posthoc observational study. A more statistically rigorous, although still posthoc, analysis was performed on more than 4000 patients from the ALARM-HF study using propensity-matching techniques. These analyses suggested that in-hospital mortality was increased 1.5-fold for dopamine or dobutamine use and greater than 2.5-fold for norepinephrine or epinephrine use compared with patients treated solely with diuretics and vasodilators.[16] Combinations of agents with different inotropic mechanisms or even vasodilators combined with positive inotropes were not considered in these analyses. The overall aims remain, first, maintaining an adequate but not excessive LV filling pressure ideally with cardiac output monitoring and, second, maintaining adequate urine flow.

Acute Inotropes: Sympathomimetics and Others

Physiologically, the basis of the acute inotropic response to an increased adrenergic drive is the rapid increase in the myocardial levels of the second messenger, cyclic adenosine monophosphate (cAMP; see Fig. 1-1). Pharmacologically, acute inotropic support uses the same principles, either by administration of exogenous catecholamines, which stimulate the β-receptor, or by inhibition of the breakdown of cAMP by phosphodiesterase (PDE) type III inhibitors (see Fig. 6-2). To give acute support to the failing circulation may require temporary peripheral vasoconstriction by β-adrenergic stimulation (Fig. 6-3). Hence there are a variety of catecholamine-like agents used for acute heart failure, depending on the combination of acute inotropic stimulation, acute vasodilation, and acute vasoconstriction that may be required (Table 6-3). Often the risk of arrhythmias must be balanced against the inotropic benefit. Countering pulmonary congestion and acute dyspnea requires intravenous furosemide and nitrates.

Cardiovascular Therapeutic Effects of Adrenergic Agents

Adrenergic effects on blood pressure. In the case of norepinephrine, the net effect is BP elevation (dominant peripheral α-effects), whereas in the case of epinephrine at physiologic doses, the vasodilatory effects of β_2-stimulation may offset the BP elevating effects of α-stimulation (see Fig. 6-2). The net effect of epinephrine is an elevation only of systolic BP (increased stroke volume) with a fall of diastolic BP (β_2-peripheral dilation). Only at high pharmacologic doses of epinephrine does α-constriction elevate diastolic BP.

β-adrenergic stimulation of the acutely failing heart. Sympathomimetic agents could thus benefit the acutely failing heart: β_1-stimulation by an inotropic effect, β_2-stimulation by afterload reduction (peripheral arterial vasodilation), and α-stimulation by restoring pressure in hypotensive states (see Table 6-2). Experimental work unfortunately shows that catecholamine stimulation, as exemplified by norepinephrine infusion, should be used with caution in the low-output state of acute myocardial infarction (AMI). β_1-effects may precipitate arrhythmias and tachycardia, which can potentially increase ischemia, and promote cell death caused by metabolic exhaustion. Excessive α-effects increase the afterload as the BP rises beyond what is required for adequate perfusion, thus increasing myocardial work. Although β_2-activation achieves beneficial vasodilation and also mediates some inotropic effect, such stimulation also causes hypokalemia with enhanced risk of arrhythmias. A further and serious problem is that prolonged or vigorous β_1-stimulation may lead to or increase receptor downgrading with a diminished inotropic response (see Fig. 1-6). Catecholamine toxicity leads to myocyte breakdown and death. These are the reasons why sympathomimetics are used only in short-term treatment of acute heart failure.

In severe acutely decompensated chronic heart failure patients, those admitted on β-blockers, and also at discharge, had a decreased 180-day mortality.[18A]

α-adrenergic effects. If the BP is low, as in low-output heart failure, a crucial decision is whether it is desired to increase the BP solely

ADRENERGIC TERMINAL NEURON
Opie 2012

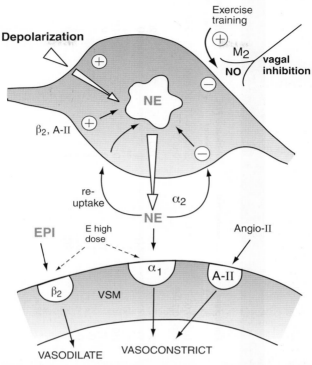

Figure 6-3 Role of adrenergic terminal neuron in regulation of vascular tone. Neuromodulation control of arteriolar constriction and dilation. *Upper panel,* terminal neuron; *lower panel,* vascular smooth muscle (VSM). Adrenergic sympathetic depolarization (*top left*) leads to release of norepinephrine (NE) from the storage granules of the terminal neurons into the synaptic cleft that separates the terminals from the arterial wall to act on postsynaptic vasoconstrictive β_1-receptors. NE also stimulates presynaptic β_2-receptors to invoke feedback inhibition of its own release, to modulate excess release of NE. By contrast, vagal cholinergic stimulation releases nitric oxide (NO), which acts on muscarinic receptors (subtype two, M_2) to inhibit the release of NE, thereby indirectly causing vasodilation. Circulating epinephrine (EPI) stimulates vascular vasodilatory β_2-receptors but also presynaptic receptors on the nerve terminal that promote release of NE. Angiotensin-II (A-II) formed in response to renin released from the kidneys in shocklike states is also powerfully vasoconstrictive, acting both by inhibition of NE release (presynaptic receptors, schematically shown to the *left* of the terminal neuron) and also directly on arteriolar receptors. (Figure © L.H. Opie, 2012.)

by inotropic support or by a combination of inotropic and peripheral vasoconstrictory effects, or only by peripheral vasoconstriction. Although the latter aim can be achieved by pure α-*stimulants,* such as *phenylephrine* (5 to 20 mg in 500 mL slow infusion) or *methoxamine* (5 to 10 mg at 1 mg/min), this option is not logical, because heart failure automatically invokes reflex adrenergic vasoconstriction. Both these α-stimulants may nonetheless be useful in anesthetic hypotension.

Combined inotropic and vasoconstrictor effects. Combined inotropic and vasoconstrictor effects are occasionally required, as may be achieved by high-dose dopamine. Furthermore, there are often defects in the rate of formation of cAMP in chronically failing hearts, such that a potentially useful combination becomes dopamine plus a PDE

Table 6-3

Sympathomimetic Inotropes for Acute Cardiac Failure Therapy

Drugs and Mediating Receptors	Dobutamine $\beta_1 > \beta_2 > \alpha$	Dopamine (Dopaminergic $> \beta$; High Dose α)	Norepinephrine $\beta_1 > \alpha > \beta_2$	Epinephrine $\beta_1 = \beta_2 > \alpha$	Isoproterenol $\beta_1 > \beta_2$	Milrinone PDE inhibitor	Phenylephrine α-agonist
Dose infusion mcg/kg/min	2-15	2-5 renal effect 5-10 inotropic 10-20 SVR ↑	0.01-0.03 max. 0.1	0.01-0.03 max. 0.1-0.3	0.01-0.1	Bolus 50-75 (10 min) Drip 0.375-0.75	0.2-0.3
Elim t½ minutes	2.4	2.0	3.0	2.0	2.0	150	20
Inotropic effect	↑↑	↑↑	←	↑↑	↑↑↑	←	0
Arteriolar vasodilation	HD ↑	↑↑	0	←	←	↑↑	→↑↑
Vasoconstriction	←	HD ↑↑	↑↑	HD ↑	0	0	0
Chronotropic effect	←	0, ↑	←	↑↑	↑↑↑	0	→↑↑
Blood pressure effect	0	HD ↑	←	0, ↑	←	→, ↓	→0
Diuretic effect (direct)	0	↑	←	0	0	0	
Arrhythmia risk	↑↑	HD ↑	←	↑↑	↑↑↑	←	0

Elim t½, Elimination half-life; *HD,* high dose; *PDE,* phosphodiesterase; *SVR,* systemic vascular resistance. ↑, increase; 0, no change; ↓, decrease.

inhibitor such as milrinone. If only inotropic stimulation is required, dobutamine is the agent of choice, although there is the risk of mild decreases in the diastolic BP by its peripheral β_2 effect. If inotropic stimulation plus peripheral vasodilation is required, then dobutamine and a vasodilator, low-dose dopamine, or milrinone is appropriate.

Mixed adrenergic intravenous inotropes. Mixed adrenergic intravenous inotropes ($\beta > \alpha$-adrenergic stimulation) have as their common property the stimulation of both β- and α-adrenergic receptors to a varying degree. α-adrenergic stimulation also results in some modest positive inotropic response in the human heart, probably of greater importance when α-receptors are relatively upgraded as in severe CHF. Included in this group of mixed adrenergic agents is dobutamine, previously considered as highly selective for β_1-receptors, but now thought also to stimulate β_2 and α-receptors (see Table 6-2).

Dobutamine

Dobutamine, a synthetic analog of dopamine, is a competitive β-adrenergic stimulating agent ($\beta_1 > \beta_2 > \alpha$). Its major characteristic is a potent inotropic effect (Fig. 6-4). However, its β_2 stimulatory effect may lead to hypotension and sometimes to a fall in diastolic pressure with reflex tachycardia. Furthermore, long-term mortality may be increased,[19] as well as increasing cardiac sympathetic activity in heart failure patients

Pharmacokinetics, dose, and indications. An infusion is rapidly cleared (half-life 2.4 minutes). The standard intravenous dose is 2.5 to 10 mcg/kg/min, with lower doses (2.5-5 mcg/kg/min) frequently sufficient, and rarely up to 40 mcg/kg/min. The drug can be infused for up to 72 hours with monitoring. There is no oral preparation. *Indications* are acute-on-chronic refractory heart failure, severe AMI (after cardiac surgery), cardiogenic shock, and excess β-blockade.

Dobutamine use, side effects, and precautions. The ideal candidate for dobutamine therapy is the patient who has severely depressed

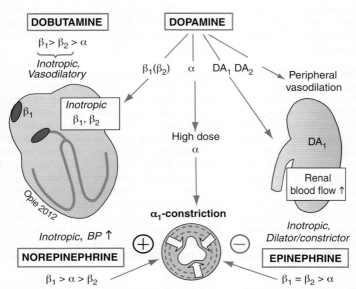

Figure 6-4   Catecholamine therapy. Receptor-specific effects of physiologic and pharmacologic agents. *BP,* Blood pressure; *DA,* dopaminergic. (Figure © L.H. Opie, 2012.)

LV function with a low cardiac index and elevated LV filling pressure, but in whom extreme hypotension is not present (mean arterial BP < 70 mm Hg but no clinical shock). Currently a major use of dobutamine is in *stress echocardiography*. The potential disadvantages of dobutamine are that (1) in severe CHF the β-receptors may be downgraded or therapeutically blocked so that dobutamine may not be as effective as anticipated,[20] (2) BP may decrease or stay unchanged and not increase, and (3) sinus tachycardia or other more serious arrhythmias may occur.[19] Although there are less arrhythmias and tachycardia than with isoproterenol, all inotropic agents increasing cytosolic calcium have the risk of enhanced arrhythmias. Tolerance to the inotropic effect may develop after prolonged infusion. A *precaution* is to dilute in sterile water or dextrose or saline, not in alkaline solutions. Use within 24 hours. Hemodynamic or careful clinical monitoring of the patient is required. Check blood potassium to minimize arrhythmias.

Dopamine

Dopamine is a catecholamine-like agent used for therapy of severe heart failure and cardiogenic shock. Physiologically, it is both the precursor of norepinephrine and releases norepinephrine from the stores in the nerve-endings in the heart (see Fig. 6-4). However, in the periphery this effect is overridden by the activity of the prejunctional dopaminergic-2 receptors, inhibiting norepinephrine release and thereby helping to vasodilate. Therefore overall dopamine stimulates the heart by both β- and α-adrenergic responses and causes vasodilation through dopamine receptors. Theoretically, dopamine has the valuable property in severe CHF or shock of specifically increasing blood flow to the renal, mesenteric, coronary, and cerebral beds by activating the specific postjunctional dopamine DA_1-receptors, although clinical data conflict on the utility of this effect.[21] At high doses dopamine causes α-receptor stimulation with peripheral vasoconstriction; the peripheral resistance increases and renal blood flow falls. The dose should therefore be kept as low as possible to achieve the desired ends.

Properties and use of dopamine. Dopamine, a "flexible molecule," also fits into many receptors to cause direct $β_1$- and $β_2$-receptor stimulation, as well as α-stimulation. The latter explains why in high doses dopamine causes significant vasoconstriction. *Pharmacokinetics*: Dopamine is inactive orally. Intravenous dopamine is metabolized within minutes by dopamine β-hydroxylase and monoamine oxidase (MAO).

Dose and indications. Dopamine can only be given intravenously, which restricts its use to short-term treatment. The dose starts at 0.5 to 1 mcg /kg/min and is increased until an acceptable urinary flow, BP, or heart rate is achieved; vasoconstriction begins at approximately 10 mcg/kg/min and becomes marked at higher doses, occasionally necessitating the addition of an α-blocking agent or sodium nitroprusside. In a few patients vasoconstriction can begin at doses as low as 5 mcg/kg/min. In cardiogenic shock or AMI, 5 mcg/kg/min of dopamine is enough to give a maximum increase in stroke volume, whereas renal flow reaches a peak at 7.5 mcg/kg/min, and arrhythmias may appear at 10 mcg/kg/min. In septic shock, dopamine has an inotropic effect and increases urine volume. Dopamine is widely used after cardiac surgery. Worsening renal function and hypokalemia related to diuretic use for acute decompensated heart failure are common and associated with poor prognosis. Low-dose dopamine infusion improves renal perfusion.

Combination with furosemide. In acute heart failure patients, the combination of low-dose furosemide (5 mg/h) and low-dose dopamine (5 mcg/kg/min) as a continuous infusion for 8 hours was equally effective as high-dose furosemide but associated with improved renal function profile and potassium homeostasis.[22]

"Renoprotective" doses. Dopamine is sometimes given for renal protection or for diuresis in critically ill patients at a typical dose of 0.5 to 2.5 mcg/kg/min. This dose did not work in an intensive care setting, arguing against the renoprotective concept.[21] However, in a carefully titrated dose-response study using intravascular ultrasound in patients with severe chronic heart failure, a dose of 3-5 mcg/kg/min increased renal blood flow, and the higher dose increased cardiac output.[23] This study reinstates the "renal dose" and forms the basis for other ongoing studies. In critically ill hypoxic patients, dopamine may have undesirable side effects such as depression of ventilation and increased pulmonary shunting, which may require supplemental oxygen.[24] "Renal dose" dopamine has not been demonstrated to prevent *contrast-dye nephropathy*,[25] and *intermittent outpatient dopamine* for chronic heart failure does not work[26] and may do harm.

Precautions, side effects, and interactions. Dopamine must not be diluted in alkaline solutions. BP, electrocardiogram, and urinary flow are monitored constantly with intermittent measurements of cardiac output and pulmonary wedge pressure if possible. For oliguria, first correct hypovolemia; try furosemide. Dopamine is contraindicated in ventricular arrhythmias, and in pheochromocytoma. Use with care in aortic stenosis. Extravasation can cause sloughing, prevented by infusing the drug into a large vein through a plastic catheter, and treated by local infiltration with phentolamine. If the patient has recently taken a MAO inhibitor, the rate of dopamine metabolism by the tissue will fall and *the dose should be cut to one tenth* of the usual.

Comparison of dopamine and dobutamine. Dopamine is the preferred inotrope in the patient who requires both a pressor effect (high-dose α-effect) and increase in cardiac output, and who does not have marked tachycardia or ventricular irritability. In cardiogenic shock, infusion of equal concentrations of dopamine and dobutamine may afford more advantages than either drug singly. The key to the effective use of these (and all intravenous inotropes) is careful monitoring of the clinical and hemodynamic response in the individual patient.

Epinephrine (Adrenaline)

Epinephrine gives mixed β_1- and β_2-stimulation with some added α-mediated effects at a high dose (see Table 6-2). A low physiologic infusion rate (<0.01 mcg/kg/min) decreases BP (vasodilator effect), whereas more than 0.2 mcg/kg/min increases peripheral resistance and BP (combined inotropic and vasoconstrictor effects). It is used chiefly when combined inotropic-chronotropic stimulation is urgently needed, as in cardiac arrest (see Fig. 12-10), in which the added α-stimulatory effect of high-dose epinephrine helps maintain the BP and overcomes the peripheral vasodilation achieved by β_2-receptor stimulation. The acute *dose* is 0.5 mg subcutaneously or intramuscularly (0.5 mL of 1 in 1000), or 0.5 to 1 mg into the central veins, or 0.1 to 0.2 mg intracardiac. The *terminal half-life* is 2 minutes. *Side effects* include tachycardia, arrhythmias, anxiety, headaches, cold extremities, cerebral hemorrhage and pulmonary edema. *Contraindications* include late pregnancy because of risk of inducing uterine contractions.

Use in septic shock. In 330 mechanically ventilated patients with septic shock and a mean arterial BP of 70 mm Hg, epinephrine 0.2 mcg/kg/min gave similar outcome and mortality results to norepinephrine 0.2 mcg/kg/min plus dobutamine 5 mcg/kg/min.[27] However, as there was no placebo group, epinephrine could have caused as much harm (or benefit) as norepinephrine plus dobutamine.

Norepinephrine (Noradrenaline)

Norepinephrine is given in an *intravenous dose* of 8 to 12 mcg/min with a terminal half-life of 3 minutes. This catecholamine has prominent β_1- and α-effects with less β_2-stimulation. Norepinephrine chiefly stimulates α-receptors in the periphery (with more marked α-effects than epinephrine) and β-receptors in the heart. Logically, norepinephrine should be of most use when a shocklike state is accompanied by peripheral vasodilation ("*warm shock*"). In the future, drugs inhibiting the formation of vasodilatory nitric oxide (NO) will probably be of greater use in such patients. *Side effects* of norepinephrine include headache, tachycardia, bradycardia, and hypertension. As with all of the catecholamines and vasodilators, note the risk of necrosis with extravasation. *Combination therapy* with PDE inhibitors helps to avoid the hypotensive effects of the PDE inhibitors. *Contraindications* include late pregnancy (see "Epinephrine" earlier in chapter) and preexisting excess vasoconstriction.

Isoproterenol (Isoprenaline)

This relatively pure β-stimulant ($\beta_1 > \beta_2$) is still sometimes used. Its cardiovascular effects closely resemble those of exercise, including a positive inotropic and vasodilatory effect. Theoretically, it is most suited to situations in which the myocardium is poorly contractile and the heart rate slow, yet the peripheral resistance high as, for example, after cardiac surgery in patients with prior β-blockade. Another ideal use is in β-blocker overdose. The intravenous dose is 0.5 to 10 mcg/min, the plasma half-life is approximately 2 minutes, and the major problem lies in the risk of tachycardia and arrhythmias. Furthermore, it may drop the diastolic BP by its β_2-vasodilator stimulation. Other side effects are headache, tremor, and sweating. Contraindications include myocardial ischemia, which can be exacerbated, and arrhythmias.

β_2-agonists

In healthy volunteers, β_2-receptors mediate chronotropic, inotropic, and vasodilator responses. Although not well tested in CHF in which there is known cardiac β_2-receptor uncoupling, some evidence suggests clinical benefit in patients already treated by diuretics and digoxin. The drugs used are basically bronchodilators (terbutaline; albuterol = salbutamol) and should therefore theoretically be ideal for the combination of chronic obstructive airways disease and CHF. By inducing hypokalemia and prolonging the QT-interval, β_2-agonists may increase the risk of arrhythmias. The pharmacologic characteristics of some of the newer β_2 agonists are complex. *Clenbuterol* has been used in patients on LV assist devices and any advantage may be attributable to hemodynamic effects or to metabolic actions.

Calcium Sensitizers

When using calcium sensitizers the principle is that there is no attempt to increase cell calcium, the common mechanism of action of the conventional inotropes with the inevitable risk of arrhythmias. Rather the contractile apparatus is sensitized to the prevailing level of calcium. Theoretically these agents should increase contractile force without the risk of calcium-induced arrhythmias. This expectation has not been met in the case of several members of this group that also have PDE inhibitory properties with arrhythmogenic risks. *Levosimendan* is licensed in some European countries but not in the United States. It sensitizes troponin C to calcium, without impairing diastolic relaxation.[28] In addition, it has vasodilatory effects mediated by opening of vascular adenosine triphosphate–sensitive potassium channels.[28] Vasodilation, which may promote reflex tachycardia, may also result from PDE 3 inhibition. In the LIDO study of 103 patients in severe low-output heart failure, levosimendan (infused at 0.1 mcg/kg/min for 24 hours after a loading dose of 24 mcg/kg over 10 min) compared well with dobutamine (5-10 mcg/kg/min) in that hemodynamic improvement was accompanied by reduced mortality up to 180 days.[28] No placebo group was included so that the difference could have been caused by harmful effects of dobutamine. In SURVIVE, in acute decompensated heart failure in 1327 patients, levosimendan had a similar primary outcome (all-cause mortality at 180 days) to dobutamine.[29] Levosimendan was better at reducing heart failure (quicker early fall in plasma B-type natriuretic peptide [BNP], less heart failure at 180 days) at the cost of more atrial fibrillation and hypokalemia. In the REVIVE II trial, patients treated with levosimendan had shorter hospital length of stay and lower cost for the initial hospital admission relative to patients treated with standard of care.[30] Based on subgroup analysis of patients administered per the current label, levosimendan appears cost-effective relative to standard of care.

Agents with Both Inotropic and Vasodilator Properties

Although *inodilation* is a term coined by Opie in 1986,[31] the rationale goes back at least to 1978 when Stemple et al.[32] combined the advantages of the vasodilator effects of nitroprusside with the inotropic effect of dopamine, thereby reducing both afterload and preload. Strictly speaking, dobutamine and low-dose dopamine should also be included as inodilators. Nonetheless, it is the PDE type III inhibitors that are the prototypical agents (Fig. 6-5). As a group, the inodilators have not improved mortality or morbidity in trials, and their use should be reserved for very serious hemodynamic situations such as LV failure with an inadequate low cardiac output despite adequate LV filling pressure.[33]

Phosphodiesterase Type III Inhibitors

PDE type III inhibitors, epitomized by milrinone, inhibit the breakdown of cAMP in cardiac and peripheral vascular smooth muscle, resulting in augmented myocardial contractility and peripheral arterial and venous vasodilation (see Fig. 6-5). Milrinone can substantially increase heart rate and decrease BP. The added dilator component may explain relative conservation of the myocardial oxygen consumption. Nonetheless, the increased levels of myocardial cAMP predispose to atrial and ventricular arrhythmias, which could explain the findings in the Milrinone-Digoxin trial in which milrinone was no better than digoxin and led to an increase in ventricular arrhythmias.[34] The only inotropic dilator currently licensed in the United States is milrinone, although both milrinone and enoximone are available in the United Kingdom.

Milrinone. Milrinone is approved for intravenous use in the United States and United Kingdom. Its pharmacologic mechanism of action is by PDE type III inhibition. The package insert gives a prominent warning that there is no evidence for efficacy or safety when given for longer than 48 hours. The further warning is that long-term oral use increased ventricular arrhythmias[34] and mortality.[35] In the large OPTIME-CHF trial on 949 patients with acute exacerbations of heart failure on a background of chronic heart failure, milrinone gave no additional benefit beyond placebo, yet caused more complications such as new atrial fibrillation and sustained hypotension without any overall mortality benefit.[36] A later analysis revealed a trend of worse outcomes in the outcome benefit in the ischemic patients.[37] There is no evidence that long-term continuous or intermittent infusion imparts benefit without potentially serious hazards.

INOTROPIC DILATORS

Opie 2012

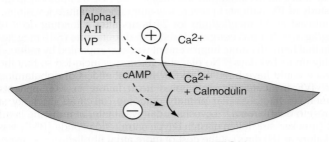

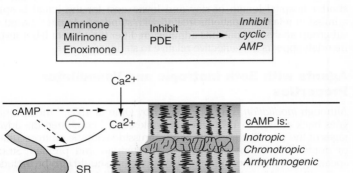

MYOCARDIAL CONTRACTION ↑

Figure 6-5 Inotropic dilators ("inodilators") have as their mechanism of action an increase of cyclic adenosine monophosphate in vascular smooth muscle (*top*) and in myocardium (*bottom*). *Alpha₁*, alpha₁-adrenergic stimulation; *A-II*, Angiotensin-II; *PDE*, phosphodiesterase; *SR*, Sarcoplasmic reticulum; *VP*, vasopressin. (Figure © L.H. Opie, 2012.)

Indications and doses are as follows. Milrinone is licensed only for intravenous use in patients with low output heart failure who are closely monitored, with facilities to treat any acute life-threatening ventricular arrhythmias that may arise. There is no clinical trial experience with infusions longer than 48 hours. A slow intravenous loading dose (over 10 minutes, diluted before use, 50 mcg/kg) may be used, although many clinicians omit the initial load to avoid hypotensive effects, followed by an intravenous infusion at a rate of 0.375 to 0.750 mcg/kg/min, usually for up to 12 hours following surgery or up to 48 hours in acute heart failure; the maximum daily dose is 1.13 mg/kg. Reduce the dose in renal failure according to the creatinine clearance (see package insert). For example, a clearance of 20 mL/min/1.73 m² gives an infusion rate of 0.28 mcg/kg/min. *Contraindications* are AMI, severe aortic stenosis, or hypertrophic obstructive subaortic stenosis. *Short-term inotropic support* by milrinone on top of the otherwise optimal management of exacerbations of chronic heart failure cannot be recommended unless there is clear clinical need for inotropes or pressor agents.

Combination therapy and drug interactions are as follows. Milrinone gives added hemodynamic benefit to patients already receiving angiotensin-converting enzyme (ACE) inhibitors, with, however, a high risk of vasodilatory side effects. Milrinone may be combined with modest doses of dobutamine, enhancing the inotropic effects and lowering filling pressures. When the BP is low, milrinone may be combined with high-dose dopamine. Other than increased tachycardia and arrhythmias, there appear to be few or no adverse drug interactions.

Enoximone. Enoximone is an investigational agent not available in the United States that is licensed for intravenous use in the United Kingdom (loading dose: 90 mcg/kg/min over 10 to 30 minutes, then 5-20 mcg/kg/min, decrease doses in renal failure). Although licensed for CHF in cases in which cardiac output is reduced and filling pressures increase, in practice it should ideally be used for acute, not chronic, heart failure or in bridging situations such as for patients awaiting transplantation. It seems that enoximone has not overcome the common problem of PDE inhibitors, namely enhancement of cAMP levels with a consequent risk of serious arrhythmias. The latter might explain why enoximone increased mortality in severe heart failure, whereas the central stimulatory effects of cAMP might explain why physical mobility and quality of life improved.[38] This unexpected paradox triggered a debate, not yet resolved, about whether it is more important to improve the quality or quantity of life in chronic, severe, end-stage heart failure.

Novel Approaches to Increasing Cardiac Performance

As noted previously, all of the currently available inotropes and inodilators operate via a mechanism that increases intracellular cAMP and calcium with resultant increases in heart rate and myocardial oxygen demand with consequent increases in ischemia, arrhythmias, and death. Multiple new approaches have been developed to improve cardiac performance potentially without these liabilities. One promising approach includes the direct activation of cardiac myosin, and two human studies report the effects of the cardiac myosin activator, omecamtiv mecarbil, in volunteers or in patients with systolic heart failure. The first-in-man (34 healthy men) study showed highly dose-dependent increased LV systolic function in response to intravenous omecamtiv mecarbil and supported potential clinical use of the drug in patients with heart failure.[39]

In an associated article on 45 patients with stable guideline-treated systolic heart failure, intravenous omecamtiv mecarbil gave concentration-dependent increases in LV ejection time (up to an 80 ms) and stroke volume (up to 9·7 mL), with a small fall in heart rate (up to 2·7 beats per min; $p < 0.0001$ for all three measures).[40] A dose-finding study in patients with acute heart failure (ATOMIC-AHF) is currently enrolling, and the high bioavailability of oral omecamtiv mecarbil presents the potential for chronic oral administration of this therapy.

Other potential new inotropic mechanisms include sodium–potassium–adenosine triphosphatase (ATPase) inhibition with SERCA activation (istaroxime), SERCA activation with vasodilation (nitroxyl donors such as CXL-1020), ryanodine receptor stabilization (S44121), and energetic modulation (etomoxir; pyruvate).[41]

Load Reduction and Vasodilation

Principles of Load Reduction

Once a specialized procedure, vasodilation is now commonplace in the therapy of heart failure and hypertension, as the peripheral circulation has become one of the prime sites of cardiovascular drug action. Vasodilators may be classified according to the site of action in the circulation (see Fig. 2-3). Preload reducers (predominantly venodilators) may be separated from those primarily reducing the afterload (predominantly arteriolar dilators), whereas mixed agents act on both pre- and afterload and are combined veno-arteriolar dilators. ACE inhibitors can be regarded as specialized vasodilators that have many other additional properties (see Chapter 5). Whereas other vasodilators, especially the arteriolar dilators, reflexly activate the renin-angiotensin axis, ACE inhibitors both vasodilate and inhibit this system, besides having sympatholytic properties.

Preload reduction. Normally as the preload (the LV filling pressure) increases, so does the peak LV systolic pressure, and the cardiac output rises (ascending limb of the Frank-Starling curve). In diseased hearts the increase in cardiac output is much less than normal, and the output fails to rise and may even fall as the filling pressure rises (the apparent descending limb of Frank-Starling curve). However, the optimal filling pressure for the diseased heart is extremely variable, not always being higher than normal. Reduction of the preload is generally but not always useful. Clinically, the major drugs that reduce the preload in heart failure are (1) furosemide by its diuretic effect, and (2) the nitrates that dilate the systemic veins to reduce the venous return and thus the filling pressure in both the right and left heart chambers.

Afterload reduction. The therapeutic aim of afterload reduction is to decrease the peripheral vascular resistance to lessen the load on the heart, improve renal function, and improve skeletal muscle perfusion. Reduction of the systemic (peripheral) vascular resistance is not the same as BP reduction because in heart failure a compensatory increase in the cardiac output tends to maintain the arterial pressure during afterload reduction. Specific afterload reducers are few and limited in practice to two. First, hydralazine is a nonspecific agent with a cellular mode of action that is still undetermined, although it may well act as a potassium channel opener. Second, the calcium channel blockers (CCBs) are afterload reducers and widely used in hypertension. They often have a negative inotropic effect, thereby restricting their use in heart failure, in which they are as a group contraindicated. Amlodipine and other long-acting CCBs may be an exception, although with severe restrictions (see Chapter 3).

Combined preload and afterload reduction. Sodium nitroprusside, used for very severe hypertension or CHF, must be given intravenously under close supervision and careful monitoring. The *α-adrenergic blockers* give combined pre- and afterload reduction, the latter explaining their antihypertensive effect. Theoretically, they should also work in CHF but do not. Rather, as a group they increase the incidence of heart failure when given as monotherapy for hypertension (see Chapter 7, p. 251). Of the two combined α- and β-blockers, labetalol and carvedilol, only the latter is well tested in heart failure (see Fig. 1-10). The β-blocking component of these drugs should be able to inhibit β-mediated myocardial toxicity resulting from neuroadrenergic activation in heart failure, and the α-blocking component to reduce peripheral vasoconstriction.

Nitroprusside: The Prototype Balanced Vasodilator

Nitroprusside is a donor of NO that vasodilates by formation of cyclic guanosine monophosphate (GMP) in vascular tissue (Fig. 6-6). Intravenous sodium nitroprusside remains the reference vasodilator for severe low output left-sided heart failure, provided that the arterial pressure is reasonable, because it acts rapidly and has a balanced effect on the afterload and preload (see Fig. 2-3), dilating both arterioles and veins. Nitroprusside, an ultra-rapid agent, seems particularly useful for increasing LV stroke work in acute severe refractory heart failure caused by mitral or aortic regurgitation. Hemodynamic and clinical improvements are also observed in patients with severe pump failure complicating AMI, in heart failure after cardiac surgery, and in patients with acute exacerbation of chronic heart failure. Because of the need for careful, continuous monitoring and its light sensitivity, as well as the risk of cyanide toxicity,[42] nitroprusside is being replaced in severe acute-on-chronic

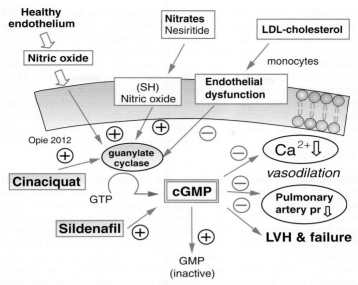

Figure 6-6   Nitric oxide, nitroprusside, and nesiritide stimulate guanylate cyclase to form cyclic guanosine monophosphate with vasodilatory properties. Note possible role of sildenafil and related compounds (see Fig. 2-6). *cGMP,* Cyclic guanosine monophosphate; *LDL,* low-density lipoprotein; *LVH,* left ventricular hypertrophy; *SH,* Sulfhydryl. (Figure © L.H. Opie, 2012.)

heart failure by nitrates, and in hypertensive crises by intravenous nicardipine, fenoldopam, or labetalol (see Table 7-4). However, at many specialized heart failure centers, nitroprusside remains a frequently used agent, supported by the results of a nonrandomized study in 175 patients with acute decompensated heart failure and a cardiac index of 2 L/min/m^2 or less admitted for intensive medical therapy including vasoactive drugs. The nitroprusside-treated patients had greater hemodynamic improvement and lower rates of all-cause mortality than the control patients.[43]

Properties, precautions, and cyanide toxicity. With infusion of nitroprusside, the hemodynamic response (direct vasodilation) starts within minutes and stops equally quickly. Nitroprusside given intravenously is converted to cyanmethemoglobin and free cyanide in the red cells; the free cyanide is then converted to thiocyanate in the liver and is cleared by the kidneys (half-life of 7 days). Extravasation must be avoided. The solution in normal saline (avoid alkaline solutions) must be freshly made and then shielded from light during infusion; it should be discarded when 4 hours old, or before if discolored. *Toxicity* is a special problem with nitroprusside particularly when given at high doses or for long periods and especially if there is liver or renal failure to limit cyanide metabolism and excretion of end products.

Cyanide toxicity: Cyanide accumulation can kill cells by inhibition of oxidative metabolism, which leads to anaerobic metabolism with lactic acidosis. This sequence is potentially fatal. However, the latter may be a terminal event more related to circulatory failure. The clinical picture is variable and ranges from abdominal pain to unexplained death. Nervous system features are prominent and include changed mental status, unexplained encephalopathy, focal lesions, convulsions (cyanide apoplexy), and even brain death.[42] Cyanide toxicity can be avoided by (1) keeping the infusion dose as low and as short as possible, and no longer than 10 minutes at top dose in the treatment of severe hypertension; (2) maintaining clinical suspicion; (3) giving concomitant sodium thiosulfate; and (4) searching for indirect evidence of toxicity such as increasing blood lactate and blood thiocyanate levels. Using the latter, it is sometimes permissible to use low-dose nitroprusside for up to 3 days when using this agent as a bridge to a mechanical assist device or to transplantation (see "Nitroprusside: Doses, Indications, and Contraindications" later in this chapter). However, thiocyanate levels only indirectly reflect cyanide toxicity and give imperfect guidance. *Thiocyanate toxicity* is another hazard (toxic thiocyanate level 100 mcg/mL). Thiocyanate is relatively nontoxic, but can become so in the presence of renal failure, giving a variety of gastrointestinal (GI) and central nervous features, some of which overlap with cyanide toxicity.

Nitroprusside: doses, indications, and contraindications. The usual dose is 0.5-10 mcg/kg/min, but infusion at the maximal rate should never last for more than 10 minutes. The package insert gives a boxed warning that, except when used briefly or at very low rates (<2 mcg/kg/min), toxic cyanide can reach potentially lethal levels. The infusion rate needs careful titration against the BP, which must be continuously monitored to avoid excess hypotension, which can be fatal. When treating severe hypertension, the package insert warns that if the BP has not been adequately controlled after 10 minutes of infusion at the maximal rate, the drug should be stopped immediately. Conversely, nitroprusside must not be abruptly withdrawn during the treatment of heart failure because of the danger of rebound hypertension.

Indications include the following situations: (1) severe acute-on-chronic heart failure, especially with regurgitant valve disease, to "rescue" the patient or to act as a bridge to transplantation or to a mechanical assist device; (2) in hypertensive crises (see Table 7-4); (3) in dissecting aneurysm; (4) for controlled hypotension in anesthesia (maximum dose 1.5 mcg/kg/min); and (5) after coronary bypass surgery, when patients frequently have reactive hypertension as they are removed from hypothermia, so that nitroprusside or nitrates may be given for 24 hours provided that hypotension is no problem. *Contraindications* are as follows: preexisting hypotension (systolic < 90 mm Hg, diastolic < 60 mm Hg). All vasodilators are contraindicated in severe obstructive valvular heart disease (aortic or mitral or pulmonic stenosis, or obstructive cardiomyopathy). Unexpectedly, carefully monitored nitroprusside can improve cardiac output in very tight aortic stenosis with severe heart failure, acting as a bridge to valve replacement and showing that an increased total vascular resistance contributes to the load on the suffering left ventricle.[44] AMI is not a contraindication, provided that excess hypotension is avoided. Nitroprusside is contraindicated in hepatic or real failure because clearance of toxic metabolites is depressed.

Side effects of nitroprusside. Side effects of nitroprusside besides cyanide toxicity, are as follows. Overvigorous treatment may cause an excessive drop in LV end-diastolic pressure, severe hypotension, and myocardial ischemia. Fatigue, nausea, vomiting, and disorientation caused by toxicity tend to arise especially when treatment continues for more than 48 hours. In patients with renal failure, thiocyanate accumulates with high-dose infusions and may produce hypothyroidism after prolonged therapy. Hypoxia may result from increased ventilation-perfusion mismatch with pulmonary vasodilation.

Treatment of cyanide toxicity. First, be vigilant to avoid cyanide toxicity. Discontinue the infusion once the diagnosis is suspected (blood thiocyanate levels are only an indirect guide). Give sodium nitrite 3% solution at less than 2.5 mL/min to total dose of 10 to 15 mL/min, followed by an injection of sodium thiosulfate, 12.5 g in 50 mL of 5% dextrose water over 10 min. Repeat if needed at half these doses.

Nitrates

Nitrates are now used in the therapy of both acute and chronic heart failure (see Chapter 2, p. 50). They work increasing vasodilatory vascular cyclic GMP. Their major effect is venous rather than arteriolar dilation, thus being most suited to patients with raised pulmonary wedge pressure and clinical features of pulmonary congestion. Nitrates produce a "pharmacologic phlebotomy." Intravenous nitrates are usually chosen instead of nitroprusside for acute pulmonary edema of MI because of the extensive experience with nitrates in large trials. Besides acting as vasodilators, nitrates may oppose the harmful growth-promoting effects of norepinephrine, raised in heart failure, on cardiac myocytes and fibroblasts.[45] As noted previously, intravenous nitrates were demonstrated to be superior to diuretics alone in patients with heart failure and acute pulmonary edema.[15] In the VMAC trial, very low doses of intravenous nitroglycerin showed no significant difference from placebo in early dyspnea relief or reduction in pulmonary capillary wedge pressure (PCWP).[46] However, a small subgroup analysis from VMAC in which nitroglycerin was more aggressively up-titrated[47] demonstrated that higher-dose intravenous nitroglycerin significantly improved PCWP, although tachyphylaxis was evident at 24 hours.[47] Intravenous nitroglycerin is probably underused in the United States. When administered for acute heart failure, starting doses should be from 20-40 mcg/min with rapid up-titration every 5-10 minutes to the desired hemodynamic or symptom effect up to approximately 200 mcg/min. The main side effects are headache and hypotension, both of which respond to decrease or cessation of the infusion.

Nesiritide

Nesiritide is the first of a new drug class of therapeutic NPs to be approved in the United States. It is a recombinant preparation of the human B-type natriuretic peptide identical to the endogenous hormone produced by the ventricles in response to increased wall stress and volume overload. In an early study, nesiritide, when added to standard therapy of acute heart failure by intravenous or oral diuretics, gave greater relief of dyspnea than did nitroglycerin.[46] Nesiritide increased peak expiratory flow rate with acute heart failure treatment during the first 24 hours.[48]

A metaanalysis of five studies in 2005 raised the risk of worsening renal function,[49] as well as increased mortality.[50] The definitive, randomized trial (ASCEND-HF) compared nesiritide to placebo in addition to standard therapy in 7141 patients and showed that patients treated with nesiritide had minimal improvement in dyspnea and no beneficial effect on hospitalizations for heart failure or death within 30 days. Although there was an increased incidence of symptomatic hypotension in the nesiritide group, there were no differences in the rates of worsening renal function.[51]

Investigational Vasodilators

Given the central role of vasodilator therapy in acute heart failure, there has been considerable enthusiasm for developing other types of vasodilator therapies, including other chimeric NPs (e.g., cenderitide) and soluble guanylate cyclase activators or stimulators (e.g., cinaciguat). Another novel investigational agent is relaxin, a pleiotropic neurohormone with vasodilating and potentially renoprotective effects, which had encouraging results in early studies[52] and is currently in Phase III trials.[53]

Vasopressin and "Vaptans"

Vasopressin receptors. Vasopressin, or antidiuretic hormone (ADH), is synthesized in the hypothalamus and is crucial for osmoregulation, cardiovascular tone, and homeostasis (Fig. 6-7). Previous clinical studies

VASOPRESSIN AND ACUTE HF
Opie 2012

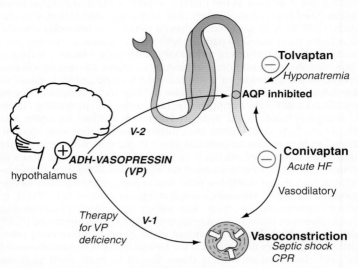

Figure 6-7   Vasopressin and heart failure. Note use of V-1 agonists for selected types of acute heart failure, and of V-2 antagonists for aquaporin (AQP) inhibition and vasodilation. *ADH*, antidiuretic hormone; *AQP*, Aquaporin; *CPR*, cardiopulmonary resuscitation. (Figure © L.H. Opie, 2012.)

have highlighted the role of vasopressin and its analogues in cardiopulmonary resuscitation (CPR), septic shock, and intraoperative hypotension.[54,55] Recently, emphasis has shifted to syndrome of inappropriate antidiuretic hormone hypersecretion (SIADH), as reviewed by Gassanov and colleagues.[56]

ADH is released in response to increased plasma osmolality, decreased arterial pressure, and reduced cardiac filling. Human ADH contains arginine, and is called *arginine vasopressin* (AVP) to distinguish it from other vasopressin analogues. Three subtypes of vasopressin receptors have been identified: V_1, V_2, and V_3. V_1 receptors are G-coupled proteins that operate via the phosphoinositide signaling pathway, causing release of intracellular calcium and vasoconstriction. V_2 receptors are also coupled to G proteins, but operate via adenylyl cyclase, using cAMP as a secondary messenger. V_2 receptors are found in renal tubules, and mediate water retention. V_3 receptors in the anterior pituitary gland are associated with corticotropin (adrenocorticotropic hormone) release and are not discussed here.

At present, no enzymes have been specifically linked to vasopressin formation or degradation. Thus most research into pharmacologic manipulation of vasopressin has focused on identifying vasopressin receptor agonists and antagonists (see Fig. 6-4).

Effects of arginine vasopressin on vascular tone. Intravenous administration of AVP has rapid onset (minutes) and is quickly distributed from the plasma to extracellular volume. Most clearance occurs as a result of liver and kidney metabolism, and a small portion of clearance is due to renal elimination. The half-life is brief (4-20 minutes), and AVP must therefore be given as a continuous intravenous infusion to maintain physiologic effects. The effects of the vasopressin system are mitigated when the sympathetic nervous system, the renin-angiotensin system (RAS), and the neurohormonal systems are intact. AVP release appears to be more tightly related to maintenance of circulating blood volume than to preserving arterial pressure. Severe increases in plasma AVP levels usually occur with profound hypotension, hemorrhagic shock, and cardiac arrest. Yet comparatively low AVP levels have been reported in patients with septic shock and in hemodynamically unstable organ donors, suggesting that clinical states of "relative vasopressin deficiency" may exist, and that these might respond to exogenous vasopressin administration. AVP has thus been relatively recently introduced in clinical practice as a vasopressor for several specific settings: intraoperative hypotension, vasodilatory shock, septic shock, and during CPR (see later). Adverse outcomes have included GI ischemia, renal ischemia, biventricular dysfunction,[57] reduced cardiac index, reduced total oxygen delivery, and reduced oxygen uptake.

Arginine vasopressin for cardiopulmonary resuscitation and shock. In both human and animal models, administration of exogenous AVP during CPR results in increased coronary perfusion pressure and improved resuscitation outcomes. Vasopressin is superior to epinephrine in increasing vital organ blood flow and improving resuscitation outcomes. The previous American Heart Association (AHA) Guidelines for CPR recommended either repeated 1-mg boluses of epinephrine or replacing the first or second dose of epinephrine with one bolus of 40 U of vasopressin or using vasopressin preferentially for asystole (see seventh edition Figs. 12-10 and 12-11). AVP has been used to treat hypotension after cardiopulmonary bypass, which appears to be associated with low circulating vasopressin levels. In doses of 0.1 U/min, vasopressin improves postcardiotomy shock in both adults and children.

Vaptans for hyponatremia. Two vasopressin antagonists ("vaptans") are now in the market for the treatment of euvolemic (Europe) or euvolemic and hypervolemic (United States) hyponatremia: conivaptan for intravenous use and tolvaptan for oral application. Both drugs are approved for (1) the treatment of hyponatremia caused by SIADH, and (2) hyponatremia caused by CHF and hepatic cirrhosis.[58] Gross and Wagner pose three questions.[59] (1) Do these drugs decrease the high mortality associated with hyponatremia? (2) Is it justifiable to use them to prevent relapse of hyponatremia in chronic SIADH? (3) Can the cost of chronic vaptan therapy be justified? They comment that the optimal vaptan regimen (dose, timing of controls) to treat SIADH is currently not established, nor is the best procedure to avoid over-rapid correction of chronic hyponatremia. Thus these authors "are hesitant to consider vaptans a treatment of choice (even) for the appropriate hyponatremias."

Conivaptan for hyponatremia in heart failure. Conivaptan (Vaprisol) is a renal V_2 receptor antagonist approved in the United States for treatment of *euvolemic hyponatremia* (serum sodium <135 mEq/L) in hospitalized patients with underlying heart failure. The expected clinical benefit of raising serum sodium might outweigh the increased risk of adverse events, including infusion site phlebitis, hypokalemia, headache, and neurologic deficits (from over-rapid correction of hyponatremia), although this hypothesis has not been adequately demonstrated in clinical trials. Dosing of conivaptan: an intravenous 20-mg loading dose over 30 minutes is followed if needed by a 20 mg continuous intravenous infusion over 24 hours. This may be titrated to 40 mg/day if serum sodium does not rise at the desired rate.

Tolvaptan for hyponatremia in heart failure. Tolvaptan (15-60 mg daily) is an oral V_2 antagonist that increased serum sodium on days 4 and 30 of administration in the SALT study.[60] In heart failure patients with signs of volume overload and on a low-sodium diet, tolvaptan monotherapy, without concomitant loop diuretic therapy, reduced body weight when compared with placebo without adverse changes in serum electrolytes, while on background medications including ACE inhibitors and β-blockers.[61] However, in the EVEREST study, despite short-term beneficial weight loss and mild improvement in dyspnea,[62] there was no long-term benefit on mortality or morbidity in heart failure.[63] The Food and Drug Administration (FDA)–approved indication is for hyponatremia (<125 mEq/L) that is symptomatic and resistant to fluid restriction. The black box warns against too-rapid correction that can cause osmotic demyelination.

Other vaptans. Other vaptans include mozavaptan, lixivaptan, and satavaptan, all acting on the V_2 receptor.

Future Directions

In addition to the new approaches noted previously, a number of intriguing therapeutic directions are currently under development. Therapies directed toward cardioprotection and *improved metabolic status* of the myocardium (e.g., pyruvate, etomoxir) are emerging as potential drugs for acute heart failure. Glucose-insulin-potassium (GIK) treatment was compared with placebo in 217 patients undergoing aortic valve replacement for critical aortic stenosis and evidence of LV hypertrophy.[64] GIK treatment reduced the incidence of low cardiac output (odds ratio, 0.22; P = 0.0001) and reduced inotrope use 6 to 12 hours postoperatively (odds ratio, 0.30; 95% confidence interval [CI], 0.15 to 0.60; P = 0.0007) and LV biopsies showed increased molecular markers of cardioprotection (adenosine monophosphate kinase, Akt phosphorylation, and O-linked N-acetylglucosamine [O-GlcNAc]-ylation of selected protein bands). Long-term studies are underway with this and other therapies to provide cardioprotection during acute heart failure. *Neurohumoral activation* includes activation of the inflammatory and immune system, as suggested by elevated levels of C-reactive protein, interleukin-6, and tissue plasminogen activator levels, all of which correlated with 180-day mortality.[65]

Novel Approaches to Increasing Cardiac Performance

As noted previously, all of the currently available inotropes and inodilators operate via a mechanism that increases intracellular cAMP and calcium with resultant increases in heart rate, myocardial oxygen demand with consequent increases in ischemia, arrhythmias, and death. Multiple new approaches have been developed to improve cardiac performance potentially without these liabilities. *Aliskiren,* the direct renin inhibitor, is under test in the ASTRONAUT study, the hypothesis being that it will oppose the abnormal neurohumoral abnormalities present in acute heart failure.

Direct activation of cardiac myosin is one promising approach. Two human studies report the effects of the cardiac myosin activator, *omecamtiv mecarbil,* in volunteers or in patients with systolic heart failure. The first-in-man (34 healthy men) study showed highly dose-dependent increased LV systolic function in response to intravenous omecamtiv mecarbil and supported potential clinical use of the drug in patients with heart failure.[39]

In an associated article on 45 patients with stable, guideline-treated systolic heart failure, intravenous omecamtiv mecarbil gave concentration-dependent increases in LV ejection time (up to an 80 ms) and stroke volume (up to 9.7 mL), with a small fall in heart rate (up to 2.7 beats per min; p < 0.0001 for all three measures). A dose-finding study in patients with acute heart failure (ATOMIC-AHF) is currently enrolling, and the high bioavailability of oral omecamtiv mecarbil indicates a potential use in chronic oral administration.[40]

Other potential new inotropic mechanisms include sodium-potassium-ATPase inhibition with SERCA activation (istaroxime), SERCA activation with vasodilation (nitroxyl donors such as CXL-1020), ryanodine receptor stabilization (S44121), and energetic modulation (etomoxir, pyruvate).[41]

Cardiogenic Shock

In cardiogenic shock the major goals are load reduction, preservation of cardiac function, and maintenance of an optimal BP so as to promote renal perfusion. Preload reduction by urgent reduction of pulmonary capillary pressure and right atrial filling pressure is sought along with a positive inotropic effect. Depending on the BP, the afterload might either have to be reduced by vasodilation, or sometimes increased by peripheral vasoconstriction. These aims can be achieved by a variety of intravenous inotropes, including dopamine, dobutamine, milrinone, and others. Some of these, such as high-dose dopamine and norepinephrine, cause α-mediated vasoconstriction to increase the BP in shocklike states. The inotropic dilators, such as milrinone, and low-dose dopamine, have a prominent vasodilator component to their inotropic action that is desired if the BP is relatively well maintained. Cardiogenic shock carries a poor prognosis despite the use of any or many drug treatments. Assist systems such as intraaortic balloon pumping (IABP-SHOCKII trial) are increasingly used and are under trial.

Chronic Heart Failure

Chronic heart failure differs from acute failure in the emphasis of therapy. In acute heart failure, the aim is to provide immediate symptomatic relief, and to rescue the patient from imminent and short-term cardiorespiratory death by optimizing the hemodynamic and neurohormonal status, and to prevent acute myocardial, renal, and other end organ damage. The emphasis is on agents given intravenously. In chronic heart failure, the objectives are to prevent chronic progressive damage to the myocardium (prevention), to prevent or reverse further enlargement of the heart (reverse remodeling), to improve the quality of life by relief of symptoms, and to prolong life. Reduction of hospitalization is an important goal for health providers because that is the major determinant of cost relating to the management of heart failure. The origin of symptoms in chronic heart failure is still not well understood.

Successive pivotal trials have now established, first, the disabling nature of conventionally treated CHF if left to run its natural course, and, second, that certain agents can partially reduce the increased mortality. The most effective drugs act largely by modulating the neurohumoral responses in heart failure (see Fig. 5-8). The key drugs are diuretics, ACE inhibitors, β-blockers, aldosterone inhibitors (spironolactone and eplerenone), and angiotensin receptor blockers (ARBs), as well as the combination of hydralazine and nitrates in select patients. Diuretics provide symptomatic relief from fluid overload. A second group of drugs comprises agents that have positive inotropic effects and generally increase cell cAMP and calcium levels, which tend to increase mortality. Most of these agents increase mortality in chronic heart failure probably as a result of worsening myocardial damage, promotion of apoptosis, and arrhythmogenesis. Digoxin has characteristics of both groups, because it both inhibits the neurohumoral response and has a positive inotropic effect. These properties might explain why it had an overall neutral effect on mortality in some studies.

Therapy of Chronic Severe Heart Failure

When the acute phase is over, the patient is often left with chronic severe heart failure that requires a different management policy. That policy is almost the same as in patients presenting initially with chronic heart failure. The diagnosis must be established with certainty, the causal factors determined, concomitant disease identified and treated, and an assessment of symptom severity and prognosis made. Symptomatic therapy is aimed at achieving optimal diuresis to treat or prevent sodium and water retention. The intention is to restore body fluid volumes and distribution to normal and not to over-diurese the patient. The disadvantageous neurohumoral response is inhibited by ACE inhibition, ARBs, β-blockade and aldosterone inhibitors (spironolactone or eplerenone) (see Fig. 5-8). Digoxin may be used for the control of heart rate in atrial fibrillation and might contribute in sinus rhythm by acting as a sympathoinhibitory agent (but see major reservations in "Digoxin in Perspective" later in this chapter). Drugs should be used in the lower doses effective in the major trials.

Current trends. Although the myocardium might be largely destroyed, symptomatic improvement is still possible using a judicious mixture of diuretics, ACE inhibition, β-adrenergic blockade, spironolactone-eplerenone, ARBs, and vasodilators such as isosorbide-hydralazine for selected patients (see Figs. 2-7 and 6-10). Overall, the strategy is to rest the feeble myocardium and to avoid stimulation. Drugs such as the ACE inhibitors, β-blockers, spironolactone-eplerenone, and isosorbide-hydralazine improve prognosis, whereas diuretics relieve fluid retention and dyspnea, and yet others may be harmful (Table 6-4). The most significant recent change to therapy of chronic heart failure is the increasing addition of aldosterone blockers after ACE inhibitors and β-blockers. Ivabradine may be emerging as another important additional therapy on top of the maximally tolerated three-drug regimen. Multiple other approaches are being investigated, including metabolic therapies (e.g., perhexiline and trimetazidine) and sildenafil (see Fig. 6-6). The many exciting recent advances in the domains of device and gene therapy are beyond the scope of this chapter.

Incremental therapy. Incremental therapy can counter the full downward evolution of progressive heart failure by matching drugs to the stage of heart failure (Table 6-5). Stage A is largely preventative. Stage B adds more active neurohumoral inhibition. Stage C includes diuretic therapy, aldosterone inhibitors, biventricular pacing (cardiac resynchronization therapy [CRT]) and implantable cardioverter defibrillators (ICDs) (see Fig. 8-16). Intervention increases in stage D to include left ventricular assist devices (LVADs) and heart transplantation, with the increasing exploration of stem-cell therapy.

Heart Failure: Therapy Specifics

General measures and lifestyle modification. General measures and lifestyle modification include mild salt restriction, water restriction in the presence of poor renal perfusion, and aspirin.[66] Warfarin gave equal overall benefit, with better reduction of stroke at the cost of more GI hemorrhage. Although periodic bed rest may be required to achieve optimal diuresis (the patient returning to bed for 1 to 2 hours of supine rest after taking the diuretic), in principle physical activity should be maintained; there is strong evidence that an exercise rehabilitation program should be undertaken if possible.[67] Exercise training for 12 months in those with well-treated chronic heart failure of median age 59 years was associated with modest 11%-15% reductions for both all-cause mortality or hospitalization, and cardiovascular mortality or heart failure hospitalization at 30 months.[68] There were similar modest reductions in patient-reported health status.[69] One of the most cost-effective of the new approaches to CHF is *home-based intervention* by a cardiac nurse, which reduced hospitalization and improved event-free survival.[70] Such home nursing visits give advice and support and oversee drug therapy, which is often very complex in advanced heart failure. A further example of the value of excellent nursing is the multidisciplinary nurse-coordinated

Table 6-4

Chronic Heart Failure: Drugs That Reduce Mortality, Improve Symptoms, or Might Harm

Reduce Mortality; Must Try to Use

1. ACE inhibitors or ARBs
2. β-blockers
3. Spironolactone or eplerenone
4. Isosorbide-hydralazine (well tested in black patients)

Improve Symptoms; Use According to Clinical Judgment

1. Diuretics
2. Nitrates
3. Iron for anemia
4. Metabolically active agents (if available: trimetazidine, perhexiline)
5. Ivabradine

May be Harmful; Use Cautiously after Due Consideration

1. Inotropes and inotropic dilators
2. Antiarrhythmics, except β-blockers and amiodarone
3. Calcium channel blockers
4. Digoxin, after checking levels of potassium and creatinine, only in low doses aiming at blood levels of 0.65-1.3 nmol/L (0.5-1 ng/mL). High-dose digoxin, with blood levels of 1.3 to 2.6 nmol/L (1-2 ng/mL), previously acceptable, no longer is.

ACE, Angiotensin-converting enzyme; *ARB,* angiotensin receptor blocker.
Table created by P.J. Commerford, modified by L.H. Opie.

Table 6-5

ACC-AHA Recommended Treatment of Chronic HF

STAGE A:
• Treat hypertension
• Quit smoking
• Treat lipids
• Exercise
• Discourage alcohol intake and illicit drug use
• ACE inhibitors or ARBs

↓ **Structural Heart Disease Develops**

STAGE B:
• Stage A therapy
• ACE inhibitors or ARBs
• β-blockers

↓ **Heart Failure Symptoms Develop**

STAGE C:
• Stage A therapy
• Diuretics
• ACE inhibitors or ARBs
• β-blockers
• Digoxin
• Aldosterone antagonist
• Hydralazine, nitrates
• Salt restriction
• Biventricular pacing, ICD

↓ **Refractory Symptoms at Rest**

STAGE D:
• Stage C therapy
• Mechanical assist devices
• Heart transplantation
• Continuous inotropic infusions
• Hospice care

ACC, American College of Cardiology; *ACE,* angiotensin-converting enzyme; *AHA,* American Heart Association; *ARB,* angiotensin receptor blocker; *HF,* heart failure; *ICD,* implantable cardiac defibrillator.

heart failure management program that reduced mortality risk and surrogate markers of well being.[71]

Advice should be given on flu immunization, alcohol consumption, cessation of smoking, sexual activity, diet, drug interactions, exercise, flying, lifestyle, and risk factors. *Anemia* is now recognized as an adverse risk prognostic factor[72] and may warrant therapy, as ongoing trials will assess the benefit of erythropoietin-stimulating agents and iron (see later).

Diuretic doses. Diuretic doses must be carefully adjusted to steer the course between optimal relief of edema and excess diuresis, polydiuresis, ionic disturbances, and prerenal azotemia. In older adults, excess use of diuretics can lead to tiredness and fatigue. Following the principle of sequential nephron blockade (see Fig. 4-2) combination diuretic therapy is often required and is usually more comfortable for patients. In those unusual patients who have severe heart failure with major reduction of the glomerular filtration rate (GFR; less than 15 to 20 mL/min), high doses of furosemide alone or more often combined with a thiazide diuretic are used. In severe fluid overload, intravenous loop diuretics may be used more often.[8,73] Metolazone is a powerful diuretic used in difficult resistant cases. Potassium-sparing diuretics, such as spironolactone and eplerenone, are often combined with those diuretics that do not spare potassium. In diuretic-resistant patients, first check for interacting drugs, especially nonsteroidal antiinflammatory drugs (see Fig. 4-5). Oral furosemide has variable absorption characteristics and occasionally the patient may benefit by a change to the better-absorbed torsemide.[74]

β-blockers. Historically coming after the ACE inhibitors, β-blockers have reduced mortality substantially. Standard heart failure therapy is diuretics, renin-angiotensin-aldosterone system (RAAS) inhibition, and β-blockers. In early heart failure β-blockade may be considered as early therapy, even before an ACE inhibitor,[75,76] the logic being that the earliest neurohumoral adaptation in is baroreflex-induced adrenergic stimulation (see Fig 5-8). The specific agents tested in chronic heart failure are bisoprolol (CIBIS I and II), metoprolol succinate (MERIT-HF), and carvedilol (US Carvedilol Study, Australia-New Zealand Study, COPERNICUS, and CAPRICORN), with doses as given in Table 1-2. Nebivolol given to older adults in heart failure reduced hospitalization but not mortality.[77] All patients with chronic heart failure and significantly reduced LV systolic function should be considered for a β-blocker. The patient should be hemodynamically stable when treatment is initiated. β-blockade is not a "rescue" treatment for more severe heart failure. Even class IV patients can substantially benefit from a β-blocker with improved morbidity and mortality, specifically carvedilol (COPERNICUS).[78] It is essential to start with a very low dose of the β-blocker, and then to titrate the dose upward slowly and steadily over many weeks. Incremental increases of dose should not be undertaken in less than 2 weeks. Doses should be titrated to the maximally tolerated dose up to the target doses from the relevant clinical trials (see Table 1-3). Many patients may have mild increases in fatigue with initiation of β-blockers, but this effect is usually transient and with proper counseling and preparation, they are generally well tolerated.[79]

Which β-blocker? The appropriate β-blocker remains under debate, but we are impressed with the overall positive data for carvedilol,[80] including its antioxidant properties.[81] At present the standard therapy is that a β-blocker is added to earlier treatment with an ACE inhibitor. However, given that increasing ACE inhibitor doses improved hospitalizations but had less effect on mortality,[82] whereas β-blocker in addition to ACE inhibitors had dramatic effects on reducing mortality, many clinicians initiate a low dose of ACE inhibitor followed by full up-titration of a β-blocker prior to up-titrating the ACE inhibitor. In addition, some emerging evidence suggests that the order of initial ACE inhibitor or β-blocker therapy may not matter.[75]

Added heart rate reduction: ivabradine. Higher heart rates are a risk factor for adverse outcomes in heart failure.[83] Ivabradine is a first-in-class specific inhibitor of the sinus node I_f current, which selectively decreases heart rate with no known off-target myocardial, vascular, or other adverse effects. This unique agent allowed the investigators of SHIFT to test the effect of solely reducing heart rate on outcomes. In the 6558-patient SHIFT study, ivabradine, added to standard therapy of chronic heart failure patients with a persistent heart rate of 70 bpm or higher, reduced the combined endpoint of cardiovascular death or hospital admission for heart failure (hazard ratio [HR] 0.82; CI: 0.75-0.90; $p < 0.0001$) compared with placebo, but had no significant effect on cardiovascular or all-cause mortality.[84] Ivabradine was titrated to a maximum of 7.5 mg twice daily. Side effects were excess bradycardia in 5% versus 1% of patients with placebo; visual side effects (phosphenes) occurred in 3% of patients versus 1% with placebo.

In the *Lancet* editorial, Teerlink expressed the concern that despite the admonitions of the SHIFT investigators, clinicians might be tempted to substitute ivabradine for β-blockers or fail to aggressively uptitrate β-blocker therapy prior to initiating ivabradine.[85] β-blockers have demonstrated marked improvement in survival in many trials with mortality risk reductions of 24%-65%, whereas ivabradine did not demonstrate improved survival in either the 10,917 patient BEAUTIFUL trial or in the 6558-patient SHIFT trial. These trial data suggest that β-blockers confer a survival benefit that may not be provided by ivabradine. Only 23% of the patients in SHIFT were at target dose and only half were receiving 50% or more of the targeted β-blocker dose. In a recent publication from SHIFT, it was noted that the beneficial effect of ivabradine progressively decreased in patients on increasing baseline doses of β-blocker, such that in the 1488 patients at target dose β-blocker, there was no benefit of ivabradine on the combined endpoint of cardiovascular mortality or heart failure hospitalization (HR 0.99, CI 0.79-1.24, $p = 0.91$) and certainly no indication of a beneficial effect on all-cause mortality (HR 1.08, 0.78-1.48, $p = 0.65$).[86] Therefore we agree that ivabradine should only be considered in patients in whom β-blocker therapy has been titrated to the maximally tolerated dose and who have a persistently elevated heart rate.

Heart rate and quality of life. In patients with systolic heart failure, a low health-related quality of life is associated with increased rates of cardiovascular death or hospital admissions for heart failure. In SHIFT, the magnitude of heart rate reduction with added ivabradine (about 10 bpm) was associated with an improved quality of life compared with placebo ($P < 0.001$).[87,88] Results from the small, unblinded CARVIVA-HF study suggest that ivabradine alone or in combination with carvedilol is safe and effective for improving exercise capacity and quality of life in heart failure patients on optimized ACE-inhibitor therapy.[89]

Registration of ivabradine in the European Union. On March 16, 2012, the European Union extended the indication of ivabradine to the treatment of chronic heart failure New York Heart Association (NYHA) classes II to IV with systolic dysfunction in patients in sinus rhythm whose heart rate is 75 bpm or more, in combination with standard therapy, including β-blockade, or when β-blockers are contraindicated or not tolerated.

Renin-angiotensin-aldosterone system inhibitors: ACE inhibitors, ARBs, and aldosterone blockade. *The key concept is that ACE inhibitors and β-blockers should be used or at least considered for use in* *all patients.* They should be titrated upward to the doses used in clinical trials unless hypotension or symptoms such as dizziness manifest themselves. When an ACE inhibitor is introduced for the first time to a patient already receiving high-dose diuretics (and therefore with intense renin-angiotensin activation), the diuretic dose must first be reduced and care taken to minimize or avoid first-dose hypotension. When an ACE inhibitor is truly not tolerated because of, for example, severe coughing, first ensure that worsening heart failure is not the cause of the cough, preferably with a rechallenge after complete resolution of the cough, and then change to an ARB on the basis of three large trials (CHARM, Val-HeFT, and VALIANT, see Chapter 5, p. 201). Aldosterone blockade is now increasing established as the next step to achieve dual RAAS inhibition. Pregnancy warnings against the use of all the RAAS blockers must be heeded.

Worsening renal function during renin-angiotensin system inhibition. In an editorial, Konstam points out, "It is reasonable to conclude that inhibiting the RAS reduces GFR through a mechanism that does not convey an adverse prognosis," based on the SOLVD (Studies of Left Ventricular Dysfunction) study, in which early reduction in GFR was associated with increased mortality within the placebo group but not in the enalapril group.[90] Greater survival benefit of enalapril versus placebo was observed in patients with early worsening of renal function, which suggests that "GFR reduction is a marker of greater RAS inhibitory effect with a resulting greater survival benefit." Thus modest reduction of GFR could be a marker of benefit rather than harm.

Aldosterone antagonism. *Spironolactone* reduces mortality in post-AMI class III and IV patients otherwise optimally treated.[91,92]

Eplerenone. Eplerenone causes less gynecomastia than spironolactone, yet with either agent added to ACE inhibition or ARB therapy, plasma potassium needs intense monitoring. The Eplerenone Post–Acute Myocardial Infarction Heart Failure Efficacy and Survival Study (EPHESUS) demonstrated that the addition of the low-dose mineralocorticoid receptor antagonist eplerenone to standard medical therapy in patients with AMI and heart failure with LV systolic dysfunction improved survival by 15%, with reductions in cardiovascular death, sudden death, and hospitalization for heart failure.[92] In EPHESUS, the doses were eplerenone 25 mg daily for the first month and up-titrated to 50 mg/day, with careful potassium monitoring, and great caution in the presence of renal failure. The mechanisms whereby eplerenone confers benefit on long-term survival and cardiovascular outcomes are independent from early potassium-sparing or diuretic effects, suggesting that mineralocorticoid receptor antagonism provides cardiovascular protection beyond its diuretic and potassium-sparing properties.[93]

EMPHASIS-HF trial. *In the EMPHASIS-HF trial* eplerenone was compared with placebo in well-treated patients with post-MI systolic heart failure (mean ejection fraction 26%) and mild symptoms.[94] Eplerenone reduced both the risk of all-cause death (HR 0.76, CI 0.62-0.93; P = 0.008) and the risk of hospitalization (HR 0.77; CI 0.76-0.88; P < 0.001) while carefully monitoring the serum potassium level (see Chapter 5, p. 159). Additionally, the incidence of new-onset atrial fibrillation or flutter was reduced.[95] Can eplerenone safely be given in post-MI heart failure without impairing renal function in heart failure with mild renal impairment? Despite a modest early decline in estimated glomerular filtration rate, eplerenone retained its prognostic benefits.[96]

The role of ARBs. ACE inhibitors are generally considered superior to ARBs for patients with CHF and LV systolic dysfunction (ELITE II, OPTIMAAL), and cost and length of clinical experience also favors ACE inhibitors. However, for ACE inhibitor–intolerant patients, there is strong evidence for an ARB, such as valsartan in the Val-HeFT trial,[97] and candesartan.[98] There is also strong evidence that the trial-tested ARB, candesartan, can be used in CHF patients who remain symptomatic on standard therapy such as ACE inhibitors and β-blockers in patients.[99]

Which RAAS blockers and when? There are now at least three ways in which the renin-angiotensin-aldosterone pathway may be inhibited: an ACE inhibitor, an ARB or aldosterone blockade, or various combinations of these. β-blockade also indirectly blocks the system. Which combination of drugs is best for which patient remains uncertain, as discussed in Chapter 5. The most difficult question relates to a patient already treated with diuretics, an ACE inhibitor, and a β-blocker. Should an ARB, an aldosterone antagonist, or both be added? Given that all three of the major outcomes trials with mineralocorticoid receptor antagonists (RALES, EPHESUS, EMPHASIS) demonstrated improved survival, the overall data and cost considerations usually decide in favor of aldosterone blockade. There is now emerging evidence for "quadruple therapy" (i.e., an ACE inhibitor, a β-blocker, spironolactone, and an ARB might benefit some carefully selected patients, but renal dysfunction and hyperkalemia must be strictly monitored). In addition, in self-identified black patients, isosorbide-hydralazine demonstrated significant reductions in all-cause mortality.[100]

Phosphodiesterase-5 inhibitors. PDE-5 inhibitors, best known for improving erectile function, also vasodilate the pulmonary and systemic vasculature (see Fig. 6-6). Initial evidence suggests that PDE-5 inhibitors benefit patients with CHF and secondary pulmonary hypertension (PH). "Cumulative data indicate that inhibition of PDE-5 is a promising approach for the treatment of ventricular remodeling induced by pressure or volume overload and heart failure."[101] In seven small trials on CHF, on a total of 199 patients, there were consistent improvements in measures such as the cardiac index.[102] In one of the trials depression score decreased and quality of life improved. However, there are no large-scale, long-term placebo-controlled trials.

Digoxin. Digoxin, as considered in detail later in this chapter, is no longer regarded as an essential drug but rather an optional choice, only carefully and selectively given in lower doses than before, on the grounds that it may give symptomatic improvement. Its many drug interactions and contradictions also limit its use. To achieve heart rate reduction beyond that obtained by β-blockade, ivabradine is a safer choice.[103]

Antiarrhythmics. Antiarrhythmics may be required. Ventricular tachyarrhythmias are a major cause of fatalities in CHF. It is important to avoid predisposing factors such as hypokalemia, digoxin excess, or chronic use of PDE inhibitors. Class I agents should be avoided. Long-term amiodarone may be considered in a low dose, and where there are facilities and there are good indications, an ICD may be chosen (see Fig. 8-16). Atrial fibrillation is a common and serious problem, and requires one of two policies: either conversion to sinus rhythm and thereafter probably low-dose amiodarone, or rate control both at rest and during exercise (see Fig. 8-13). The AF-CHF trial demonstrated that a rhythm-control strategy or the presence of sinus rhythm were not associated with better outcomes in 1376 patients with atrial fibrillation and CHF,[104] so many clinicians opt for a rate-control strategy. β-blockers, digoxin, and amiodarone are commonly used for these effects, whereas CCBs are relatively contraindicated because of their negative inotropic properties.

Short-term inotropic support. Short-term inotropic support by sympathomimetics or inotropic dilators cannot be lightly undertaken. Yet milrinone or others may give dramatic symptomatic relief as a rescue operation, when inotropic support is essential. In patients with exacerbation of heart failure, and not needing urgent inotropic or pressor support, there may be modest benefit at the risk of adverse effects.

Vasodilator therapy. In patients who remain symptomatic despite full therapy (diuretics, ACE inhibitors, β-blockers, spironolactone, ARBs, and probably digoxin) isosorbide dinitrate with hydralazine is worth trying. The FDA approved the combination of isosorbide dinitrate and hydralazine as add-on treatment for CHF in self-defined black subjects, largely on the basis of the 43% reduction in all-cause mortality among the 1050 self-identified blacks in the A-HeFT trial.[100] Whether this combination in addition to standard therapy is effective in non-black populations has not been directly tested. *Hydralazine* is predominantly an arteriolar dilator probably acting as a vascular potassium channel opener. Hydralazine may potentiate nitrates by retarding the development of nitrate tolerance (see Fig. 2-7). The role of hydralazine alone in heart failure patients already treated by diuretics, ACE inhibitors, and other effective agents is not clear and not recommended.

Novel drugs. *Aquaretics* or "vaptans" antagonize the vasopressin type 2 receptors in the kidney, thereby promoting free water clearance and lessening hyponatremia (see Fig. 4-5). In the long term, their use has been relatively disappointing (see Chapter 4, p. 107). *Perhexiline* acts metabolically to inhibit adverse myocardial fatty acid oxidation, but requires monitoring of blood levels to avoid hepatic or neural toxicity.[105] Perhexiline may be particularly useful in patients with both refractory angina and heart failure.[106] *Trimetazidine,* another partial fatty acid inhibitor that has minimal side effects and is available in some European countries, improves LV function and insulin sensitivity in idiopathic dilated or ischemic cardiomyopathy.[107] Other reports show benefit in ischemic or diabetic cardiomyopathy,[108] and a recent meta-analysis of 884 patients suggested beneficial effects on multiple clinical outcomes, including LV remodeling.[109] *Sildenafil,* already erotically famous, is emerging under another guise as a possible aid to the failing myocardium by increasing cyclic GMP (see Fig. 6-6). *Pentoxyfylline* is a complex agent that decreases the synthesis of tumor necrosis factor–α (TNFα) and improves the ejection fraction, yet it also has PDE activity and outcome data are missing.[110] Vasopressin (ADH) antagonists are logical, but the results with *tolvaptan* in the EVEREST trial were disappointing in terms of their ability to improve long-term outcomes.[62,63] Many other agents to improve cardiac performance are under investigation as well.[41] Of these prospects, the only agents that are already available and licensed, albeit not for use in CHF, are tolvaptan, pentoxifylline, and sildenafil. Those that should work but have been disappointing include (1) endothelin (ET) antagonists, which should unload the heart by vasodilation and improve coronary endothelial integrity; and (2) cytokine antagonists, including etanercept that decoys TNFα from its receptor.

Gene therapy. Impaired contraction is now firmly established as a key feature of advanced heart failure, so that the current interest in upregulation of the cardiac sarcoendoplasmic calcium-transporting ATPase (SERCA2a) is clinically relevant (see Fig. 6-8).[111] SERCA2a has been upregulated in human heart failure by adeno-associated virus type 1/SERCA transfer delivered by antegrade epicardial coronary artery infusion with clear benefit over 12 months in a small phase 2 human trial.[112] Furthermore, there is now the theoretical possibility of molecular upregulation of SERCA2 by SUMOylation, in which SUMO represents the small ubiquitin-related modifier type 1.[113]

Stem cell therapy. An initial study suggests that intracoronary infusion of autologous cardiac stem cells improves LV systolic function and

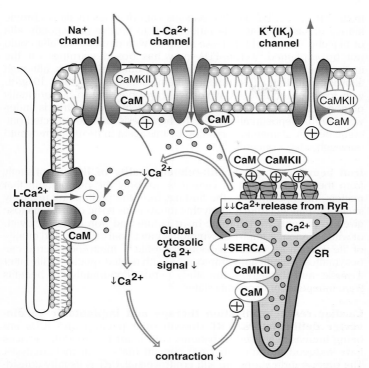

Figure 6-8   Gene therapy to promote intracellular calcium ion movements in heart failure. Sites of action. The regulation of Ca^{2+} changes in heart failure from the normal pattern (see Fig. 1-1) to a diminished and restricted flow of Ca^{2+}. Gene therapy, still in early development, aims to upregulate the activity of sarcoplasmic endoplasmic reticulum calcium-ATPase (SERCA), the key enzyme in regulation of Ca^{2+} uptake into the sarcoplasmic reticulum (SR), hence increasing release of Ca^{2+} from the SR into the cytosol via the ryanodine receptors (RyR). The overall effect is to enhance the Ca^{2+} signal to contraction. Upregulation of SERCA by gene therapy *would not* directly correct other ion abnormalities, such as diminished Ca^{2+} entry via the L-calcium channel, the enhanced entry of sodium ions, and increased potassium ion loss. Thus far there is no specific therapy to correct these ionic abnormalities. For acute heart failure, the catecholamine inotropes (see Fig. 6-4) and inodilators (see Fig. 6-6) increase the depleted intracellular Ca^{2+} stores. For chronic HF, β-blockers (see Figs. 1-7 and 1-8) and ivabradine act by totally different ionic currents to reduce calcium ion influx, therefore being additive in effects (see Fig. 8-4). Digoxin also acts differently to inhibit the sodium-potassium pump followed by sodium-Ca^{2+} exchange to increase intracellular Ca^{2+}, thus indirectly promoting contractility with an added and separate vagomimetic effect (see Fig. 6-11). (Figure © L.H. Opie, 2012.)

reduces infarct size in patients with heart failure after MI,[114] and another study using intracoronary autologous cardiosphere-derived cells demonstrated reductions in scar mass, increases in viable heart mass and regional contractility, and regional systolic wall thickening, but no associated changes in ventricular volumes.[115] Additional studies with mesenchymal precursor cells have also been encouraging, so that further larger, phase 2 studies with these different approaches will follow.

Therapy of anemia: erythropoietin-stimulating agents. Chronic heart failure is often accompanied by anemia, which may be a new therapeutic target in heart failure. Intravenous iron, erythropoietin, and erythropoietin-stimulating agents such as darbepoetin alfa can increase hemoglobin, but that in itself gives no clinical benefit.[116] In some, ACE inhibition contributes or even causes the anemia (see Chapter 5, p. 133).

In the TREAT STUDY on 4038 patients with diabetes mellitus, chronic kidney disease, and anemia randomized to receive darbepoetin alfa or placebo, the twofold increase in stroke with darbepoetin alfa could not be explained.[117] The FDA now has boxed warnings on the erythropoietin-stimulating agents pointing out the dangers, although allowing initiation of treatment if hemoglobin is less than 10 g/dL, with focus on transfusion avoidance, corresponding to the originally demonstrated benefit approved in 1989. Nonetheless, one trial is underway with darbepoetin alfa to test the hypothesis that the expected outcome benefit of anemia correction by this agent in heart failure would outweigh safety concerns.[118]

Iron hemostasis and health-related quality of life. Surprisingly, from the patients' point of view, it is not only the hemoglobin that matters. More positive are the findings from the preliminary, relatively small, 459-patient FAIR-HF study that intravenous ferric carboxymaltose given to patients with chronic heart failure and iron deficiency, with or without anemia, improves symptoms, functional capacity, and quality of life with an acceptable side-effect profile.[119] Intravenous ferric carboxymaltose significantly improved health-related quality of life after 4 weeks and throughout the study period. Importantly, the benefits were independent of anemia status.[120]

Cardiac resynchronization therapy and implantable cardioverter defibrillators. CRT (biventricular pacing) and ICDs are being increasingly used in patients with heart failure. Both devices have reduced mortality in large clinical trials or in metaanalyses. The precise indications are still controversial. CRT is usually considered when there is QRS prolongation as a sign of impaired intraventricular conduction. These treatments may be life-saving but are expensive, which raises serious problems in relation to national medical budgets.

Cardiac surgery. Cardiac surgery must be considered when valve defects are present, there is clear evidence of myocardial ischemia, or a remodeling procedure is indicated. The utility of ventricular reconstruction surgery remains debated, although the results of the hypothesis 2 component of the STICH trial suggests that this role may be very limited.[121] The hypothesis 1 component of STICH also suggested that there was no significant difference between medical therapy alone and medical therapy plus coronary artery bypass graft (CABG) with respect to death from any cause in patients with coronary artery disease and LV dysfunction.[122] Furthermore, the assessment of myocardial viability did not identify patients with a differential survival benefit from CABG, as compared with medical therapy alone.[123]

Last resorts. Severe heart failure refractory to furosemide may benefit from *extracorporeal ultrafiltration* for the removal of intravascular fluid.[124] *Cardiac transplantation* or *destination therapy with an LVAD* are measures of last resort, although better outcomes are emerging with improved technologies[125,126] and better patient selection.[127] The number of transplants is falling partly because of the lack of donors and the improvement of medical and device therapy. The indications are now more stringent than previously. There are no controlled trials of transplantation. Mechanical assist devices are also being considered for lifetime treatment.

Maximal Heart Failure Therapy Summarized

As the severity of heart failure progresses, so does the need for established and novel therapies (Fig. 6-9). Fully fledged heart disease is a complex phenomenon, starting with the heart and involving the lungs,

Progressive chronic heart failure, NYHA classes

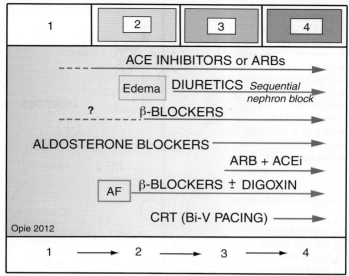

Figure 6-9 Schematic therapy of progressive chronic heart failure. Note early use of angiotensin converting enzyme (ACE) inhibitors, and increasingly early use of β-blockers. The role of diuretics is fundamental in relief of edema and fluid retention, using the principle of sequential nephron block. Angiotensin receptor blocker (ARB) + ACE inhibitor (ACEi): the combination of these agents was used in some trials with benefit. However, this combination is controversial. Cardiac resynchronization therapy (CRT), also called *biventricular* (Bi-V) pacing, is used later. *AF,* Atrial fibrillation; *NYHA,* New York Heart Association class of severity of heart failure. (Figure © L.H. Opie, 2012.)

the kidneys, and the peripheral vasculature (Fig. 6-10). Maximal therapy includes both the established therapies as shown on the top left of Fig. 6-10, with the novel therapies below. Of the latter, the I_f blocker ivabradine is approved for addition to β-blockade in the European Union for patients with a persistent tachycardia. Specific drugs are required to act on pulmonary edema (see "Acute Heart Failure" earlier in chapter), the kidneys, and the peripheral arteries. For the latter two sites of therapy, RAAS blockade remains fundamental.

Digoxin in Perspective

The combined inotropic-bradycardic actions of digoxin (Fig. 6-11) are unique when compared with the many sympathomimetic inotropes that all tend to cause tachycardia. Besides its weak positive inotropic effect, it slows the ventricular rate, which allows better ventricular filling in CHF, especially with atrial fibrillation. Digoxin also decreases the sympathetic drive generated by the failing circulation, which provides a rationale for its use in CHF in sinus rhythm. Nonetheless, this use is now controversial, especially because a trial on 6800 patients failed to show any mortality benefit for digoxin, despite the absence of treatment with β-blockers, aldosterone antagonists, and devices.[128] Consequently, its use in sinus rhythm remains optional and controversial with some strong arguments against its use.[129] The optimal use of digoxin requires a thorough knowledge of the multiple factors governing its efficacy and toxicity, including numerous drug interactions. Because the effects of digoxin in the acutely ill patient with hypoxia and electrolyte disturbances are often difficult to predict and because there is a lack of evidence of efficacy, digoxin is now very seldom justified in acute heart failure and is much less used in chronic heart failure.

MAXIMAL THERAPY FOR SEVERE CHF

Opie 2012

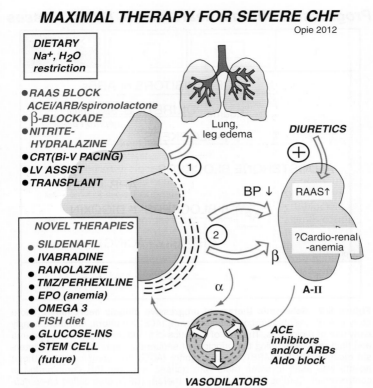

Figure 6-10 Principles of maximum therapy for congestive heart failure (CHF). Diuretics are given for back pressure into the lungs with edema (1) yet stimulate the renin-angiotensin-aldosterone system (RAAS). Poor left ventricular (LV) function also activates this system (2) by a low blood pressure with decreased renal perfusion or by reflex β-adrenergic (β) baroreceptor activation. Vasoconstriction results from formation of angiotensin-II (A-II) or from α-adrenergic activity. Logically, angiotensin-converting enzyme inhibitors (ACEi) and angiotensin receptor blockers (ARBs) are an integral part of the therapy, as are β-blockers. Aldosterone (Aldo) blockers are also essential. Among other therapies, ivabradine is the best tested. Nitrate-hydralazine benefited self-declared black patients in the United States, but may well relieve vasoconstriction in others. Trimetazidine (TMZ) and perhexiline inhibit myocardial fatty acid oxidation to improve ejection fraction. Sildenafil should help by increasing cyclic guanosine monophosphate (see Fig. 6-7). Biventricular pacing (Bi-V), also called *cardiac resynchronization therapy* (CRT), is especially used when there is delayed ventricular conduction (long QRS). LV assist devices are regarded as a bridge to transplantation. Stem cells are for the future. (Figure © L,H, Opie, 2012.)

Nonetheless it remains the only drug for chronic heart failure that inhibits the sodium pump.

Sodium pump inhibition. Sodium pump inhibition explains the myocardial cellular effect of digitalis. As the sodium pump (Na/K-ATPase) is inhibited, there is a transient increase in intracellular sodium close to the sarcolemma, which in turn promotes calcium influx by the sodium-calcium exchange mechanism to enhance myocardial contractility (Fig. 6-11), with arrhythmogenic risk. However, digoxin is still inotropic at lower doses and blood levels than previously standard.[130-132]

Direct calcium uptake. Digoxin toxicity, studied with digitoxin, promotes calcium entry into heart cells though new transmembrane calcium channels.[133]

INOTROPIC, VAGAL AND SYMPATHETIC EFFECTS OF DIGOXIN

Opie 2012

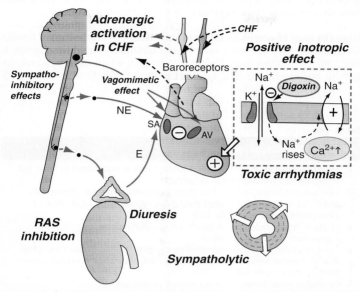

Figure 6-11   Digoxin has both neural and myocardial cellular effects. The inotropic effect of digoxin is due to inhibition of the sodium pump in myocardial cells. Slowing of the heart rate and inhibition of the atrioventricular (AV) node by vagal stimulation and the decreased sympathetic nerve discharge are important therapeutic benefits. Toxic arrhythmias are less well understood, but may be caused by calcium-dependent afterpotentials. *CHF,* Congestive heart failure; *E,* epinephrine; *NE,* norepinephrine; *RAS,* renin-angiotensin system; *SA,* sinoatrial. (Figure © L.H. Opie, 2012.)

Autonomic and renin-angiotensin effects. Sinus slowing and atrioventricular (AV) nodal inhibition results from *parasympathetic activation.* A modest direct depression of nodal tissue may account for those effects of digoxin still found after vagal blockade. The action of digoxin on AV conduction, which it slows, and on the AV refractory period, which it prolongs, is primarily dependent on increased vagal tone, rather than the direct effect of digoxin. Part of the toxic symptoms of digitalis may be explained by parasympathomimetic effects, such as nausea, vomiting, and anorexia. *Sympathetic inhibition* may play an important role in the effects of digitalis in CHF. Digitalis inhibits sympathetic nerve discharge, an effect that occurs before any observed hemodynamic changes.[131] *Renin release* from the kidney is inhibited because digoxin decreases the activity of the renal sodium pump with a natriuretic effect. Less renin release should lead to vasodilation to help offset the direct vasoconstrictor mechanism of digoxin.

Pharmacokinetics of digoxin (Table 6-6). The serum half-life of digoxin is 1.5 days. Approximately one third of the body stores are lost daily, mostly as unchanged digoxin by the kidneys. Approximately 30% is excreted by nonrenal routes (stools, hepatic metabolism) in those with normal renal function. In digitalized subjects, approximately half of the digoxin is bound to skeletal muscle receptors accounting (with blood) for most of the volume of distribution. The "fit" between digitalis and the receptor is much less "tight" for skeletal muscle than for the myocardium, which remains the major site of action. Multiple pharmacokinetic factors influence the blood level obtained with a given dose of digoxin (see Tables 6-6 and 6-7 in Drugs for the Heart, 7th edition) and the sensitivity to digoxin (Table 6-7). In *renal impairment*, excretion is decreased and the maintenance dose is lower. The loading dose may also be lower (next section).

Digoxin use: changes in clinical practice. (1) *Chronic atrial fibrillation without overt CHF* may now be the condition for which digoxin is probably most often used. Unfortunately even when used by cardiologists in well-organized trial studies for atrial fibrillation, as in PALLAS,

Table 6-6

Digoxin Pharmacokinetics

1. Rapid absorption of 75% of oral dose; the rest is inactivated in lower gut to digoxin reduction products by bacteria.
2. Circulates in blood, unbound to plasma proteins; previous "therapeutic level" 1-2 ng/mL, current ideal level 0.5-1 ng/mL* (0.65-1.3 nmol/L); blood half-life approximately 36 h.
3. Binds to tissue receptors in heart and skeletal muscle.
4. Lipid-soluble; brain penetration.
5. Most of absorbed digoxin excreted unchanged in urine (tubular excretion and glomerular filtration). Approximately 30% undergoes nonrenal clearance, more in renal failure.
6. In chronic renal failure, reduced volume of distribution.
7. With small lean body mass, reduced total binding to skeletal muscle.

*Optimal range 0.5 to 0.8 ng/mL in men.[136]

Table 6-7

Factors Altering Sensitivity to Digoxin at Apparently Therapeutic Levels

Physiologic effects

Enhanced vagal tone (increased digoxin effect on SA and AV nodes)
Enhanced sympathetic tone (opposite to vagal effect)

Systemic factors or disorders

Renal failure (reduced volume of distribution and excretion)
Low lean body mass (reduced binding to skeletal muscle)
Chronic pulmonary disease (hypoxia, acid-base changes)
Myxedema (? prolonged half-life)
Acute hypoxemia (sensitizes to digitalis arrhythmias)

Electrolyte disorders

Hypokalemia (most common; sensitizes to toxic effects)
Hyperkalemia (protects from digitalis arrhythmias)
Hypomagnesemia (caused by chronic diuretics; sensitizes to toxic effects)
Hypercalcemia (increases sensitivity to digitalis)
Hypocalcemia (decreases sensitivity)

Cardiac disorders

Acute myocardial infarction (may cause increased sensitivity)
Acute rheumatic or viral carditis (danger of conduction block)
Thyrotoxic heart disease (decreased sensitivity)

Concomitant drug therapy

Diuretics with K+ loss (increased sensitivity via hypokalemia)
Drugs with added effects on SA or AV nodes (verapamil, diltiazem, β-blockers, clonidine, methyldopa, or amiodarone)

AV, Atrioventricular; *SA,* sinoatrial.

the mean levels were in the toxic range and could, hypothetically, have contributed to a higher incidence of heart failure.[134] Digoxin may be combined with verapamil, diltiazem, or β-blocking drugs to control the ventricular rate during exercise. However, note that the optimal heart rate remains moot. Note the verapamil-digoxin interaction whereby verapamil decreases nonrenal clearance. (2) In *chronic atrial fibrillation with heart failure* there are no good outcome studies[129] so that its dosage and effects are still judged clinically. A logical combination is with a β-blocker that not only slows the ventricular rate but improves exercise tolerance and the ejection fraction.[135] Note the absence of any hard event outcome data. (3) In *CHF with sinus rhythm* the limited benefits found in the large DIG trial,[128,136] the very narrow therapeutic-toxic window,[130] and numerous drug interactions (see Tables 6-6 and 6-7 in Drugs for the Heart, 7th edition) have cast major doubts on the ideal dose and blood levels. *These problems have relegated digoxin to an optional and potentially dangerous extra in the management of CHF*, if not carefully given in lower doses than before. In 2009 the American College of Cardiology and AHA gave digitalis a level of evidence B, but this appears not to be based on any current outcome trial. Digitalis can be beneficial in patients with current or prior symptoms of heart failure and reduced LV ejection fraction to decrease hospitalizations for heart failure.[137] Note that the hard data for the benefits of heart rate reduction in heart failure are strong for ivabradine (see page 195) and weak for digoxin.

Digoxin for ambulatory patients. Going back to data based on the DIG trial 1997, in ambulatory patients with chronic heart failure and low serum digoxin concentrations (SDCs), mortality and hospitalizations were reduced.[138] Low-dose digoxin (< or = 0.125 mg/day) was the strongest independent predictor of low SDC (adjusted odds ratio, 2.07; 95% CI 1.54-2.80). Thus digoxin in a lower dose might be best for those already on it, or for those who cannot access effective modern agents.

Digoxin not for advanced heart failure. In patients with advanced heart failure referred for cardiac transplantation and otherwise optimally treated, digoxin was associated with a higher risk for the primary outcomes (chiefly death) with a hazard ratio 2.28 (p < 0.001). There was deterioration in major outcomes (combined death, urgent transplant or insertion of LV assist device) and increased hospitalization rates.[139]

Doses and blood levels of digoxin. There is general agreement that the therapeutic-toxic window of digoxin is narrow. Previously, the ideal blood level was pragmatically regarded as 1-2 ng/mL (1.3-2.6 nmol/L). Currently lower doses and lower blood levels are finding strong spokesmen. Supportive data come from a retrospective analysis of the large DIG trial on 3782 heart failure patients followed up for 3 years.[136] All-cause mortality was modestly decreased, albeit by only 6% in the tertile with digoxin levels in the previously "low" range, 0.5 to 0.8 ng/mL or 0.6 to 1 nmol/L. The next tertile of digoxin levels (0.9-1.1 ng/mL) had no effect on mortality, whereas higher levels (1.2 ng/mL or more) were associated with a mortality increase of 12%.[136] *The hypothesis, based on the "old" trials, is that digoxin has bidirectional effects on mortality, with the "turn around" level being approximately 1 ng/mL,*[130] giving a practical therapeutic range of 0.5 to 1.0 ng/mL (Fig. 6-12).

Digitalization. First check renal function and then consider the age of the patient. Currently the trend is toward lower digoxin dose, commonly initiated at 0.25 mg per day, followed by 0.125 mg daily, and even lower doses if the patient is older than 70 years old or in renal impairment.[26] *Blood digoxin levels* are still valuable to allow for variable GI absorption, variable cardiac responses, and possible drug interactions.

PRESENT and PAST TOXIC DIGOXIN LEVELS

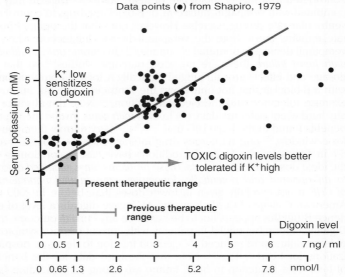

Figure 6-12   Possible therapeutic and toxic serum digoxin levels. As the serum potassium falls, the heart is sensitized to the arrhythmias of digitalis toxicity. Conversely, as the serum potassium rises, a higher serum digoxin level is tolerated. Note current lower "therapeutic" levels of digoxin. There are no good prospective data linking digoxin levels to outcome. (Potassium data modified from Shapiro W. *Am J Cardiol* 1978;41:852–859.)

Steady-state plasma and tissue concentrations are achieved in 5 to 7 days.

Digoxin contraindications. Contraindications include *hypertrophic obstructive cardiomyopathy,* some cases of *Wolff-Parkinson-White syndrome* with atrial fibrillation (see Fig. 8-14), significant *AV nodal heart block, and diastolic dysfunction.* Relative contraindications are *renal failure* and *older age* (reduce doses).

Digoxin in women. In the DIG trial, only 22% of participants were women, in whom there was an unexplained increased 23% risk of all-cause mortality.[140] Speculatively, the authors thought that there could be a renal interaction with hormone replacement therapy, commonly used at that time.

Digoxin and breast cancer. Two studies show an increased risk of breast cancer with digoxin use in women. The larger study relates to use at any time,[141] and the other to continuous use for at least 2 years and to invasive cancer.[142]

Digoxin in older adults. Decreased skeletal muscle, lean body mass, and renal function increase digoxin levels (see Table 6-7). Digoxin half-life may be prolonged up to 73 hours, depending on renal function. The *digoxin dose* is often lower than 0.125 mg daily, such as 0.125 mg every second day. The exact dose required can be calculated from the total body weight, serum creatinine, age, presence of heart failure, concomitant CCBs (verapamil, diltiazem, or nifedipine), gender, and trough digoxin concentration.[143]

Drug interactions. The most recent interaction is a potentially lethal interaction with dronaderone.[134] The *verapamil-digoxin* interaction is also important, with blood digoxin levels rising by approximately 50% to 75%. *Amiodarone* and *propafenone* (for Amiodarone see p. 289; for propafenone see p. 284) also elevate serum digoxin levels. *Diuretics* may induce hypokalemia, which (1) sensitizes the heart to digoxin toxicity (see Fig. 6-12), and (2) shuts off the tubular secretion of digoxin when the plasma potassium falls to below 2-3 mEq/L.

Digoxin toxicity. In April 2008, 800 million digoxin tablets (Digitek) were recalled by the manufacturer as possibly containing double the labeled amount of drug.[144] The typical patient with digoxin toxicity (see Table 6-7) is an older adult woman with advanced heart disease and bradycardia, and abnormal renal function.[145] Hypokalemia is common (see Fig. 6-10). Digitalis toxicity should be considered in any patient receiving digoxin who presents with new GI, ocular, or central nervous system complaints, or new arrhythmia or AV conduction disturbance. The *cellular mechanism* of toxicity includes (1) intracellular calcium overload that predisposes to calcium-dependent delayed afterdepolarizations (see Fig. 6-11); (2) excess vagal stimulation, predisposing to sinus bradycardia and AV block; and (3) an added "direct" depressive effect of digoxin on nodal tissue.

   Treatment of digoxin toxicity. The diagnosis of digoxin toxicity is confirmed if the digoxin blood level is inappropriately high for the patient in the presence of suspicious clinical features. With only suggestive symptoms, *withdrawal of digoxin* is sufficient while awaiting confirmation by elevated plasma levels. With dangerous arrhythmias and a low plasma potassium, potassium chloride may be infused intravenously very cautiously as 30 to 40 mEq in 20 to 50 mL of saline at 0.5 to 1 mEq/min into a large vein through a plastic catheter (infiltration of potassium solution can cause tissue necrosis and infusion into small veins causes local irritation and pain). *Phenytoin* reverses high-degree AV block, possibly acting centrally. *Dose:* Stop β-blockers and any drugs elevating the blood digoxin levels (verapamil). Because of its very long half-life, don't stop amiodarone. *Oral potassium* (4 to 6 g potassium chloride, 50 to 80 mEq) may be given orally in divided doses when arrhythmias are not urgent (e.g., premature ventricular contractions). Potassium is contraindicated if AV conduction block or hyperkalemia are present, because potassium further increases AV block. *Activated charcoal* (50 to 100 g) enhances GI clearance of digoxin. *Cholestyramine* has a similar but less powerful effect.

   Digoxin-specific antibodies (Digibind). Digoxin-specific antibodies (Digibind) can be strikingly effective therapy for life-threatening digoxin intoxication, especially when there is severe ventricular tachycardia or significant hyperkalemia (>5.5 mEq/L). To calculate doses, work out the total body digoxin load from the blood level; each vial binds approximately 0.5 mg of digoxin.

Digoxin: Summary. Digoxin is an extremely complex drug with unique properties and is increasingly seen as having a limited role that requires expert initiation and supervision.

Heart Failure With Preserved Systolic Function: Diastolic Heart Failure

Definitions. In standard descriptions of heart failure therapy, it is often forgotten that approximately half of those with clinical heart failure are not suffering from predominant heart failure with reduced systolic function (HFrEF), but rather systolic function is relatively preserved and diastolic failure dominates. The current term for this situation is *heart failure with preserved ejection fraction* (HF-Preserved EF, or HFpEF), which, however, gives no mechanistic insight. The definition of preserved ejection fraction varies, often being equal to or more than 50%,[146] but different cut-off values are taken in various studies, such as 45%,[147] 40%,[148] or even 35%.[149] Overall, the condition is serious, with a long-term prognosis very similar to that of systolic failure.[146,150] Besides the problem of the differing levels of ejection fraction for diagnosis, there are no accepted mechanistic explanations. Those proposed include increased muscle stiffness (as, for example, from fibrosis) with greater sensitivity to volume overload, and LV remodeling and dilation with volume-dependent increased LV filling pressures.[151]

The closely related condition of *diastolic heart failure* is a syndrome with signs and symptoms of heart failure, which in addition has echocardiographic evidence of LV diastolic dysfunction,[152] thus being more precise. For example, in a subset of patients with HFpEF in the CHARM-preserved study with a mean ejection fraction of 50%, one-third did not have objective diastolic dysfunction, suggesting a deficiency in either the specificity of the clinical criteria or the sensitivity of the echocardiographic criteria, or some combination. Moderate and severe diastolic dysfunction were important predictors of adverse outcome in less than one half of these patients.[153] Conversely, diastolic dysfunction even in the absence of heart failure is also a serious condition. It progresses to a combined incidence of mortality and overt heart failure of 20% over 3 years.[152] To diagnose diastolic dysfunction requires expert echocardiography, including at least mitral valve and pulmonary vein inflow pattern by pulse-wave Doppler and mitral annular velocities by tissue Doppler imaging.

The pathophysiologic characteristics of HFpEF is incompletely understood. In patients with clinical diastolic heart failure (DHF), there were significant abnormalities in LV relaxation and increased LV chamber stiffness as assessed by invasive hemodynamics and echocardiography.[154] Magnetic resonance imaging (MRI) studies confirm that concentric geometry and hypertrophy resulting from LV systolic pressure overload as in hypertension is one underlying cause of left ventricular hypertrophy with preserved ejection fraction.[155] In a group of older adult patients with concentric hypertrophy with heart failure at the start, only 25% developed LV systolic dysfunction over 7 years.[156] Those with heart failure and preserved ejection fractions have more noncardiac comorbidities (four on average) and *more* noncardiovascular hospitalizations and fewer heart failure–related hospitalizations than those with reduced ejection fraction.[157] Non–heart failure hospitalizations, which dominate, are three times greater in patients with HFpEF. The strong implication is that all these comorbidities, which may be the chief problem, need assessment and therapy.[157]

Incidence. HFpEF is the most common form of HF in the population, being dominant among older adults.[157] HFpEF is more common in older adults and in women and is becoming more common as the population ages.[146] The major predisposing causes are obesity, hypertension, coronary artery disease, and diabetes.[146,148,150] Obesity leading to hypertension and hypertensive heart failure is of particular importance in black patients.[158] In those black patients presenting with hypertension, the mean LV ejection fraction was 55%, and diastolic dysfunction was echocardiographically diagnosed in 24%.[159] The 10-year analysis from the Copenhagen Hospital Heart Failure study showed that among patients with a clinical diagnosis of heart failure, 61% had a preserved ejection fraction,[160] but when the added requirement for heart failure diagnosis was an elevated N-terminal pro B-type natriuretic peptide (NT-proBNP), only 29% had "true" HFpEF.

Therapy. The underlying cause should be vigorously treated (control hypertension, prevent myocardial ischemia, reduce LV hypertrophy) and particular attention paid to the avoidance of tachycardia and the control or prevention of atrial fibrillation. Fluid retention is treated with diuretics, but then what? Treatment strategies for HFpEF remain unproven despite several large-scale trials. Holland et al. undertook a metaanalysis of the effects of pharmacologic interventions on exercise capacity, diastolic function, and mortality in 20 randomized controlled trials, with β-blockers (7); ACE inhibitors (8); CCBs (2); and one each of statins, diuretics, and ACE inhibitor–ARBs.[161] They also analyzed 12 observational studies. Exercise tolerance was improved (n = 183; CI: 27.3 to 75.7; p < 0.001), but not the early-to-late diastolic filling ratio, an index of diastolic dysfunction. All-cause mortality was unchanged.

Specific trials.

Angiotensin receptor blockers. Candesartan was added in CHARM-Preserved,[148] to prior therapy by diuretics (75%), β-blockers (56%), CCBs or other vasodilators (68%), or digoxin (28%), with prior ACE inhibition in only 19%. After a mean follow up of 3 years, only one combined secondary endpoint was positive, namely cardiovascular death, hospitalization for CHF, MI, or stroke (p = 0.037). Total mortality and total hospitalizations were unchanged. Using a new index of the efficacy of heart failure therapy, days alive and out of hospital, candesartan was better than placebo by 24.1 days over the length of the study (P < 0.001).[162] In the I-PRESERVE trial, 4128 patients with heart failure and LV ejection fraction of 45% or more were randomized to *irbesartan* or placebo and followed for more than 4 years.[163] There were no significant differences in the primary endpoint of all-cause mortality or cardiovascular hospitalizations (heart failure, MI, arrhythmia, or stroke) or any of the other prespecified outcomes. Paradoxically, irbesartan showed unexpected benefit in lower-risk patients with HFpEF.[164] "Lower risk" was defined by the lower-range plasma concentrations of NPs, suggesting benefits of early, but not later, higher-risk stages of the disease. As this was a posthoc analysis, prospective studies are required to further investigate this potential benefit.

ACE inhibitors for HFpEF. In the PEACE trial, 8290 apparently low-risk patients with stable coronary artery disease and preserved LV ejection fraction (≥40%; mean 59%) were randomized to either *trandolapril* or placebo and followed for more than 6 years with no significant difference in death from cardiovascular causes, MI, or coronary revascularization between the treatments.[165] Although these patients did not have HFpEF, there was an outcome benefit detected over 6 years, including reduced risk of cardiovascular death or heart failure in those subgroups initially identified by novel biomarkers.[166] In contrast to previous results with other biomarkers such as NT-proBNP, elevated levels of two or three of these selected biomarkers (midregional pro-A-type natriuretic peptide, midregional proadrenomedullin, and C-terminal proendothelin-1) identified the patients at high risk. In this subset, only 14 patients would have to be treated for 6 years to prevent one cardiac death or hospitalization for heart failure. *Perindopril* was compared with placebo in the PEP-CHF trial in older adult subjects with a diagnosis of heart failure, treated with diuretics and an echocardiogram suggesting diastolic dysfunction and excluding substantial LV systolic dysfunction or valve disease.[167] Although there was no significant difference in the primary endpoint of all-cause mortality or unplanned heart failure–related hospitalization, possibly attributable to high drop-out and cross-over to open label ACE inhibitor rates, there were trends at 1 year to improvements in hospitalization for heart failure, functional class, and 6-minute corridor walk test in patients treated with perindopril. Given these results and the beneficial effects of ACE inhibitors in other studies of cardiovascular disease (e.g. HOPE; EUROPA), we believe that ACE inhibitors should be considered as therapy in these patients, especially in the presence of other indications like hypertension.

β-blockade for HFpEF. The effect of *nebivilol* on outcomes was compared with placebo in 2128 patients with a history of heart failure and a wide range of LV systolic function (LV ejection fraction ≥ 35%) in the SENIORS study.[77] The primary endpoint of all-cause mortality or cardiovascular hospital admission was significantly improved by nebivolol, although mortality was statistically unchanged. Interestingly, there was no difference of note between the beneficial effect of nebivolol between patients with ejection fractions of less than or more than 35%, suggesting that there may have been an improvement in outcomes in patients with less severe LV dysfunction. Also note that the mean systolic BP in the preserved ejection fraction group was 145 mm Hg versus 135 mm Hg in the lower ejection fraction group,[149] so that BP reduction might in part explain the positive result.

Role of aldosterone blockers. Increasing evidence suggests that enhanced aldosterone signaling plays a key role in the onset and progression of HFpEF and in DHF. Aldosterone, a potent stimulator of myocardial and vascular fibrosis, may be a key mediator of heart failure progression in this population and is therefore an important therapeutic target. The effects of eplerenone were tested in a small, randomized, double-blind, placebo-controlled trial of only 44 patients with HFpEF.[156] There were no changes in the 6-minute walk distance, the primary endpoint. Nonetheless, there was a possible benefit on fibrous tissue as measured by serum markers of collagen turnover, which decreased, and diastolic function improved (E/E', p = 0.01). Whether these favorable effects will translate into morbidity and mortality benefit in a larger trial remains to be determined.

Trials in progress. TOPCAT is designed to evaluate the effect of spironolactone on morbidity, mortality, and quality of life in patients with HFpEF.[147] The Aldo-DHF trial will test whether aldosterone receptor blockade by spironolactone 25 mg daily will improve exercise capacity and diastolic function in patients with DHF. Inclusion criteria are age 50 years or older, NYHA type II or III, preserved LV ejection fraction ($\geq$50%), and echocardiographic diastolic dysfunction.[168] The two primary endpoints are changes in exercise capacity (peak VO_2, spiroergometry) and in diastolic function (E/é, echocardiography) after 12 months.

Further trials are in progress to assess the effect of angiotensin receptor inhibition by the angiotensin receptor blocker, neprilysin, combine with valsartan on HF with preserved ejection fraction,[168A] and on hypertension already treated by valsartan.[168B]

Overall interpretation. While awaiting outcome trials, our view is that persisting clinical heart failure, whatever the ejection fraction, requires added therapy by appropriately increased diuretics, renin-angiotensin inhibition, or β-blockade, and that BP reduction may play a role. Vasodilators may also benefit by afterload reduction.[169]

Right Ventricular Failure

"For a long time, the importance of right ventricle ... function has been neglected."[170] Right ventricular (RV) physiology is characterized by its close relationship with the pulmonary circuit. The right ventricle can accommodate significant changes in preload, but is highly sensitive to increases in afterload. Progressive dilatation and dysfunction can initiate a cycle of oxygen supply-demand mismatch that ultimately leads to RV failure. Echocardiography and cardiac MRI are the primary modalities used for noninvasive assessment of RV function.[171] The management of RV failure centers on the optimization of preload, afterload, and contractility. Few targeted therapies exist, although novel agents have shown promise in early studies.

LV dysfunction predisposes to RV dysfunction, as after anterior MI.[170] The right ventricle is the most anterior cardiac chamber, has a triangular shape, and its free wall is thinner than the left ventricle because the right ventricle contracts in a low-impedance system. Importantly, the shape, location, and contraction conditions make the RV chamber assessment by echo technically challenging. RV dysfunction can now be assessed by RV fractional area change of 35% or less.

RV afterload represents the load that the right ventricle has to overcome during ejection. Compared with the left ventricle, the right ventricle demonstrates a heightened sensitivity to afterload change (see Fig. 6-12). Although in clinical practice, pulmonary vascular resistance (PVR) is the most commonly used index of afterload, PVR may not reflect the complex nature of ventricular afterload.

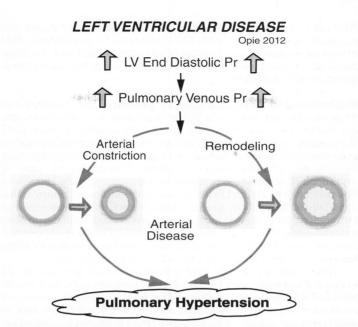

LEFT VENTRICULAR DISEASE
Opie 2012

⇧ LV End Diastolic Pr ⇧

⇧ Pulmonary Venous Pr ⇧

Arterial Constriction

Remodeling

Arterial Disease

Pulmonary Hypertension

Figure 6-13 How left ventricular (LV) disease can evolve into secondary pulmonary hypertension. First, the LV end-diastolic pressure (Pr) increases, leading to an indirect increase in the pulmonary venous pressure. Arterial constriction and remodeling both predispose to pulmonary arterial hypertension. (Figure © L.H. Opie, 2012.)

The evidence that guides the management of isolated RV failure is not nearly as well established as the evidence that guides the management of chronic heart failure resulting from LV systolic dysfunction.[172] Most recommendations are based on either retrospective or small randomized studies.[173] However, RV failure usually is a component of LV failure except when pulmonary arterial hypertension (PAH) is the underlying cause. Because of ventricular interdependence, RV dysfunction in turn worsens LV dysfunction.[172] Experimentally, high doses of bisoprolol (10 mg/kg) and carvedilol (15 mg/kg) given to rats have delayed the progression from PH to RV failure[174] or improved RV function.[175] Clinically, even after PAH-targeted therapy, RV function can deteriorate despite a reduction in PVR. Such loss of RV function is associated with a poor outcome, irrespective of any changes in PVR.[176] Pulmonary capacitance in relation to pulmonary vascular resistance (PVR).

Specific treatment goals. Specific treatment goals[173] include optimization of preload, afterload, and contractility. The use of β-blockers, standard in LV failure, has not been well explored in RV failure. Maintenance of sinus rhythm and AV synchrony is especially important in RV failure because atrial fibrillation and high-grade AV block may have profound hemodynamic consequences. Ventricular interdependence also is an important concept to consider when tailoring therapy. Excessive volume loading may increase pericardial constraint and decrease LV preload and cardiac output through the mechanism of ventricular interdependence. Alternatively, hypovolemia may decrease RV preload and cardiac output. In acute RV failure, every effort should be made to avoid hypotension, which may lead to a vicious cycle of RV ischemia and further hypotension.

Pulmonary Hypertension

Secondary pulmonary hypertension. Although guidelines contain detailed recommendations regarding PAH, they contain only a relatively short paragraph on the other, much more frequent forms of PH, including PH secondary to left heart disease (Fig. 6-13). PH is present in

68% to 78% of patients with chronic severe LV systolic dysfunction and is commonly associated with RV dysfunction.[177] In contrast, PAH focuses on a relatively small subset of all patients with PH, a condition that most commonly occurs secondary to pulmonary venous hypertension in patients with CHF.

Measurement of pulmonary artery pressure. The prevalence of PH in chronic heart failure is highly dependent on patient selection and the threshold of pulmonary artery (PA) systolic pressure used. PA pressure can be measured invasively by right heart catheterization (gold standard) or noninvasively by Doppler echocardiography. Using the definition of a RV pressure gradient of more than 35 mm Hg (equivalent to an estimated PA systolic pressure >45 mm Hg), 7% of 1380 patients with HF had PH.[178] In that situation, prime therapy is that of LV failure. But what is specific therapy for PAH? The presence of PAH remains an important independent predictor of mortality, despite powerful associations with other well-established markers of poor outcome such as mitral regurgitation, plasma markers, or elevated LV filling pressure such as NT-proBNP, as well as LV and RV dysfunction.

Drugs currently used to treat patients with PAH (prostanoids, ET receptor antagonists, and PDE-5 inhibitors) have not been well investigated in PH secondary to LV disease (Fig. 6-14).[179] Clearly more studies are needed in this common situation. However, despite such lack of evidence-based efficacy data, a current trend is toward the use of targeted PAH drugs in patients with PH associated with left heart disease. This trend is supported by a small study showing that sildenafil lowered PVR and improved exercise capacity and quality of life in patients with heart failure complicated by PH.[177] These patients also had prior therapy by diuretics and β-blockers (100%), ACE inhibitor or ARB (77%), spironolactone (76%), digoxin (65%), and an implantable cardiac defibrillator (83%). Mechanistically, short-term cyclic GMP-enhancing treatment with sildenafil and BNP infusions improved LV diastolic distensibility in vivo, in part by phosphorylating titin.[180] The proposal is that these agents might act directly on cardiac proteins in addition to vasodilating.

Pulmonary Arterial Hypertension

PAH is a rare and incurable progressive disease, including idiopathic PAH, heritable PAH, and PAH secondary to other diseases. Idiopathic PAH is panvasculopathy in which clones of endothelial cells proliferate and give rise to plexiform lesions, the pathologic hallmark of this condition, thereby promoting complex vascular lesions with near-total or total lumen obliteration[181,182] acting by multiple mechanisms including increased serotonin release. Thus there is increasing vascular smooth muscle damage.[182] The functional consequences include decreased endothelial NO production and increased PDE-5 expression and activity in both PA and in the RV muscle cells. The overall result is an increase in PVR in a disease that affects both the PA and the right ventricle.

These obstructive proliferative changes in the lung microcirculation promote RV hypertrophy, eventually leading to right heart failure and premature death. PAH can occur in isolation (primary pulmonary hypertension), or be related to other diseases such as human immunodeficiency virus (HIV) infection, congenital heart disease, connective tissue disorders like scleroderma[183] and systemic lupus erythematosus, or idiopathic pulmonary fibrosis. PAH can also be induced by substance abuse with appetite suppressants, cocaine, or other drugs. Optimal therapy remains undecided.[184]

Catheter diagnosis. Heart catheterization is required to diagnose PAH: a mean PA pressure of 25 mm Hg or more and a PVR greater than 3 Wood units.[181] As this is a pulmonary vascular disease, the diagnosis

PULMONARY ARTERIAL HYPERTENSION

Opie 2012

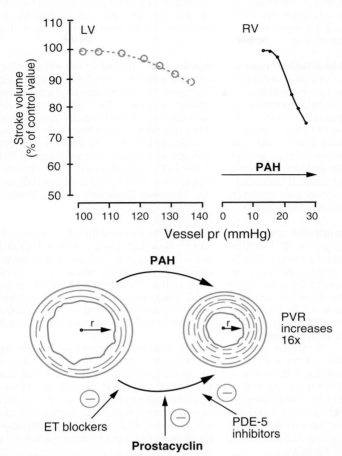

Figure 6-14 Increased intaarterial pressure in pulmonary arterial hypertension (PAH) leads to a much sharper fall in stroke volume than does increased left ventricular (LV) pressure (*upper panel*). To decrease the intraarterial pressure in PAH, the major vasodilator drugs are endothelin (ET) blockers and prostacyclin and phosphodiesterase (PDE)-5 inhibitors (*bottom panel*). *PVR*, pulmonary vascular resistance; *RV*, right ventricle. (Figure © L.H. Opie, 2012.)

also requires exclusion of underlying LV dysfunction (PCWP less than 15 mm Hg). Further exclusions are thromboembolism and parenchymal lung disease.[181]

In PAH, the RV adaptation to chronic pressure overload is related not only to the levels of vascular resistance (steady afterload), but also to PA stiffness (pulsatile load). Indexes of PA stiffness (elasticity, distensibility, capacitance, stiffness index beta, and pulse pressure) were independently associated with the degree of RV dysfunction, dilation, and hypertrophy in PH. Such increased PA stiffness is associated with reduced survival in PH.[185]

Therapeutic options. There is no cure for PAH, but treatment options include prostanoids, PDE-5 inhibitors, and ET-receptor antagonists. A metaanalysis including all therapy types in 21 trials on 3140 patients found a reduction in all-cause mortality of 43% (RR 0.57; CI 0.35-0.92; P = 0.023).[186] Vasodilators as a group give a 39% mortality reduction.[184]

Prostacyclins. Epoprostenol (Flolan) is the only PAH-specific therapy with demonstrated survival benefit in a randomized, prospective clinical trial.[187] Although continuous infusions of intravenous epoprostenol or subcutaneous treprostinil give benefit, both are limited by the need for meticulous catheter care, continuous infusion, and daily preparation.

Phosphodiesterase-5 inhibitors. PDE-5 inhibitors vasodilate by acting on PDE-5 in the pulmonary and systemic vasculature. Furthermore, vascular remodeling can be promoted by decreased proliferation and increased apoptosis of PA smooth muscle cells.[181] RV inotropy also increases.[181] There is also a direct action on the lungs, in which expression of PDE-5 is suppressed. Thus sildenafil also preferentially improves blood flow to well-ventilated regions of the lung in patients with lung disease such as idiopathic pulmonary fibrosis, another cause of PAH, with symptomatic benefit.[188] The PDE-5 inhibitors sildenafil (Revatio) and tadalafil (Adcirca) are FDA approved for the treatment of PAH, with sildenafil also approved by the European Medicines Agency. Mortality trials are not available.

Endothelin receptor antagonists. The first oral therapy approved for therapy of PAH was bosentan.[189] Bosentan gives combined ET_A/ET_B receptor antagonism. Selective ET_A antagonists (sitaxsentan approved in Europe; ambrisentan approved in the United States) theoretically preserve the vasodilatory action of the ET_B receptor. However, no trial data show whether selective ET_A antagonism is better than combined ET_A and ET_B antagonism (also see macitentan, next section). Furthermore, there are no robust trial data to indicate improved survival with any of these agents.[182]

Macitentan is a dual ET_A/ET_B receptor antagonist with high lipophilic affinity with inhibitory constants in nanomolar range.[190] Experimentally, it improves survival in monocrotaline-induced pulmonary hypertensive rats and protects against end-organ damage in diabetes. ET-1 can change tissue structure and induce fibrosis. Tissue ET-1 acts via binding to the two G protein-coupled receptors (ET_A/ET_B) located on a large variety of cell types such as endothelial cells and macrophages. Blockage of both is required to oppose the overall pathologic effects of ET-1 stimulation.

SERAPHIN study. On April 30, 2012, Actelion (SIX: ATLN) announced the initial analysis of the event-driven study SERAPHIN with macitentan in 742 patients with PAH and treated for up to 3.5 years.[191] Macitentan decreased the risk of a morbidity-mortality event during the treatment period versus placebo by 45% in the 10 mg–dose group ($p < 0.0001$) and 30% ($p = 0.01$) in the 3-mg group.

Combination therapy. In patients with primary PAH the addition of sildenafil to long-term intravenous epoprostenol therapy improved exercise capacity, time to clinical worsening, hemodynamic measurements, and quality of life.[192] Conversely, the addition of epoprostenol to sildenafil after 2 years of sildenafil treatment did not improve a group of Japanese patients.[193]

Therapies in evolution. The evolution of therapies is very active. Listed alphabetically, the major drugs in development are as follows. *Cicletanine* counters endothelial dysfunction in PAH by coupling to endothelial nitric oxide synthase.[194] *Fasudil* is an Rho-kinase inhibitor that counters calcium sensitization and vasoconstriction. Experimentally, PAH was more improved by fasudil than by bosentan or sildenafil, whereas combining bosentan or sildenafil with fasudil had no synergistic effect.[195] *Imatinib* is an inhibitor of the activity of the vasculopathic protease-activated receptor–2 found on mast cells and platelets (see Fig. 9-3) and increased in PAH.[196] *Riociguat* activates soluble guanylate cyclase that in turn improves endothelial function and lessens fibrous tissue remodelling.[197] *Selexipag* is a direct and highly prostaglandin receptor agonist that significantly decreased PVR in a phase 2 study.[198] *Terguride*, a dopamine agonist with antiserotonergic and antifibrotic properties,[199] is entering clinical studies.

Pulmonary arterial hypertension in scleroderma. PAH in scleroderma (progressive systemic sclerosis) is an example of PAH secondary to connective tissue diseases. Survival depends on severity of RV dysfunction, the degree of renal impairment, and the cardiac adaptation to pulmonary vascular disease.[200] The PAH is trigged by circulating autoantibodies that damage the endothelium and activate fibroblasts. Approved therapies include prostacyclins, ET antagonists, and PDE-5 inhibitors. *Prostacyclins* (continuous infusions of intravenous epoprostenol or subcutaneous treprostinil) give benefit but are limited by the need for meticulous catheter care, continuous infusion, and daily preparation. *Selective ET receptor A antagonists* (sitaxsentan approved in Europe; ambrisentan approved in the United States; bosentan) preserve the vasodilatory action of the ET B receptor. The *PDE-5 inhibitors* sildenafil (three times daily) and tadalafil (once daily) are approved for use in PAH (including PAH-systemic sclerosis) in the United States. However, the response to all such therapies is limited.[183]

Drug-induced pulmonary arterial hypertension. There are many drugs that have been linked to PAH. Among the best-known are Fen-Phen, fenfluramine, and fenfluramine derivatives, which are associated with PAH, heart valve disease, and cardiac fibrosis. Fenfluramine was withdrawn from the US market in 1997 but lingered on in Europe. It induces gene dysregulation in human PA smooth muscle and endothelial cells.[201] HIV infection and treatment with highly active antiretroviral therapy including HIV protease inhibitor ritonavir (RTV) may be associated with endothelial dysfunction and PAH. Dasatinib (Sprycel) is an anticancer drug that can induce severe precapillary PAH when given for certain acute and chronic leukemias.[202] In a large French Registry of approximately 3000 patients, there were 64 reports of PAH.[202] The FDA warned in October 2011 that symptoms of heart failure might arise any time after initiation of therapy, even after 1 year. Thereupon the drug should be stopped, and if required, diagnostic right heart catheterization undertaken.

Heart Failure in Women

Menopause influences the pattern of disease, with the incidence of coronary heart disease increasing thereafter. Nonetheless, women have a lower baseline risk for CHD at all ages except perhaps beyond 80 years. Thus it is not a simple issue of being pre- or postmenopausal.

Patterns of heart failure are different. Women are relatively neglected in clinical trials, although the DIG study warned of increased mortality of unknown cause in women with heart failure compared with men (Table 6-8). Women are more likely to have HFpEF with a better prognosis than men. On the other hand, in HFrEF, women are older with a lower quality life, and more often with concomitant diabetes. Device therapy is underused.

Management of heart failure and treatment of cardiomyopathies in pregnant women and postpartum requires special consideration (Table 6-8). During pregnancy, ACE inhibitors, ARBs, spironolactone, eplerenone, and renin inhibitors are contraindicated because of fetotoxicity. Therefore such medication ideally needs be terminated and replaced. Nonetheless, there are isolated reports that eplerenone is less antiandrogenic than spironolactone when used in pregnancy for primary aldosteronism without the expected potent antiandrogenic

Table 6-8

Gender and Cardiovascular Differences

Estrogen vascular effects: Favorable lipid profile, lower LDL, higher HDL; facilitates NO-vasodilation; antifibrotic.

Pregnancy may precipitate or worsen HF; physiologic 30%-50% increase in CO. Peripartum cardiomyopathy*: defined as deterioration in cardiac function between the last month of pregnancy and up to 5 months postpartum with no other cause evident.

Therapy for HF in pregnancy: ACE inhibitors, ARBs and spironolactone-eplerenone contraindicated in all trimesters (this C/I is not mentioned by Shin et al.).

Menopause: Risk of HF rises, estrogen deprivation.

Failure of HRT to give CV protection in prospective trials.

HRT in HF may vasodilate and block inflammatory cytokines, but no prospective trials.

Patterns of HF: Women more likely to have HFpEF; better prognosis than in men. In HF with reduced EF, women older, lower QOL, diabetes more often associated.

HF management: Women underrepresented in all trials, also in Dig trial (22%).

Digoxin for HF:[140] ↑ risk of all-cause death in women (HR, 1.23). ? Interaction with HRT.

Device therapy: Underused, women have more LBBB, a criterion for CRT.

ACE, Angiotensin-converting enzyme; *ARB,* angiotensin receptor blocker; *C/I,* confidence interval; *CO,* cardiac output; *CRT,* cardiac resynchronization therapy; *CV,* cardiovascular; *EF,* ejection fraction; *HDL,* high-density lipoprotein; *HF,* heart failure; *HFpEF,* heart failure with preserved ejection fraction; *HR,* hazard ratio; *HRT,* hormone replacement therapy; *LBBB,* left bundle branch block; *LDL,* low-density lipoprotein; *NO,* nitric oxide; *QOL,* quality of life.

*See section on page 216.

Based on review data in Shin JJ, et al. Heart failure in women. *Clin Cardiol* 2012; 35:172–177.

effects that can cause ambiguous genitalia in a male fetus.[203] Diuretics should be used sparingly as they may decrease blood flow to the placenta and have an effect on lactation.[204]

Peripartum Cardiomyopathy

PPCM is a not-so-rare (up to 1:1000) yet serious type of idiopathic heart failure without any underlying determinable heart disease during the last month of pregnancy or the first 5 months postpartum. The incidence varies worldwide but is high in developing nations; the cause of the disease might be a combination of environmental and genetic factors.[205] In Turkey, of 42 consecutive women with PPCM only 47.6% had a full recovery, with an average time to complete recovery of 19.3 months after initial diagnosis.[206] The cause of PPCM is uncertain but one proposal is that mutations associated with familial dilated-cardiomyopathy genes overlap with those found in PPCM, thus suggesting a clinical overlap of these two diseases. More specifically, proinflammatory factors and autoimmune processes may play a role.[207] There is increasing evidence that the disease occurs as a result of the consequences of imbalanced oxidative stress leading to proteolytic cleavage of prolactin into a potent angiostatic factor with inhibition of cardioprotective STAT-3.[208] This study suggested that inhibition of prolactin release could be a novel therapeutic strategy for PPCM.

Peripartum cardiomyopathy–targeted therapies. Intravenous immunoglobulin, pentoxifylline, and bromocriptine have all been used in small trials.[205] These all need further extended controlled studies. *Immunoglobulin* is most logical if given for patients with proven myocarditis. In a small retrospective study, women treated with immune globulin had a greater improvement in ejection fraction during early follow-up than patients treated conventionally.[209] *Pentoxifylline* 400 mg three times daily, added to prior conventional therapy in 30 patients was the only independent predictor of outcome (P = 0.04).[210] However, the control and pentoxifylline groups were studied sequentially. *Bromocriptine* is a dopamine-2D agonist that inhibits prolactin release and thus specifically acts on the disease molecular mechanism. A recent small prospective randomized pilot study showed that bromocriptine added to standard heart failure therapy had beneficial effects on ventricular ejection fraction and clinical outcome in patients with acute severe PPCM.[204,211] Bromocriptine was given as 2.5 mg twice daily for 2 weeks followed by 2.5 mg daily for 6 weeks.

SUMMARY

1. *Heart failure is a complex, potentially fatal condition.* It includes acute heart failure, often needing therapy by intravenous diuretics, vasodilators and possibly inotropes; and chronic heart failure, which may present as classic systolic failure that requires neurohumoral antagonism by ACE inhibitors (or ARBs), β-blockers, and aldosterone blockers, besides diuretics. Equally frequently, heart failure may present with a preserved ejection fraction and diastolic dysfunction, and with less clear therapeutic options.

2. *Acute heart failure with pulmonary edema.* Acute heart failure with pulmonary edema is not a uniform entity. The problem is the many different causes and varying clinical presentations. Intravenous furosemide remains fundamental, yet the dose should be limited. New agents acting on specific mechanisms are a promising approach.

3. *Cardiogenic shock with or without pulmonary edema.* β-receptor stimulatory inotropes are often used in the acute therapy of severe heart failure, but these drugs may further damage the myocardium. The problem of β-receptor downregulation may require added PDE inhibition. Available drugs include dobutamine and dopamine. Vasopressin helps in septic or perianesthetic shock. Epinephrine gave similar outcomes to norepinephrine plus dobutamine in septic shock.

4. *Inotropic-dilators (PDE inhibitors).* Intravenous preparations with their inotropic and vasodilator effects should be especially useful in patients with β-receptor downgrading, as in acute-on-chronic severe CHF or during prolonged therapy with dobutamine or other β₁-stimulants, or after chronic β-blockade. Thus milrinone has a limited place in the management of short-term therapy of heart failure.

5. *Load reduction and vasodilators.* These are often chosen in severe acute heart failure, especially when the BP is relatively well maintained, to relieve the burden on the failing myocardium. Such agents include furosemide, nitrates, and nitroprusside. They may be carefully combined with agents that give inotropic or pressure support such as dobutamine or dopamine.

6. *Five current approaches to chronic heart failure.* The five major approaches to the management of CHF are, first, elimination and prevention of fluid retention; second, the use of ACE inhibitors as standard therapy; third, inhibition of the β-adrenergic response by β-blockers initially given in low doses but up-titrated to maximally tolerated doses; fourth, inhibition of aldosterone effects by spironolactone and eplerenone; and, fifth, the use of

ARBs. The combination of nitrates and hydralazine is also a useful adjunct in select patients, including self-identified blacks. In addition, metabolic modulators, if available, may give added benefit. The "vaptans" are registered for use in symptomatic heart failure resistant to fluid restriction. Gene therapy is not yet available. General measures include intense disease-management programs, exercise training, and correction of anemia. Mechanical and electrical devices (ICDs, CRT, and mechanical assist devices) are increasingly used with substantial trial support.

7. *Digoxin reappraised.* In the past, digoxin was standard therapy in CHF, at a time when inotropic therapy was regarded as desirable. Digoxin use in patients already optimally treated by a combination of mortality-reducing drugs such as β-blockers, ACE inhibitors and ARBs, and aldosterone blockers has never been tested. A small unproven mortality benefit may exist at blood levels less than 1 ng/mL, converting to a substantially increased mortality at higher blood levels. Inexplicably, women in the large DIG study had an increased mortality whereas men did not. In view of many uncertainties and without clear outcome trials in the current era, and in the light of new therapies, we do not recommend digoxin for heart failure. In ambulatory patients already receiving digoxin, the best prognosis is with low blood levels (low-dose digoxin ≤ 0.125 mg/day).

8. *Preserved systolic function.* Preserved systolic function despite clinical heart failure is a common and serious condition echocardiographically, and is the result of *DHF*. This condition is relatively more common in women. In one large trial, adding the ARB candesartan to prior therapy reduced the secondary endpoint (cardiovascular death or hospitalization for CHF, MI, or stroke). However, only 19% were receiving prior ACE inhibition. Renin-angiotensin inhibition should be considered for all patients with heart failure, whatever the ejection fraction. In general, the major benefit of drug treatment of heart failure with preserved systolic function is improved exercise tolerance, a major positive for the patient, yet without mortality decrease in a metaanalysis.

9. *PAH.* The presence of PAH secondary to chronic left heart failure is an important independent predictor of mortality. Therapy is not well defined but may include sildenafil and related compounds. Primary PAH is much rarer yet much better studied. It may occur secondary to various pulmonary vascular diseases, including scleroderma (systemic sclerosis), or as an idiopathic event. In the latter case, therapy is well defined and includes prostanoids, PDE-5 inhibitors, and ET blockers. New agents are in development. Nonetheless, the prognosis remains grave.

10. *Pregnancy.* During pregnancy ACE inhibitors, ARBs, spironolactone, eplerenone, and renin inhibitors are contraindicated because of fetotoxicity. Diuretics should be used sparingly as they may decrease blood flow to the placenta and have an effect on lactation. Molecular therapy in the form of bromocriptine may be specific therapy for peripartum cardiomyopathy.

11. *Women and heart disease.* The influence of menopause and of aging in women is under increasing study. There appear to be lifelong biological differences in cardiovascular disease patterns. There are still deficiencies in knowledge of the ideal therapy of heart failure in women.

12. *The future therapy of heart failure.* It is dangerous to be a prophet. Advances are emerging. New drugs are based on new mechanisms. Ultimately heart failure is a biological problem and the solution will lie in the prevention of the causes of the disorder and in the ability to replace or repair the myocardial cells using gene therapy or stem cell regeneration.

References*

*The complete reference list is available online at www.expertconsult.com.

2. Editorial. *Lancet* 2011;378:637.
3. Felker GM, et al. Clinical trials of pharmacological therapies in acute heart failure syndromes: lessons learned and directions forward. *Circ Heart Fail* 2010;3:314–325.
4. Metra M, et al. The pathophysiology of acute heart failure—it is a lot about fluid accumulation. *Am Heart J* 2008;155:1–5.
7. Peacock WF, et al. Morphine and outcomes in acute decompensated heart failure: an ADHERE analysis. *Emer Med J* 2008;25:205–209.
8. Felker GM, et al. Diuretic strategies in patients with acute decompensated heart failure. *N Engl J Med* 2011;364:797–805.
9. Yilmaz MB, et al. Impact of diuretic dosing on mortality in acute heart failure using a propensity-matched analysis. *Eur J Heart Fail* 2011;13:1244–1252.
11. Damman K, et al. Increased central venous pressure is associated with impaired renal function and mortality in a broad spectrum of patients with cardiovascular disease. *J Am Coll Cardiol* 2009;53:582–588.
12. Mullens W, et al. Importance of venous congestion for worsening of renal function in advanced decompensated heart failure. *J Am Coll Cardiol* 2009;53:589–596.
13. Cotter G, et al. Fluid overload in acute heart failure—re-distribution and other mechanisms beyond fluid accumulation. *Eur J Heart Fail* 2008;10:165–169.
14. Fallick C, et al. Sympathetically mediated changes in capacitance: redistribution of the venous reservoir as a cause of decompensation. *Circ Heart Fail* 2011;4:669–675.
16. Mebazaa A, et al. Short-term survival by treatment among patients hospitalized with acute heart failure: the global ALARM-HF registry using propensity scoring methods. *Intensive Care Med* 2011;37:290–301.
22. Giamouzis G, et al. Impact of dopamine infusion on renal function in hospitalized heart failure patients: results of the Dopamine in Acute Decompensated Heart Failure (DAD-HF) trial. J Card Fail 2010;16:922–930.
23. Elkayam U, et al. Renal vasodilatory action of dopamine in patients with heart failure: magnitude of effect and site of action. *Circulation* 2008;117:200–205.
30. de Lissovoy G, et al. Hospital costs for treatment of acute heart failure: economic analysis of the REVIVE II study. *Eur J Health Econ* 2010;11:185–193.
39. Teerlink JR, et al. Dose-dependent augmentation of cardiac systolic function with the selective cardiac myosin activator, omecamtiv mecarbil: a first-in-man study. *Lancet* 2011;378:667–675.
40. Cleland JG, et al. The effects of the cardiac myosin activator, omecamtiv mecarbil, on cardiac function in systolic heart failure: a double-blind, placebo-controlled, crossover, dose-ranging phase 2 trial. *Lancet* 2011;378:676–683.
41. Hasenfuss G, et al. Cardiac inotropes: current agents and future directions. *Eur Heart J* 2011;32:1838–1845.
43. Mullens W, et al. Sodium nitroprusside for advanced low-output heart failure. *J Am Coll Cardiol* 2008;52:200–207.
48. Ezekowitz JA, et al. Assessment of dyspnea in acute decompensated heart failure: insights from ASCEND-HF (Acute Study of Clinical Effectiveness of Nesiritide in Decompensated Heart Failure) on the contributions of peak expiratory flow. *J Am Coll Cardiol* 2012;59:1441–1448.
51. O'Connor CM, et al. Effect of nesiritide in patients with acute decompensated heart failure. *N Engl J Med* 2011;365:32–43.
52. Teerlink JR, et al. Relaxin for the treatment of patients with acute heart failure (Pre-RELAX-AHF): a multicentre, randomised, placebo-controlled, parallel-group, dose-finding phase IIb study. *Lancet* 2009;373:1429–1439.
53. Ponikowski P, et al. Design of the RELAXin in acute heart failure study. *Am Heart J* 2012;163:149–155.
54. Bauer SR, et al. Arginine vasopressin for the treatment of septic shock in adults. *Pharmacotherapy* 2010;30:1057–1071.
56. Gassanov N, et al. Arginine vasopressin (AVP) and treatment with arginine vasopressin receptor antagonists (vaptans) in congestive heart failure, liver cirrhosis and syndrome of inappropriate antidiuretic hormone secretion (SIADH). *Eur J Clin Pharm* 2011;67: 333–346.
57. Elzouki AN, et al. Terlipressin-induced severe left and right ventricular dysfunction in patient presented with upper gastrointestinal bleeding: case report and literature review. *Am J Emer Med* 2010;28:540.

58. Narayen G, Mandal SN. Vasopressin receptor antagonists and their role in clinical medicine. *Indian J Endocrinol Metab* 2012;16:183–191.

59. Gross PA, et al. Vaptans are not the mainstay of treatment in hyponatremia: perhaps not yet. *Kidney Int* 2011;80:594–600.

61. Udelson JE, et al. A multicenter, randomized, double-blind, placebo-controlled study of tolvaptan monotherapy compared to furosemide and the combination of tolvaptan and furosemide in patients with heart failure and systolic dysfunction. *J Card Fail* 2011; 17:973–981.

64. Howell NJ, et al. Glucose-insulin-potassium reduces the incidence of low cardiac output episodes after aortic valve replacement for aortic stenosis in patients with left ventricular hypertrophy: results from the Hypertrophy, Insulin, Glucose, and Electrolytes (HINGE) trial. *Circulation* 2011;123:170–177.

65. Milo-Cotter O, et al. Neurohormonal activation in acute heart failure: results from VERITAS. *Cardiology* 2011;119:96–105.

66. Homma S, et al. For the WARCEF Investigators. Warfarin and aspirin in patients with heart failure and sinus rhythm. *N Engl J Med* 2012;366:1859–1869.

68. O'Connor CM, et al. For the HF-ACTION Investigators. Efficacy and safety of exercise training in patients with chronic heart failure: HF-ACTION randomized controlled trial. *JAMA* 2009;301:1439–1450.

69. Flynn KE, et al. Effects of exercise training on health status in patients with chronic heart failure: HF-ACTION randomized controlled trial. *JAMA* 2009;301:1451–1459.

71. Angermann CE, et al. on behalf of the Competence Network Heart Failure Mode of Action and Effects of Standardized Collaborative Disease Management on Mortality and Morbidity in Patients With Systolic Heart Failure: the Interdisciplinary Network for Heart Failure (INH) Study. *Circ Heart Fail* 2012;5:25–35.

75. Funck-Brentano C, et al. CIBIS-III investigators. Influence of order and type of drug (bisoprolol vs. enalapril) on outcome and adverse events in patients with chronic heart failure: a post hoc analysis of the CIBIS-III trial. *Eur J Heart Fail* 2011;13:765–772.

83. Castagno D, et al. Association of heart rate and outcomes in a broad spectrum of patients with chronic heart failure: results from the CHARM (Candesartan in Heart Failure: assessment of Reduction in Mortality and morbidity) program. *J Am Coll Cardiol* 2012;59:1785–1795.

84. Swedberg K, et al. Ivabradine and outcomes in chronic heart failure (SHIFT): a randomised placebo-controlled study. *Lancet* 2010;376:875–885. Erratum in *Lancet* 2010; 376:1988.

85. Teerlink JR. Ivabradine in heart failure—no paradigm SHIFT yet. *Lancet* 2010;376: 847–849.

86. Swedberg K, et al. Effect on outcomes of heart rate reduction by ivabradine in patients with congestive heart failure: is there an influence of beta-blocker dose? *J Am Coll Cardiol* 2012;59:1785–1795.

87. Ekman I, et al. Heart rate reduction with ivabradine and health related quality of life in patients with chronic heart failure: results from the SHIFT study. *Eur Heart J* 2011; 32:2395–2404.

88. Böhm M, et al. Heart rate as a risk factor in chronic heart failure (SHIFT): the association between heart rate and outcomes in a randomised placebo-controlled trial. *Lancet* 2010;376:886–894.

89. Volterrani M, et al. Effect of carvedilol, ivabradine or their combination on exercise capacity in patients with Heart Failure (the CARVIVA HF trial). *Int J Cardiol* 2011;151: 218–224.

90. Konstam MA. Renal function and heart failure treatment: when is a loss really a gain? *Circ Heart Fail* 2011;4:677–679.

93. Rossignol P, et al. Eplerenone survival benefits in heart failure patients post-myocardial infarction are independent from its diuretic and potassium-sparing effects: insights from an EPHESUS (Eplerenone Post-Acute Myocardial Infarction Heart Failure Efficacy and Survival Study) substudy. *J Am Coll Cardiol* 2011;58 58:1958–1966.

94. Zannad F, et al. For the EMPHASIS-HF Study Group. Eplerenone in patients with systolic heart failure and mild symptoms. *N Engl J Med* 2011;364:11–21.

95. Cleland JG, et al. Clinical trials update from the ESC Heart Failure meeting 2011: TEHAF, WHICH, CARVIVA, and atrial fibrillation in GISSI-HF and EMPHASIS-HF. *Eur J Heart Fail* 2011;13:1147–1151.

96. Rossignol P, et al. Determinants and consequences of renal function variations with aldosterone blocker therapy in heart failure patients after myocardial infarction: insights from the Eplerenone Post-Acute Myocardial Infarction Heart Failure Efficacy and Survival Study. *Circulation* 2012;125:271–279.

101. Dai W, et al. Is inhibition of phosphodiesterase Type 5 by sildenafil a promising therapy for volume-overload heart failure? *Circulation* 2012;125:1341–1343.

102. Schwartz BG, et al. Cardiac uses of phosphodiesterase-5 inhibitors. *J Am Coll Cardiol* 2012;59:9–15.

103. Swedberg K, et al. The beat goes on: on the importance of heart rate in chronic heart failure. *Eur Heart J* 2012;33:1044–1045.

104. Talajic M, et al. Maintenance of sinus rhythm and survival in patients with heart failure and atrial fibrillation. *J Am Coll Cardiol* 2010;55:1796–1802.

106. Phan TT, et al. Multi-centre experience on the use of perhexiline in chronic heart failure and refractory angina: old drug, new hope. *Eur J Heart Fail* 2009;11:881–886.

107. Tuunanen H, et al. Effects of trimetazidine, a metabolic modulator, on cardiac function and substrate metabolism in idiopathic cardiomyopathy. *Circulation* 2008; [Submitted].

109. Zhang L, et al. Additional use of trimetazidine in patients with chronic heart failure: a meta-analysis. *J Am Coll Cardiol* 2012;59:913–922.

111. McMurray JJ, et al. Calcium handling in the failing heart and SUMO—weighing the evidence. *N Engl J Med* 2011;365:1738–1739.
112. Jessup M, et al. for the Calcium Upregulation by Percutaneous Administration of Gene Therapy in Cardiac Disease (CUPID) Investigators. Calcium upregulation by percutaneous administration of gene therapy in cardiac disease (CUPID): a phase 2 trial of intracoronary gene therapy of sarcoplasmic reticulum Ca2+-ATPase in patients with advanced heart failure. *Circulation* 2011;124:304–313.
113. Kho C, et al. SUMO1-dependent modulation of SERCA2a in heart failure. *Nature* 2011;477:601–605.
114. Bolli R, et al. Cardiac stem cells in patients with ischaemic cardiomyopathy (SCIPIO): initial results of a randomised phase 1 trial. *Lancet* 2011;378:1847–1857.
115. Makkar RR, et al. Intracoronary cardiosphere-derived cells for heart regeneration after myocardial infarction (CADUCEUS): a prospective, randomised phase 1 trial. *Lancet* 2012;379:895–904.
116. Ghali JK, et al. Study of Anemia in Heart Failure Trial (STAMINA-HeFT) Group. Randomized double-blind trial of darbepoetin alfa in patients with symptomatic heart failure and anemia. *Circulation* 2008;117:526–535.
117. Skali H, et al. TREAT Investigators. Stroke in patients with type 2 diabetes mellitus, chronic kidney disease, and anemia treated with darbepoetin alfa: the trial to reduce cardiovascular events with Aranesp therapy (TREAT) experience. *Circulation* 2011;124:2903–2908.
118. McMurray JJ, et al. RED-HF Committees and Investigators. Design of the Reduction of Events with Darbepoetin alfa in Heart Failure (RED-HF): a Phase III, anaemia correction, morbidity-mortality trial. *Eur J Heart Fail* 2009;11:795–801.
119. Anker SD, et al. FAIR-HF Trial Investigators. Ferric carboxymaltose in patients with heart failure and iron deficiency. *N Engl J Med* 2009;361:2436–2448.
120. Comin-Colet J, et al. The effect of intravenous ferric carboxymaltose on health-related quality of life in patients with chronic heart failure and iron deficiency: a subanalysis of the FAIR-HF study. *Eur Heart J* Jan 31, 2012.
121. Jones RH. Coronary bypass surgery with or without surgical ventricular reconstruction: STICH Hypothesis 2 Investigators. *N Engl J Med* 2009;360:1705–1717.
122. Velazquez EJ, et al. STICH Investigators. Coronary-artery bypass surgery in patients with left ventricular dysfunction. *N Engl J Med* 2011;364:1607–1616.
123. Bonow RO, et al. STICH Trial Investigators. Myocardial viability and survival in ischemic left ventricular dysfunction. *N Engl J Med* 2011;364:1617–1625.
125. Slaughter MS, et al. HeartMate II Investigators. Advanced heart failure treated with continuous-flow left ventricular assist device. *N Engl J Med* 2009;361:2241–2251.
126. Strueber M, et al. HeartWare Investigators. Multicenter evaluation of an intrapericardial left ventricular assist system. *J Am Coll Cardiol* 2011;57:1375–1382.
127. Kirklin JK, et al. Third INTERMACS Annual Report: the evolution of destination therapy in the United States. *J Heart Lung Transplant* 2011;30:115–123.
129. Opie LH. Dilated cardiomyopathy and potentially deadly digoxin. *S Afr Med J* 2011;101:388–390.
133. Arispe N, et al. Digitoxin induces calcium uptake into cells by forming transmembrane calcium channels. *Proc Nat Acad Sci USA* 2008;105:2610–2615.
134. Opie LH, et al. Dronaderone in high-risk permanent atrial fibrillation. *New Engl J Med* 2012;366:1159.
137. Jessup M, et al. 2009 focused update: ACCF/AHA guidelines for the diagnosis and management of heart failure in adults: a report of the American College of Cardiology Foundation/American Heart Association Task Force on Practice Guidelines: developed in collaboration with the International Society for Heart and Lung Transplantation. *Circulation* 2009;119:1977–2016.
138. Ahmed A, et al. Effects of digoxin at low serum concentrations on mortality and hospitalization in heart failure: a propensity-matched study of the DIG trial. *Int J Cardiol* 2008;123:138–146.
139. Georgiopoulou VV, et al. Digoxin therapy does not improve outcomes in patients with advanced heart failure on contemporary medical therapy. *Circ Heart Fail* 2009;2:90–97.
141. Biggar RJ, et al. Digoxin use and the risk of breast cancer in women. *J Clin Oncol* 2011;29:2165–2170.
142. Ahren TP, et al. Digoxin treatment is associated with an increased incidence of breast cancer: a population-based case-control study. *Breast Cancer Res* 2008;10:R102.
143. Yukawa M, et al. Determination of digoxin clearance in Japanese elderly patients for optimization of drug therapy: a population pharmacokinetics analysis using nonlinear mixed-effects modelling. *Drugs Aging* 2011;28:831–841.
144. Nordt SP, et al. Retrospective review of digoxin exposures to a poison control system following recall of Digitek® tablets. *Am J Cardiovasc Drugs* 2010;10:261–263.
145. Pita-Fernández S, et al. Clinical manifestations of elderly patients with digitalis intoxication in the emergency department. *Arch Gerontol Geriatr* 2011;53:e106–e110.
147. Desai AS, et al. The TOPCAT study. Rationale and design of the treatment of preserved cardiac function heart failure with an aldosterone antagonist trial: a randomized, controlled study of spironolactone in patients with symptomatic heart failure and preserved ejection fraction. *Am Heart J* 2011;162:966–972.
149. van Veldhuisen DJ, et al. Beta-blockade with nebivolol in elderly heart failure patients with impaired and preserved left ventricular ejection fraction: data From SENIORS (Study of Effects of Nebivolol Intervention on Outcomes and Rehospitalization in Seniors With Heart Failure). *J Am Coll Cardiol* 2009;53:2150–2158.
152. Vogel MW, et al. The natural history of preclinical diastolic dysfunction: a population-based study. *Circ Heart Fail* 2012;5:144–151.

155. Gaasch WH, et al. Left ventricular structural remodeling in health and disease: with special emphasis on volume, mass, and geometry. *J Am Coll Cardiol* 2011;58: 1733–1740.
156. Deswal A, et al. Results of the Randomized Aldosterone Antagonism in Heart Failure With Preserved Ejection Fraction Trial (RAAM-PEF). *J Card Fail* 2011;17:634–642.
157. Kitzman DW. Outcomes in patients with heart failure with preserved ejection fraction: it is more than the heart. *J Am Coll Cardiol* 2012;59:1006–1007.
158. Sliwa K, et al. Hypertension—a global perspective. *Circulation* 2011;123:2892–2896.
159. Stewart S, et al. The clinical consequences and challenges of hypertension in urban-dwelling black Africans: insights from the Heart of Soweto Study. *Int J Cardiol* 2011;146:22–27.
160. Carlsen MC, et al. Prevalence and prognosis of heart failure with preserved ejection fraction and elevated N-terminal pro brain natriuretic peptide: a 10-year analysis from the Copenhagen Hospital Heart Failure Study. *Eur J Heart Failure* 2012;14:240–247.
161. Holland DJ, et al. Effects of treatment on exercise tolerance, cardiac function, and mortality in heart failure with preserved ejection fraction: a meta-analysis. *J Am Coll Cardiol* 2011;57:1676–1686.
162. Ariti CA, et al. Days alive and out of hospital and the patient journey in patients with heart failure: insights from the candesartan in heart failure: assessment of reduction in mortality and morbidity (CHARM) program. *Am Heart J* 2011;162:900–906.
163. Massie BM, et al.; I-PRESERVE Investigators. Irbesartan in patients with heart failure and preserved ejection fraction. *N Engl J Med* 2008;359:2456–2467.
164. Anand IS, et al. Prognostic value of baseline plasma amino-terminal pro-brain natriuretic peptide and its interactions with irbesartan treatment effects in patients with heart failure and preserved ejection fraction: findings from the I-PRESERVE trial. *Circ Heart Fail* 2011;4:569–577.
166. Sabatine MS, et al. Evaluation of multiple biomarkers of cardiovascular stress for risk prediction and guiding medical therapy in patients with stable coronary disease. *Circulation* 2012;125 :233–240.
168. Edelmann F, et al. Rationale and design of the aldosterone receptor blockade in diastolic heart failure trial: a double-blind, randomized, placebo-controlled, parallel group study to determine the effects of spironolactone on exercise capacity and diastolic function in patients with symptomatic diastolic heart failure (Aldo-DHF). *Eur J Heart Fail* 2010;12:874–882.
168A. Solomon SD, et al.; for the PARAMOUNT Investigators. The angiotensin receptor neprilysin inhibitor LCZ696 in heart failure with preserved ejection fraction: a phase 2 double-blind randomised controlled trial. *Lancet* 2012;380:1387–1395.
168B. Ruilope LM, et al. Blood-pressure reduction with LCZ696, a novel dual-acting inhibitor of the angiotensin II receptor and neprilysin: a randomised, double-blind, placebo-controlled, active comparator study. *Lancet* 2010;375:1255–1266.
169. Schwartzenberg S, et al. Effects of vasodilation in heart failure with preserved or reduced ejection fraction implications of distinct pathophysiologies on response to therapy. *J Am Coll Cardiol* 2012;59:442–451.
170. Azevedo PS, et al. Predictors of right ventricle dysfunction after anterior myocardial infarction. *Can J Cardiol* Mar 13, 2012. [Epub ahead of print]
171. Sayer GT, et al. Right ventricular performance in chronic congestive heart failure. *Cardiol Clin* 2012;30:271–282.
172. Haddad F, et al. Right ventricular function in cardiovascular disease. Part I. Anatomy, physiology, aging and functional assessment of the right ventricle. *Circulation* 2008; 117:1436–1448.
173. Haddad F, et al. Right ventricular function in cardiovascular disease. Part II: pathophysiology, clinical importance, and management of right ventricular failure. *Circulation* 2008;117:1717–1731.
174. De Man FS, et al Bisoprolol delays progression towards right heart failure in experimental pulmonary hypertension. *Circ Heart Fail* 2012;5:97–105.
175. Bogaard HJ, et al. Adrenergic receptor blockade reverses right heart remodeling and dysfunction in pulmonary hypertensive rats. *Am J Respir Crit Care Med* 2010;182: 652–660.
176. Van de Veerdonk MC, et al. Progressive right ventricular dysfunction in patients with pulmonary arterial hypertension responding to therapy. *J Am Coll Cardiol* 2011;58: 2511–2519.
178. Damy T, et al. Determinants and prognostic value of pulmonary arterial pressure in patients with chronic heart failure. *Eur Heart J* 2010;31:2280–2290.
179. Rosenkranz S, et al. Pulmonary hypertension due to left heart disease: updated Recommendations of the Cologne Consensus Conference 2011. *Int J Cardiol* 2011;154 (Suppl 1):S34–S44.
180. Bishu K, et al. Sildenafil and B-type natriuretic peptide acutely phosphorylate titin and improve diastolic distensibility in vivo. *Circulation* 2011;124:2882–2891.
181. Archer SL, et al. Phosphodiesterase type 5 inhibitors for pulmonary arterial hypertension. *N Engl J Med* 2009;361:1864–1871.
182. Archer SL, et al. Basic science of pulmonary arterial hypertension for clinicians: new concepts and experimental therapies. *Circulation* 2010;121:2045–2066.
183. Sweiss NJ, et al. Diagnosis and management of pulmonary hypertension in systemic sclerosis. *Curr Rheumatol Rep* 2010;12:8–18.
184. Macchia A, et al. Systematic review of trials using vasodilators in pulmonary arterial hypertension: Why a new approach is needed. *Am Heart J* 2010;159:245–257.
185. Stevens GR, et al. RV dysfunction in pulmonary hypertension is independently related to pulmonary artery stiffness. *JACC Cardiovasc Imaging* 2012;5:378–387.

186. Galiè N, et al. A meta-analysis of randomized controlled trials in pulmonary arterial hypertension. *Eur Heart J* 2009;30:394–403.
188. Zisman DA, et al. Idiopathic Pulmonary Fibrosis Clinical Research Network: a controlled trial of sildenafil in advanced idiopathic pulmonary fibrosis. *N Engl J Med* 2010;363:620–628.
190. Iglarz M, et al. Pharmacology of macitentan, an orally active tissue-targeting dual endothelin receptor antagonist. *J Pharmacol Exp Ther* 2008;327:736–745.
191. Levin J. SERAPHIN trial, Actelion Release April 30, 2012. [Available on Google]
192. Simonneau G, et al. PACES Study Group. Addition of sildenafil to long-term intravenous epoprostenol therapy in patients with pulmonary arterial hypertension: a randomized trial. *Ann Intern Med* 2008;149:521–530.
193. Yanagisawa R, et al. Impact of first-line sildenafil monotreatment for pulmonary arterial hypertension. *Circ J* 2012;76:1245–1252.
194. Waxman AB, et al. Cicletanine for the treatment of pulmonary arterial hypertension. *Arch Intern Med* 2008;168:2164–2166.
195. Mouchaers KT, et al. Fasudil reduces monocrotaline-induced pulmonary arterial hypertension: comparison with bosentan and sildenafil. *Eur Respir J* 2010;36:800–807.
196. Kwapiszewska G, et al. PAR-2 Inhibition reverses experimental pulmonary hypertension. *Circ Res* 2012;110:1179–1191.
197. Geschka S, et al. Soluble guanylate cyclase stimulation prevents fibrotic tissue remodeling and improves survival in salt-sensitive Dahl rats. *PLoS One* 2011;6:e218–e253.
198. Simonneau G, et al. Selexipag, an oral, selective IP receptor agonist for the treatment of pulmonary arterial hypertension. *Eur Respir J* 2012;40:874–880
199. Kekewska A, et al. Antiserotonergic properties of terguride in blood vessels, platelets, and valvular interstitial cells. *J Pharmacol Exp Ther* 2012;340:369–376.
200. Campo A, et al. Hemodynamic predictors of survival in scleroderma-related pulmonary arterial hypertension. *Am J Respir Crit Care Med* 2010;182:252–260.
201. Yao W, et al. Fenfluramine-induced gene dysregulation in human pulmonary artery smooth muscle and endothelial cells. *Pulm Circ* 2012;1:405–418.
202. Montani D, et al. Pulmonary arterial hypertension in patients treated by dasatinib. *Circulation* 2012;125:2128–2137.
203. Cabassi A, et al. Eplerenone use in primary aldosteronism during pregnancy. *Hypertension* 2012;59:e18–e19.
204. Regitz-Zagrosek V, et al. ESC Guidelines on the management of cardiovascular diseases during pregnancy. *Eur Heart J* 2011;32:3147–3197.
205. Bhattacharyya A, et al. Peripartum cardiomyopathy: a review. *Tex Heart Inst J* 2012;39: 8–16.
206. Biteker M, et al. Delayed recovery in peripartum cardiomyopathy: an indication for long-term follow-up and sustained therapy. *Eur J Heart Fail* 2012;14: 895–901.
207. Sliwa K, et al. Current status on knowledge on aetiology, diagnosis, management, and therapy on peripartum cardiomyopathy: a position statement from the Heart Failure Association of the European Society of Cardiology Working Group on peripartum cardiomyopathy. *Eur J Heart Fail* 2010;12:767–778.
211. Sliwa K, et al. Evaluation of bromocriptine in the treatment of acute severe peripartum cardiomyopathy: a proof of concept pilot study. *Circulation* 2010;121:1465–1473.

7

Antihypertensive Therapies

LIONEL H. OPIE · HENRY KRUM
· RONALD G. VICTOR · NORMAN M. KAPLAN

"On the basis of current evidence, it can be recommended that blood pressure is lowered at least below 140/90 mm Hg in all hypertensive patients and that lower values be pursued if tolerated."

2007 Guidelines of the European Societies of Hypertension and Cardiology[1]

"Comprehensive hypertension control strategies might address overall cardiovascular disease risk rather than an exclusive focus on blood pressure."

Kotchen 2010[2]

The blood pressure (BP) is the product of the cardiac output (CO) and the peripheral vascular resistance (PVR):

$$BP = CO \times PVR$$

Hence, as shown in Fig. 7-1, all antihypertensive drugs must act either by reducing the CO (β-blockers and diuretics) or the PVR (all the others, and perhaps a late effect of diuretics and β-blockade). Diuretics act chiefly by volume depletion, thereby reducing the CO, and also as indirect vasodilators. Most of the antihypertensive drugs, including diuretics, β-blockers, α-blockers, angiotensin-converting enzyme (ACE) inhibitors, angiotensin-II receptor blockers (ARBs), and calcium channel blockers (CCBs), but excluding the centrally active agents and ganglion blockers, have other uses and are therefore also discussed elsewhere in this book. Although hypertension is easy to treat, it is often difficult to manage optimally, as most patients will require lifestyle modification plus combination therapy with two, three, or more antihypertensive drugs of different mechanisms of action (Table 7-1). Asymptomatic patients often will not stay on therapy, particularly if it makes them feel weak, sleepy, forgetful, or impotent. In this regard, the ACE inhibitors and especially the ARBs seem very well tolerated. Fortunately, with most currently used modern antihypertensive agents, the quality of life (QOL) improves rather than deteriorates and cognitive function is preserved.[3,4] A small proportion of patients have resistant hypertension (RH) that only responds to multiple therapies after excluding poor adherence or secondary cause. It must constantly be considered that hypertension is usually multifactorial in cause, that different drugs act on different mechanisms (Fig. 7-2), and that the aim is to match the drugs to the patient. In the future such matching should be much more efficient, especially if genetic profiling ever becomes feasible.[5]

HYPERTENSION MECHANISMS
Opie 2012

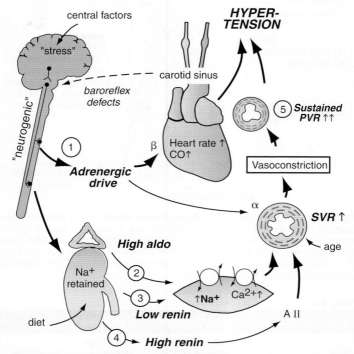

Figure 7-1 Multifactorial origin of hypertension. Note major mechanisms: **1,** Increased adrenergic drive as found especially in younger hypertensives. **2-4,** Renal-adrenal mechanisms, including (**2** and **3**) low renin hypertension as in those with inherently higher aldosterone (aldo) levels or renal sodium retention (sodium epithelial channel). **4,** High-renin hypertension, as in renal dysfunction. **5,** Increased systemic vascular resistance (SVR) or peripheral vascular resistance (PVR), the end result of all of these mechanisms. *CO,* cardiac output. (Figure © L.H. Opie, 2012.)

Principles of Treatment

Despite the fact that hypertension remains the most common diagnosis of patients seen in practitioners' offices[6] and the most common indication for prescription drugs,[7] it remains poorly controlled in all developed nations.[8] The reasons are multiple, perhaps the most obvious being its nature as a common, incurable, persistent, but usually asymptomatic disease with a treatment that provides no obvious short-term benefit. The complications of hypertension (Fig. 7-3) will not change, but closer attention to the principles to be described could markedly improve its control. As will be noted, prevention should be our primary goal but, lacking that, effective treatment can slow if not stop its insidious damage to the heart, brain, and kidneys.

Ascertainment of Hypertension

BP constantly changes over short and long intervals. Therefore more than a few measurements in the office are almost always needed to establish its level and range. Mean office readings are often recommended.[9] A novel proposal is that the maximum office systolic blood pressure

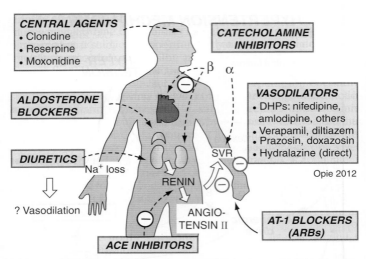

Figure 7-2   Different types of antihypertensive agents act at different sites.
Because hypertension is frequently multifactorial in origin, it may be difficult
to find the ideal drug for a given patient and drug combinations are often used.
ACE, Angiotensin-converting enzyme; *ARBs,* angiotensin receptor blockers;
AT-1, angiotensin II subtype 1; *DHP,* dihydropyridine; *SVR,* systemic vascular
resistance. (Figure © L.H. Opie, 2012.)

Table 7-1

Specifics About Additional Oral Antihypertensives			
Drug	**Registered Trade Name (in US)**	**Dose Range (mg/day)**	**Doses/Day**
α-Blockers			
Prazosin	Minipress	2-20	2
Terazosin	Hytrin	1-20	1
Doxazosin	Cardura XL	1-16	1
Direct Vasodilators			
Hydralazine	Apresoline	50-200	2-3
Minoxidil	Loniten	5-40	1
Nonreceptor Adrenergic Inhibitors			
Reserpine	Serpasil	0.05-0.25	1
Rauwolfia root	Raudixin	50-100	1
Centrally Active			
Methyldopa	Aldomet	500-1500	2
Clonidine	Catapres	0.5-1.5	2-3
Clonidine transdermal	Catapres-TTX	1 patch	(Once weekly)
Guanabenz	Wytensin	8-64	2
Guanfacine	Tenex	1-3	1
Peripheral			
Guanethidine	Ismelin	10-150	1
Guanadrel	Hylorel	10-75	2

For diuretics, see Tables 4-3 and 4-5; β-blockers, see Table 1-3; combined α- and
β-blockers, see Table 1-3; angiotensin-converting enzyme inhibitors, see Table 5-4;
angiotensin receptor blockers, see Table 5-12; calcium antagonists (calcium channel
blockers), see Tables 3-2 and 3-5.

(SBP), often ascribed to anxiety and thus ignored, is a strong predictor of
cardiovascular events, independently of the mean SBP level.[10] For multiple reasons, out-of-office readings provide more accurate assessment
of the future course of the disease.[11] The prognostic superiority of out-
of-office readings largely reflects the larger number of readings taken,
both by machine and by self-measured home readings. Despite the many

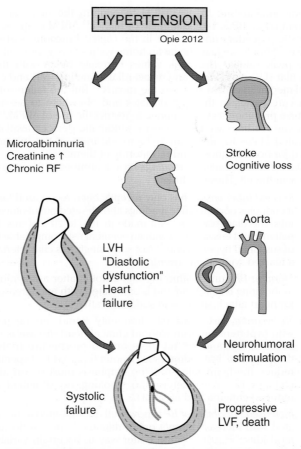

Figure 7-3 Hypertension and cardiovascular complications. Cardiac complications are the most common cause of death. Hypertension also kills by renal failure and cerebral complications such as stroke. The two major cardiovascular events are left ventricular hypertrophy (LVH) and promotion of aortic and coronary artery disease. LVH often first manifests symptoms as diastolic dysfunction, then progresses to systolic left ventricular failure (LVF) which, if allowed to progress, can lead to death. *RF, renal failure.* (Figure © L.H. Opie, 2012.)

different and increasingly sophisticated ways of obtaining the "true" BP, the office BP remains standard, and repeated values of *greater than* 140/90 mm Hg are taken as evidence of hypertension and major guidelines recommend lowering SBP to less than 140 mm Hg in all hypertensive patients. But how valid is this cut-off point?

There are two relevant trials. The MRC mild hypertension trial included very low-risk hypertensive patients (8.2% cardiovascular events over 10 years on placebo), and found that lowering SBP/diastolic blood pressure (DBP) to mean values of 138/86 rather than 149/91 mm Hg significantly reduced stroke and all cardiovascular events, but not coronary events or mortality.[12] Likewise in Chinese hypertensive patients treated by a daily small dose of felodipine (5 mg), a mean SBP of less than 140 mm Hg reduced major clinical events in those with a prior mean SBP of 153 mm Hg.[13] For every 100 patients treated for 3.3 years, 2.1 cardiovascular events were prevented in uncomplicated hypertension and 5.2 events in older adult hypertensive patients.

Ambulatory blood pressure monitoring. Ambulatory blood pressure monitoring (ABPM) is the easiest and quickest way to establish the diagnosis (and to monitor its therapy). In the United Kingdom, the current recommendations are to use ABPM to confirm the diagnosis when the mean office BP is 140/90 mm Hg or higher.[14] ABPM is an excellent diagnostic procedure and, at least in the United Kingdom, is also cost effective.[15] Should we take the mean home values or pay more attention to the peak values? The peak values correlate better with the left ventricular (LV) mass index and myocardial infarction (MI) and carotid intimal-medial thickness than do the means.[16] But the failure of most health care payers in the United States and elsewhere to adequately reimburse practitioners will continue to restrict the use of ABPM.[17]

Home readings with inexpensive automatic devices, available in the United States for less than $40, provide most of the information needed for both diagnosis and monitoring of therapy.

Out-of-office ambulatory readings have a number of the vagaries of BP measurements. These include:

- *Masked hypertension* has only recently been recognized because it connotes normal office readings and elevated out-of-office read-ings. The diagnosis has been made in 10% to 20% of unselected patients and is associated with an eventual risk comparable to that of sustained hypertension.[11] Not surprisingly, it is characterized by a marked sympathetic overdrive.[18]

- *Morning BP* surge within the first 2 hours after awakening and ambulating is common and is associated with an increased risk for heart attack, stroke, and sudden death.[19]

- *Tachycardia*, fast heart rate frequenty found among patients with hypertension even without clinical heart disease, is not an innocent bystander.[20] Yet there are no prospective trials with drugs such as ivabradine (see Chapter 6, p. 195) that specifically reduce the heart rate. Thus the emphasis must be on lifestyle changes (aerobic exercise, no smoking, no stimulant drugs, reduced caffeine and alcohol).

- *Increased variability of BP* is now well documented to be associ-ated with increased target organ damage[21] and cardiovascular morbidity.[22,23] ABPM is the better way to ascertain variability[24] but monitoring in clinic or home over a longer period can pro-vide useful information.[24] CCBs as a group are more effective than other agents in reducing blood pressure variability (BPV).[23] The X-CELLENT study compared four parallel treatment arms (placebo, candesartan, indapamide sustained release, and amlo-dipine).[25] The best reduction in BPV was by amlodipine, associ-ated with decreased BP ($P < 0.006$) and reduced heart rate (HR) variability ($P < 0.02$).

J-shaped curve. The J-shaped curve remains a tricky problem. "Alive and well," says Norman Kaplan.[26] John Chalmers writes, "It is clear that there must be a J-curve relating blood pressure to cardiovascular risk because, at pressures below the lower limits for autoregulation, perfu-sion of vital organs must fail." However, he questions whether "any such J-curve is related to the patients' inherent risk profile or directly to blood pressure–lowering treatment."[27] In a large prospective outcome study in patients with manifest vascular disease, with end points of cardiovascular events and all-cause mortality, there were clear J-shaped curves with the nadirs at 140-143/82-84 mm Hg.[28] The J-curve is thus an independent risk factor for recurrent events. Association is not causality, providing a strong rationale for future trials evaluating BP treatment targets.

What is the diastolic cut off point? When the DBP drops below a certain value, perhaps at approximately 65 mm Hg (fifth Korotkoff sound), cardiovascular events increase, but what is the reason?[26] Others state that the cut off point is approximately 70-80 mm Hg, which may actually increase mortality in those with coronary artery disease.[29] Another study places the turn-around BP value at less than 60 mm Hg.[30]

The European guidelines comment that a similar J-curve phenomenon occurs in placebo-treated groups of several trials.[31] Also noted is that several post hoc analyses consistently showed that the nadir of cardiovascular outcome incidence had a rather wide range, between 120 and 140 mm Hg SBP and between 70 and 80 mm Hg DBP, and that within this low BP range the differences in achieved cardiovascular protection are small (Figs. 7-4 and 7-5).[32]

What practical policy must be followed if the proposed critical DBP of 65 mm Hg is reached? Presumably but without trial data, the BP-lowering medication should be reduced when the diastolic BP drops to less than 65 mm Hg until the level rises to 65-70 mm Hg. That leaves the likely increase in systolic BP to look after itself. A few outcome studies would be helpful.

Sleep apnea hypertension. In a consecutive series of 125 patients with RH, sleep apnea was the commonest cause (64%) (see page 258).

Central blood pressure. Central BP obtained from carotid and radial distension waves and a validated transfer function will increasingly be used in clinical practice[24] because the central pressure is more closely related to vascular outcomes than is the brachial pressure.[33]

Aortic stiffness. Arterial stiffness is an independent predictor of cardiovascular events and mortality in hypertensive patients, especially in older adults (see Fig. 7-11). It is calculated from the carotid-femoral wave velocity.[34] An analysis of 15 trials from one center showed that antihypertensive therapy improved arterial stiffness beyond the effect on BP.[35]

Pulse wave velocity. Carotid-femoral pulse wave velocity is now considered the gold standard for arterial stiffness assessment in daily practice.

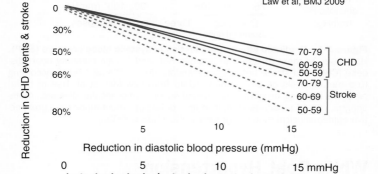

EFFECT OF DBP REDUCTION ON CHD & STROKE

Figure 7-4   Predicted effects of reduction of diastolic blood pressure (DBP). Half-doses of three drugs could improve DBP and reduce coronary heart disease (CHD) and stroke better than standard doses of single drugs according to a meta analysis of 147 studies. (Data from Law MR, et al. Use of blood pressure lowering drugs in the prevention of cardiovascular disease: meta-analysis of 147 randomised trials in the context of expectations from prospective epidemiological studies. *Br Med J* 2009;338:b1665.)

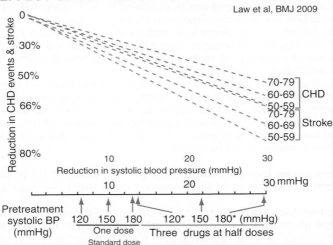

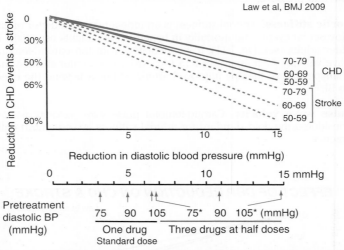

Figure 7-5 Predicted effects of reduction of systolic blood pressure (SBP). Half-doses of three drugs could improve SBP and reduce coronary heart disease (CHD) and stroke better than standard doses of single drugs according to a metaanalysis of 147 studies. (Data from Law MR, et al. Use of blood pressure lowering drugs in the prevention of cardiovascular disease: meta-analysis of 147 randomised trials in the context of expectations from prospective epidemiological studies. *Br Med J* 2009;338:b1665.)

White-Coat Hypertension and Prehypertension

White-coat hypertension. White-coat hypertension (i.e., persistently elevated office readings but persistently normal out-of-office readings) is present in up to 20% of patients. Although its short-term danger is minimal, it eventually poses a hazard with the likelihood for cardiovascular events that is 68% of that seen with sustained hypertension.[11] White-coat hypertension may masquerade as RH, which is an uncontrolled office BP of 140/90 mm Hg or more, despite the use of three or more antihypertensive drugs, including a diuretic. Following this diagnosis, the use of ABPM is crucial to split up two different groups, those with true and those with white-coat RH. ABPM then classifies RH patients into two groups: true uncontrolled RH (office BP and 24-hour BP ≥130/80 mm Hg) and white-coat (controlled) RH (white-coat RH: office BP ≥140/90 mm Hg and 24-hour BP <130/80 mm Hg).[36] White-coat hypertension may account for as much as 40% of all apparently resistant patients as detected by the office BP.[11] For follow up, to avoid white-coat creeping up to sustained hypertension, ABPM is required every 6-12 months.

Prehypertension. *Does a BP of less than 140/90 mm Hg warrant drugs?* A radical change in approach to modestly or even minimally elevated BP has resulted from two mega-meta-analyses on approximately 1 million adults.[32,37] Any increase in BP to more than 115/75 mm Hg increases cardiovascular risk, which doubles with every rise of 20/10 mm Hg. The previously normal and high-normal BP ranges of 120 to 139 mm Hg systolic and 80 to 89 mm Hg diastolic are now considered *prehypertensive*, with calls for active lifestyle changes to avoid moving into the overtly hypertensive category, which remains 140/90 mm Hg or more.[38] These stricter views have led to more active antihypertensive intervention at lower BP levels, sometimes even giving drugs where there are no solid trial data as in those with BP levels less than 140/90 mm Hg in whom only lifestyle modification is presently appropriate. Contrariwise, a more radical view is that prehypertension may warrant drug therapy, as supported by the epic metaanalysis by 147 studies on nearly 1 million people (see Figs. 7-4 and 7-5).[32]

Determination of Overall Cardiovascular Risk

After accurate ascertainment of the usual level of BP, the other major contributors to cardiovascular risk should be assessed by history, physical examination, and routine laboratory testing, including an electrocardiogram.[39] Thereby a number of levels of risk can be calculated from Framingham or other databases. With knowledge of overall risk, appropriate therapy for hypertension and the need for additional treatments for other risk factors can be determined (Table 7-2). For some patients, testing beyond the routine (e.g., echocardiography) may be used to decide on the need to start active antihypertensive drug therapy. The presence of target organ damage generally mandates faster and more intensive therapy.

Lifetime Risk versus Current Risk

In a very large study, 61,585 American men and women were followed from age 55 for 700,000 person-years. Life-time risk for cardiovascular disease (CVD) was 53% for men and 40% for women. Life-time risk for CVD increased with increasing BP at index age. Individuals who maintained or decreased their BP to normal levels at index age had the lowest remaining life-time risk for CVD, 22%-41%, as compared with individuals who had or developed hypertension by the age of 55, 42%-69%. These data support a dose-response adverse effect for the length of time at high BP levels.[40]

The Goals of Therapy

The goal of therapy is to provide maximal protection against cardiovascular consequences with minimal bother to the patient. Currently available medications should cause little if any bother (except financial) to the patient, but there remains uncertainty regarding how to provide maximal protection.

Table 7-2

Risk Stratification in Treatment of Hypertension

Other Risk Factors and Disease History	Normal SBP 120-129 or DBP 80-84	High Normal SBP 130-139 or DBP 85-89	Grade 1 SBP 140-159 or DBP 90-99	Grade 2 SBP 160-179 or DBP 100-109	Grade 3 SBP ≥ 180 or DBP ≥ 110
			Blood Pressure (mm Hg)		
No other risk factors	Average risk	Average risk	<15% 10-year risk	15%-20% 10-year risk	20%-30% 10-year risk
1-2 risk factors	<15% 10-year risk	<15% 10-year risk	15%-20% 10-year risk	15%-20% 10-year risk	>30% 10-year risk
3 or more risk factors or TOD or diabetes mellitus	15%-20% 10-year risk	20%-30% 10-year risk	20%-30% 10-year risk	20%-30% 10-year risk	>30% 10-year risk
Associated clinical conditions	20%-30% 10-year risk	>30% 10-year risk	>30% 10-year risk	>30% 10-year risk	>30% 10-year risk

DBP, Diastolic blood pressure; *SBP,* systolic blood pressure; *TOD,* target organ damage.

Based on and modified from recommendations of European Societies of Cardiology and Hypertension.[39] 10-year risk of cardiovascular disease according to Framingham criteria.

Risk factors for coronary heart disease (note slight differences from adenosine triphosphate III in Chapter 10): blood pressure as previously; cholesterol level >250 mg/dL, low-density lipoprotein >155 mg/dL, high-density lipoprotein cholesterol <40 mg/dL in men, <48 mg/dL in women; family history of premature coronary heart disease; smoking, age (men >55, women >65), abdominal obesity, C-reactive protein ≥1 mg/dL.

TOD, target organ damage: left ventricular hypertrophy; ultrasound evidence of arterial disease, increased serum creatinine up to 1.5 mg/dL (133 μmol/L) in men, slightly lower in women, microalbuminuria up to 300 mg/24 h.

Associated clinical conditions: cerebrovascular disease including transient ischemic attack, angina or myocardial infarction, congestive heart failure, renal impairment, proteinuria, peripheral vascular disease, and advanced retinopathy.

Reduction of all-cause mortality. As sustained reduction of BP in established hypertension lessens the overall risk of CVD, including strokes and heart failure, it is not surprising that a large US study (based on data in the Third National Health and Nutrition Examination) has linked BP control to decreased all-cause mortality.[41] Conversely, mortality risk linearly increased with SBP although not with DBP.

Lower blood pressures for higher-risk and black patients? In patients with diabetes or renal damage 130/80 is a generally accepted goal that should be upheld[27] even though disputed.[42] For non-Hispanic black patients, the International Society for Hypertension in Blacks (ISHIB) has recently lowered the definition of uncomplicated hypertension to 135/85 mm Hg (for primary prevention), recognizing the greater rate of progression to established hypertension, and dropping the definition of complicated hypertension even lower to 130/80 mm Hg (for secondary prevention). These recommendations are based on the greater CVD risk in blacks;[43] however, these new recommendations are controversial because of limited evidence.[44]

Lifestyle Modifications

Seeing that cardiovascular risk starts at only 115/75 mm Hg, and considering the shocking statistic that middle-aged American adults have a 90% lifetime risk of developing hypertension,[45] the real recommendation should be "lifestyle modification for all." If lifestyles can be improved, BP will fall[46] and, probably, cardiovascular events prevented.[47] The problem is how to change lifetime habits in a meaningful way. Counseling of those who are overweight is of minimal value over time[48] and, for the increasing number who are markedly obese, bariatric surgery may be the only hope.[49]

Our attention should therefore turn to children and their parents to help prevent the adoption of unhealthy habits. Intermittent external counseling by itself does not seem to work to prevent weight gain[50] or to increase physical activity,[51] and perhaps only a program that integrates home, school, and community would work.

Sodium reduction. Approximately 5% to 15% of all strokes and 10% to 20% of all heart attacks in the United States would be prevented if the food industry could be pressured to reduce the sodium content of processed food so that daily NaCl intake fell gradually over a decade from 10 g to 7; black persons would benefit the most, thus reducing racial disparity in CVD.[52]

Nondrug therapies. Meanwhile, to optimally protect those who are hypertensive, nondrug therapies should be standard in all hypertensive patients, particularly *weight reduction* for obese patients and moderate dietary *sodium reduction* from the usual level of approximately 10 g of sodium chloride per day down to approximately 5 g or 88 mmol or 2 g sodium, which will reduce the BP by approximately 7/4 mm Hg in hypertensive patients.[46] In the DASH-sodium study, further sodium reduction to approximately 1.4 g per day (urinary sodium of 65 mmol/day), enhanced the BP-lowering benefits of the high-fruit, high-vegetable DASH diet to give a total reduction of approximately 7 mm Hg lower than the standard diet, a degree of BP fall approximately the same as seen with an effective antihypertensive agent. The *ideal diet* is low in calories, rich in fresh rather than processed foods, and high in fruits and vegetables (and hence high in potassium) besides being low in fat and sodium.[53] Better than an approach directed to an individual, a reduction in the amount of sodium added to canned and packaged foods by food processors would be more effective.[54] *Weight loss* reduces BP, improves the QOL, and specifically benefits those with left ventricular hypertrophy (LVH).[55]

Multifactorial intervention with both weight loss and sodium restriction should be used before drug therapy is instituted, especially in older adults and in those with marginal BP elevations. Other measures include increased *aerobic exercise,* cessation of smoking, and moderation of alcohol. Smoking is an independent risk factor for coronary heart disease and stroke, besides increasing the risk of malignant hypertension.

Correction of Other Risk Factors

The efficacy of antihypertensive treatment depends not only on the control of the BP, but also on the control of co-existing risk factors, especially those for CVD, which is the major cause of mortality in hypertension (see Fig. 7-3). Whereas in low-risk groups, many hundreds of patients must be treated to prevent one stroke, in very high-risk groups, such as older adults, only 20 to 25 patients need to be treated for 1 year to prevent one cardiovascular event, including stroke. The well-known Framingham tables and several websites aid the assessment of risk factors. Explaining the exact risk over 10 years to a specific patient often helps in achieving a desirable lifestyle and reaching BP goals. The new European guidelines show color-coded tables, with the highest risk of 10-year fatality being in red and the lowest in green.[1]

In addition, risk assessment charts have been adopted for use in low-income countries.[56] The patient can readily grasp that reaching a specific BP goal means moving from a "bad" color, say orange, to a better one, say yellow, with less risk of stroke or heart attack to the best, green. Another approach is to shock the patient by calculating from the risk factor profile the age of the cardiovascular system which could be 5-20 years older that the patient's actual age. The evidence for additional protection in hypertensive patients by improvements in blood lipids and other features of the metabolic syndrome is presented in Chapters 11 (Fig. 11-1; p. 441).

Systolic versus diastolic versus pulse pressure. Although all recommendations for treatment in the past were based on a cut-off DBP level, there are two important new developments. First, the BP level must be seen as part of an overall risk profile. Second, systolic levels should be considered, particularly in older adults. At all ages, there are more predictive or risk values than diastolic values[57] and the Seventh Report of the Joint National Committee on Prevention, Detection, Evaluation, and Treatment of High Blood Pressure (JNC 7) states that SBP is a "much more important" cardiovascular risk factor than the diastolic in those older than 50 years.[38] A wide pulse pressure, largely reflecting a high systolic level and increased vascular stiffness, may be the most accurate predictor of all.

Overall Aims of Treatment

Reducing cardiovascular risk safely is the sole aim of therapy. Some trials have suggested a *J-shaped curve* indicating an increase of coronary complications in patients whose DBP was reduced to lower than 70 mm Hg.[30] The HOT trial attempted to disprove the presence of a J-curve with treatment.[58] Despite a less than desired separation of BP in the three groups assigned to reach a diastolic of 90, 85, or 80 mm Hg, the lowest incidence of endpoints was seen at a DBP of 83 mm Hg and a small but apparent increase in cardiovascular mortality occurred when the DBP was lowered to less than 70 mm Hg. In other studies of older adults with isolated systolic hypertension, a decrease of diastolic pressure to less than 65 mm Hg increased the risk of stroke and coronary heart disease. Patients with concomitant renal disease seem particularly susceptible to systolic levels less than 130 mm Hg.[59] Patients with coronary disease are susceptible to diastolics less than 80 mm Hg.[29] Therefore caution remains advisable.

Preservation of the brain. Preservation of the brain is now recognized as of paramount importance. Prevention of major and minor strokes by BP control starting in midlife is one imperative. Unexpectedly, factors that contribute to albuminuria may contribute to cognitive decline, suggesting that both conditions share a common microvascular pathogenesis.[60]

Guidelines: choice of initial and subsequent drugs. For many years, a great deal of attention, energy, and money has been spent in deciding which drug is the best choice for initial therapy and which combination is best for eventual therapy. "Drugs targeting the sympathetic nervous system are no longer considered as first-line antihypertensives. Central sympatholytics are limited by their side effects, and outcome trials have shown that α- and β-blockers are inferior in lowering the incidence of heart failure and strokes, respectively, compared with other drugs."[61] However, this restriction may not apply to more current vasodilating β-blockers.

The most recent "ACD" guidelines come from The British Society of Hypertension acting together with the UK National Institute of Excellence (NICE). They chose three outcomes-based groups of agents that are evidenced based: A is for ACE inhibitors and ARBs, C is for CCBs, and D is for diuretics.[9] The missing "B" is for β-blockers and indicates the gap from their previous recommendations, as these agents are now downgraded (nebivolol may be an exception; see later). These authorities also distinguish between thiazide-like diuretics such as chlorthalidone and indapamide slow release and the standard thiazides such as hydrochlorothiazide (HCTZ) with preference for the thiazide-like diuretics. The major reasons are that the standard thiazides have no outcome studies in hypertension when used at the presently recommended doses, whereas the thiazide-like agents are evidence based as in ALLHAT and HYVET.

These issues are open to debate. For initial therapy JNC 7[38] advocated a low-dose thiazide diuretic for most patients. The expectation is that the eighth report due soon will support chlorthalidone as the low-dose diuretic of choice. The European Hypertension Society[39] recommends whatever class seems most appropriate for the patient, whereas the World Health Organization[29] states that any class may be used but a diuretic is preferred. Thus two out of the three major guidelines suggest a low-dose diuretic as the first choice for uncomplicated patients; this recommendation is reinforced when cost is factored into the equation. However, in most developed countries, including the United States, diuretics are used in only approximately 30% of patients.[62] The reasons include the delayed response to diuretic therapy and the possible metabolic complications. However, diuretics combine well with all other antihypertensive classes.

As to the eventual therapy needed to reach the lower goals of BP now advocated by all experts, there is agreement to add whatever is appropriate for the individual patient—in other words, a "compelling" indication or a "favored" choice—to a diuretic and to add additional drugs from other classes to reach the goal.

Although the details vary somewhat, the tabulation based on the 2007 European guidelines fits most situations very nicely (Table 7-3). All classes have their place.

If these various guidelines are followed, the use of low-dose diuretic therapy should markedly increase. On the other hand, the β-blockers will almost certainly be used less overall,[63] but more so in those patients who need them because of MI or heart failure. CCBs have been better than other classes for prevention of stroke[64] and for reduction of BP variability.[25] ACE inhibitors received good marks in black patients only when used with a diuretic[65] or when used in older adult

Table 7-3

Guidelines for Selecting Drug Treatment for Hypertension

Class of Drug	Favored Indications	Possible Indications	Compelling Contraindications	Possible Contraindications
Diuretics (low-dose thiazides)	Congestive heart failure Older adults with hypertension Systolic hypertension African origin subjects	Obesity	Gout	Pregnancy Dyslipidemia Metabolic syndrome Sexually active men
Diuretics (loop)	Congestive heart failure Renal failure		Hypokalemia	Diabetic renal disease
Diuretics (antialdo)	Congestive heart failure Postinfarct Aldosteronism (First or second degree)	Refractory hypertension	Hyperkalemia Renal failure	
CCBs	Angina, effort Older adults Systolic hypertension	Peripheral vascular disease Diabetes African origin	Heart block* Clinical heart failure (possible exception: amlodipine, but needs care)	Preexisting ankle edema
ACE inhibitors	Left ventricular dysfunction or failure Postinfarct Nephropathy, type 1 diabetic or nondiabetic Proteinuria	CV protection (BP already controlled) Type 2 nephropathy	Pregnancy Hyperkalemia Bilateral renal artery stenosis	Severe cough Severe aortic stenosis

Angiotensin-II Antagonists (ARBs)	ACE inhibitor cough Diabetes type 2 nephropathy including micro-albuminuria LVH Heart failure	Postinfarct	Pregnancy Bilateral renal artery stenosis Hyperkalemia	Severe aortic stenosis
β-Blockers	Angina Tachyarrhythmias Post-MI Heart failure (uptitrate)	Pregnancy Diabetes	Asthma, severe COPD Heart block†	Obesity Metabolic syndrome Athletes and exercising patients Erectile dysfunction Peripheral vascular disease

ACE, Angiotensin-converting enzyme; Aldo, aldosterone; ARB, angiotensin receptor blocker; BP, blood pressure; CCB, calcium channel blocker; COPD, chronic obstructive pulmonary disease; CV, cardiovascular; LVH, left ventricular hypertrophy; MI, myocardial infarction.

*Grade 2 or 3 atrioventricular block with verapamil or diltiazem.

†Grade 2 or 3 atrioventricular block.

white patients.[66] Ideally, ACE inhibitors should be combined with their natural partners, the diuretics, or with their new suitors, the CCBs (see "ACCOMPLISH" later in this chapter). ARBs, the fastest growing class, are no better than other classes in protection against stroke, heart attack, or heart failure.[64] However, in hypertension there are no good comparative head-to-head outcome studies of ARBs with their cheaper siblings, the ACE inhibitors.

Resistant hypertension and aldosterone antagonists. "Resistant hypertension is almost always multifactorial in origin."[67] Therapy requires strong advice on adverse lifestyles, detection and therapy of secondary causes of hypertension, and the use of effective multidrug regimens. The standard definition is the failure to control the BP on three or more agents including a diuretic at target or at least at the highest tolerated doses. In fact, most studies on RH have studied patients on four or more drugs. Thus adherence and excellent physician-patient relationships become essential, as repeated studies show that as the number of drugs that should be taken increases, the number of drugs actually taken decreases. Building on the three basic drug classes— namely a diuretic, an ACE inhibitor (or ARB), and a CCB—there is a good case to regard aldosterone blockade as the next logical step. One old drug, *spironolactone,* has been revitalized for use in heart failure[68] and RH.[69,70] *Eplerenone* is a congener that provides more selective aldosterone blockade, and may become another major player in RH without the sexual side effects of spironolactone, although it is currently priced higher. Serum potassium levels should be measured before initiating eplerenone and then monitored regularly to avoid hyperkalemia. (Similar monitoring for hyperkalemia is required for spironolactone.) Eplerenone is considerably weaker than spironolactone, but the Food and Drug Administration (FDA) limits the maximum daily dose to 100 mg because higher doses increase the risk of hyperkalemia.

Relative efficacy. As seen in Table 7-3, certain drugs are favored in certain patients (e.g., diuretics and CCBs in blacks and older adults and ACE inhibitors or ARBs in diabetics with nephropathy). Moreover, all drugs have certain limitations and contraindications. However, it should be noted that in the overall hypertensive population, the response rate (i.e., BP lowered to less than 140/90 mm Hg) to each of the five major groups of agents as monotherapy may be no more than 30% to 40% depending on the severity of the hypertension and the drug chosen, so that combination therapy is usually required in addition to lifestyle modification. Finally, financial considerations may be crucial. Diuretics, reserpine, and hydralazine are inexpensive, as are generic β-blockers, ACE inhibitors, and verapamil. Of the CCBs, amlodipine is the best tested and generic in many countries. Newer agents can be much more expensive.

Compliance and Adherence

There are two different yet complementary approaches, the first to target known high-risk patients, and the second to achieve better adherence of the wider population with less severe but more common hypertension levels in the community.[2] In Spain a three-pronged intervention helped to control their "high-risk" hypertensive patients: (1) counting pills during physician visits, (2) designating a family member to support adherence behavior, and (3) providing patients with an information sheet about their BP medications.[2] In Canada a hypertension education program involves pharmacists,[71] and is remarkably successful with 80% in one survey using antihypertensives, and almost all of those (89%) adhering to the prescriptions.[72] However, even in Canada many persons seen in an academic family practice were not well controlled.[73] A wide community-based approach could be the start to reach the many individuals with uncontrolled hypertension, as in approximately 50% of US blacks.[2]

Combination Therapy

An interesting concept is that combination therapy by several agents, up to three, in low doses give better control of BP than larger doses of any single agent (see Figs. 7-4 and 7-5).[32] Although impressively based on a metaanalysis of 147 studies, there is little trial data to show that substantial BP outcome benefits result from treating uncomplicated hypertension at levels less than 140/90 mm Hg, which still remains the cut-off point (Fig. 7-6). Nonetheless, this study strongly argues the case for combining several agents in half doses.

Diuretics for Hypertension

Diuretics have been the basis of several impressive trials, many in older adult patients, in which hard endpoints have been reduced. Diuretics are widely recommended as first-line therapy (Fig. 7-7) and are among the three drug groups of first choice selected in the recent UK recommendations.[9] They are better at reducing coronary heart disease, heart failure, stroke, and cardiovascular and total mortality than placebo, and in at least one of these endpoints they are better than β-blockers, CCBs, ACE inhibitors (but equal to the ARBs), and α-blockers.[74] Diuretics are inexpensive and remain basic in the therapy of hypertension.[75] Thus it is not surprising that they are still widely used either as monotherapy (see Fig. 7-2) or in combination (Fig. 7-7). They combine particularly well with ACE inhibitors and ARBs. In contrast, the dihydropyridine (DHP) CCBs have inherent diuretic properties, making this combination less effective than expected. The vascular complications that are more directly related to the height of the BP per se (strokes and congestive heart failure) have been reduced more than that of the most common cause of disease and death among hypertensive patients, namely coronary heart disease.[74] Hypothetically, metabolic side effects from the high doses of diuretics used in earlier trials, particularly on lipids and

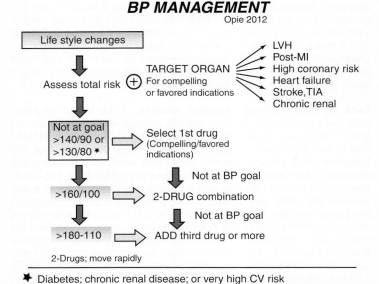

Figure 7-6 **Proposed simplified treatment algorithm for hypertension therapy.** *BP,* Blood pressure; *LVH,* left ventricular hypertrophy; *MI,* myocardial infarction; *TIA,* transient ischemic attack. (Figure © L.H. Opie, 2012.)

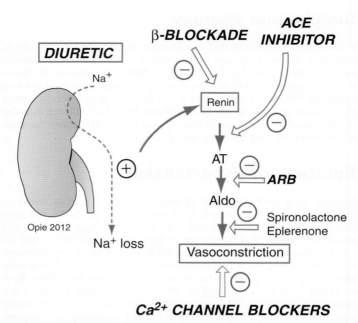

Figure 7-7   Diuretics. Diuretics, basically acting by sodium loss, cause a reactive increase in circulating renin that results in angiotensin-mediated vasoconstriction to offset the hypotensive effect. Diuretics therefore combine well with β-blockers, which inhibit the release of renin, with angiotensin-converting enzyme (ACE) inhibitors that inhibit the formation of angiotensin-II, with angiotensin receptor blockers (ARBs), and with calcium channel blockers, which directly oppose diuretic-induced vasoconstriction. Of these combinations, those of diuretic and ACE inhibitor or ARB are particularly well tested. ACE inhibitors and ARBs lessen the metabolic side effects of diuretics. *Aldo,* Aldosterone; *AT,* angiotensin. (Figure © L.H. Opie, 2012.)

insulin sensitivity,[76] as well as potassium and magnesium depletion, and increased uric acid levels, may in part explain why death from coronary disease has not decreased as much as it should have. For example, a serum potassium of 3.5 mmol/L or less increased cardiovascular events by approximately four times over a mean follow-up of 6.7 years.[77] Also on the debit side, impotence is a relatively frequent side effect of chlorthalidone—more so than with any other antihypertensive drug class.[78] Furthermore, the response in younger white patients (younger than 60 years) is poor.[79]

Lack of dose-finding outcome studies. A persistent problem with the concept of low-dose diuretic therapy is that there are no good comparative studies between the different diuretics, their "low" doses, and outcomes. Strictly speaking, we do not know that the low doses of diuretics currently used really result in patient benefit except in older adults in whom low-dose chlorthalidone (12.5 mg) was chosen as initial therapy in the SHEP study.[80] Even there, in many patients the dose was doubled and a β-blocker added. Logically, the lower the dose of diuretic, the fewer the metabolic side effects, whereas (within limits) the antihypertensive potency may still be adequately expressed. However, the available evidence suggests that the following are low doses that nonetheless are effectively and safely antihypertensive in mild to moderate hypertension: HCTZ 12.5 mg, chlorthalidone 12.5 to 15 mg, and bendrofluazide 1.25 mg.[81] If chlorthalidone has a more lasting antihypertensive effect than HCTZ, as evidence suggests,[82] then these comparisons suggest an advantage for chlorthalidone.

Diuretic dose: hydrochlorothiazide. Although a single morning dose of 12.5 mg of HCTZ or its equivalent will provide a 10 mm Hg fall in the BP of most patients with uncomplicated hypertension within several weeks, even that dose may be too high in combination therapies. Higher doses such as 25 mg increase the risk of diabetes.[83] Lower doses (6.25 mg HCTZ) may be equally effective when combined with β-blockade, ACE inhibition, or an ARB. Such low doses of HCTZ may require several weeks to act. Low-dose thiazides may be combined with all other classes, including the DHP CCBs,[84] which have their own mild diuretic capacity. Alternatively, sodium restriction may be the secret in making low-dose HCTZ work. The advantage of low-dose HCTZ (or its equivalent in other diuretics) is that adverse metabolic and lipid effects are minimized or completely avoided. Nevertheless, even 12.5 mg HCTZ may still induce potassium wastage and hypokalemia.[76,85] This trend to hypokalemia can be prevented by concomitant ACE inhibitor or ARB therapy.[76]

Chlorthalidone. A 15 mg daily dose was used in the TOMH study[86] in patients with very mild hypertension. Combined with weight loss and other measures, it was as effectively antihypertensive as other groups of agents. It gave an unexpectedly good QOL (despite the doubling of impotence) and at the end of 4 years blood cholesterol changes (elevated at 1 year) had reverted to normal.[86] Chlorthalidone 12.5 mg daily was the first-line treatment in the study on systolic hypertension in the SHEP study of older adults.[80] Thereafter the dose was doubled in about one third of patients and atenolol was added, if needed, to control BP. In SHEP, after 4.5 years, total stroke was reduced by 36%. On the debit side, the higher dose increased the risk of hypokalemia with partial loss of cardiovascular benefit.[87] In ALLHAT, chlorthalidone at a daily dose of 12.5 to 25 mg was considered the best overall drug versus the CCB amlodipine or the ACE inhibitor lisinopril, but at the cost of increased diabetes and hypokalemia.[88]

Chlorthalidone versus hydrochlorothiazide. As fully discussed in Chapter 4 (p. 102), overall data favor cardiovascular outcomes with the longer-acting chlorthalidone over HCTZ despite more metabolic problems such as hypokolemia.[89]

Bendrofluazide. Bendrofluazide is a standard thiazide in the United Kingdom, once given at 10 mg a day in a large trial, and is effective over 24 hours at a daily dose of only 1.25 mg.[90] Current UK guidelines favor its replacement whenever starting therapy by more widely used agents.

Amiloride. Among diuretics, amiloride uniquely has potassium-retaining effects. In difficult-to-treat hypertension in black patients on two drugs (thiazide and CCB), amiloride was at least as effective as spironolactone and the combination with a standard thiazide was not much more effective than amiloride alone.[91]

Indapamide. The modified thiazide *indapamide (Lozol, Natrilix SR)* may be more lipid neutral than standard thiazides and is promoted in some countries as a vasodilating diuretic. The previous standard dose of 2.5 mg once daily has been dropped by the manufacturers to 1.5 mg daily in a sustained-release formulation. Yet the potassium may fall, and the blood glucose and uric acid rise, as warned in the package insert. Indapamide induces regression of LVH and was better than enalapril 20 mg once daily.[92] A large indapamide-based antihypertensive trial in much older adults, HYVET, had to be stopped because of reduced mortality.[93]

Loop diuretics for hypertension. Furosemide is not ideal as it is short acting and needs to be given at least twice a day to be adequately antihypertensive. Torasemide is free of metabolic and lipid side–effects, yet is antihypertensive when used in the subdiuretic dose of 2.5 mg once daily.[94] At the higher daily doses registered for hypertension in the United States, namely 5 to 10 mg, it becomes natriuretic with greater risk of metabolic changes.

Potassium-sparing combination diuretics. Potassium-sparing combination diuretics may add a few cents to the cost but save a good deal more by the prevention of diuretic-induced hypokalemia and hypomagnesemia. The risk of torsades-related sudden death should also be reduced.[95] A small observational study suggests better retention of cognitive function in older adults.[96] To be effectively antihypertensive, the potassium-sparing agents are combined with another diuretic, generally a thiazide. Fixed-dose combinations of *triamterene (Dyazide, Maxzide)* or *amiloride (Moduretic)* with HCTZ are available. The general problem is that the thiazide dose is too high. The dose of HCTZ in one tablet of Dyazide is 25 mg, but only approximately half is absorbed. Maxzide contains 25- or 50-mg HCTZ. Standard Moduretic contains 50 mg (far too much), but in Europe, a "mini-Moduretic" *(Moduret)* with half the standard thiazide dose is now marketed to overcome this objection. However, even these doses are probably too high. *Aldactazide* combines 25-mg spironolactone with 25-mg thiazide. Note that in general, thiazides are relatively ineffective with poor renal function as compared with loop diuretics.

Combinations of diuretics with other antihypertensives. Diuretics may add to the effect of all other types of antihypertensives. Combination with ACE inhibition or an ARB is logical and part of the ACD concept (see p. 235) but may not be as good a combination as A and C (see Chapter 5, p. 134). A number of well-designed factorial studies have varied the dose of HCTZ from 6.25 mg to 25 mg and studied the interaction with a β-blocker,[97] diltiazem,[98] or an ACE inhibitor.[99] In general, somewhat greater antihypertensive effects were obtained with 25-mg HCTZ, yet the difference between the high and the low doses of thiazide were negligible when the alternate agent was given at higher doses. Thus there is a good argument for starting combination therapy with 6.25-mg HCTZ, a dose that effectively avoids hypokalemia. A combination that has trial support in much older adults is that of indapamide with an ACE inhibitor.[93]

Diuretics: conclusions. Despite reservations about metabolic side effects such as new-onset diabetes at higher doses, low-dose diuretics remain among the preferred initial treatments, especially in older adults, the obese, and black patients. Compared with placebo, low-dose diuretics reduce stroke and coronary disease in older adults and achieve outcome benefit, including mortality reduction, in patients with mild to moderate hypertension.[76] Diuretics appear to work particularly well in older black patients while being much less effective in younger white patients.[64] Two large positive outcome studies with diuretics have been in older adults, with the mean age well older than 60 years even at the start of the trial.[80,88] Of note, in these trials the diuretic dose was often uptitrated, whereas a better course would probably be to keep the diuretic dose low and to add another agent, as in HYVET, in which an ACE inhibitor was added.[93] In this trial there was an early mortality benefit, so that the trial had to be stopped.

Calcium Channel Blockers

CCBs (calcium antagonists) compare well in their antihypertensive effect with other classes and are more effective than the others in protection against stroke.[100] CCBs act primarily to reduce PVR, aided by at least an initial diuretic effect, especially in the case of the short-acting DHPs. No negative inotropic effect can be detected in patients with initially normal myocardial function. Regarding the effects on plasma

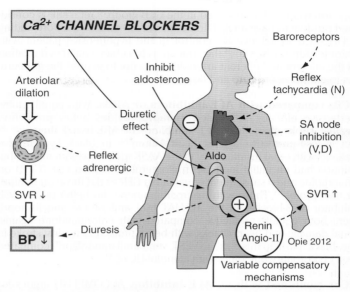

Figure 7-8 Calcium channel blockers (CCBs). CCBs act largely by peripheral arterial dilation, with a lesser diuretic effect. They also evoke counterregulatory mechanisms that depend on stimulation of renin and formation of angiotensin, as well as on reflex release of norepinephrine. Such acute adrenergic stimulation with short-acting nifedipine (N) may precipitate myocardial ischemia in the presence of coronary disease (see Fig. 3-6). Currently only long-acting CCBs are used in the treatment of hypertension. The inhibition of aldosterone release obviates overall fluid retention. *Aldo,* Aldosterone; *BP,* blood pressure; *D,* diltiazem; *SA,* sinoatrial; *SVR,* systemic vascular resistance; *V,* verapamil. (Figure © L.H. Opie, 2012.)

catecholamines, DHPs must be distinguished from non-DHPs such as verapamil and diltiazem. As a group, DHPs reflexly stimulate the adrenergic system to increase plasma catecholamines modestly,[101] with a borderline elevation of plasma renin activity caused by the counterregulatory effect (Fig. 7-8). Non-DHPs tend to decrease catecholamine levels. There are several long-term outcome studies available with CCBs in hypertension and the consistent message is that CCBs are safe and effective, particularly for prevention of stroke.[100] Amlodipine, often combined with an ACE inhibitor, provided greater antihypertensive efficacy and better protection against cardiovascular events, mortality, and the development of new diabetes than did atenolol-based therapy in the ASCOT trial.[102] CCBs are particularly effective in older adult patients and are equally effective in blacks as in nonblacks. They act independently of sodium intake. CCBs may be selected as initial monotherapy, especially if there are other indications for these agents such as angina pectoris or Raynaud phenomenon or supraventricular tachycardia (non-DHPs). Previous ungrounded fears that CCBs increased MI have now been laid to rest and replaced by data suggesting superior protection against MI by amlodipine.[100,102]

CCBs compared with diuretics. Compared with diuretics (also advocated for older adult and black patients), generic CCBs are becoming less expensive, with generic amlodipine now being widely available and being added to many $4 formularies; moreover, CCBs cause no metabolic disturbances in potassium, glucose, uric acid, or lipid metabolism. Patients on CCBs do not require intermittent blood chemistry checks. In a study on South African black patients with hypertension, a CCB regimen was better able to reduce DBP to less than 90 mm Hg than HCTZ 12.5 to 25 mg.[103] There is no evidence that CCBs cause impairment of renal function. On the contrary, in ALLHAT indices of renal function were better preserved in the CCB group.[88] Yet it still is considered prudent to have an ACE inhibitor or ARB on board before adding a DHP-CCB to achieve BP control in the hypertensive patient with chronic kidney disease;[104] the concept is to achieve balanced dilation of the afferent and efferent arterioles so as not to expose the glomerulus to excessive pressure and flow.

CCBs compared with ACE inhibitors or ARBs. With equal antihypertensive efficacy, CCB-based therapy provides better protection against stroke than does ACE inhibitor– or ARB-based therapy,[88,100] but is less protective against heart failure.[105] In black hypertensive patients with renal insufficiency in the AASK trial, those with microalbuminuria had an initial increase in glomerular filtration rate (GFR) on amlodipine and a subsequent equal fall in GFR as did those on ramipril or metoprolol.[106] Those with macroalbuminuria did better on the ACE inhibitor or β-blocker. In the ALLHAT trial, amlodipine and lisinopril were both equally protective compared with chlorthalidone against renal damage and heart attacks, with better protection against stroke in the black participants.[88] In INVEST, verapamil-trandolapril compared well on coronary outcomes with atenolol-HCTZ.[83]

CCBs combined with an ACE inhibitor. ACCOMPLISH argues for the ACE inhibitor–CCB combination versus the ACE inhibitor–thiazide as the preferred initial therapy in a high-risk hypertensive population.[107] Importantly, initial antihypertensive treatment with benazepril plus amlodipine slowed progression of nephropathy to a greater extent than did benazepril plus HCTZ.[108]

Metaanalysis of outcome studies with CCBs. Taking together the available studies in 2007, CCBs compared with placebo reduced stroke, coronary heart disease, major cardiovascular events, and cardiovascular death with, however, a trend to increased heart failure.[105] Compared with conventional therapy by diuretics and β-blockers, CCBs had the same effect on cardiovascular death and total mortality, increased heart failure, with a strong trend to decreased stroke. In addition, there was a lower rate of new diabetes with CCBs, including verapamil,[109] than with β-blocker or diuretic therapy.[88,110]

Lacidipine, a new CCB. Lacidipine, available in Europe, is claimed to cause less ankle edema than amlodipine. In the ELSA trial on 2334 hypertensives over 4 years, lacidipine was superior to atenolol in restraining carotid atherosclerosis and limiting development of new metabolic syndrome.[111]

Present assessment of CCBs. The questions previously relating to the long-term safety of CCBs have been resolved in that only very high doses of short-acting agents may cause ischemic events, probably by precipitously lowering the BP, whereas long-acting CCBs are safe. CCBs may be better at cardiovascular and stroke prevention than some other choices.[100,102] Thus CCBs are now accorded a position among the first-line choices by the NICE group.[112] ACE inhibitor plus amlodipine combinations may also be considered as first-line therapy, having performed very well in both ASCOT and ACCOMPLISH. Many pharmaceutical companies recently have branded fixed-dose combinations of amlodipine with almost every ACE inhibitor or ARB.

ACE Inhibitors for Hypertension

Captopril was the first ACE inhibitor, but multiple others are now available. All are antihypertensive, with few practical differences, except for duration of action (see Table 5-4). ACE inhibitors have few side effects (principally cough and rarely angioedema), are simple to use, have a flat dose-response curve, and have a virtual absence of contraindications except for bilateral renal artery stenosis and pregnancy. By preferentially relaxing the renal efferent arterioles and thereby reducing the intraglomerular pressure, they usually cause the serum creatinine to rise initially. They may precipitate hyperkalemia, especially in the presence of preexisting renal dysfunction, diabetes complicated by type 4 renal tubular acidosis, or when combined with potassium-retaining agents such as spironolactone. They readily combine with other modalities of treatment—with the exception of ACE inhibitors or the direct renin inhibitor—and are well accepted by older adults. Furthermore, a strong case has been made for their preferential use in diabetic hypertensive patients, in postinfarction follow-up, and in renal or heart failure. The HOPE study[113] emphasizes their role in cardiovascular protection in high-risk patients.

Mild to moderate hypertension. ACE inhibitors can be used as monotherapy in patients with mild to moderate hypertension, even in low-renin patients, or in combination with other standard agents. For monotherapy, moderate dietary salt restriction is especially important.[114] Differences in sodium intake and the relative activity of the renin-angiotensin mechanism may explain why only a variable percentage of mild to moderate hypertensive patients respond to monotherapy with ACE inhibition. *Monotherapy = use of a single drug to treat disease or condition*

Metaanalysis of outcome studies. ACE inhibitor–based therapy was better than placebo against stroke, coronary heart disease, heart failure, major cardiovascular events, cardiovascular death, and total mortality.[115] When compared to a diuretic with or without β-blocker–based therapy, ACE inhibitor therapy was exactly equal, although there was a trend toward lesser benefit in stroke. When compared with CCB-based therapy, ACE inhibitor therapy was equivalent for coronary heart disease, cardiovascular death, and total mortality; clearly better for prevention of heart failure; and marginally worse for prevention of stroke.

Coronary disease and ACE inhibitors. In the HOPE trial of patients at high risk of coronary heart disease, the addition of ramipril provided substantial cardioprotection.[113] However, uncertainty exists as to whether this was related to the extra antihypertensive effect provided by the ACE inhibitor, especially throughout the night, because the ramipril was given as 10 mg at night with substantial BP differences in the ABPM substudy.[116] In the EUROPA study, perindopril given in a high dose of 8 mg to patients with established coronary disease but with other otherwise relatively low risk, gave substantial cardiovascular protection especially by reducing MI.[117] Here, too, there was substantial BP reduction. In addition, a large body of experimental evidence supports the notion that there are direct vascular protective effects and in three trials of heart failure, an additional BP-independent effect of ACE inhibitors has been shown.[115]

Combination therapy. In ACCOMPLISH, the ACE inhibitor benazepril plus amlodipine gave better reduction in morbidity and mortality than did amlodipine plus HCTZ. This superiority was only found when the estimated glomerular filtration rate (eGFR) was more than 60 mL/min.[108]

Renal Disease and ACE Inhibitors

In *renovascular hypertension,* in which circulating renin is high and a critical part of the hypertensive mechanism, ACE inhibition is logical first-line therapy. Because the hypotensive response may be dramatic, a low test dose is essential. With standard doses of ACE inhibitors, the GFR falls acutely to largely recover in cases of unilateral, but not bilateral, disease. However, blood flow to the stenotic kidney may remain depressed after removal of the angiotensin-II support, and progressive ischemic atrophy is possible. Careful follow-up of renal blood flow and function is required. Angioplasty or surgery is preferable to chronic medical therapy, but only now is a comparison between medical therapy versus angioplasty being performed in patients with unilateral disease.

In *acute severe hypertension,* sublingual (chewed) captopril rapidly brings down the BP, but it is not clear how bilateral renal artery stenosis can be excluded quickly enough to make the speed of action of captopril an important benefit. Furthermore, the safety of such sudden falls of BP in the presence of possible renal impairment (always a risk in severe hypertension) has not been evaluated. But we know the risk of leaving the BP so high. Thus the best option is slow reduction of BP in hospital.

In *diabetic hypertensive patients* with nephropathy and proteinuria, ACE inhibitors and ARBs provide preferential dilation of the renal efferent arterioles, immediately reducing intraglomerular pressure and thereby protecting against progressive glomerulosclerosis.[118] Although the use of ACE inhibitors and ARBs in both diabetic and nondiabetic nephropathy has become routine, two disquieting reports question their efficacy. First, Kent et al.[118] found no benefit in nondiabetic nephropathy in those with less than 500 mg/day proteinuria. Second, in a nested case-control analysis of the long-term outcome of 6102 hypertensive diabetic patients, the use of ACE inhibitors was protective of progression to renal failure up to 3 years, but the risk increased to 4.2-fold greater after 3 years.[119]

Although in the past ACE inhibitors and ARBs have often been used together for extra renal protection in proteinuric patients, ONTARGET[120] showed that combining ACE inhibitor plus ARB therapy in patients at high cardiovascular risk, including diabetics, increased serious renal outcomes and hyperkalemia when compared with monotherapy with either agent. Similar risks are seen when an ACE inhibitor or ARB is combined with the direct-renin inhibitor,[121,122] causing the FDA to issue a black-box warning and to take the fixed-dose combination off the market. Moreover, the COOPERATE trial, which had provided the earlier evidence supporting the practice of "dual renin-angiotensin system (RAS) blockade," has been retracted by the editors of Lancet on the basis of scientific misconduct.[123]

Special Groups of Patients

Older adults. In those younger than 80 years old, the aim still remains to maintain BP at less than 140/90 mm Hg.[124] In *older adults with hypertension,* the BP aim should be 150/80 mm Hg.[93] Large outcome studies have documented the efficacy and outcome benefit of therapy based on diuretic therapy,[93] ACE inhibition in white patients,[66] with good evidence for responsiveness to ARBs.[125] The aortic pressure is markedly abbreviated and peaked, in keeping with the clinical findings of increasing systolic and decreasing diastolic pressure with age. The likelihood of multisystem disease means that older adults need more time for a careful history, clinical examination, and basic investigations, although, on the other hand, it is easy to over investigate.

Older black hypertensive men. In older black men with hypertension captopril was no better than placebo,[64] perhaps because there were two factors (ethnic group and age) both predisposing to a low-renin state. Similarly, in the ALLHAT trial lisinopril afforded less stroke protection than chlorthalidone or amlodipine for *black patients,*[88] probably because the trial design did not allow combination with either a diuretic or a DHP CCB.

Hypertension with heart failure. In patients who have hypertension with heart failure ACE inhibitors with diuretics have been automatic first-line therapy with equivalent results from the ARBs such as telmisartan.[126]

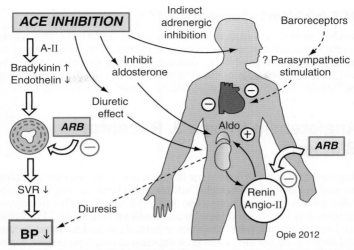

Figure 7-9   Angiotensin-converting enzyme (ACE) inhibitors and angiotensin receptor blockers (ARBs). Proposed mechanisms whereby these agents may have their antihypertensive effects. Note that the major effect is on the peripheral arterioles causing vasodilation and a fall in the systemic vascular resistance (SVR), also called the *peripheral vascular resistance*. Indirect inhibition of adrenergic activity also promotes arteriolar dilation. Several ancillary mechanisms are at work, including renal and indirect adrenal effects, as well as possible central inhibition. Parasympathetic activity may also be stimulated. *All & Angio-I,* angiotensin II; *Aldo,* aldosterone; *BP,* blood pressure. (Figure © L.H. Opie, 2012.)

Pregnancy hypertension. ACE inhibitors are totally contraindicated for pregnant patients with hypertension because fetal growth is impaired.

Combinations with ACE Inhibitors

ACE inhibitors are often combined with *thiazide diuretics* to enhance hypotensive effects (see Fig. 7-7) and to lessen metabolic side effects. This combination is logical because diuretics increase renin, the effects of which are antagonized by ACE inhibitors. The addition of a thiazide is better from the BP point of view than increasing the dose of the ACE inhibitor. When combined with potassium-retaining thiazide diuretics *(Dyazide, Moduretic, Maxzide)*, and especially spironolactone, there is a *risk of hyperkalemia* because ACE inhibitors decrease aldosterone secretion and hence retain potassium (Fig. 7-9). Nonetheless, in the RALES heart failure study, low-dose spironolactone was added to ACE inhibition and diuretic with little hyperkalemia, yet these patients were carefully monitored and the dose of ACE inhibitor reduced if necessary.[68] *ACE-inhibition plus β-blockade* is theoretically not a combination of choice except in heart failure. *ACE inhibitors plus CCBs* are now increasingly used in the therapy of hypertension.[102,127] This combination attacks both the RAS and the increased PVR. The ACE inhibitor reduces the ankle edema of the DHPs and both types of agents are free of metabolic and central nervous system side effects. In the ASCOT trial,[102] wherein the initial CCB arm was supplemented with an ACE inhibitor in 60% of patients, BP was lowered modestly more with the CCB–ACE inhibitor combination, which might have contributed to the better outcomes. As mentioned later (see page 253), in ACCOMPLISH this combination was superior to an ACE inhibitor–diuretic in reducing major events.

ACE Inhibitors: Summary

In addition to BP lowering, the overall evidence is that these agents also confer some added vascular protection, especially in diabetics and in renal disease. ACE inhibitors combine well with diuretics and CCBs, and have relatively infrequent side effects. The practice of combining ACE inhibitors with ARBs ("dual RAS blockade") should be stopped.

Angiotensin-II Type 1 Receptor Blockers

Angiotensin-II subtype 1 receptor blockers act on the specific receptor for angiotensin-II that has highly adverse roles in promoting cardiovascular pathologic conditions (see Table 5-1; Fig. 7-9). The prototype, losartan, has now been joined by many others (see Table 5-11). ARBs are being used more and more for hypertension and for heart failure and they are, by far, the fastest growing class of antihypertensive drugs in the United States and Europe[100] because they are virtually free of side effects, in particular the cough that occurs in approximately 10% of patients given an ACE inhibitor and because they are so heavily marketed since they all remain patent-protected. There is increasing evidence of their capacity to reduce hard endpoints.[128] ARBs are superior to β-blockade in patients with LVH[128] and to alternate therapies in type 2 diabetics with nephropathy,[129] but are not better than ACE inhibitors in heart failure in postinfarct patients.[115]

ARBs were thought to be better than ACE inhibitors in protection against stroke.[130] This contention is strengthened by experimental and clinical evidence that agents that reduce circulating angiotensin-II (e.g., ACE inhibitors) are less effective in protecting the cerebral circulation than are agents that increase circulating A-II levels by blocking the AT_1 receptor (e.g., ARBs). The argument is based on increased activation of the AT_2-receptor when the AT_1 receptor is blocked, which "would facilitate the recruitment of collateral vessels or increase neuronal resistance to anoxia."[131] However, the large ONTARGET study on more than 25,000 persons at high cardiovascular risk shows that the ACE inhibitor ramipril and the ARB telmisartan are equally good in reducing cardiovascular outcomes, including stroke.[132]

Current and future role of ARBs in hypertension. ARBs block the same RAS as the ACE inhibitors, with much the same effects but presently at greater cost. Thus an ACE inhibitor remains the more cost-effective solution, with an ARB substituted only if ACE inhibitor side effects, chiefly cough, develop. Another view is that ARBs have an excellent record in comparative studies showing better or similar cardiovascular outcome benefit,[88,132] virtually without the major side effects of ACE inhibitors, and provide relatively symptom-free control of hypertension. ARBs are better tolerated than ACE inhibitors and all other antihypertensive drug classes, and thus promote adherence.[133]

Direct Renin Inhibitor

As the only new antihypertensive class introduced in more than a decade, the first direct renin inhibitor, aliskiren, was heavily promoted at first, although enthusiasm may be starting to wane. It clearly lowers BP as well as other RAS blockers[134] and according to one 24-hour ABPM study, it adds to the antihypertensive effect of a full dose of an ARB.[135] It provides dose-dependent and sustained 24-hour efficacy, which is enhanced by concomitant diuretic.[136] The possible downside is production of excess potentially pathogenic renin,[137] which might help to explain the adverse effects noted in the ALTITUDE study (see Chapter 5, p. 162).

ACCELERATE was a small study in which hypertensive persons were given either aliskiren (150-300 mg) or amlodipine (5-10 mg) or the combination, with approximately equal BP reduction in both arms and a larger drop when combined.[138] In the future aliskiren might be promoted as part of a polypill (see Chapter 5, p. 163).

Aldosterone Blockers

Spironolactone and eplerenone. There is a special argument for spironolactone and eplerenone in primary aldosteronism but also in those subjects with RH.[69,70] Based on ASPIRANT[70] and the ASCOT-BPLA[69] studies, spironolactone is an attractive fourth-line agent. The ASPIRANT study was the first proper randomized controlled trial with spironolactone, when spironolactone 25 mg or placebo was given to patients with RH. In this small, 8-week trial on 111 patients with RH, 75% or more were taking four agents (ACE inhibitor, β-blocker, CCB, including a diuretic [100%]). The ABP nighttime systolic, 24-hour systolic, and the office systolic BP values all fell with spironolactone (difference of −8.6, −9.8, and −6.5 mm Hg; P = 0.011, 0.004, and 0.011), but the diastolic changes were not significant. Maybe higher doses would have dropped the diastolic values further. Based on the RALES trial (see Chapter 5, p. 159), spironolactone is finding wider use in hypertensive patients with congestive heart failure, provided that serum K is carefully monitored.

Eplerenone. *Eplerenone (Inspra)* is a more specific congener with much less risk of gynecomastia. Unlike spironolactone, eplerenone does not have an active metabolite. It has a half-life of 3.5 to 5 hours and is excreted in urine (66%) and in feces. Because eplerenone metabolism is predominantly by hepatic CYP3A4, eplerenone must not be used with drugs that are strong inhibitors of CYP3A4 (such as ketoconazole, clarithromycin, nefazodone, ritonavir and nelfinavir). The starting dose of eplerenone is 50 mg daily, increased if needed to 50 mg twice daily. The full antihypertensive effect may need 4 weeks.

Besides improving survival in post-MI heart failure in EPHESUS,[139] eplerenone is now used for hypertension, either alone or in combination with other agents. The antihypertensive effect of eplerenone 50 mg daily was equal in black and white patients and was superior to losartan 50 mg daily in black patients.[140] Mechanistically, eplerenone improves the impaired endothelial function in hypertensive persons, which losartan does not.[141] Eplerenone may apparently be used instead of spironolactone in RH (see preceding paragraph). Nonetheless, there are no formal outcome trials on eplerenone for RH. There are strict FDA warnings about contraindications that include hyperkalemia of more than 5.5 mEq/L, a reduced creatinine clearance of 30 mL/min or less, type 2 diabetics with early renal involvement, and the use of other K-retaining agents or K-supplements.

The future. An aldosterone synthase inhibitor is undergoing early testing.[142]

Decreased sympathetic activity. In a small but provocative study, aldosterone blockers as first-line agents (in patients of mean age 68 years) unexpectedly reduced sympathetic activity as measured by serum norepinephrine (NE) levels, whereas the diuretic did not, thus giving an additional mechanism of action.[143] Furthermore, the BP levels fell more with the aldosterone blocker. In another small study, skeletal muscle sympathetic nerve activity as measured directly with intraneural microelectrodes increased and glucose tolerance worsened when antihypertensive therapy was initiated with chlorthalidone, but both

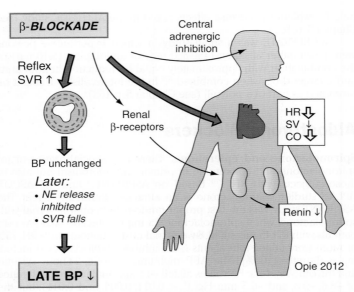

Figure 7-10 Proposed antihypertensive mechanisms of β-blockade. An early fall in heart rate (HR), stroke volume (SV), and cardiac output (CO) does not lead to a corresponding fall in blood pressure (BP) because of baroreflex-mediated increased peripheral α-adrenergic vasoconstriction, with a rise in systemic vascular resistance (SVR). Within a few days β-blockade of prejunctional receptors on the terminal neuron, with consequent inhibition of release of norepinephrine (NE), may explain why the SVR reverts to normal. The BP now falls. In the case of vasodilatory β-blockers (see Fig. 1-10) there is an early decrease in SVR and a more rapid fall in BP. (Figure © L.H. Opie, 2012.)

sympathetic activity and glucose tolerance were unchanged when therapy was initiated with spironolactone.[144]

β-Blockers for Hypertension

β-blockers act by multiple mechanisms (Fig. 7-10). As first recognized by Messerli et al. in 1998,[145] proven by Carlberg et al. in 2004,[146] and amply confirmed since,[63,147] β-blockers do not protect against heart attack better than other classes and are associated with a 14% increase in the risk of stroke. β-blockers are no longer recommended for primary prevention and are now often relegated to specific concomitant conditions for secondary prevention (see Table 7-3). Their relative ineffectiveness for primary prevention can be attributed to multiple adverse effects: loss of insulin sensitivity with resultant increased risk of diabetes; increase in plasma triglyceride and lowering of high-density lipoprotein (HDL) cholesterol; increase in body weight; easy fatigability, which reduces the ability to perform physical activity; as noted in a substudy of the ASCOT trial, a lesser reduction in central as opposed to peripheral BP[148]; and finally an increase in BP variability.[148A] Furthermore, β-blockers differ from other standard antihypertensive agents in reducing aortic pressure less for a given fall in brachial pressure.[149] Their reservations may apply less or not at all to the vasodilating β-blockers, especially not to nitric oxide (NO)–generating nebivolol. At the same time, there is another strong point of view, based on an analysis of more than 200,000 persons with more than 20,000 outcome events in the BP Trialists' Collaboration, that there were no differences in the proportionate risk reductions achieved with different BP-reducing regimens.[150] In other words, the basic message remains, "Get the BP down."

Vasodilating β-blockers. Labetalol, carvedilol,[151] and nebivolol (in SENIORS for HF), cause less metabolic mischief and logically should be used in place of metoprolol or atenolol, although there are no good outcome data for their use as antihypertensives. Nebivolol has NO-producing properties. Are these specifically protective? One claim is that nebivolol reduced central aortic pressure and LVH better than metoprolol.[152] However, in relation to the wider use of nebivolol on this basis, the caution is that "the real paradigm shift will only come if and when studies demonstrate that selective reduction in central pressure reduces cardiovascular events."[149] A strong proposal is that nebivolol is superior to metoprolol in effects on insulin sensitivity and fibrinolytic balance. At doses that were equipotent with respect to reductions in BP, heart rate, and renin activity, metoprolol treatment decreased insulin sensitivity, increased plasminogen activator inhibitor–1 antigen concentrations, and increased oxidative stress, whereas nebivolol treatment did not.[153] The real question is whether expensive nebivolol offers any real advantage over generic carvedilol, which now is included on standard formularies. In the GEMINI study, carvedilol was superior to metoprolol in limiting insulin resistance.[154]

Pharmacokinetics of β-blockers. Dose adjustment is more likely to be required with more lipid-soluble (lipophilic) agents, which have a high "first-pass" liver metabolism that may result in active metabolites: the rate of formation depends on liver blood flow and function. The ideal β-blocker for hypertension is long acting, cardioselective (see Fig. 1-9), metabolically favorable (see previous comments on nebivolol), and usually effective in a standard dose. Simple pharmacokinetics may be an added advantage (no liver metabolism, little protein binding, no lipid solubility, and no active metabolites). Sometimes added vasodilation should be an advantage, as in older adults or in black patients. The ideal drug would also be "lipid neutral," as is claimed for some agents (see Table 10-5) and glucose neutral. In practice, once-a-day therapy is satisfactory with many β-blockers, but it is important to check early morning predrug BP to ensure 24-hour coverage (as with all agents). Combinations of β-blockers with one or another agent from all other classes have been successful in the therapy of hypertension. Nonetheless, combination with another drug suppressing the RAS, such as an ACE inhibitor or an ARB, is not logical, nor did it work well in ALLHAT.[88]

Diuretics plus β-blockers. Diuretics plus β-blockers in combination should ideally contain no more than 12.5 mg HCTZ, 1.25 mg bendrofluazide, or preferably a similar low dose of chlorthalidone. Diuretic–β-blocker combinations should be avoided whenever diabetes risk is a consideration.

α-Adrenergic Blockers

Of the α_1-receptor blockers, *prazosin (Minipress), terazosin (Hytrin),* and *doxazosin (Cardura)* are available in the United States. Their advantages are freedom from metabolic or lipid side effects, but some patients develop other troublesome side effects: drowsiness, diarrhea, postural hypotension, and occasional tachycardia. Tolerance, related to fluid retention, may develop during chronic therapy with α_1-blockers, requiring increased doses or added diuretics. Fluid retention may explain why the doxazosin arm of the ALLHAT study was terminated because of an excess of heart failure, compared with reference diuretic.[155] Thus these agents now have a lesser place in initial monotherapy. Nonetheless, in the TOMH study on mild hypertension,[86] doxazosin 2 mg/day given over 4 years and combined with lifestyle changes reduced the BP as much as agents from other groups. The QOL improved as much as with placebo, although not quite as much as with acebutolol; blood cholesterol fell; and the incidence of impotence was lowest in the doxazosin group.[78]

Thus despite the disappointing ALLHAT result, α-blockers may still be chosen especially in those with features of the metabolic syndrome or in the many men with benign prostatic hypertrophy in whom α-blockers provide symptomatic relief.[156] α-blockers combine well with other drugs and doxazosin, and when used as the third line of therapy in the ASCOT trial, provided an impressive lowering of BP by 12/7 mm Hg in those patients who had not responded to full doses of their initial two drugs.[157] Phenoxybenzamine and phentolamine are combined α_1 and α_2-blockers used only for *pheochromocytoma*. Labetalol and carvedilol have limited α-blocking activity.

Direct Vasodilators

Hydralazine used to be a standard third-line drug, its benefits enhanced and side effects lessened by concomitant use of a diuretic and an adrenergic inhibitor. Being inexpensive, hydralazine is still widely used in the developing world. Elsewhere fear of lupus (especially with continued doses of more than 200 mg daily) and lack of evidence for regression of LVH has led to its replacement by the CCBs. Nonetheless, hydralazine has undergone a facelift for use in heart failure, combined with isosorbide dinitrate (BiDil, see Chapter 2, p. 50), particularly for black patients. *Minoxidil* is a potent long-acting vasodilator acting on the potassium channel. In addition to inciting intense renal sodium retention that requires large doses of loop diuretics to overcome, it often causes profuse hirsutism, so its use is usually limited to men with severe RH or renal insufficiency (it dilates renal arterioles). Occasionally minoxidil causes pericarditis. In one series, LV mass increased by 30%.

Central Adrenergic Inhibitors

Of the centrally acting agents, *reserpine* is easiest to use in a low dose of 0.05 mg/day, which provides almost all of its antihypertensive action with fewer side effects than higher doses. Onset and offset of action are slow and measured in weeks. When cost is crucial, reserpine and diuretics are the cheapest combination. *Methyldopa*, still used despite adverse central symptoms and potentially serious hepatic and blood side effects, acts like clonidine on central α_2-receptors, usually without slowing the heart rate. *Clonidine, guanabenz,* and *guanafacine* provide all of the benefits of methyldopa with none of the rare but serious autoimmune reactions (as with methyldopa, sedation is frequent). In the VA study,[64] clonidine 0.2 to 0.6 mg/day was among the more effective of the agents tested. It worked equally well in younger and older age groups and in black and white patients. The major disadvantage in that trial was the highest incidence of drug intolerance. A particular problem is clonidine rebound. A *transdermal form of clonidine* (Catapres-TTS) provides once-a-week therapy, likely minimizing the risks of clonidine rebound. *Guanabenz* resembles clonidine but may cause less fluid retention and reduces serum cholesterol by 5% to 10%. *Guanfacine* is a similar agent that can be given once daily (at bedtime for less daytime somnolence), with less risk of rebound hypertension if abruptly discontinued. *Imidazole receptor blockers* (e.g., moxonidine, rilmenidine) are available in Europe, but not in the United States.

Combination Therapy

Background. In general, guidelines suggest that therapy for mild hypertension (BP <160/100 mm Hg) should start with one drug, with combinations of drugs for more severe hypertension. Guidelines also recommend initial drug combinations as first-step treatment strategy in high-risk hypertension. However, the hard evidence that this policy is associated with cardiovascular benefits compared with initial monotherapy is limited. Does a combination of antihypertensive drugs provide a greater cardiovascular protection in daily clinical antihypertensive monotherapy?

Initial combination therapy. In a population-based, nested case-control study involving 209,650 patients from Lombardy, Italy, and using logistic regression to model the cardiovascular risk associated with starting on or continuing with combination therapy, those started on combination therapy had an 11% cardiovascular risk reduction with respect to those starting on monotherapy.[158] Compared with patients who maintained monotherapy also during follow-up, those who started on combination therapy and kept it all along had 26% reduction of cardiovascular risk (95% confidence interval [CI]: 15% to 35%). Thus the authors argue that indications for using combinations of BP drugs should be broadened. However, as pointed out in the accompanying editorial,[159] the study remains observational as the patients were not randomized. To correctly assess initial combination versus initial monotherapy would require much larger randomized trials. In the meantime, we note that the concept of low doses of two drugs being better than high doses of one receives support from the Law metaanalysis of 147 trials (see Figs. 7-4 and 7-5): addition of the starting dose of a second drug causes a fivefold greater reduction in BP than doubling the dose of the first drug.[32] In addition, low-dose combination therapy reduces the risk of dose-dependent side effects.

CCB–ACE inhibitor combination. CCB–ACE inhibitor combination therapy had a resounding success in ASCOT,[102] which paved the way for ACCOMPLISH. The amlodipine-perindopril–based combination regimen was much better than the atenolol-diuretic regimen. After a mean of 5.5 years of follow-up, major decreases were in total cardiovascular events (HR 0.84; p < 0.0001), stroke (HR 0.77; p = 0.0003), all-cause mortality (HR 0.89: p = 0.025) and new diabetes (HR 0.70; p < 0.0001).

ACCOMPLISH. The Avoiding Cardiovascular Events through Combination Therapy in Patients Living with Systolic Hypertension (ACCOMPLISH) trial showed that initial antihypertensive therapy with benazepril plus amlodipine was superior to benazepril plus HCTZ in reducing cardiovascular morbidity and mortality in high-risk hypertensive patients.[160] Benazepril is a prodrug that is rapidly converted to an active metabolite, benazeprilat, with an elimination half-life of 22 hours. In ACCOMPLISH benazepril was used once daily and was successfully combined with the long-acting DHP-CCB amlodipine in the double-blind, randomized trial on 11,506 patients with hypertension at high risk for cardiovascular events. Doses were benazepril (20 mg) plus amlodipine (5 mg) or benazepril (20 mg) plus HCTZ (12.5 mg), orally once daily. Both primary outcome events (P < 0.001) and secondary endpoints (death from cardiovascular causes, nonfatal MI, and nonfatal stroke [P = 0.002]) were reduced by approximately 20% more in the benazepril-amlodipine group.[160] ACCOMPLISH argues for the ACE inhibitor–CCB combination versus the ACE inhibitor–thiazide combination as the preferred initial therapy in a high-risk hypertensive population. Of note is the longer half-life of amlodipine versus HCTZ. Nonetheless, with exactly similar rates of 24-hour BP control,[107] there must be explanations other than better BP reduction for the superior results in the ACE inhibitor–CCB group.

Renal effects. Progression of chronic kidney disease, a prespecified endpoint in ACCOMPLISH,[108] was defined as doubling of serum creatinine concentration or end-stage renal disease (eGFR <15 mL/min/1.73 m^2) or need for dialysis. Events of renal progression in the benazepril-amlodipine

AORTIC WAVE WITH AGE

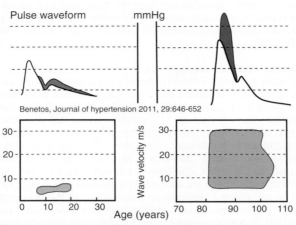

Benetos, Journal of hypertension 2011, 29:646-652

Figure 7-11   Changes in aortic pressure wave in older adults. Note abrupt rise and fall in older adults (*upper panel, right side*) and marked differences in wave velocity patterns (older adults *right lower panel*). These are direct invasive arterial measurements.[164] The associated carotid-femoral delay can be measured noninvasively.[34] *m/s*, meters/seconds.

group equalled 2% compared with 3.7% in the benazepril-HCTZ group (HR 0.52; CI: 0.41-0.65, p < 0.0001). Thus initial antihypertensive treatment with benazepril-amlodipine should be considered in preference to benazepril-HCTZ because it slows progression of nephropathy to a greater extent. Extrapolation to the broader picture is that slower ACE inhibitor plus CCB therapy should be considered as first line for patients with high-risk hypertension rather than the usual ACE inhibitor plus thiazide.

Polypill. The polypill concept is gaining ground,[161-163] in support of the Law and Wald[32] concept that several drugs at low doses are better able to drop BP than high doses of single drugs (see Figs. 7-4 and 7-5).

Patient Profiling: The Elderly

As lifespan now extends, more and more patients are falling into the older adult category. The algorithm provided in the current guidelines of the British Hypertension Society[9] is rational in giving preferential benefit of C (CCB) drugs. In much older adults, therapy is diuretic based as in HYVET.[93] Note the resounding success of CCB–ACE inhibitor combination in ASCOT[102] and in ACCOMPLISH.[160] As most patients require two or more drugs to achieve adequate BP control, the issue as to which should be chosen for initial therapy has almost become moot. Nonetheless, as noted in Table 7-3, certain choices are more appropriate for many concomitant conditions.

Changes with aging. With aging, there is inevitable aortic stiffening (Fig. 7-11),[164] which explains the inevitable rise of systolic BP with age. The resulting carotid-femoral delay can be measured noninvasively.[34] Multiple trials have documented even better protection against stroke and other outcome measures by treatment of older adults than reported in the middle aged.[165] Thus an equivalent BP reduction will produce a greater benefit in older adults than in younger patients,[32] especially if there are other risk factors such as diabetes mellitus. Dementia is delayed or prevented.[166] In older adults, evidence for the benefit of β-blockers has "not been convincing," whereas CCBs match the needs of the older adult patient typically with "increasing arterial stiffness and diastolic dysfunction secondary to decreased atrial and ventricular compliance."[167] For combination therapy, this massive American College of Cardiology–American Heart Association review notes that in ACCOMPLISH (mean age 67 years), amlodipine plus the ACE inhibitor benazepril gave better reduction in morbidity and mortality than did amlodipine plus HCTZ 12-25 mg daily. Note that this superiority was only found when the eGFR was more than 60 mL/min.[108]

Treating patients older than 80. Patients older than 80 should be treated, with care, and with a BP target of 150/80 mm Hg.[93]

Blood pressure limits. There is compelling evidence to suggest that sustained SBP elevations of more than 160 mm Hg require treatment,[93,165] and that the systolic rather than the diastolic pressure is of greater importance in this age group. Therefore *isolated systolic hypertension* (with DBP of less than 90) should be actively treated. In the presence of end-organ damage, including abnormalities of the thoracic or abdominal aorta, or diabetes, BP values of more than 140 mm Hg should be taken as reason for active therapy. Less commonly, there is *isolated diastolic hypertension* with sustained DBP values of 90 mm Hg and systolic values that are not elevated. These levels should be treated as in younger patients.

Lifestyle changes. Again, whenever possible, treatment includes non-pharmacological measures, including exercise training. Even walking sharpens cognitive skills in older adult patients.[168] Older women are especially sodium-sensitive. Besides sodium restriction, increased dietary potassium may be protective.[169] The combination of sodium restriction, loss of weight, and walking is especially desirable.

How low to go. In the decisive HYVET trial in much older adults, the aim was 150/80 mm Hg.[93] The *J-shaped curve* (see "J-shaped curve" earlier in chapter) is of particular significance in hypertensive patients with myocardial ischemia or LVH, or in older adults with an increased pulse pressure and low diastolic BP to start with. Is the damage caused by excessively dropping the diastolic BP mitigated or exceeded by the benefit of dropping the systolic BP? Here there are no prospective trial data.

Drugs for older adult hypertensive patients. *Low-dose diuretics* remain the first-line drug choice for older adults because they were used in the SHEP study[82] and several other major trials, including HYVET,[93] and perhaps, equally important, because they help to lessen osteoporosis (see Chapter 4, p. 105) and dementia,[166] conditions that are often disabling in older adults.

Calcium channel blockers. CCBs are able to reduce morbidity and mortality in older adults, the agents used being nitrendipine in the Syst-Eur and Syst-China trials, and nifedipine in older adult Chinese patients with hypertension, all being long-acting DHPs. Amlodipine was equal to a diuretic or an ACE inhibitor in coronary protection in the ALLHAT trial.[88]

β-blockers. β-blockers are at a disadvantage compared with diuretics in older adults, but may be indicated for secondary prevention of MI or for heart failure. Risks of β-blockade in older adults include excess sinus or atrioventricular node inhibition and a decreased CO, which in the senescent heart could more readily precipitate failure.

ACE inhibitors and ARBs. ACE inhibitors and ARBs are also often used in older adults. The STOP-2 trial provides evidence that they are as good as conventional treatment and perhaps better than CCBs[170] and in the men in the Australian trial, better than a diuretic.[90] Logically, ACE inhibitors and ARBs are more effective with dietary sodium restriction, or low-dose diuretics, or both. ACE inhibitors improve insulin sensitivity in older adults, which may help protect from adverse metabolic effects of concurrent diuretics. So far SCOPE has been the only study with an ARB in older adults.[171]

Combination treatment. Combination treatment is often required, as was the case in nearly two thirds of older adult patients with hypertension in ALLHAT.[88] ACE inhibitor or ARB plus diuretics, and CCBs plus ACE inhibitors or ARBs all seem to work equally well, using mortality and cardiovascular events as outcome measures.

Two cautions are needed for treating older adults: they may experience cardiac or cerebral ischemia if the diastolic pressure is lowered to less than 70 mm Hg[30] and they often have orthostatic hypotension (and postprandial hypotension), which may be worsened by addition of antihypertensive therapy.[172]

Patient Profiling: Other Special Groups

Angina and hypertension. The only antianginal antihypertensive agents are β-blockers and CCBs. A direct comparison between atenolol and verapamil showed equality of major outcomes with some other advantages for verapamil such as fewer anginal attacks and less new diabetes.[83] Despite this trial result, verapamil is little used, mainly because constipation is a particularly limiting side effect. Diuretics, α-blockers, ACE inhibitors, and ARBs do not have direct antianginal effects, although indirect improvements in the myocardial oxygen balance by regression of LVH and reduction of BP have been shown by use of an ACE inhibitor in the HOPE trial[113] and an ARB in the LIFE trial.[128]

Black patients. In ALLHAT, the risk for stroke was greater with the ACE inhibitor lisinopril, but the control of BP also was poorer, probably because of the trial design, which prohibited the combination of the ACE inhibitor with a thiazide or with amlodipine.[88] Of note, angioedema in black patients was much more common with lisinopril (0.7%) than seen in usual practice. Black patients respond better to monotherapy with a diuretic or to a CCB than to monotherapy with an ACE inhibitor or ARB or β-blocker. The common denominator might be the low renin status of older black patients taken as a group. Overall evidence suggests that combination with diuretic increases sensitivity to a β-blocker or an ACE inhibitor or an ARB likely because the diuretic increases renin. In a direct comparison, CCB therapy was more effective than a low-dose diuretic as first-line therapy in South African black patients,[103] perhaps because sodium intake was not controlled.

Diabetic hypertensive patients. Based largely on expert opinion only, previous guidelines have recommended that antihypertensive therapy should be started in diabetics at a BP of more than 130/80 mm Hg and the goal of therapy is to lower systolic pressure to less than 130 mm Hg.[38] In the recent ACCORD trial, further BP reduction reduced strokes, but did not afford further protection against heart attack or other cardiovascular complications and caused more adverse drug reactions[173]; however, the benefit of more intense BP lowering may have been underestimated as the diabetic study cohort had a surprisingly low CVD event rate.

Diabetics with nephropathy. In type 1 diabetic nephropathy, ACE inhibitors have repeatedly been shown to reduce proteinuria and protect against progressive glomerular sclerosis and loss of renal function.[174] In type 2 diabetic nephropathy, trials with ARBs have shown similar renal protection.[175] In those with type 2 diabetes the relative resistance of the renal renin response to RAS blockade supports the concept of an activated RAS in diabetes, and implies that diabetic patients might require higher doses of RAS blockers to fully suppress RAS.[176]

Evidence for specific renoprotection is stronger for ACE inhibitors for type I and ARBs for type 2 diabetic renal disease. Using the combined data of the RENAAL and IDNT trials, a progressively lower cardiovascular risk was observed with a lower albuminuria level particularly evident in those reaching the SBP target of 130 mm Hg or less. Because the SBP and albuminuria responses to ARB therapy are variable and discordant, there should be a dual target of reducing both BP and albuminuria.[177] Nonetheless, in practice ACE inhibitors may be used whenever ARBs cannot be afforded.[178]

Dyslipidemias. For patients with established dyslipidemias, a statin will be needed, particularly in view of the impressive coronary and stroke protection with 10 mg atorvastatin in the ASCOT-LLA trial where the mean cholesterol level was only modestly elevated (see Chapter 10, p. 420). Although the higher doses of *diuretics* previously used increased plasma cholesterol, with modern low-dose treatment the problem is less. Regarding β-blockade, many had assumed that the protection β-blockers provide against recurrent heart attacks may serve to prevent initial coronary events in hypertensive patients, but the evidence shows poor comparison and no benefit compared with other drugs.[179] Because earlier generation β-blockers raise serum triglycerides, lower HDL cholesterol levels, impair insulin sensitivity, and may precipitate type 2 diabetes while providing less protection against stroke, they are no longer recommended for primary prevention. The *α-blockers* clearly improve the blood lipid profile, whereas the ACE inhibitors, ARBs, and CCBs are "lipid neutral" in most studies. All of these agents also allow a better exercise performance than β-blockers.

Exercising hypertensive patients. Low- to moderate-intensity aerobic exercise training lowers the resting BP, so that increased exercise is part of lifestyle modification in the treatment of hypertension. Lack of exercise is an independent risk factor for coronary heart disease. When, besides lifestyle modification and exercise, drug treatment is required, then the best category of drug might be that which leaves the increased CO of exercise unchanged while blunting the simultaneous BP rise. This goal is best attained by the ACE inhibitors or ARBs or by DHP-CCBs. β-blockade, in contrast, limits the CO by decreasing the heart rate, even in the case of vasodilatory β-blockers.

Metabolic syndrome. Hypertension is present in 50% of type 1 diabetes, mostly secondary to renal damage; in type 2 diabetes, hypertension is present in 80%, often as a component of the *metabolic syndrome* (see Chapter 11, Fig. 11-1). Among treated hypertensive patients, diabetes developed over 25 years in 20.4%, related both to weight gain and use of β-blockers.[180] In diabetes, the BP aims have been stricter than in nondiabetics. JNC 7 recommended a goal BP of 130/80 mm Hg. In the ADVANCE study[181] the BP in high-risk diabetic patients already treated to mean BP levels of 140/77 mm Hg was further reduced by the addition of an ACE inhibitor, perindopril, together with a diuretic, indapamide. Mean BP reductions were 5.6/2.2 mm Hg. All-cause mortality fell by 14% (p = 0.03). In diabetics with isolated systolic hypertension, the systolic BP should drop to approximately 140 mm Hg. Again, treatment starts with lifestyle modification including control of hyperglycemia. It makes sense to avoid high-dose diuretics and β-blockers as initial therapy in those prone to diabetes because of a personal or family history or by the metabolic syndrome.[110] Rather, there are arguments for initial ACE inhibitors or ARBs. CCBs generally leave diabetic control unaltered and in the Syst-Eur trial the long-acting DHP nitrendipine protected the diabetics better than did the diuretic in SHEP.[182] A logical sequence (although not trial based) would be an ACE inhibitor or ARB, a CCB as the second drug, and either a metabolically neutral vasodilating β-blocker or a very low-dose thiazide as the third drug. α-blockers may also be appropriate.

Obese hypertensive patients. The characteristics of obesity hypertension are an increased plasma volume, a high CO (explicable by Starling's law), and a low PVR. The basic mechanisms are complex but include an increased tubular reabsorption of sodium and increased sympathetic outflow. Weight reduction is not easy to achieve and even harder to maintain, but even small degrees of weight loss, if maintained, help keep BP down. For every 1 kg of weight loss, there is a BP reduction of approximately 1 mm Hg.[183] Because of the association between insulin resistance and obesity, and the potential adverse effects of high doses of diuretics on insulin, the dose of diuretic should be kept low. LVH is a particular hazard, which obesity and insulin resistance promote independently of the BP. Regarding further drug choice, in the absence of good trial data, a logical selection is an agent that is metabolically beneficial and known to combine well with a diuretic such as an ACE inhibitor or an ARB. An ACE inhibitor–DHP–CCB combination avoids the diabetogenic potential of a thiazide. In general, β-blockers should be avoided.[184]

Postinfarct hypertensive patients. In patients with hypertension, acute myocardial infarction (AMI) often drops the BP, which may then creep back in the postinfarct months. There has been no adequate prospective study to determine the best treatment of postinfarct hypertension, but β-blockers and ACE inhibitors (or ARBs) are in any case indicated post-MI and should also handle the hypertension.

Smokers. It is *imperative* that the patient stops smoking. Smoking, besides being an independent risk factor for coronary artery disease and for stroke, also interacts adversely with hypertension. First, smoking helps to promote renovascular and malignant hypertension. Second, smoking damages the vascular endothelium, the integrity of which is now thought to be important in maintaining a normal BP and erectile function. Third, heavy smoking results in a sustained rise in BP or intense swings to high systolic values, as revealed by ambulatory measurements.[185] Normal casual office BP values while the patient is not smoking mask the adverse effects of smoking on the BP.

Pregnancy hypertension. The best tested drug is methyldopa (Category B; see Table 12-10). ACE inhibitors and ARBs are totally contraindicated.

Sleep apnea in hypertensive patients. In a consecutive series of 125 patients with RH, sleep apnea was the commonest cause (64%). Age older than 50 years, large neck circumference measurement, and snoring were good predictors of obstructive sleep apnea.[186] Catheter-based renal sympathetic denervation lowered BP and decreased indices of sleep apnea in patients with refractory hypertension and obstructive sleep apnea. Interestingly, there are also accompanying improvements in glucose tolerance.[187]

Specific Aims of Antihypertensive Therapy

Regression of left ventricular hypertrophy. Preferably diagnosed by echocardiography rather than electrocardiogram, LVH is increasingly seen as an important complication of hypertension. Apart from being an independent cardiovascular risk factor, LVH is associated with abnormalities of diastolic function, which can result in dyspnea or even overt LV failure. An important point is that reduction of the BP does not rapidly result in decreased LVH so that prolonged therapy, up to 3 years, may be needed to achieve full regression. Several important retrospective analyses support the concept that the most effective agents in achieving LV regression are those that interrupt the growth pathways that make myocytes hypertrophy such as the ACE inhibitors, ARBs, or CCBs.[39] The LIFE study gave a decisive advantage to the ARB losartan versus a β-blocker, atenolol.[128] In the LIFE study, both protection against sudden death[188] and the incidence of new diabetes were related to the regression of LVH.[189] Of interest is the concept that it is not only the daytime BP that governs LVH, but also the absence of a normal nocturnal BP fall. A novel aim is reduction of central aortic pressure. The hypertrophic response to catecholamines is mediated by α-adrenoreceptors, not β-adrenoreceptors. Vasodilating β-blockers should theoretically be better than standard β-blockers. Thus nebivolol reduced LVH better than metoprolol.[152]

Atrial fibrillation. LVH caused by hypertension predisposes to left atrial enlargement and thus to atrial fibrillation (see Fig. 8-11). Control of ventricular rate is one viable strategy, as achieved by a number of antihypertensive drugs: verapamil, diltiazem, and β-blockers. Going further back, LVH itself must be tackled by strict control of the BP. A recent editorial reviews the evidence in favor of choosing ARBs as class 1 level A agents in the prevention of atrial fibrillation in hypertension, on the basis of the prespecified secondary analyses from two large trials with double-blind design (valsartan in VALUE; telmisartan in ONTARGET/TRANSCEND).[190] ACE inhibitors, although without such solid data, are likely to have much the same effects.

Early morning blood pressure rise. The highest BP found in the early morning hours soon after rising is strongly associated with sudden death, AMI, and stroke. Logically, there has been a drive for the use of ultra–long acting agents to blunt this early morning rise. In reality, the optimal management of early morning hypertension is still not clear and only one comparative prospective trial addressed this point. The drug used was time-released verapamil *(Covera HS)*, which showed no benefit of the CCB over β-blocker-based therapy.[191] However, this trial was prematurely terminated. Presently, the ideal policy, especially in those at risk of cardiac complications, is to achieve a normal BP in the morning, as measured at home, either by the patient or by ambulatory monitoring.

Ventricular arrhythmias. Often associated with LVH, ventricular ectopic activity can be relatively harmless or can be indicative of underlying systolic dysfunction, the latter being due to hypertensive heart disease alone or in combination with coronary disease. β-blockade is often successful in suppression of harmless but irritating arrhythmias. Persistent and significant ventricular tachycardia may reflect accompanying coronary artery disease. Severe life-threatening arrhythmias in high-risk hypertensive patients may require class III agents, such as the β-blocker sotalol or amiodarone (see Chapter 8, p. 288), taking care to avoid diuretic-induced hypokalemia with risk of torsades.

Sildenafil to treat erectile dysfunction and hypertension. Sexual dysfunction, especially in men, has been reported with almost every antihypertensive drug, probably a consequence of reduction of blood flow through genital vessels already having endothelial damage from the ravages of smoking, hypercholesterolemia, and diabetes. In addition, erectile dysfunction can reflect early systemic vascular disease even in the absence of CVD. One study found an ARB to be better in maintenance of male sexual function when compared with β-blockade.[192] In the TOMH study, the incidence of impotence was lowest in those receiving the α-blocker doxasozin.[78] When needed, sildenafil or one of its successors can be used in hypertensive patients without angina and therefore not taking nitrates. It is important to note that sildenafil mainly promotes formation of vascular cyclic guansine monophosphate but also cyclic adenosome monophosphate to decrease peripheral BP, which accounts both for the well-known adverse interaction with nitrates (Fig. 2-6) and significant fall in BP.[193]

Optimal intellectual activity. In general, antihypertensives, with the exception of centrally active agents such as clonidine and methyldopa, should be free of central side effects. Nevertheless, β-blockers may have subtle effects on the intellect. Although propranolol is the major culprit, even the lipid-insoluble agent atenolol is not blameless. To be totally sure of unimpaired intellectual activity, CCBs, ACE inhibitors, or ARBs seem to be the agents of choice. With control of hypertension, dementia may be delayed or prevented.[166]

Overall quality of life. In general, all categories of antihypertensive agents improve the QOL except for propranolol and methyldopa, and probably other centrally active agents such as clonidine. Caution is advised in the interpretation of QOL studies because patients who drop out as a result of adverse effects are often not included. Nonetheless, impaired exercise capacity or lessened sexual performance, both occurring with β-blockers, clearly are bad news for the active male hypertensive patient. Conversely, a sufferer from anxiety-driven hypertension and tachycardia can achieve dramatic subjective relief from a β-blocker.

Cost effectiveness in the developing world. Worldwide, expensive drugs often are a luxury, and the principles of choice are governed by economic necessity. True trial outcome data are lacking.[194] Much can be said for low-dose thiazide diuretics as initial therapy, or a CCB depending on costs. A diuretic-based therapy is logical in black patients, and when combined with enalapril and a CCB, controlled the BP in 78% of black South African hypertensive patients. With LVH as endpoint, the CCB was much more effective than the diuretic. The price of generic CCBs in a country like India is very low.

Acute Severe Hypertension

First, it is important to consider whether the patient is suffering from a hypertensive urgency (BP very high, must come down but not necessarily rapidly) or emergency (complicated by acute heart failure papilledema or hypertensive encephalopathy) before choosing any of the drugs listed in Table 7-4. For urgency, careful use of rapidly acting oral agents such as furosemide and captopril is appropriate for imitation, with other agents added under tight supervision. For a true emergency, hospitalization is essential with careful administration of one of several agents (see Table 7-4). However, a rapid reduction of hypertension may have adverse end organ effects on brain and heart. *Thus it is prudent to consider whether rapid pressure reduction is really desirable in the presence of cerebral symptoms or symptoms of MI.* Therefore carefully titrated *intravenous nitroprusside, nicardipine,* or *labetalol* is preferable. Intravenous fenoldopam, a dopamine DA$_1$-selective agent, has the advantage of improving renal blood flow and the disadvantage of causing a reflex tachycardia. For acute LV failure, enalaprilat or sublingual captopril is first choice (see Table 7-4), together with a loop diuretic. For acute coronary syndromes, intravenous nitroglycerin is first choice, often with esmolol.

Table 7-4

Drugs Used in Hypertensive Urgencies and Emergencies

Clinical Requirement	Mechanism of Antihypertensive Effect	Drug Choice	Dose
Urgent reduction of severe acute hypertension	NO donor	Sodium nitroprusside infusion (care: cyanide toxicity)	0.3-2 mcg/kg/min (careful monitoring)
Hypertension plus ischemia (± poor LV)	NO donor	Infusion of nitroglycerin 20-200 mcg/min or isosorbide dinitrate 1-10 mg/h	Titrate against BP
Hypertension plus ischemia plus tachycardia	β-blocker (especially if good LV)	Esmolol bolus or infusion	50-250 mcg/kg/min
Hypertension plus ischemia plus tachycardia	α-β-blocker	Labetalol bolus or infusion	2-10 mg
			2.5-30 mcg/kg/min
Hypertension plus heart failure	ACE inhibitor (avoid negative inotropic rugs)	Enalaprilat (IV)	0.5-5 mg bolus
		Captopril (sl)	12.5-25 mg sl
Hypertension without cardiac complications	Vasodilators, including those that increase heart rate	Hydralazine	5-10 mg boluses
		Nifedipine (see text)*	1-4 mg boluses
			5-10 mg sl (care)
		Nicardipine : bolus : infusion	5-10 mcg/kg/min
			1-3 mcg/kg/min
Severe or malignant hypertension, also with poor renal function	Dopamine (DA-1) agonist; avoid with β-blockers	Fenoldopam†	0.2-0.5 mcg/kg/min
Hypertension plus pheochromocytoma	α-β-or combined α-β-blocker (avoid pure β-blocker)	Phentolamine	1-4 mg boluses
		Labetalol : bolus : infusion	2-10 mg
			2.5-30 mcg/kg/min

ACE, Angiotensin-converting enzyme; *BP,* blood pressure; *IV,* intravenous; *LV,* left ventricular; *NO,* nitric oxide; *sl,* sublingual.
Modified from Foex, et al. *Cardiovascular drugs in the perioperative period.* New York: Authors' Publishing House; 1999, with permission. Nitrate doses from Table 6, Niemenen MS, et al. *Eur Heart J* 2005;266:384.
*Not licensed in the United States; oral nifedipine capsules contraindicated.
†Licensed as *Corlopam* for use in severe or malignant hypertension in the United States; for detailed infusion rates, see package insert. Note tachycardia as side effect must not be treated by β-blockade (package insert).

Nitroprusside. Nitroprusside is still used extensively, but requires careful monitoring to avoid overshoot. Nitroprusside reduces preload and afterload. The package insert warns against continuing a high-dose infusion for more than 10 minutes if the BP dose not drop, because of the danger of cyanide toxicity (see Chapter 6, p. 186). *Labetalol* does not cause tachycardia and gives a smooth dose-related fall in BP; the side effects of β-blockade, such as bronchospasm, may be countered by the added α-blockade of labetalol. Hydralazine and dihydralazine may cause tachycardia and are also best avoided, especially in angina, unless there is concomitant therapy with a β-blocker or in preeclampsia for which it is the only approved parenteral agent in pregnancy.

Acute stroke with hypertension. In acute stroke with hypertension, the benefits of BP reduction remain conjectural, and most neurologists would only reduce the BP if the diastolic level exceeds 120 mm Hg.

Maximal Drug Therapy

When confronted with the occasional patient who appears to be refractory to all known forms of therapy, the following points are worth considering: (1) Is the patient really adherent with the therapy? (2) Exclude white-coat hypertension. Are the BP values taken in the doctor's office really representative of those with which the patient lives? There can be striking differences. (3) Has the patient developed some complications such as atherosclerotic renal artery stenosis or renal failure? (4) Has the patient increased sodium or alcohol intake, or taken sympathomimetic agents or nonsteroidal antiinflammatory agents? (5) Are there temporary psychological stresses? (6) Could a cause of secondary hypertension be inapparent? For example, a high plasma aldosterone and low plasma rennin may be a clue to inapparent hyperaldosteronism that requires either replacing the thiazide by an aldosterone antagonist, or a combination of the two. Resistance may be overcome by aldosterone blockers even in the absence of hyperaldosteronism.[195] Then, finally, is the therapy really maximal, particularly regarding the diuretic dose? Overfilling of dilated vasculature by reactive sodium retention may also preclude a fall in the peripheral resistance. (Note that the concept of low-dose diuretic therapy must be abandoned at this stage).

Drugs for truly resistant hypertension. RH is still an understudied clinical condition with a high cardiovascular morbidity and mortality, in which ABPM is established to guide diagnosis, therapy, and prognosis.[36] This means that the PVR or the CO or both has failed to fall. Generally, the emphasis should be on vasodilator therapy, acting on every conceivable mechanism: CCB, α-blockade, ACE inhibition, angiotensin receptor blockade, K^+ channel-induced vasodilation by *minoxidil*, high-dose diuretics, and aldosterone blockers. Severe hypertension often has a volume-dependent component and reactive sodium retention often accompanies the fall in BP induced by vasodilatory drugs and especially minoxidil; therefore the addition of more diuretics, particularly the loop agents, is an important component of maximal therapy. Of the loop diuretics, torsemide is registered for once-daily use in hypertension. Of the others, metolazone is equally effective as torsemide and even more certain to provide 24-hour efficacy. The *ganglion blockers* (guanethidine and guanadrel), now decidedly out of fashion because of frequent orthostatic hypotension and interference with sexual activity, should therefore be reserved for the last resort. The present trend is to emphasize the three basic drugs, namely a CCB like amlodipine, an ACE inhibitor–ARB, and a diuretic, and then to add two more, spironolactone and α-blockade, and only then to aim for renal artery denervation if available.

Renal Artery Denervation for Hypertension

Catheter-based renal artery denervation is under intense investigation for the treatment of drug-resistant hypertension.[196] The US pivotal trial, Simplicity HTN-3, is recently underway. In an uncontrolled initial study of 153 patients with RH (mean: 176/98 ± 17/15 mm Hg on a mean of 5 BP agents) catheter-based renal sympathetic denervation gave a substantial reduction in BP of approximately 25/12 mm Hg sustained to 2 years or more of follow-up, without significant adverse events.[197] In SIMPLICITY HTN-2, in which patients were randomized to continued five-drug therapy alone or to continued five-drug therapy plus renal artery denervation, the 6-month data are quite promising[198] but need to be confirmed independently in the newly started SIMPLICITY HTN-3 trial that has a larger sample, a sham denervation arm, and mandatory 24-hour ABPM.

Renal artery denervation destroys both renal sympathetic (efferent) nerves, which stimulate renal vasoconstriction and renin release while blocking natriuresis, and afferent renal nerves (i.e., nerve trafficking to brain from kidney), which can trigger generalized reflex sympathetic overactivity and thus contribute to hypertension,[199] and raises the possibility that renal denervation (RDN) may exert systemic effects beyond just lowering of BP. Specifically, RDN has in early phase studies improved in measures of insulin sensitivity in diabetics with hypertension[200] and parameters of sleep apnea.[187] But an editorial in *Hypertension*[61] asks whether these patients really have drug-resistant hypertension, stating that there was almost no treatment with central sympatholytics or with α-blockers and few were treated by aldosterone antagonists. The counterargument is that many patients would prefer a one-time intervention to continuing with complex multiple medications.

Baroreflex Activation Therapy for Hypertension

Implantation of a carotid baroreceptor pacemaker is another device-based approach being investigated for RH. Prolonged baroreflex activation by sustained electrical stimulation of the carotid sinus nerves in dogs lead to sustained reductions in arterial pressure, heart rate, and plasma NE concentrations.[201] The first US pivotal trial randomized patients with RH to an experimental condition of bilateral carotid baroreflex activation for 12 months or to a comparison condition of sham activation for the first 6 months followed by actual carotid baroreflex activation for the next 6 months; the results showed benefit for some but not all efficacy endpoints and too many adverse events (facial nerve palsy) related to the surgical procedure.[202] A second-generation device using a much smaller unilateral stimulating electrode (Barostim Neo, CVRx Inc) is currently being tested in Europe.

SUMMARY

1. *Major advances* in the recent past include the following. The BP goals have become lower, but strongly related to the degree of risk. Therefore risk factor stratification is now an important part of the evaluation of hypertension. Blood lipid profiles should always be obtained and a statin given if indicated. Clinical examination should establish target organ damage prior to multifactorial lifestyle intervention.

2. *Older adults and diabetics* have emerged as two major high-risk groups. In older adults, treatment of systolic hypertension reduces stroke, cardiovascular events, and all-cause mortality. In diabetic patients, BP should ideally be reduced to 130/80 mm Hg in addition to statin therapy.

3. *As agents of first choice,* several national guidelines including those of the Joint National Committee in the United States recommend low-dose diuretics for uncomplicated hypertension in patients lacking specific indications for other agents because diuretics reduce a variety of important endpoints, including all-cause mortality. The British Society of Hypertension recommends one of three first-line choices: CCBs, ACE inhibitors–ARBs, or diuretics (chlorthalidone or indapamide). By contrast, the European Society of Hypertension proposes that any of five categories of drugs should be suitable, namely low-dose diuretics, β-blockers, CCBs, ACE inhibitors, or ARBs. The recent appreciation of a lesser protection against stroke by β-blockers has largely relegated them to secondary protection.

4. *In diabetics,* ACE inhibitors or ARBs are almost always the first choice. Diuretics, CCBs, and β-blockers may all be needed to bring down the BP to the low levels required.

5. *In older adults,* agents that have been primarily used in trials are low-dose diuretics and long-acting DPE calcium blockers. CCBs are logical therapy to counter impaired vasodilation in the aging arteries. In much older adults, the HYVET trial using initial diuretic therapy by indapamide was stopped because of a mortality reduction. The BP aim was 150/100 mm Hg. Caution is needed in further lowering already low diastolic pressure in those with isolated systolic hypertension, with data suggesting that the drop should not be less than 65-70 mm Hg.

6. *In coronary disease* in hypertensive patients, optimal management should control both BP and blood lipids, thereby potentially helping to reduce coronary mortality. No particular group of antihypertensive agents seems particularly effective in reducing coronary mortality. By contrast, statins are achieving increasing success.

7. *In severe emergency hypertension,* selection should be made from the available intravenous agents according to the characteristics of the patient. For those with severe hypertension but no acute target organ damage, fast-acting oral agents such as furosemide and captopril should be used.

8. *In refractory hypertension,* it is important to ensure compliance; to exclude a secondary cause, including aldosteronism; to think of white-coat hypertension; to check the 24-hour BP pattern; and only then to increase the medication.

9. *In drug-refractory hypertension,* renal artery sympathetic denervation is increasingly regarded as an option, although further data are needed for mechanical baroreceptor activation therapy.

10. *As a general approach,* we recommend a patient-guided approach together with a consideration of the major outcome trials and guidelines as the most appropriate way to treat hypertension. Improved control of hypertension is responsible for approximately 20% of the decline in coronary mortality noted in the United States from 1980 to 2000.[203] Even better effects can be achieved with more adequate control of BP.

References

1. Mancia G, et al. 2007 guidelines for the management of arterial hypertension: the Task Force for the Management of Arterial Hypertension of the European Society of Hypertension (ESH) and of the European Society of Cardiology (ESC). *J Hypertens* 2007;25:1105–1187.
2. Kotchen TA. The search for strategies to control hypertension. *Circulation* 2010;122:1141–1143.
3. Beto JA, et al. Quality of life in treatment of hypertension: a meta-analysis of clinical trials. *Am J Hypertens* 1992;5:125–133.
4. PROGRESS Collaborative Group. Effects of blood pressure lowering with perindopril and indapamide therapy on dementia and cognitive decline in patients with cerebrovascular disease. *Arch Intern Med* 2003;163:1069–1075.
5. Turner ST, et al. Personalized medicine for high blood pressure. *Hypertension* 2007;50:1–5.
6. Burt CW, et al. *Ambulatory medical care utilization estimates for 2005: advanced data from vital and health statistics no. 388.* Hyattsville (MD): National Centre for Health Statistics; 2007.
7. Cherry D, et al. *National ambulatory medical care survey 2005 summary. Advanced data from vital and health statistics no. 387.* Hyattsville (MD): National Centre for Health Statistics; 2007.
8. Wang YR, et al. Outpatient hypertension treatment, treatment intensification, and control in Western Europe and the United States. *Arch Intern Med* 2007;167:141–147.
9. Krause T, et al. For the Guideline Development Group. Management of hypertension: summary of NICE guidance. *Br Med J* 2011;343:d48–d91.
10. Matsui Y, et al. Maximum value of home blood pressure: a novel indicator of target organ damage in hypertension. *Hypertension* 2011;57:1087–1093.
11. Hansen TW, et al. Prognostic superiority of daytime ambulatory over conventional blood pressure in four populations: a meta-analysis of 7,030 individuals. *J Hypertens* 2007;25:1554–1564.
12. Medical Research Council Working Party. MRC trial of treatment of mild hypertension: principal results. *Br Med J* 1985;291:97–104.
13. Zhang Y, et al. FEVER Study Group. Is a systolic blood pressure target <140 mmHg indicated in all hypertensives? Subgroup analyses of findings from the randomized FEVER trial. *Eur Heart J* 2011;32:1500–1508.
14. Krause T, et al. For the Guideline Development Group. Management of hypertension: summary of NICE guidance. *Br Med J* 2011 Aug 25;343:d48–d91.
15. Lovibond K, et al. Cost-effectiveness of options for the diagnosis of high blood pressure in primary care: a modelling study. *Lancet* 2011;378:1219–1230.
16. Matsui Y, et al. Maximum value of home blood pressure: a novel indicator of target organ damage in hypertension. *Hypertension* 2011;57:1087–1093.
17. O'Brien E. Is the case for ABPM as a routine investigation in clinical practice not overwhelming? *Hypertension* 2007;50:284–286.
18. Grassi G, et al. Neurogenic abnormalities in masked hypertension. *Hypertension* 2007;50:537–542.
19. Kario K, et al. Morning surge in blood pressure as a predictor of silent and clinical cerebrovascular disease in elderly hypertensives: a prospective study. *Circulation* 2003;107:1401–1406.
20. Palatini P. Role of elevated heart rate in the development of cardiovascular disease in hypertension. *Hypertension* 2011;58:745–750.
21. Tatasciore A, et al. Awake systolic blood pressure variability correlates with target-organ damage in hypertension subjects. *Hypertension* 2007;50:325–332.
22. Mancia G, et al. Blood pressure control and improved cardiovascular outcomes in the International Verapamil SR-Trandolapril Study. *Hypertension* 2007;50:299–305.
23. Webb AJS, et al. Effect of dose and combination of antihypertensives on interindividual blood pressure variability: a systematic review. *Stroke* 2011;42:2860–2865.
24. Bilo G, et al. A new method for assessing 24-h blood pressure variability after excluding the contribution of nocturnal blood pressure fall. *J Hypertens* 2007;25:2058–2066.
25. Zhang Y, et al. Effect of antihypertensive agents on blood pressure variability: the Natrilix SR versus candesartan and amlodipine in the reduction of systolic blood pressure in hypertensive patients (X-CELLENT) study. *Hypertension* 2011;58:155–160.
26. Kaplan NM. The diastolic J curve: alive and threatening. *Hypertension* 2011;58:751–753.
27. Chalmers J. Is a blood pressure target of <130/80 mm Hg still appropriate for high-risk patients? *Circulation* 2011;124:1700–1702.
28. Dorresteijn JA, et al. On behalf of the Secondary Manifestations of Arterial Disease Study Group. Relation between blood pressure and vascular events and mortality in patients with manifest vascular disease: J-curve revisited. *Hypertension* 2012;59:14–21.
29. Messerli FH, et al. Dogma disputed: can aggressively lowering blood pressure in hypertensive patients with coronary artery disease be dangerous? *Ann Intern Med* 2006;144:884–893.
30. Protogerou AD, et al. Diastolic blood pressure and mortality in the elderly with cardiovascular disease. *Hypertension* 2007;50:172–180.
31. Mancia G, et al. For the European Society of Hypertension. Reappraisal of European guidelines on hypertension management: a European Society of Hypertension Task Force document. *J Hypertens* 2009;27:2121–2158.
32. Law MR, et al. Use of blood pressure lowering drugs in the prevention of cardiovascular disease: meta-analysis of 147 randomised trials in the context of expectations from prospective epidemiological studies. *Br Med J* 2009;338:b16–b65.
33. Roman MJ, et al. Central pressure more strongly relates to vascular disease and outcome than does brachial pressure: the Strong Heart Study. *Hypertension* 2007;50:197–203.

34. Van Bortel LM, et al. Artery Society, European Society of Hypertension Working Group on Vascular Structure and Function, and European Network for Noninvasive Investigation of Large Arteries: Expert consensus document on the measurement of aortic stiffness in daily practice using carotid-femoral pulse wave velocity. *J Hypertens* 2012;30:445–448.

35. Ong KT, et al. Aortic stiffness is reduced beyond blood pressure lowering by short-term and long-term antihypertensive treatment: a meta-analysis of individual data in 294 patients. *J Hypertens* 2011;29:1034–1042.

36. Muxfeldt ES, et al. Appropriate time interval to repeat ambulatory blood pressure monitoring in patients with white-coat resistant hypertension. *Hypertension* 2012;59:384–389.

37. Lewington S, et al. Age-specific relevance of usual blood pressure to vascular mortality: a meta-analysis of individual data for one million adults in 61 prospective studies. *Lancet* 2002;360:1903–1913.

38. Chobanian AV, et al. The seventh report of the Joint National Committee on Prevention, Detection, Evaluation and Treatment of High Blood Pressure. *JAMA* 2003;289:2560–2572.

39. The Task Force for the Management of Arterial Hypertension of the European Society of Hypertension (ESH) and of the European Society of Cardiology (ESC), Mancia G, et al. 2007 guidelines for the management of arterial hypertension. *J Hypertens* 2007;25: 1105–1187.

40. Allen N, et al. Impact of blood pressure and blood pressure change during middle age on the remaining lifetime risk for cardiovascular disease: the cardiovascular lifetime risk pooling project. *Circulation* 2012;125:37–44.

41. Gu O, et al. Association of hypertension treatment and control with all-cause and cardiovascular disease mortality among US adults with hypertension. *Am J Hypertens* 2010; 23:38–45.

42. Mancia G, et al. Blood Pressure Targets Recommended by Guidelines and Incidence of Cardiovascular and Renal Events in the Ongoing Telmisartan Alone and in Combination With Ramipril Global Endpoint Trial (ONTARGET). *Circulation* 2011;124:1727–1736.

43. Flack JM, et al. International Society on Hypertension in Blacks. Management of high blood pressure in blacks: an update of the International Society on Hypertension in Blacks consensus statement. *Hypertension* 2010;56:780–800.

44. Wright Jr JT, et al. New recommendations for treating hypertension in black patients: evidence and/or consensus? *Hypertension* 2010;56:801–803.

45. Vasan RS, et al. Residual lifetime risk for developing hypertension in middle-aged women and men: the Framingham Heart Study. *JAMA* 2002;287:1003–1010.

46. He FJ, et al. Effect of modest salt reduction on blood pressure: a meta-analysis of randomized trials: implications for public health. *J Hum Hypertens* 2002;16:761–770.

47. Cook NR, et al. Long term effects of dietary sodium reduction on cardiovascular disease outcomes: observational follow-up of the trials of hypertension prevention (TOHP). *Br Med J* 2007;334:885.

48. Dansinger ML, et al. Meta-analysis: the effect of dietary counseling for weight loss. *Ann Intern Med* 2007;147:41–50.

49. Sjöström L, et al. Effects of bariatric surgery on mortality in Swedish obese subjects. *N Engl J Med* 2007;357:741–752.

50. James J, et al. Preventing childhood obesity: two year follow-up results from the Christchurch obesity prevention programme in schools (CHOPPS). *Br Med J* 2007;335:762.

51. van Sluijs EM, et al. Effectiveness of interventions to promote physical activity in children and adolescents: systematic review of controlled trials. *Br Med J* 2007;335:703.

52. Bibbins-Domingo K, et al. Projected effect of dietary salt reductions on future cardiovascular disease. *N Engl J Med* 2010;362:590–599.

53. Sacks FM, et al. For the DASH-Sodium Collaborative Research Group. Effects on blood pressure of reduced dietary sodium and the Dietary Approaches to Stop Hypertension (DASH) diet. *N Engl J Med* 2001;344:3–10.

54. Havas S, et al. The urgent need to reduce sodium consumption. *JAMA* 2007;298:1439–1441.

55. Schillaci G, et al. Effect of body weight changes on 24-hour blood pressure and left ventricular mass in hypertension: a 4-year follow up. *Am J Hypertens* 2003;16:634–639.

56. Mendis S, et al. World Health Organization (WHO) and International Society of Hypertension (ISH) risk prediction charts: assessment of cardiovascular risk for prevention and control of cardiovascular disease in low and middle-income countries. *J Hypertens* 2007;25:1578–1582.

57. Benetos A, et al. Prognostic value of systolic and diastolic blood pressure in treated hypertensive men. *Arch Intern Med* 2002;162:577–581.

58. HOT Study, Hansson L, et al. Effects of intensive blood-pressure lowering and low-dose aspirin in patients with hypertension: principal results of the Hypertension Optimal Treatment (HOT) randomised trial. *Lancet* 1998;351:1755–1762.

59. Weiner DE, et al. Lowest systolic blood pressure is associated with stroke in stages 3 to 4 chronic kidney disease. *J Am Soc Nephrol* 2007;18:960–966.

60. Barzilay JI, et al. ONTARGET and TRANSCEND Investigators. Albuminuria and decline in cognitive function: the ONTARGET/TRANSCEND studies. *Arch Intern Med* 2011;171:142–150.

61. Biaggioni I. Interventional approaches to reduce sympathetic activity in resistant hypertension: to ablate or stimulate? *Hypertension* 2012;59:194–195.

62. WHO/ISH Writing Group. 2003 World Health Organisation (WHO)/ International Society of Hypertension (ISH) statement on management of hypertension. *J Hypertens* 2003;21: 1983–1992.

63. Opie LH. Beta-blockade should not be among several choices for initial therapy of hypertension. *J Hypertens* 2008;26:161–163.

64. Materson BJ, et al. Single-drug therapy for hypertension in men: a comparison of six antihypertensive agents with placebo: the Department of Veterans Affairs Cooperative Study Group on Antihypertensive Agents. *N Engl J Med* 1993;328:914–921.

65. Middlemost SJ, et al. Effectiveness of enalapril in combination with low-dose hydrochlorothiazide versus enalapril alone for mild to moderate systemic hypertension in black patients. *Am J Cardiol* 1994;73:1092–1097.
66. Wing LM, et al. A comparison of outcomes with angiotensin-converting-enzyme inhibitors and diuretics for hypertension in the elderly. *N Engl J Med* 2003;348:583–592.
67. Calhoun DA, et al. Resistant hypertension: diagnosis, evaluation, and treatment: a scientific statement from the AHA professional education committee of the Council for High Blood Pressure Research. *Circulation* 2008;117:e510–e526.
68. RALES Study, Pitt B, et al. For the Randomized Aldactone Evaluation Study Investigators. The effect of spironolactone on morbidity and mortality in patients with severe heart failure. *New Engl J Med* 1999;341:709–717.
69. Chapman N, et al. Effect of spironolactone on blood pressure in subjects with resistant hypertension. *Hypertension* 2007;49:839–845.
70. Václavík J, et al. Addition of spironolactone in patients with resistant arterial hypertension (ASPIRANT): a randomized, double-blind, placebo-controlled trial. *Hypertension* 2011;57:1069–1075.
71. Rabi DM, et al. Canadian Hypertension Education Program: the 2011 Canadian Hypertension Education Program recommendations for the management of hypertension: blood pressure measurement, diagnosis, assessment of risk, and therapy. *Can J Cardiol* 2011;27:415–433.
72. Gee ME, et al. Antihypertensive medication use, adherence, stops, and starts in Canadians with hypertension: Outcomes Research Task Force of the Canadian Hypertension Education Program. *Can J Cardiol* 2012;28:383–389.
73. Houlihan SJ, et al. Hypertension treatment and control rates: chart review in an academic family medicine clinic. *Can Fam Phys* 2009;55:735–741.
74. Psaty BM, et al. Health outcomes associated with various antihypertensive therapies used as first-line agents. *JAMA* 2003;289:2534–2544.
75. Ernst ME, et al. Use of diuretics in patients with hypertension. *N Engl J Med* 2009;361: 2153–2164.
76. Zillich AJ, et al. Thiazide diuretics, potassium, and the development of diabetes: a quantitative review. *Hypertension* 2006;48:219–224.
77. Cohen HW, et al. High and low serum potassium associated with cardiovascular events in diuretic-treated patients. *J Hypertens* 2001;19:1315–1323.
78. Grimm RH, et al. Long-term effects on sexual function of five antihypertensive drugs and nutritional hygienic treatment in hypertensive men and women: Treatment of Mild Hypertension Study (TOMHS). *Hypertension* 1997;29:8–14.
79. Hiltunen TP, et al. Predictors of antihypertensive drug responses: initial data from a placebo-controlled, randomized, cross-over study with four antihypertensive drugs (The GENRES Study). *Am J Hypertens* 2007;20:311–318.
80. SHEP Cooperative Research Group. Prevention of stroke by antihypertensive drug treatment in older persons with isolated systolic hypertension Final results of the Systolic Hypertension in the Elderly Program (SHEP). *JAMA* 1991;265:3255–3264.
81. Reyes AJ. Diuretics in the therapy of hypertension. *J Hum Hypertens* 2002;16(Suppl 1): S78–S83.
82. Ernst ME, et al. Comparative antihypertensive effects of hydrochlorothiazide and chlorthalidone on ambulatory and office blood pressure. *Hypertension* 2006;47:352–358.
83. Pepine CJ, et al. A calcium antagonist vs a non-calcium antagonist hypertension treatment strategy for patients with coronary artery disease: the International Verapamil-Trandolapril Study (INVEST): a randomized controlled trial. *JAMA* 2003;290:2805–2816.
84. Julius S, et al. Outcomes in hypertensive patients at high cardiovascular risk treated with regimens based on valsartan or amlodipine: the VALUE randomised trial. *Lancet* 2004; 363:2022–2031.
85. Cruz MN, et al. Acute responses to phytoestrogens in small arteries from men with coronary heart disease. *Am J Physiol Heart Circ Physiol* 2006;290:H1969–H1975.
86. TOMH Study, Neaton JD, et al. Treatment of Mild Hypertension study (TOMH): final results. *JAMA* 1993;270:713–724.
87. Franse LV, et al. Hypokalemia associated with diuretic use and cardiovascular events in the Systolic Hypertension in the Elderly Program. *Hypertension* 2000;35:1025–1030.
88. ALLHAT Collaborative Research Group. Major outcomes in high-risk hypertensive patients randomized to angiotensin-converting enzyme inhibitor or calcium channel blocker vs diuretic: the Antihypertensive and Lipid-Lowering Treatment to Prevent Heart Attack Trial (ALLHAT). *JAMA* 2002;288:2981–2997.
89. Dorsch MP, et al. Chlorthalidone reduces cardiovascular events compared with hydrochlorothiazide: a retrospective cohort analysis. *Hypertension* 2011;57:689–694.
90. Wiggan MI, et al. Low dose bendrofluazide (1.25 mg) effectively lowers blood pressure over 24 h: results of a randomized, double-blind, placebo-controlled crossover study. *Am J Hypertens* 1999;12:528–531.
91. Saha C, et al. Improvement in blood pressure with inhibition of the epithelial sodium channel in blacks with hypertension. *Hypertension* 2005;46:481–487.
92. Gosse P, et al. On behalf of the LIVE investigators. Regression of left ventricular hypertrophy in hypertensive patients treated with indapamide SR 1.5 mg versus enalapril 20 mg: the LIVE study. *J Hypertens* 2000;18:1465–1475.
93. Beckett N, et al. for the HYVET Study Group. Treatment of hypertension in patients 80 years of age or older. *N Engl J Med* 2008;358:1887–1898.
94. Baumgart P. Torasemide in comparison with thiazides in the treatment of hypertension. *Cardiovasc Drugs Ther* 1993;7(Suppl 1):63–68.
95. Siscovick DS, et al. Diuretic therapy for hypertension and the risk of primary cardiac arrest. *New Engl J Med* 1994;330:1852–1857.

96. Yasar S, et al. For the Ginkgo Evaluation of Memory (GEM) Study Investigators. Diuretic use is associated with better learning and memory in older adults in the Ginkgo Evaluation of Memory study. *Alzheimer's Dement* 2012;8:188–195.

97. Frishman WH, et al. A multifactorial trial designed to assess combination therapy in hypertension. *Arch Intern Med* 1994;154:1461–1468.

98. Thulin T, et al. Diltiazem compared with metoprolol as add-on-therapies to diuretics in hypertension. *J Human Hypertens* 1991;5:107–114.

99. Elliott WJ, et al. Equivalent antihypertensive effects of combination therapy using diuretic + calcium antagonist compared with diuretic + ACE inhibitor. *J Human Hypertens* 1990;4:717–723.

100. Wang JG, et al. Prevention of stroke and myocardial infarction by amlodipine and angiotensin receptor blockers: a quantitative overview. *Hypertension* 2007; 50:181–188.

101. Grossman EH, et al. Effect of calcium antagonists on plasma norepinephrine levels, heart rate and blood pressure. *Am J Cardiol* 1997;80:1453–1458.

102. Dahlöf B, et al. Prevention of cardiovascular events with an antihypertensive regimen of amlodipine adding perindopril as required versus atenolol adding bendroflumethiazide as required, in the Anglo-Scandinavian Cardiac Outcomes Trial-Blood Pressure Lowering Arm (ASCOT-BPLA): a multicentre randomised controlled trial. *Lancet* 2005; 366:895–906.

103. Sareli P, et al. Efficacy of different drug classes used to initiate antihypertensive treatment in black subjects: results of a randomized trial in Johannesburg, South Africa. *Arch Intern Med* 2001;161:965–971.

104. Nakamura T, et al. Comparison of renal and vascular protective effects between telmisartan and amlodipine in hypertensive patients with chronic kidney disease with mild renal insufficiency. *Hypertens Res* 2008;31:841–850.

105. BP Trialists. Effects of different blood-pressure-lowering regimens on major cardiovascular events: results of prospectively-designed overviews of randomised trials. *Lancet* 2003;362:1527–1535.

106. Wright Jr JT, et al. for the African American Study of Kidney Disease and Hypertension Study Group (AASK). Effect of blood pressure lowering and antihypertensive drug class on progression of hypertensive kidney disease. *JAMA* 2002:2421–2431.

107. Jamerson KA, et al. Efficacy and duration of benazepril plus amlodipine or hydrochlorothiazide on 24-hour ambulatory systolic blood pressure control. *Hypertension* 2011; 57:174–179.

108. Bakris GL, et al. Renal outcomes with different fixed-dose combination therapies in patients with hypertension at high risk for cardiovascular events (ACCOMPLISH): a prespecified secondary analysis of a randomised controlled trial. *Lancet* 2010; 375:1173–1181.

109. Cooper-Dehoff R, et al. INVEST Investigators Predictors of development of diabetes mellitus in patients with coronary artery disease taking antihypertensive medications (findings from the INternational VErapamil SR-Trandolapril STudy [INVEST]). *Am J Cardiol* 2006;98:890–894.

110. Lam SK, et al. Incident diabetes in clinical trials of antihypertensive drugs. *Lancet* 2007;369:1513–1514; author reply 1514–1515.

111. Zanchetti A, et al. Prevalence and incidence of the metabolic syndrome in the European Lacidipine Study on Atherosclerosis (ELSA) and its relation with carotid intima-media thickness. *J Hypertens* 2007;25:2463–2470.

112. McManus RJ, et al. National Institute for Health and Clinical Excellence NICE hypertension guideline 2011: evidence based evolution. *Br Med J* 2012;344:e181.

113. HOPE Investigators, Yusuf S, et al. Effects of an angiotensin-converting enzyme inhibitor, ramipril, on cardiovascular events in high-risk patients. *N Engl J Med* 2000;342:145–153.

114. Chrysant SG, et al. Effects of isradipine or enalapril on blood pressure in salt-sensitive hypertensives during low and high dietary salt intake. MIST II Trial Investigators. *Am J Hypertens* 2000;3:1180–1188.

115. Blood Pressure Lowering Treatment Trialists' Collaboration. Blood pressure-dependent and independent effects of agents that inhibit the renin-angiotensin system. *J Hypertens* 2007;25:951–958.

116. Svensson P, et al. Comparative effects of ramipril on ambulatory and office blood pressures: a HOPE substudy. *Hypertension* 2008;31:38:E28–E32.

117. EUROPA Trial, Fox KM, et al. The European trial on reduction of cardiac events with perindopril in stable coronary artery disease (EUROPA). *Eur Heart J* 1998;19: J52–J55.

118. Kent DM, et al. Progression risk, urinary protein excretion, and treatment effects of angiotensin-converting enzyme inhibitors in nondiabetic kidney disease. *J Am Soc Nephrol* 2007;18:1959–1965.

119. Suissa S, et al. ACE-inhibitor use and the long-term risk of renal failure in diabetes. *Kidney Int* 2006;69:913–919.

120. Mann JF, et al. ONTARGET investigators. Renal outcomes with telmisartan, ramipril, or both, in people at high vascular risk (the ONTARGET study): a multicentre, randomised, double-blind, controlled trial. *Lancet* 2008;372:547–553.

121. Harel Z, et al. The effect of combination treatment with aliskiren and blockers of the renin-angiotensin system on hyperkalaemia and acute kidney injury: systematic review and meta-analysis. *Br Med J* Jan 9,2012;344:e42. doi: 10.1136/bmj.e42.

122. McMurray JJ, et al. Aliskiren, ALTITUDE, and the implications for ATMOSPHERE. *Eur J Heart Fail* 2012;14:341–343.

123. *Lancet*. Retraction—Combination treatment of angiotensin-II receptor blocker and angiotensin-converting-enzyme inhibitor in non-diabetic renal disease (COOPERATE): a randomised controlled trial. *Lancet* Oct 10, 2009;374(9697):1226.

124. Aronow WS, et al. ACCF/AHA 2011 Expert consensus document on hypertension in the elderly. *J Am Coll Cardiol* 2011;57:2037–2114.

125. Mallion JM, et al. Systolic blood pressure reduction with olmesartan medoxomil versus nitrendipine in elderly patients with isolated systolic hypertension. *J Hypertens* 2007; 25:2168–2177.

126. ONTARGET Investigators, Yusuf S, et al. Telmisartan, ramipril, or both in patients at high risk for vascular events. *N Engl J Med* 2008;358:1547–1559.

127. Weir MR. Targeting mechanisms of hypertensive vascular disease with dual calcium channel and renin-angiotensin system blockade. *J Hum Hypertens* 2007;21:770–779.

128. LIFE Study Group, Dahlöf B, et al. Cardiovascular morbidity and mortality in the Losartan Intervention for Endpoint reduction in hypertension study (LIFE): a randomised trial against atenolol. *Lancet* 2002;359:995–1003.

129. Berl T, et al. Cardiovascular outcomes in the Irbesartan diabetic nephropathy trial of patients with type 2 diabetes and overt nephropathy. *Ann Intern Med* 2003;138:542–549.

130. Boutitie F, et al. Does a change in angiotensin II formation caused by antihypertensive drugs affect the risk of stroke? A meta-analysis of trials according to treatment with potentially different effects on angiotensin II. *J Hypertens* 2007;25:1543–1553.

131. Fournier A, et al. Is the angiotensin II Type 2 receptor cerebroprotective? *Curr Hypertens Rep* 2004;6:182–189.

132. ONTARGET Investigators, Yusuf S, et al. Telmisartan, ramipril, or both in patients at high risk for vascular events. *N Engl J Med* 2008;358:1547–1559.

133. Kronish IM, et al. Meta-analysis: impact of drug class on adherence to antihypertensives. *Circulation* 2011;123:1611–1621.

134. Jordan J, et al. Direct renin inhibition with aliskiren in obese patients with arterial hypertension. *Hypertension* 2007; 49:1047–1055.

135. Oparil S, et al. Efficacy and safety of combined use of aliskiren and valsartan in patients with hypertension: a randomised, double-blind trial. *Lancet* 2007; 370:221–229.

136. Oh BH, et al. Aliskiren, an oral renin inhibitor, provides dose-dependent efficacy and sustained 24-hour blood pressure control in patients with hypertension. *J Am Coll Cardiol* 2007; 49:1157–1163.

137. Sealey JE, et al. Aliskiren, the first renin inhibitor for treating hypertension: reactive renin secretion may limit its effectiveness. *Am J Hypertens* 2007; 20:587–597.

138. Brown MJ, et al. Aliskiren and the calcium channel blocker amlodipine combination as an initial treatment strategy for hypertension control (ACCELERATE): a randomised, parallel-group trial. *Lancet* 2011;377:312–320.

139. Pitt B, et al. For the Eplerenone post-acute myocardial infarction heart failure efficacy and survival study investigators. Eplerenone, a selective aldosterone blocker, in patients with left ventricular dysfunction after myocardial infarction. *N Engl J Med* 2003;348: 1309–1321.

140. Flack JM, et al. Efficacy and tolerability of eplerenone and losartan in hypertensive black and white patients. *J Am Coll Cardiol* 2003;41:1148–1155.

141. Fujimura N, et al. Mineralocorticoid receptor blocker eplerenone improves endothelial function and inhibits Rho-associated kinase activity in patients with hypertension. *Clin Pharmacol Ther* 2012;91:289–297.

142. Calhoun DA, et al. Effects of a novel aldosterone synthase inhibitor for treatment of primary hypertension: results of a randomized, double-blind, placebo- and active-controlled phase 2 trial. *Circulation* 2011;124:1945.

143. Wray DW, et al. Impact of aldosterone receptor blockade compared with thiazide therapy on sympathetic nervous system function in geriatric hypertension. *Hypertension* 2010;55:1217–1223.

144. Menon DV, et al. Differential effects of chlorthalidone versus spironolactone on muscle sympathetic nerve activity in hypertensive patients. *J Clin Endocrinol Metab* 2009;94: 1361–1366.

145. Messerli FH, et al. Are beta-blockers efficacious as first-line therapy for hypertension in the elderly? A systematic review. *JAMA* 1998;279:1903–1907.

146. Carlberg B, et al. Atenolol in hypertension: is it a wise choice? *Lancet* 2004;364: 1684–1689.

147. Bangalore S, et al. Cardiovascular protection using beta blockers. *JACC* 2007;50.

148. Williams B, et al. Differential impact of blood pressure-lowering drugs on central aortic pressure and clinical outcomes: principal results of the Conduit Artery Function Evaluation (CAFE) study. *Circulation* 2006;113:1213–1225.

148A. Rothwell, PM et al. Effects of beta blockers and calcium-channel blockers on within-individual variability in blood pressure and risk of stroke. *Lancet Neurol* 2010;9:469–480.

149. Tomlinson LA, et al. Rate-limiting step: can different effects of antihypertensives on central blood pressure be translated into outcomes? *Hypertension* 2011;57:1047–1048.

150. Czernichow S, et al. Blood Pressure Lowering Treatment Trialists' Collaboration: the effects of blood pressure reduction and different blood pressure-lowering regimens on major cardiovascular events according to baseline blood pressure: meta-analysis of randomized trials. *J Hypertens* 2011;29:4–16.

151. Torp-Pedersen C, et al. Effects of metoprolol and carvedilol on pre-existing and new onset diabetes in patients with chronic heart failure: data from the Carvedilol Or Metoprolol European Trial (COMET). *Heart* 2007;93:968–973.

152. Kampus P, et al. Differential effect of nebivolol and metoprolol on central aortic pressure and left ventricular wall thickness. *Hypertension* 2011;57:1122–1128.

153. Ayers K, et al. Differential effects of nebivolol and metoprolol on insulin sensitivity and plasminogen activator inhibitor in the metabolic syndrome. *Hypertension* 2012; 59:893–898.

154. Phillips RA, et al. GEMINI Investigators. Demographic analyses of the effects of carvedilol vs metoprolol on glycemic control and insulin sensitivity in patients with type 2 diabetes and hypertension in the Glycemic Effects in Diabetes Mellitus: Carvedilol-Metoprolol Comparison in Hypertensives (GEMINI) study. *J Cardiometab Syndr* 2008; 3:211–217.

155. Einhorn PT, et al. The Antihypertensive and Lipid Lowering Treatment to Prevent Heart Attack Trial (ALLHAT) Heart Failure Validation Study: diagnosis and prognosis. *Am Heart J* 2007;153:42–53.

156. McConnell JD, et al. The long-term effect of doxazosin, finasteride, and combination therapy on the clinical progression of benign prostatic hyperplasia. *N Engl J Med* 2003;349:2387–2398.

157. Chang C, et al. The effect on blood pressure and lipid profiles of doxazosin GITS as a third-line antihypertensive agent in the Anglo-Scandinavian Cardiac Outcomes Trial (ASCOT). *J Hypertens* 2006;24:S3.

158. Corrao G, et al. Cardiovascular protection by initial and subsequent combination of antihypertensive drugs in daily life practice. *Hypertension* 2011;58:566–572.

159. Kotchen TA. Expanding role for combination drug therapy in the initial treatment of hypertension? *Hypertension* 2011;58:550–551.

160. Jamerson K, et al. ACCOMPLISH Trial Investigators. Benazepril plus amlodipine or hydrochlorothiazide for hypertension in high-risk patients. *N Engl J Med* 2008;359: 2417–2428.

161. Yusuf S, et al. Effects of a polypill (Polycap) on risk factors in middle-aged individuals without cardiovascular disease (TIPS): a phase II, double-blind, randomised trial. *Lancet* 2009;18(373):1341–1351.

162. Lonn E, et al. The polypill in the prevention of cardiovascular diseases: key concepts, current status, challenges, and future directions. *Circulation* 2010;122:1078–1088.

163. Sanz G, et al. The Fixed-dose Combination Drug for Secondary Cardiovascular Prevention project: improving equitable access and adherence to secondary cardiovascular prevention with a fixed-dose combination drug. Study design and objectives. *Am Heart J* 2011;162:811–817.

164. Benetos A, et al. Blood pressure regulation during the aging process: the end of the "hypertension era"? *J Hyperten* 2011;29:646–652.

165. Staessen JA, et al. Risks of untreated and treated isolated systolic hypertension in the elderly: meta-analysis of outcome trials. *Lancet* 2000;355:865–872.

166. Staessen JA, et al. Less atherosclerosis and lower blood pressure for a meaningful life perspective with more brain. *Hypertension* 2007;49:389–400.

167. Aronow WS, et al. ACCF/AHA 2011 Expert consensus document on hypertension in the elderly. *J Am Coll Cardiol* 2011;57:2037–2114.

168. Larkin M. Walking sharpens some cognitive skills in elderly. *Lancet* 1999;354:401.

169. He FJ, et al. Potassium intake and blood pressure. *Am Heart J* 1999;12:849–851.

170. STOP-2 Study. Randomised trial of old and new antihypertensive drugs in elderly patients: cardiovascular mortality and morbidity in the Swedish Trial in Old Patients with Hypertension-2 study. *Lancet* 1999;354:1751–1756.

171. SCOPE Study, Lithell H, et al. The Study on Cognition and Prognosis in the Elderly (SCOPE): principal results of a randomised double-blind intervention trial. *J Hypertens* 2003;21:875–886.

172. Gupta V, et al. Orthostatic hypotension in the elderly: diagnosis and treatment. *Am J Med* 2007;120:841–847.

173. ACCORD Study Group, Cushman WC, et al. Effects of intensive blood-pressure control in type 2 diabetes mellitus. *N Engl J Med* 2010;362:1575–1585.

174. Lewis E, et al. For the Collaborative Study Group. The effect of angiotensin-converting enzyme inhibition on diabetic nephropathy. *N Engl J Med* 1993;329: 1456–1462.

175. Rossing K, et al. Enhanced renoprotective effects of ultrahigh doses of irbesartan in patients with type 2 diabetes and microalbuminuria. *Kidney Int* 2005;68:1190–1198.

176. Hollenberg NK, et al. Renal responses to three types of renin-angiotensin system blockers in patients with diabetes mellitus on a high-salt diet: a need for higher doses in diabetic patients? *J Hypertens* Oct 13, 2012 [Epub ahead of print].

177. Holtkamp FA, et al. Albuminuria and blood pressure, independent targets for cardioprotective therapy in patients with diabetes and nephropathy: a post hoc analysis of the combined RENAAL and IDNT trials. *Eur Heart J* 2011;32:1493–1499.

178. Ruggenenti P, et al. Preventing microalbuminuria in type 2 diabetes. *N Engl J Med* 2004;351:1941–1951.

179. Lindholm LH, et al. Should beta blockers remain first choice in the treatment of primary hypertension? A meta-analysis. *Lancet* 2005;366:1545–1553.

180. Almgren T, et al. Diabetes in treated hypertension is common and carries a high cardiovascular risk: results from a 28-year follow-up. *J Hypertens* 2007;25:1311–1317.

181. Patel A, et al. Effects of a fixed combination of perindopril and indapamide on macrovascular and microvascular outcomes in patients with type 2 diabetes mellitus (the ADVANCE trial): a randomised controlled trial. *Lancet* 2007;370:829–840.

182. Tuomilehto J, et al. Effects of calcium-channel blockade in older patients with diabetes and systolic hypertension. *N Engl J Med* 1999;340:677–684.

183. Neter JE, et al. Influence of weight reduction on blood pressure: a meta-analysis of randomized controlled trials. *Hypertension* 2003;42:878–884.

184. Williams B. The obese hypertensive: the weight of evidence against beta-blockers. *Circulation* 2007;115:1973–1974.

185. Minami J, et al. Is it time to regard cigarette smoking as a risk factor in the development of sustained hypertension? *Am J Hypertens* 1999;12:948–949.

186. Pedrosa RP, et al. Obstructive sleep apnea: the most common secondary cause of hypertension associated with resistant hypertension. *Hypertension* 2011;58:811–817.
187. Witkowski A, et al. Effects of renal sympathetic denervation on blood pressure, sleep apnea course, and glycemic control in patients with resistant hypertension and sleep apnea. *Hypertension* 2011;58:559–565.
188. Wachtell K, et al. Regression of electrocardiographic left ventricular hypertrophy during antihypertensive therapy and reduction in sudden cardiac death: the LIFE Study. *Circulation* 2007;116:700–705.
189. Okin PM, et al. In-treatment resolution or absence of electrocardiographic left ventricular hypertrophy is associated with decreased incidence of new-onset diabetes mellitus in hypertensive patients: the Losartan Intervention for Endpoint Reduction in Hypertension (LIFE) Study. *Hypertension* 2007;50:984–990.
190. Kjeldsen SE, et al. Prediction and prevention of atrial fibrillation in patients with high blood pressure or history of hypertension. *J Hypertens* 2012;30:887–889.
191. Black HR, et al. Principal results of the Controlled Onset Verapamil Investigation of Cardiovascular End Points (CONVINCE) trial. *JAMA* 2003;289:2073–2082.
192. Fogari R, et al. Sexual activity in hypertensive men treated with valsartan or carvedilol: A crossover study. *Am J Hypertens* 2001;14:27–31.
193. Taddei S, et al. Phosphodiesterase 5 inhibition to treat essential hypertension: is this the beginning of the story? *Hypertension* 2006;48:546–548.
194. Opie LH, et al. Cardiovascular disease in sub-Saharan Africa. *Circulation* 2005;112: 3536–3540.
195. Hood SJ, et al. The spironolactone, amiloride, losartan, and thiazide (SALT) double-blind crossover trial in patients with low-renin hypertension and elevated aldosterone-renin ratio. *Circulation* 2007;116:268–275.
196. Esler MD, et al. Renal sympathetic denervation in patients with treatment-resistant hypertension. *Lancet* 2010;376:1903–1909.
197. SIMPLICITY HTN-1 Investigators. Catheter-based renal sympathetic denervation for resistant hypertension: durability of blood pressure reduction out to 24 months. *Hypertension* 2011;57:911–917.
198. Krum H, et al. Catheter-based renal sympathetic denervation for resistant hypertension: a multicentre safety and proof-of-principle cohort study. *Lancet* 2009;373:1275–1281.
199. Converse Jr RL, et al. Sympathetic overactivity in patients with chronic renal failure. *N Engl J Med* 1992;327:1912–1918.
200. Mahfoud F, et al. Effect of renal sympathetic denervation on glucose metabolism in patients with resistant hypertension: a pilot study. *Circulation* 2011;123:1940–1946.
201. Lohmeier TE, et al. Chronic lowering of blood pressure by carotid baroreflex activation: mechanisms and potential for hypertension therapy. *Hypertension* 2011;57:880–886.
202. Bisognano JD, et al. Baroreflex activation therapy lowers blood pressure in patients with resistant hypertension: results from the double-blind, randomized, placebo-controlled Rheos pivotal trial. *J Am Coll Cardiol* 2011;58:765–773.
203. Ford ES, et al. Explaining the decrease in U.S. deaths from coronary disease, 1980-2000. *N Engl J Med* 2007;356:2388–2398.

8

Antiarrhythmic Drugs and Strategies

STANLEY NATTEL · BERNARD J. GERSH · LIONEL H. OPIE

"Devices and radiofrequency ablation have revolutionized the therapy of life-threatening and highly symptomatic arrhythmias."

Authors of this chapter, 2004

Overview of New Developments

There have been several major trends since the last edition of this book: (1) The persistent imperfections of current antiarrhythmic drugs and rapidly expanding technologies have led to a continued explosion in the use of devices and ablative techniques for both supraventricular and ventricular arrhythmias. (2) Atrial fibrillation (AF) has become a very active focus of research, with the recognition that with our aging population it is now a major health hazard, yet with persisting problems in management such as the continuing controversy regarding rate versus rhythm control with an ever increasing trend toward intervention by ablation. (3) There has been increasing interest in the use of so-called upstream therapy in arrhythmia management, particularly AF. Upstream therapy involves the targeting of processes leading to the development of the arrhythmia substrate, with the hope of preventing initial arrhythmia occurrence (primary prevention) or reducing the likelihood of arrhythmia recurrence after initial presentation (secondary prevention). (4) Stroke is recognized as the principal clinically significant complication of AF and the introduction of new antithrombotic agents, so that stroke prevention has become one of the primary considerations in the science of AF management. (5) Important gender differences in cardiac electrophysiology exist. Compared with men, women have higher resting heart rates and longer QT intervals with greater risk of drug-induced torsades de pointes. Women with AF are at a higher risk of stroke, and they are less likely to receive anticoagulation and ablation procedures. Women have a better response to cardiac re-synchronization therapy (CRT) in terms of reduced numbers of hospitalizations and more robust reverse ventricular remodeling. Further studies are required to elucidate the underlying pathophysiologic characteristics of these sex differences in cardiac arrhythmias.[1]

Antiarrhythmic Drugs

Antiarrhythmic drugs are used either to alleviate significant symptoms or to prolong survival. The wisdom of treating arrhythmias "prophylactically" has been severely questioned by a large trial (Cardiac Arrhythmia Suppression Trial)[2] and by a metaanalysis of nearly 100,000 patients with acute myocardial infarction (AMI) treated with antiarrhythmic drugs.[3] These studies stress that arrhythmias should be treated with antiarrhythmic drugs only when their power to prevent hard negative outcomes outweighs the adverse effect potential, which appears to be the case for only a few drugs and indications such as β-blockers following myocardial infarction (MI).[4] Interestingly, evidence for sudden-death prevention in ischemic heart disease and heart failure has been obtained for drugs like aldosterone antagonists, angiotensin-converting enzyme (ACE) inhibitors, angiotensin-receptor blockers, statins, and omega-3 fatty acids,[4] whereas most antiarrhythmic agents have not demonstrated such properties. These observations reinforce the notion that lethal arrhythmias are not simply an "electrical accident" and that effective therapy must target upstream causes.[5] The only antiarrhythmic agent that does appear to prevent sudden cardiac death (SCD) is amiodarone,[6] a drug acting on multiple ionic channels, which is effective against a wide spectrum of arrhythmias. However, even amiodarone is inferior to implantable cardioverter defibrillators (ICDs) for sudden-death prevention in the patients at highest risk.[7]

Classification. There are four established classes of antiarrhythmic action (Table 8-1). The original Vaughan Williams classification with four classes now incorporates ionic mechanisms and receptors as the basis of the more complex Sicilian Gambit system for antiarrhythmic drug classification (Fig. 8-1).[8] Another descriptive division is into those drugs used only in the therapy of supraventricular tachycardias (VTs; Table 8-2) and those used chiefly against VTs (Table 8-3).

Class IA: Quinidine and Similar Compounds

Historically, quinidine was the first antiarrhythmic drug used, and its classification as a class IA agent (the others being disopyramide and procainamide) might suggest excellent effects with superiority to other agents. That is not so, and now that the defects and dangers of quinidine are better understood, it is used less and less. Class IA agents are those that act chiefly by inhibiting the fast sodium channel with depression

Table 8-1

Antiarrhythmic Drug Classes			
Class	**Channel Effects**	**Repolarization Time**	**Drug Examples**
1A	Sodium block Effect + +	Prolongs	Quinidine Disopyramide Procainamide
1B	Sodium block Effect +	Shortens	Lidocaine Phenytoin Mexiletine Tocainide
1C	Sodium block Effect + + +	Unchanged	Flecainide Propafenone
II	I_f, a pacemaker and depolarizing current; indirect Ca^{2+} channel block	Unchanged	β-blockers (excluding sotalol that also has class III effects)
III	Repolarizing K^+ currents	Markedly prolongs	Amiodarone Sotalol Ibutilide Dofetilide
IV	AV nodal Ca^{2+} block	Unchanged	Verapamil Diltiazem
IV-like	K^+ channel opener (hyperpolarization)	Unchanged	Adenosine

AV, Atrioventricular.
    + = inhibitory effect; + + = markedly inhibitory effect; + + + = major inhibitory effect.

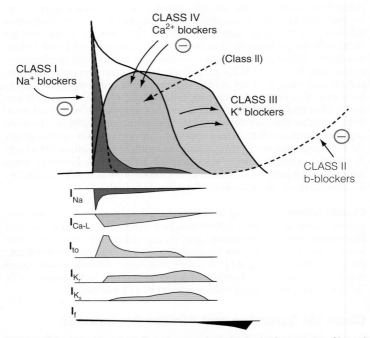

CLASSES OF ANTIARRYTHMIC DRUGS
Opie 2012

Figure 8-1   The classical four types of antiarrhythmic agents. Class I agents decrease phase zero of the rapid depolarization of the action potential (rapid sodium channel). Class II agents, β-blocking drugs, have complex actions including inhibition of spontaneous depolarization (phase 4) and indirect closure of calcium channels, which are less likely to be in the "open" state when not phosphorylated by cyclic adenosine monophosphate. Class III agents block the outward potassium channels to prolong the action potential duration and hence refractoriness. Class IV agents, verapamil and diltiazem, and the indirect calcium antagonist, adenosine, all inhibit the inward calcium channel, which is most prominent in nodal tissue, particularly the atrioventricular node. Most antiarrhythmic drugs have more than one action. In the *lower panel* are shown the major currents on which antiarrhythmics act, according to the Sicilian gambit. *Ca-L,* long-lasting calcium; *I,* current; If, inward funny current; K_r, rapid component of repolarizing potassium current; K_s, slow component; *Na,* sodium; t_o, transient outward. (Figure © L.H. Opie, 2012.)

of phase 0 of the action potential. In addition, they prolong the action potential duration (APD) and thereby have a mild class III action (see Fig. 8-1). Such compounds can cause proarrhythmic complications by prolonging the QT interval in certain genetically predisposed individuals or by depressing conduction and promoting reentry. There are no large-scale outcome trials to suggest that quinidine or other class I agents decrease mortality; rather there is indirect evidence that suggests increased or at best neutral, mortality. For quinidine and procainamide, see Table 8-3.

Class IB: Lidocaine

As a group, class IB agents inhibit the fast sodium current (typical class I effect; see Fig. 8-1) while shortening the APD in nondiseased tissue. The former has the more powerful effect, whereas the latter might actually predispose to arrhythmias, but ensures that QT prolongation does not occur. Class IB agents act selectively on diseased or ischemic tissue, where they are thought to promote conduction block, thereby interrupting

Text continued on p. 280

Table 8-2

Antiarrhythmic Drugs Used Only in Therapy of Supraventricular Arrhythmias

Agent	Dose	Pharmacokinetics and Metabolism	Side Effects and Contraindications	Interactions and Precautions
Adenosine (class IV-like)	For paroxysmal SVT, initial dose 6 mg by rapid IV. If the dose is ineffective within 1 to 2 minutes, 12 mg may be given and if necessary, 12 mg after a further 1 to 2 minutes. A dose of 0.0375 to 0.25 mg/kg body weight is reported to be effective in children.	$T_{1/2}$ = 10-30 seconds. Rapidly taken by active transport system into erythrocytes and vascular endothelial cells (major route of elimination) where it is metabolized to inosine and adenosine monophosphate.	Usually transient and include nausea, light-headedness, headache, flushing, provocation of chest pain, sinus or AV nodal inhibition, bradycardia, and with large dose infusion rare side effects hypotension, tachycardia, bronchospasm. Contraindication in asthmatic, second- or third-degree AV block, sick sinus syndrome.	Caution: In atrial flutter, adenosine may precipitate 1:1 conduction. Dipyridamole inhibits the breakdown of adenosine; therefore dose of adenosine should be reduced. Methylxanthines (caffeine, theophylline) antagonize the interaction of adenosine with its receptors.
Esmolol (class II)	IV 500 mcg/min loading dose over 1 minute before each titration/maintenance step. Use steps of 50, 100, 150, and 200 mcg/min over 4 minutes each, stopping at the desired therapeutic effect.	$T_{1/2}$ = 9 minutes. Following an initial bolus and infusion, onset of action occurs within 2 minutes and a 90% steady-state level is reached within 5 minutes. Following discontinuation full recovery from β-blockade properties occur at 18-30 minutes. Esmolol metabolized in red blood cells without renal or hepatic metabolism.	Hypotension, peripheral ischemia, confusion, thrombophlebitis and skin necrosis from extravasation, bradycardia, bronchospasm. Contraindicated in severe bradycardia heart block (>1 degree) cardiogenic shock, and overt heart failure.	Interactions with warfarin and catecholamine-depleting drugs. Can increase digoxin blood levels and prolong the action of succinylcholine.

Continued

Table 8-2

Antiarrhythmic Drugs Used Only in Therapy of Supraventricular Arrhythmias (Continued)

Agent	Dose	Pharmacokinetics and Metabolism	Side Effects and Contraindications	Interactions and Precautions
Verapamil (class IV)	5-10 mg by slow IV push (over 2-3 minutes), which can be repeated with 10 mg in 10-15 minutes if tolerated. In US a second dose of 10 mg given after 10 minutes if required. Oral dose: 120-480 mg daily in three to four divided doses.	$T_{1/2}$ 2-8 hours after an oral dose or after IV administration. After repeated oral doses this increases to 4.5-12 hours. Verapamil acts within 5 minutes of IV administration and 1-2 hours after oral administration with a peak plasma level after 1-2 hours. Approximately 90% absorbed from the GI tract with intersubject variation and considerable first-pass metabolism in the liver. The bioavailability is only approximately 20%.	Contraindicated in hypotension, cardiogenic shock, marked bradycardia, second or third degree block, WPW syndrome, wide-complex tachycardia, VT and uncompensated heart failure. Also in sick sinus syndrome without a pacemaker.	Decreased serum concentrations of phenobarbital, phenytoin, sulfinpyrazone, and rifampin. Increased serum concentrations of digoxin, quinidine, carbamazepine, and cyclosporin. Increased toxicity with rifampin and cimetidine. Dose reduced if liver function is impaired.
Diltiazem (class IV)	Initial dose 0.25 mg/kg over 2 min, ECG, BP monitoring. Further dose of 0.35 mg/kg after 15 min if required. For AF or flutter, initial infusion of 5-10 mg/h, may increase by 5 mg/h up to 15 mg/h, up to 24 h.	$T_{1/2}$ = 3-5 hours (longer in older adults). After absorption diltiazem extensively metabolized by cytochrome P450 with bioavailability of approximately 40% with considerable interindividual variation. 80% bound to plasma protein. No effect of renal or hepatic dysfunction on plasma concentration of diltiazem.	AV block, bradycardia, and rarely asystole or sinus arrest. C/I in sick sinus syndrome, preexisting second or third degree heart block, wide QRS tachycardia, marked bradycardia, or LV failure.	Risk of bradycardia, AV block with amiodarone, β-blockers, digoxin and mefloquine. Blood diltiazem may ↑ with cimetidine and ↓ with inducers: barbiturates, phenytoin, and rifampin. Reduce doses of carbamazepine, cyclosporine. Digoxin level variable, may ↑, watch AV node.

	Dose	Pharmacokinetics	Side effects / Contraindications	Interactions
Ibutilide (class III)	IV infusion: 1 mg over 10 min, (under 60 kg: 0.1 mg/kg). If needed, repeat after 10 min.	Initial distribution $T_{\frac{1}{2}}$ is 1.5 minutes. Elimination $T_{\frac{1}{2}}$ averages 6 h (range 2-12 h). Efficacy is usually within 40 min.	Nausea, headache, hypotension, bundle branch block, AV nodal block, bradycardia, torsades de pointes, sustained monomorphic VT, tachycardia, ventricular extrasystoles. Avoid concurrent therapy with class I or III agents. Care with amiodarone or sotalol. C/I: previous torsades de pointes, decompensated heart failure.	Interactions with Class IA and other Class III antiarrhythmic drugs that prolong the QT interval (e.g., antipsychotics, antidepressants, macrolide antibiotics, and some antihistamines). Check QT (see Fig. 8-4). Correct hypokalemia and hypomagnesemia.
Dofetilide (class III)	Dose 250 mcg twice daily, maximum 500 mcg twice daily if normal renal and cardiac function. If LV dysfunction, 250 mcg twice daily. Check QT 2-3 h after dose, if QTc is >15% or >500 msec, reduce dose. If QTc >500 msec, stop.	Oral peak plasma concentration in 2.5 hours and a steady state within 48 h. 50% excreted by kidneys unchanged.	Torsades de pointes in 3% of patients which can be reduced by ensuring normal serum K, avoiding dofetilide or reducing the dose if abnormal renal function, bradycardia, or base-line QT↑. Avoid with other drugs increasing QT. C/I: previous torsades, creatinine clearance <20 mL/min.	Increased blood levels with ketoconazole, verapamil, cimetidine, or inhibitors of cytochrome CYP3 A4, including macrolide antibiotics, protease inhibitors such as ritonavir. Other precautions as previously.

AF, Atrial fibrillation; AV, atrioventricular; BP, blood pressure; C/I, contraindication; ECG, electrocardiogram; GI, gastrointestinal; IV, intravenous; LV, left ventricular; SVT, supraventricular tachycardia; $T_{\frac{1}{2}}$, plasma half-life; VT, ventricular tachycardia; WPW, Wolff-Parkinson-White.

Table 8-3

Antiarrhythmic Drugs Used in Therapy of Ventricular Arrhythmias

Agent	Dose	Pharmacokinetics and Metabolism	Side Effects and Contraindications	Interactions and Precautions
Lidocaine (class 1B)	IV 75-200 mg; then 2-4 mg/min for 24-30 h. (No oral use)	Effect of single bolus lasts only few min, then $T_{1/2}$ approximately 2 h. Rapid hepatic metabolism. Level 1.4-5 mcg/mL; toxic > 9 mcg/mL.	Reduce dose by half if liver blood flow low (shock, β-blockade, cirrhosis, cimetidine, severe heart failure). High-dose CNS effects.	β-blockers decrease hepatic blood flow and increase blood levels. Cimetidine (decreased hepatic metabolism of lidocaine).
Mexiletine (class IB)	*IV 100-250 mg at 12.5 mg/min, then 2 mg/kg/h for 3.5 h, then 0.5 mg/kg/h. Oral 100-400 mg 8-hourly; loading dose 400 mg.	$T_{1/2}$ 10-17 h. Level 1-2 mcg/mL. Hepatic metabolism, inactive metabolites.	CNS, GI side effects. Bradycardia. hypotension especially during co-therapy.	Enzyme inducers; disopyramide and β-blockade; increases the theophylline levels.
Phenytoin (class IB)	IV 10-15 mg/kg over 1 h. Oral 1 g; 500 mg for 2 days; then 400-600 mg daily.	$T_{1/2}$ 24 h. Level 10-18 mcg/mL. Hepatic metabolism. Hepatic or renal disease requires reduced doses.	Hypotension, vertigo, dysarthria, lethargy, gingivitis, macrocytic anemia, lupus, pulmonary infiltrates.	Hepatic enzyme inducers.
Flecainide (class IC)	*IV 1-2 mg/kg over 10 min, then 0.15-0.25 mg/kg/h. Oral 100-400 mg 2 times daily. Hospitalize.	$T_{1/2}$ 13-19 h. Hepatic ⅔; ⅓ renal excretion unchanged. Keep trough level below 1 mcg/mL.	QRS prolongation. Proarrhythmia. Depressed LV function. CNS side effects. Increased incidence of death postinfarct.	Many, especially added inhibition of conduction and nodal tissue.
Propafenone (class IC)	*IV 2 mg/kg then 2 mg/min. Oral 150-300 mg 3 times daily.	$T_{1/2}$ variable 2-10 h, up to 32 h in nonmetabolizers. Level 0.2-3 mcg/mL. Variable hepatic metabolism (P-450 deficiency slows).	QRS prolongation. Modest negative inotropic effect. GI side effects. Proarrhythmia.	Digoxin level increased. Hepatic inducers.

Sotalol (class III)	160-640 mg daily, occasionally higher in two divided doses.	$T_{1/2}$ 12 h. Not metabolized. Hydrophilic. Renal loss.	Myocardial depression, sinus bradycardia, AV block. Torsades if hypokalemic.	Added risk of torsades with IA agents or diuretics. Decrease dose in renal failure.
Amiodarone (class III)	Oral loading dose 1200-1600 mg daily; maintenance 200-400 mg daily, sometimes less. IV 150 mg over 10 min, then 360 mg over 6 h, then 540 mg over remaining 24 h, then 0.5 mg/min.	$T_{1/2}$ 25-110 days. Level 1-2.5 mcg/mL. Hepatic metabolism. Lipid soluble with extensive distribution in body. Excretion by skin, biliary tract, lachrymal glands.	Complex dose-dependent side effects including pulmonary fibrosis. QT prolongation. Torsades uncommon.	Class IA agents predispose to torsades. β-blockers predispose to nodal depression, yet give better therapeutic effects.

AV, Atrioventricular; *CNS*, central nervous system; *GI*, gastrointestinal; *IV*, intravenous; *LV*, left ventricular; $T_{1/2}$, plasma half-life.

*Not licensed for intravenous use in the United States.

Class IA agents (Table 8-1) are no longer recommended, and tocainide, mexiletine, and bretylium are rarely used. These agents were considered in the previous editions of this book.

Enzyme hepatic inducers are barbiturates, phenytoin, and rifampin, which induce hepatic enzymes, thereby decreasing blood levels of the drug.

reentry circuits. They have a particular affinity for binding with inactivated sodium channels with rapid onset-offset kinetics, which may be why such drugs are ineffective in atrial arrhythmias, because the APD is so short. For mexiletene, see Table 8-3.

Lidocaine

Lidocaine (Xylocaine, Xylocard) has become a standard intravenous agent for suppression of serious ventricular arrhythmias associated with AMI and with cardiac surgery. The concept of prophylactic lidocaine to prevent VT and ventricular fibrillation (VF) in AMI is now outmoded.[9,10] This intravenous drug has no role in the control of chronic recurrent ventricular arrhythmias. Lidocaine acts preferentially on the ischemic myocardium and is more effective in the presence of a high external potassium concentration. Therefore hypokalemia must be corrected for maximum efficacy (also for other class I agents). Lidocaine has no value in treating supraventricular tachyarrhythmias.

Pharmacokinetics. The bulk of an intravenous dose of lidocaine is rapidly deethylated by liver microsomes (see Table 8-3). The two critical factors governing lidocaine metabolism and hence its efficacy are liver blood flow (decreased in old age and by heart failure, β-blockade, and cimetidine) and liver microsomal activity (enzyme inducers). Because lidocaine is so rapidly distributed within minutes after an initial intravenous loading dose, there must be a subsequent infusion or repetitive doses to maintain therapeutic blood levels (Fig. 8-2). Lidocaine metabolites circulate in high concentrations and may contribute to toxic and therapeutic actions. After prolonged infusions, the half-life may be

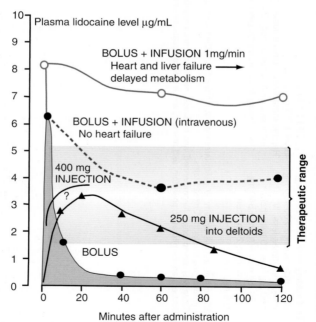

LIDOCAINE KINETICS
Opie 2012

Figure 8-2 Lidocaine kinetics. To achieve and to maintain an adequate blood level of lidocaine requires an initial bolus followed by an infusion. For an intramuscular injection to give sustained high blood levels may require a dose of 400 mg. Note that in the presence of cardiac or liver failure, delayed metabolism increases the blood level with danger of toxic effects. (Figure © L.H. Opie, 2012.)

longer (up to 24 hours) because of redistribution from poorly perfused tissues.

Dose. A constant infusion would take 5 to 9 hours to achieve therapeutic levels (1.4 to 5 mcg/mL), so standard therapy includes a loading dose of 75 to 100 mg intravenously, followed after 30 minutes by a second loading dose, or 400 mg intramuscularly. Thereafter lidocaine is infused at 2 to 4 mg/minute for 24 to 30 hours, aiming at 3 mg/minute, which prevents VF but may cause serious side effects in approximately 15% of patients, in half of whom the lidocaine dose may have to be reduced. Poor liver blood flow (low cardiac output or β-blockade), liver disease, or cimetidine or halothane therapy calls for halved dosage. The dose should also be decreased for older adult patients in whom toxicity develops more frequently and after 12 to 24 hours of infusion.

Clinical use. *Should lidocaine be administered routinely to all patients with AMI?* The question has been asked for at least 25 years. Today the answer is no. Evidence from more than 20 randomized trials and 4 metaanalyses have shown that lidocaine reduces VF but adversely affects mortality rates, presumably because of bradyarrhythmias and asystole.[10,11] *When can it be used?* Lidocaine can be used when tachyarrhythmias or very frequent premature ventricular contractions seriously interfere with hemodynamic status in patients with AMI (especially when already β-blocked) and during cardiac surgery or general anesthesia. *When should lidocaine not be used?* Lidocaine should not be used prophylactically or when there is bradycardia or bradycardia plus ventricular tachyarrhythmias, when atropine (or pacing) and not lidocaine is required.

Side effects. Lidocaine is generally free of hemodynamic side effects, even in patients with congestive heart failure (CHF), and it seldom impairs nodal function or conduction (Table 8-4). The higher infusion rate of 3 to 4 mg/minute may result in drowsiness, numbness, speech disturbances, and dizziness, especially in patients older than 60 years of age. Minor adverse neural reactions can occur in approximately half the patients, even with 2 to 3 mg/minute of lidocaine. Occasionally there is sinoatrial (SA) arrest, especially during co-administration of other drugs that potentially depress nodal function.

Drug interactions and combination. In patients receiving cimetidine, propranolol, or halothane, the hepatic clearance of lidocaine is reduced and toxicity may occur more readily, so that the dose should be reduced. With hepatic enzyme inducers (barbiturates, phenytoin, and rifampin) the dose needs to be increased. Combination of lidocaine with early β-blockade is not a contraindication, although there is no reported experience. The obvious precaution is that bradyarrhythmias may become more common because β-blockade reduces liver blood flow. Hence a standard dose of lidocaine would have potentially more side effects, including sinus node inhibition.

Lidocaine failure in AMI-related VT and VF. If lidocaine apparently fails, is there hypokalemia, severe ongoing ischemia, or other reversible underlying factor? Are there technical errors in drug administration? Is the drug really called for or should another class of agent (e.g., β-blockade, class III agent like intravenous amiodarone) be used? In a retrospective analysis of AMI patients, 6% developed sustained VT and VF, and of those who survived 3 hours, amiodarone, but not lidocaine, was associated with an increased risk of death.[12] However, it remains unclear whether the worse outcome of amiodarone-treated patients was due to an effect of the drug or to selection of sicker patients to receive amiodarone, reinforcing the need for randomized trials in this population.

Table 8-4

Effects and Side Effects of Some Ventricular Antiarrhythmic Agents on Electrophysiology and Hemodynamics

Agent	Sinus Node	Sinus Rate	A-His	PR	AV Block	H-P	WPW	QRS	QT	Serious Hemodynamic Effects	Risk of Torsades	Risk of Monomorphic VT
Lidocaine	0	0	0/↓	0	0	0	↓/0	0	0	Toxic doses	0	0
Phenytoin	0	0	↑/0	0	Lessens	0	→/0	0	↓	IV hypotension	0, +	0, +
Flecainide	0/↓	0	↓↓↓	↑	Avoid	↓↓	↓A/R	↑	↑ (via QRS)	LV ↓↓	0	+++
Propafenone	0/↓	0	↓↓↓	↑	Avoid	↓↓	↓A/R	↑	0	LV →	0	+++
Sotalol	↓↓	↓↓	→	↑	Avoid	0	A/R	0	↑↑↑↑	IV use	+	0, +
Amiodarone	→	→	→	0/→	Avoid	0/↓	A/R	0	↑↑	IV use	+/−	0, +

A, antegrade; A-His, Atria-His conduction; AV, atrioventricular; H-P, His-Purkinje conduction; IV, intravenous; LV, left ventricular; PR, PR interval; R, retrograde; VT, ventricular tachycardia; WPW, Wolff-Parkinson-White syndrome accessory pathways.

Conclusions. Lidocaine remains a reasonable initial therapy for treatment of sustained VT, predominantly because of ease of use and a low incidence of hemodynamic side effects and drug interactions. However, the efficacy of lidocaine is relatively low (15% to 20%) compared with other class I antiarrhythmic drugs (procainamide—approximately 80%). Thus the use of lidocaine allows about one fifth of monomorphic VTs to be terminated and suppressed with virtually no risk of side effects.

Phenytoin (Diphenylhydantoin)

Phenytoin (Dilantin, Epanutin) is now much less used. It may be effective against the ventricular arrhythmias occurring after congenital heart surgery. Occasionally in patients with epilepsy and arrhythmias a dual antiarrhythmic and antiepileptic action comes to the fore.

Class IC Agents

Class IC agents have acquired a particularly bad reputation as a result of the proarrhythmic effects seen in the Cardiac Arrhythmia Suppression Trial (CAST)[2] (flecainide) and the Cardiac Arrest Study Hamburg (CASH) study[13] (propafenone). Nonetheless, when carefully chosen they fulfill a niche not provided by other drugs. As a group they have three major electrophysiologic (EP) effects. First, they are powerful inhibitors of the fast sodium channel, causing a marked depression of the upstroke of the cardiac action potential, which may explain their marked inhibitory effect on His-Purkinje conduction with QRS widening. In addition they may variably prolong the APD by delaying inactivation of the slow sodium channel[14] and inhibition of the rapid repolarizing current (I_{Kr}).[15] Class IC agents are all potent antiarrhythmics used largely in the control of paroxysmal supraventricular tachyarrhythmias, especially AF and VAs resistant to other drugs. They are effective in the unusual condition of catecholaminergic polymorphic VT.[16] Their markedly depressant effect on conduction, together with prolongation of the APD, may explain the development of electrical heterogeneity and proarrhythmias. In addition, faster heart rates, increased sympathetic activity, and diseased or ischemic myocardium all contribute to the proarrhythmic effects.[17] These drugs must therefore be avoided in patients with structural heart disease (Fig. 8-3). In others, they are widely used to prevent recurrences of AF. Here the evidence is strong for propafenone and moderate for flecainide.[18]

Flecainide

Flecainide (Tambocor) is effective for the treatment of both supraventricular and ventricular arrhythmias. Its associated proarrhythmic potential limits its use, especially in the presence of structural heart disease. The drug should be started under careful observation, using a gradually increasing low oral dose with regular electrocardiograms (ECGs) to assess QRS complex duration and occasionally serum levels. Once steady-state treatment has been reached (usually five times the half-life of the drug), it is advisable to perform a 24-hour Holter analysis or a symptom-limited exercise stress test to detect potential arrhythmias.[19] For pharmacokinetics, side effects, and drug interactions see Tables 8-3 to 8-5.

Indications. Indications are (1) paroxysmal supraventricular tachycardia (PSVT) including paroxysmal atrial flutter or fibrillation and Wolff-Parkinson-White (WPW) arrhythmias, and always only in patients without structural heart disease; (2) life-threatening sustained VT in which benefit outweighs proarrhythmic risks; and (3) catecholaminergic polymorphic VT, by blocking open RyR2 channels.[16] For maintenance of sinus rhythm after cardioversion of AF, it is moderately successful.[18]

RECURRENT/PERSISTENT A FIB

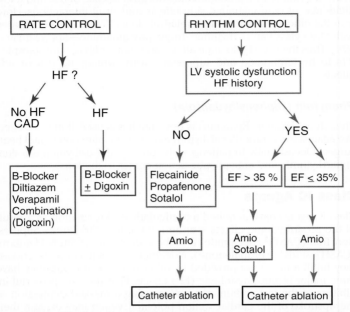

Figure 8-3 **Algorithm for drug therapy for rate control or rhythm control.** Modified from recommendations of Canadian Cardiovascular Society, with dronaderone removed in view of recent European Medicines Agency warnings about the safety of this drug and their recommendation to use it only to maintain sinus rhythm in selected patients with persistent or paroxysmal atrial fibrillation after successful restoration of sinus rhythm. *A fib,* Atrial fibrillation; *Amio,* amiodarone; *CAD,* coronary artery disease; *EF,* ejection fraction; *HF,* heart failure; *LV,* left ventricular. (Modified from Skanes AC, et al. Focused 2012 update of the Canadian Cardiovascular Society atrial fibrillation guidelines: recommendations for stroke prevention and rate/rhythm control. *Can J Cardiol* 2012;28:125–136.)

Flecainide is *contraindicated* in patients with structural heart disease and in patients with right bundle branch block and left anterior hemiblock unless a pacemaker is implanted (package insert). It is also contraindicated in the sick sinus syndrome, when the left ventricle is depressed, and in the postinfarct state. There is a boxed warning in the package insert against use in chronic sustained AF.

Cardiac proarrhythmic effects. The cardiac proarrhythmic effects of flecainide include aggravation of ventricular arrhythmias and threat of sudden death as in the CAST study.[2] The proarrhythmic effect is related to nonuniform slowing of conduction and the risk is greatest in patients with prior MI, especially those with significant ventricular ectopy. Patients at risk of AMI are probably also at increased risk. Monitoring the QRS interval is logical but "safe limits" are not established. Furthermore, as shown in the CAST study,[2] late proarrhythmic effects can occur. In patients with preexisting sinus node or atrioventricular (AV) conduction problems, there may be worsening of arrhythmia. Flecainide increases the endocardial pacing threshold. Atrial proarrhythmic effects are of two varieties. As the atrial rate falls the ventricular rate might rise. Second, VAs may be precipitated.

Propafenone

Propafenone (Rythmol in the United States, Arythmol in the United Kingdom, Rytmonorm in the rest of Europe) has a spectrum of activity

Table 8-5

Interactions (Kinetic and Dynamic) of Antiarrhythmic Drugs

Drug	Interaction With	Result
Lidocaine	β-blockers, cimetidine, halothane, enzyme inducers	Reduced liver blood flow (increased blood levels) Decreased blood levels
Flecainide	Major kinetic interaction with amiodarone	Increase of blood F levels; half-dose
	Added negative inotropic effects (β-blockers, quinidine, disopyramide)	As previously Conduction block
	Added AV conduction depression (quinidine, procainamide)	
Propafenone	As for flecainide (but amiodarone interaction not reported); digoxin; warfarin	Enhanced SA, AV, and myocardial depression; digoxin level increased; anticoagulant effect enhanced
Sotalol	Diuretics, Class IA agents, amiodarone, tricyclics, phenothiazines (see Fig. 8-4)	Risk of torsades; avoid hypokalemia
Amiodarone	As for sotalol	Risk of torsades
	digoxin	Increased digoxin levels
	phenytoin	Double interaction, see text
	flecainide	Increased flecainide levels
	warfarin	Increased warfarin effect
Ibutilide	All agents increasing QT	Risk of torsades
Dofetilide	All agents increasing QT	Risk of torsades
	Liver interactions with verapamil, cimetidine, ketoconazole, trimethoprim	Increased dofetilide blood level, more risk of torsades
Verapamil Diltiazem	β-blockers, excess digoxin, myocardial depressants, quinidine	Increased myocardial or nodal depression
Adenosine	Dipyridamole	Adenosine catabolism inhibited; much increased half-life; reduce A dose
	Methylxanthines (caffeine, theophylline)	Inhibit receptor; decreased drug effects

AV, Atrioventricular; *IV,* intravenous; *SA,* sinoatrial.

Enzyme inducers = hepatic enzyme inducers (i.e. barbiturates, phenytoin, rifampin).

For references, see Table 8-4 in 5th edition.

and some side effects that resemble those of other class IC agents, including the proarrhythmic effect. In the CASH study, propafenone was withdrawn from one arm because of increased total mortality and cardiac arrest recurrence.[13] Propafenone is regarded as relatively safe in suppressing supraventricular arrhythmias including those of the WPW syndrome and recurrent AF,[20] always bearing in mind the need to first eliminate structural heart disease.

Pharmacologic characteristics. In keeping with its class IC effects, propafenone blocks the fast inward sodium channel, has a potent membrane stabilizing activity, and increases PR and QRS intervals without effect on the QT interval. It also has mild β-blocking and calcium (L-type channel) antagonist properties. For pharmacokinetics, side effects, drug interactions, and combinations, see Tables 8-3 to 8-5. Note that in 7% of white patients, the hepatic cytochrome isoenzyme, P-450 2D6, is genetically absent, so that propafenone breakdown is much slower.

Dose. Dose is 150 to 300 mg three times daily, up to a total of 1200 mg daily, with some patients needing four daily doses and some only two. The UK trial[20] compared 300 mg twice with three times daily; the latter was both more effective and gave more adverse effects. Marked interindividual variations in its metabolism mean that the dose must be individualized.

Indications for Propafenone. In the United States (only oral form), indications are (1) life-threatening ventricular arrhythmias, and (2) suppression of supraventricular arrhythmias, including those of WPW syndrome and recurrent atrial flutter or fibrillation.[9,10] These must be in the absence of structural heart disease (risk of proarrhythymia). There is strong evidence in favor of propafenone in acute conversion of AF and for maintenance of sinus rhythm.[18] *Intravenous propafenone* (not licensed in the United Kingdom or the United States) followed by oral propafenone, is as effective as amiodarone in the conversion of chronic AF.[21] Intravenous propafenone is also effective in catecholaminergic polymorphic VT.[16] *Propafenone "on-demand,"* also called the "pill in the pocket," may be tried for paroxysmal AF although it is not licensed for this purpose, after a trial under strict observation. Oral propafenone, 500 mg, for recent-onset AF was more effective than placebo for conversion to sinus rhythm within 8 hours and had a favorable safety profile. The rate of spontaneous conversion to sinus rhythm was higher in patients without structural heart disease.[22] *Relative contraindications* include preexisting sinus, AV or bundle branch abnormalities, or depressed left ventricular (LV) function. Patients with asthma and bronchospastic disease including chronic bronchitis should not, in general, be given propafenone (package insert). Propafenone has mild β-blocking properties, especially when the dose exceeds 450 mg daily. It is estimated that the β-blockade effect is approximately $\frac{1}{40}$ that of propranolol.[23]

Class II Agents: β-Adrenoceptor Antagonists

Whereas class I agents are increasingly suspect from the long-term point of view, β-blockers have an excellent record in reducing post-MI mortality.[3,24] These agents act on (1) the current I_f, now recognized as an important pacemaker current (Fig. 8-4) that also promotes proarrhythmic depolarization in damaged heart tissue; and (2) the inward calcium current, I_{Ca-L}, which is indirectly inhibited as the level of tissue cyclic adenosine monophosphate (cAMP) falls. The general arguments for β-blockade include (1) the role of tachycardia in precipitating some arrhythmias, especially those based on triggered activity; (2) the increased sympathetic activity in patients with sustained VT and in

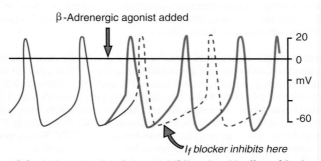

BETA & I_f EFFECTS ON SA NODE

Opie 2012

β-Adrenergic agonist added

20

0

mV

-60

I_f blocker inhibits here

Figure 8-4   Action potential of sinoatrial (SA) node, with effect of β-adrenergic stimulation and of inhibition of current I_f, relevant to recent development of a specific I_f blocker. (Figure © L.H. Opie, 2012.)

patients with AMI; (3) the fundamental role of the second messenger of β-adrenergic activity, cyclic AMP, in the causation of ischemia-related VF; and (4) the associated antihypertensive and antiischemic effects of these drugs. The mechanism of benefit of β-blockade in postinfarct patients is uncertain, but is likely to be multifactorial and probably antiarrhythmic in part.[24]

Indications. Antiarrhythmic therapy by β-blockade is indicated for the following: It is used especially for inappropriate or unwanted sinus tachycardia, for paroxysmal atrial tachycardia provoked by emotion or exercise, for exercise-induced ventricular arrhythmias, in the arrhythmias of pheochromocytoma (combined with α-blockade to avoid hypertensive crises), in the hereditary prolonged QT syndrome, in heart failure,[25] and sometimes in the arrhythmias of mitral valve prolapse. A common denominator to most of these indications is increased sympathetic β-adrenergic activity. In patients with stable controlled heart failure, β-blockers reduce all-cause, cardiovascular, and sudden death mortality rates.[25-27] β-blockers are also effective as monotherapy in severe recurrent VT not obviously ischemic in origin, and empirical β-blocker therapy seems as good as EP guided therapy with class I or class III agents. β-blocker therapy improved survival in patients with VF or symptomatic VT not treated by specific antiarrhythmics in the AVID trial.[28] β-blockers in combination with amiodarone have a synergistic effect to significantly reduce cardiac mortality.[29] β-blockers with amiodarone may be effective in treating episodes of "electrical storm."[30]

Which β-Blocker for Arrhythmias? The antiarrhythmic activity of the various β-blockers is reasonably uniform, the critical property being that of β1-adrenergic blockade,[25] without any major role for associated properties such as membrane depression (local anesthetic action), cardioselectivity, and intrinsic sympathomimetic activity (see Figs. 1-9 and 1-10). These additional properties have no major influence on the antiarrhythmic potency. *Esmolol*, a selective β1 antagonist, has a half-life of 9 minutes with full recovery from its β-blockade properties at 18 to 30 minutes.[31] Esmolol is quickly metabolized in red blood cells, independently of renal and hepatic function. Because of its short half-life, esmolol can be useful in situations in which there are relative contraindications or concerns about the use of a β-blocker. For instance, in a patient with a supraventricular tachycardia, fast AF, or atrial flutter and associated chronic obstructive airway disease or moderate LV dysfunction, esmolol would be advantageous as a therapeutic intervention.

In the United States, the β-blockers licensed for antiarrhythmic activity include propranolol, sotalol, and acebutolol. The latter is attractive because of its cardioselectivity, its favorable or neutral effect on the blood lipid profile (see Table 10-5), and its specific benefit in one large postinfarct survival trial. However, the potential capacity of acebutolol to suppress serious VAs has never been shown in a large trial. Metoprolol 25 to 100 mg twice daily, not licensed for this purpose in the United States, was the agent chosen when empirical β-blockade was compared with EP guided antiarrhythmic therapy for the treatment of ventricular tachyarrhythmias. Both sotalol (class II and III activities) and metoprolol (class II) reduce the recurrence of ventricular tachyarrhythmias and inappropriate discharges following ICD implantation.[32,33] In the CASH study, amiodarone was compared with metoprolol, propafenone, and ICDs.[13] ICDs were best. The propafenone arm was stopped prematurely because of excess mortality compared with other therapies, whereas patients on metoprolol had a survival equivalent to that of those treated with amiodarone.

Drawbacks to β-blockade antiarrhythmic therapy. There continue to be many patients with absolute or relative contraindications including pulmonary problems, conduction defects, or overt untreated severe heart failure. A large metaanalysis[34] showed that a mortality reduction of up to 40% could still be achieved despite such relative contraindications. It is important to recognize that mild to moderate LV dysfunction, already treated by ACE inhibitors and diuretics, is no longer an absolute contraindication, but rather a strong indication for β-blockers, especially if there is symptomatic heart failure (class II and III). Another drawback is that the efficacy of β-blockers against symptomatic ventricular arrhythmias is less certain. *At present, β-blockers are the closest to an ideal class of antiarrhythmic agents for general use because of their broad spectrum of activity and established safety record.* Furthermore, the use of β-blockers in combination with other antiarrhythmic agents may have a synergistic role and can reduce the proarrhythmic effects seen with some of these agents. On the other hand, β-blockers are relatively ineffective for such indications as preventing AF recurrence, promoting sinus-rhythm maintenance in AF patients, and acute termination of most sustained tachyarrhythmias.

Mixed Class III Agents: Amiodarone and Sotalol

As the evidence for increased mortality in several patient groups with class I agents mounted, attention shifted to class III agents. Two widely used agents with important class III properties, as well as actions of other drug classes, are amiodarone and sotalol. In the ESVEM trial[35] sotalol was better than six class I antiarrhythmic agents (Table 8-6).[36-43] Amiodarone, in contrast to class I agents, exerts a favorable effect on a variety of serious arrhythmias.[44] Both amiodarone and sotalol are mixed, not pure, class III agents, a quality that may be of crucial importance.

The *intrinsic problem* with class III agents is that these compounds act by lengthening the APD and hence the effective refractory period, and must inevitably prolong the QT interval to be effective. In the presence of hypokalemia, hypomagnesemia, bradycardia, or genetic predisposition, QT prolongation may predispose to torsades de pointes. This may especially occur with agents such as sotalol that simultaneously cause bradycardia and prolong the APD. By acting only on the repolarization phase of the action potential, class III agents should leave conduction unchanged. However, amiodarone and sotalol have additional properties that modify conduction—amiodarone being a significant sodium and calcium channel inhibitor and sotalol a β-blocker. Amiodarone makes the action potential pattern more uniform throughout the myocardium, thereby opposing EP heterogeneity that underlies some serious ventricular arrhythmias. The efficacy of amiodarone exceeds that of other antiarrhythmic compounds including sotalol. Furthermore, the incidence of torsades with amiodarone is much lower than expected from its class III effects. Yet amiodarone has a host of potentially serious extracardiac side effects that sotalol does not.

Amiodarone

Amiodarone (Cordarone) is a unique "wide-spectrum" antiarrhythmic agent, chiefly class III but also with powerful class I activity and ancillary class II and class IV activity. Thus it blocks sodium, calcium, and repolarizing potassium channels. In general, the status of this drug has changed from that of a "last-ditch" agent to one that is increasingly used (1) when life-threatening arrhythmias are being treated, and (2) in low doses for AF (Fig. 8-5). Its established antiarrhythmic benefits and potential for *mortality reduction*[45] need to be balanced against several considerations: First, the slow onset of action of oral therapy may require large intravenous or oral loading doses to achieve effects rapidly. Second, the many serious side effects, especially pulmonary

Table 8-6

Key Trials with Antiarrythmics or Devices for Ventricular Arrhythmias

Drug Class or Device	Acronym	Hypothesis	Key Results
Class IC	CAST—Cardiac Arrhythmia Suppression Trial[2]	PVC suppression gives benefit.	Mortality doubled in treatment group.
Class II	Steinbeck[36]	EPS guided versus empiric β-blockade with metoprolol.	Equal benefits; EPS not needed.
Class II, III (Sotalol)	ESVEM—Electrophysiological Study Versus ECG Monitoring, 1993[37]	Which drug class is better? Which selection method is better?	Sotalol better than 6 Class I agents; Holter = EPS.
Class III	EMIAT—European Myocardial Infarct Amiodarone Trial, 1997[38]	Amiodarone can reduce sudden death in post-MI with low ejection fraction.	Arrhythmia deaths decreased, total deaths unchanged.
Class III	CAMIAT—Canadian Acute Myocardial Infarction Amiodarone Trial[39]	Post-AMI with frequent VPS or nonsustained VT—? Reduced mortality.	Sudden death and mortality reduced.
ICD	MADIT—Multicenter Automatic Defibrillator Implantation Trial[40]	ICD in high-risk patients (coronary artery disease + NSVT on EPS) would improve beyond drugs.	Mortality reduced by half, trial stopped.
ICD	AVID—Antiarrhythmic Versus Implantable Defibrillators[41]	Resuscitated VF or VT (with low ejection fraction) better on ICD	26%-31% mortality reduction with ICD; trial terminated.
ICD	MUSTT—Multicenter Unsustained Tachycardia Trial[42]	EPS-guided therapy can reduce death in survivors of AMI.	Cardiac arrest or death from arrhythmia reduced by 27% in ICD group.
ICD	CIDS—Canadian Implantable Defibrillator Study[7]	VF, cardiac arrest, or sustained VT; all-cause deaths, ICD vs. amiodarone.	ICD better than amiodarone only in highest-risk patients; 50% less risk with ICD.
ICD	MADIT-2[43]	Post-MI, LV ejection fraction ≤30%.	All-cause mortality reduced by 31% by ICD.
ICD	SCD-HeFT—Sudden Cardiac Death—Heart Failure	Dilated cardiomyopathy, Class II or III symptoms ejection fraction ≤35%.	All-cause mortality reduced 23% by ICD; amiodarone no benefit.

AMI, Acute myocardial infarction; *ECG,* electrocardiogram; *EPS,* electrophysiologic stimulation; *ICD,* implanted cardioverter defibrillator; *LV,* left ventricular; *MI,* myocardial infarction; *NSVT,* nonsustained ventricular tachycardia; *PVC,* premature ventricular complex; *VF,* ventricular fibrillation; *VPS,* ventricular premature systoles; *VT,* ventricular tachycardia.

infiltrates and thyroid problems (Fig. 8-5), dictate that there must be a fine balance between the maximum antiarrhythmic effect of the drug and the potential for side effects. Third, the half-life is extremely long. Fourth, there are a large number of potentially serious drug interactions, some of which predispose to torsades de pointes, which is nonetheless

AMIODARONE FOR ATRIAL FIBRILLATION

Opie 2012

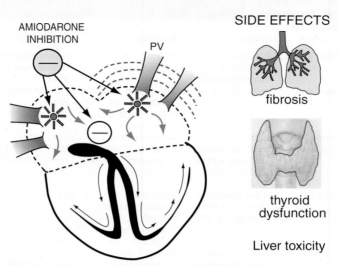

Figure 8-5 Amiodarone inhibition of atrial fibrillation. Benefits must be balanced against risks of pulmonary fibrosis, thyroid dysfunction, and other side effects. *PV,* pulmonary vein. (Figure © L.H. Opie, 2012.)

rare when amiodarone is used as a single agent. For recurrent AF, amiodarone may be strikingly effective with little risk of side effects.[46,47] Otherwise the use of amiodarone in as low a dose as possible should be restricted to selected patients with refractory ventricular arrhythmias in which an ICD is not appropriate (see later, section on ICDs, page 320, section on Secondary Prevention).

Electrophysiologic characteristics. Amiodarone is a complex antiarrhythmic agent, predominantly class III, that shares at least some of the properties of each of the other three EP classes of antiarrhythmics. The class III activity means that amiodarone lengthens the effective refractory period by prolonging the APD in all cardiac tissues, including bypass tracts. It also has a powerful class I antiarrhythmic effect inhibiting inactivated sodium channels at high stimulation frequencies. Its benefits in AF may be explained at least in part by prolongation of the refractory periods of both the left and right superior pulmonary veins,[48] and inhibition of the AV node (see Fig. 8-5). Furthermore, it is "uniquely effective" against AF in experimental atrial remodeling.[49] Amiodarone noncompetitively blocks α- and β-adrenergic receptors (class II effect), and this effect is additive to competitive receptor inhibition by β-blockers.[45] The weak calcium antagonist (class IV) effect might explain bradycardia and AV nodal inhibition and the relatively low incidence of torsades de pointes. Furthermore, there are relatively weak coronary and peripheral vasodilator actions.

Pharmacokinetics. The pharmacokinetics of this highly lipid soluble drug differ markedly from other cardiovascular agents.[45] After variable (30% to 50%) and slow gastrointestinal (GI) absorption, amiodarone distributes slowly but very extensive into adipose tissues.[50] Because of this, amiodarone must fill an enormous peripheral-tissue depot to achieve adequate blood and cardiac concentrations, accounting for its slow onset of action. In addition, when oral administration is stopped, most of the drug is in peripheral stores unavailable to elimination systems, causing very slow elimination with a very long half-life, up to 6 months.[51] The onset of action after oral administration is delayed and a steady-state drug effect (*amiodaronization*) may not be established for several months unless large loading doses are used. Even when given intravenously, its full EP effect is delayed,[52] although major benefit can be achieved within minutes as shown by its effect on shock-resistant VF.[53] Amiodarone is lipid soluble, extensively distributed in the body and highly concentrated in many tissues, especially in the liver and lungs. It undergoes extensive hepatic metabolism to the pharmacologically active metabolite, desethylamiodarone. A correlation between the clinical effects and serum concentrations of the drug or its metabolite has not been clearly shown, although there is a direct relation between the oral dose and the plasma concentration, and between metabolite concentration and some late effects, such as that on the ventricular functional refractory period. The therapeutic range is not well defined, but may be between 1 and 2.5 mg/mL, almost all of which (95%) is protein bound. Higher levels are associated with increased toxicity.[45] Amiodarone is not excreted by the kidneys, but rather by the lachrymal glands, the skin, and the biliary tract.

Dose. When reasonably rapid control of an urgent arrhythmia is needed, the initial loading regimen is up to 1600 mg daily in two to four divided doses usually given for 7 to 14 days, which is then reduced to 400 to 800 mg/day for a further 1 to 3 weeks. By using a loading dose, sustained VT can be controlled after a mean interval of 5 days. Practice varies widely however, with loading doses of as low as 600 mg daily being used in less urgent settings. Maintenance doses vary. For high-dose therapy, 400 mg daily or occasionally more is employed, but the risk of side effects is substantial over time. For prevention of recurrent AF, one loading regimen used was 800 mg daily for 14 days, 600 mg daily for the next 14 days, 300 mg daily for the first year and 200 mg thereafter.[54] Downward dose adjustment may be required during prolonged therapy to avoid development of side effects while maintaining optimal antiarrhythmic effect. Maintenance doses for atrial flutter or fibrillation are generally lower (200 mg daily or even 100 mg[55]) than those needed for serious ventricular arrhythmias. *Intravenous amiodarone* (approved in the United States) may be used for intractable arrhythmias. The aim is an infusion over 24 hours. Start with 150 mg/10 minutes, then 360 mg over the 6 next hours, then 540 mg over the remaining time up to a total of 24 hours, to give a total of 1050 mg over 24 hours, or for AF in AMI or after cardiac surgery (see next section), 5 mg/kg over 20 minutes, 500 to 1000 mg over 24 hours, then orally, and then 0.5 mg/minute. Deliver by volumetric infusion pump. Higher intravenous loading doses are more likely to give hypotension. For shock-resistant cardiac arrest, the intravenous dose is 5 mg/kg of estimated body weight, with a further dose of 2.5 mg/kg if the VF persists after a further shock.[53]

Indications. In the United States, the license is only for recurrent VF or hemodynamically unstable VT after adequate doses of other ventricular antiarrhythmics have been tested or are not tolerated, because its use is accompanied by substantial toxicity. Amiodarone is not uncommonly used for AF, especially in lower, relatively nontoxic doses and in older patents at lower risk of long-term toxicity. With the increasing use of ablation therapy for AF, amiodarone use has lately decreased considerably. In the prophylactic control of *life-threatening ventricular tachyarrhythmias* (especially post-MI and in association with congestive cardiac failure), or after cardiac surgery,[56] amiodarone has been regarded as one of the most effective agents available,[57] yet is now being replaced by ICDs. To reduce mortality in chronic LV failure, amiodarone was no better than placebo whereas an ICD was much better, reducing mortality by 23%.[58] However, in the ICD era, there is a new role for amiodarone (plus β-blockade) to inhibit repetitive, unpleasant ICD shocks.[59]

Intravenous amiodarone. Intravenous amiodarone is indicated for the initiation of treatment and prophylaxis of frequently recurring VF or destabilizing VT and those refractory to other therapies. When oral amiodarone cannot be used, then the intravenous form is also indicated. *Caution*: Be aware of the risk of hypotension with intravenous amiodarone. Generally, intravenous amiodarone is used for 48 to 96 hours while oral amiodarone is instituted. In the ARREST study amiodarone was better than placebo (44% versus 34%, $P = 0.03$) in reducing immediate mortality.[60] Similar data were obtained when amiodarone was compared with lidocaine for shock-resistant VF.[53] For the acute conversion of chronic AF, intravenous amiodarone is as effective as intravenous propafenone,[21] both having strong evidence in their favor.[18] However, amiodarone-induced conversion is often delayed beyond 6 hours, thereby limiting its usefulness.

Preventing recurrences of paroxysmal atrial fibrillation or flutter. Amiodarone is probably the most effective of the available drugs to prevent recurrences of paroxysmal AF or flutter,[18,46,47,54] and is an entirely reasonable choice for patients with structural cardiac disease or CHF.[51] Sinus rhythm is maintained much more successfully with low-dose 200 mg/day amiodarone than with either sotalol or class I agents, and in the virtual absence of torsades as found with the other agents (except for propafenone).[61] This benefit must be balanced against the cost of side effects (see following sections on side effects), which may be reduced by very low doses (100 mg daily).[55] Amiodarone is not licensed in the United States for supraventricular arrhythmias despite its very frequent use in AF, a common disease. *Contraindications* to amiodarone are severe sinus node dysfunction with marked sinus bradycardia or syncope, second- or third-degree heart block, known hypersensitivity, cardiogenic shock, and probably severe chronic lung disease.

Side effects. The most common side effects are sinus bradycardia, especially in older adults, and QT prolongation with, however, a very low incidence of torsades (<0.5%).[51] Serious adverse effects, listed in a thorough review of 92 studies, include optic neuropathy/neuritis (≤1%-2%), blue-gray skin discoloration (4%-9%), photosensitivity (25%-75%), hypothyroidism (6%), hyperthyroidism (0.9%-2%), pulmonary toxicity (1%-17%), peripheral neuropathy (0.3% annually), and hepatotoxicity (elevated enzyme levels, 15%-30%; hepatitis and cirrhosis, <3%, 0.6% annually).[62] Recommended preventative actions are baseline and 6-monthly thyroid function tests and liver enzymes and baseline and yearly ECG and chest radiograph with physical examination of skin, eyes, and peripheral nerves if symptoms develop. Corneal microdeposits (>90%) are usually asymptomatic.

Thyroid side effects. Amiodarone has a complex effect on the metabolism of thyroid hormones (it contains iodine and shares a structural similarity to thyroxin), the main action being to inhibit the peripheral conversion of T4 to T3 with a rise in the serum level of T4 and a small fall in the level of T3. In most patients, thyroid function is not altered by amiodarone. In approximately 6% hypothyroidism may develop during the first year of treatment, but hyperthyroidism only in 0.9%[45]; the exact incidence varies geographically. Hyperthyroidism may precipitate arrhythmia breakthrough and should be excluded if new arrhythmias appear during amiodarone therapy. Once established, the prognosis of amiodarone-induced thyrotoxicosis is poor so that early vigilance is appropriate.[63] In older men (mean age 67 years), subclinical hypothyroidism (thyroid-stimulating hormone 4.5-10 mU/L) can be common, up to 20% more than in controls, suggesting extra alertness (thyroid tests at 3 months) and treatment by levothyroxine.[64] Thyrotoxicosis may be much more common in iodine-deficient areas (20% versus 3% in normal iodine areas).[51]

Cardiac side effects and torsades de pointes. Amiodarone may inhibit the SA or AV node (approximately 2% to 5%), which can be serious in those with prior sinus node dysfunction or heart block. It is probably a safe drug from the hemodynamic point of view. Only 1.6% required discontinuation of amiodarone because of bradycardia in a metaanalysis.[45]

Pulmonary side effects. In higher doses, there is an unusual spectrum of toxicity, the most serious being pneumonitis, potentially leading to pulmonary fibrosis and occurring in 10% to 17% at doses of approximately 400 mg/day, which may be fatal in 10% of those affected (package insert). Metaanalysis of double-blind amiodarone trials suggests that there is an absolute risk of 1% of pulmonary toxicity per year, with some fatal cases. Of note, pulmonary toxicity may be dose-related, and very rarely occurs with the low doses of about 200 mg daily, used for prevention of recurrent AF.[47,65] Pulmonary complications usually regress if recognized early and if amiodarone is discontinued. Symptomatic therapy may include steroids.

Other extracardiac side effects. Central nervous system side effects like proximal muscle weakness, peripheral neuropathy, and other neural symptoms (headache, ataxia, tremors, impaired memory, dyssomnia, bad dreams) occur with variable incidence. *GI side effects* were uncommon in the GESICA study.[66] Yet nausea can occur in 25% of patients with CHF, even at a dose of only 200 mg daily; exclude increased plasma levels of liver function enzymes. These effects usually resolve with dose reduction. *Testicular dysfunction* may be a side effect, detected by increased gonadotropin levels in patients on long-term amiodarone. *Less serious side effects* are as follows: Corneal microdeposits develop in nearly all adult patients given prolonged amiodarone. Symptoms and impairment of visual acuity are rare and respond to reduced dosage. Macular degeneration rarely occurs during therapy, without proof of a causal relationship. A photosensitive slate-gray or bluish skin discoloration may develop after prolonged therapy, usually exceeding 18 months. Avoid exposure to sun and use a sunscreen ointment with ultraviolet A (UVA) and UVB protection. The pigmentation regresses slowly on drug withdrawal.

Drug withdrawal for side effects. When amiodarone must be withdrawn, as for pulmonary toxicity, the plasma concentration falls by 50% within 3 to 10 days, then as tissue stores deplete slowly (very long half-life).

Dose-dependency of side effects. A full and comprehensive metaanalysis of the side effects of amiodarone showed that even low doses may not be free of adverse effects.[65] At a mean dose of 152 to 330 mg/day, drug withdrawal because of side effects was 1.5 times more common than with placebo.[65] Specifically, however, low-dose amiodarone was not associated with torsades.

Drug interactions. The most serious interaction is an additive proarrhythmic effect with other drugs prolonging the QT interval, such as class IA antiarrhythmic agents, phenothiazines, tricyclic antidepressants, thiazide diuretics, and sotalol. Amiodarone may increase quinidine and procainamide levels (these combinations are not advised). With phenytoin, there is a double drug interaction. Amiodarone increases phenytoin levels while at the same time phenytoin enhances the conversion of amiodarone to desethylamiodarone. *A serious and common interaction is with warfarin.* Amiodarone prolongs the prothrombin time and may cause bleeding in patients on warfarin, perhaps by a hepatic interaction; decrease warfarin by about one-third and retest the international normalized ratio (INR). Amiodarone increases the plasma digoxin concentration, predisposing to digitalis toxic effects (not arrhythmias because amiodarone protects); decrease digoxin by approximately half and remeasure digoxin levels. Amiodarone, by virtue of its weak β-blocking and calcium antagonist effect, tends to inhibit nodal activity and may therefore interact adversely with β-blocking agents and calcium antagonists. However, the antiarrhythmic efficacy of amiodarone is generally increased by co-prescription with β-blocking drugs.[29]

Hospitalization. To initiate therapy, there is some controversy about the need for hospitalization, which is required for life-threatening VT and VF. For recurrences of AF (not licensed in the United States), low-dose therapy can be initiated on an outpatient basis. If amiodarone is added to an ICD, the defibrillation threshold is usually increased and must be rechecked prior to discharge from hospital.

Sotalol

Sotalol (Betapace in the United States, Sotacor in Europe) was first licensed in the United States for control of severe ventricular arrhythmias. It is now licensed as Betapace AF for maintenance of sinus rhythm in patients with recurrent symptomatic AF or atrial flutter. Although less effective than amiodarone,[44,46,47] sotalol is chosen, particularly when amiodarone toxicity is feared. As a mixed class II and class III agent, it also has all the beneficial actions of the β-blocker. Inevitably, it is also susceptible to the "Achilles's heel" of all class III agents, namely torsades de pointes.

Electrophysiology. Sotalol is a racemic mixture of dextro and levo isomers, and these differ in their EP effects. Although these agents have comparable class III activity, the class II activity arises from l-sotalol.[67] The pure class III investigational agent d-sotalol increased mortality in postinfarct patients with a low ejection fraction (EF) in the SWORD study.[68] This result suggests that the class III activity, perhaps acting through torsades, can detract from the positive β-blocking qualities of the standard dl-sotalol. In practice, class III activity is not evident at low doses (<160 mg/day) of the racemic drug. In humans, class II effects are sinus and AV node depression. Class III effects are prolongation of the action potential in atrial and ventricular tissue and prolonged atrial and ventricular refractory periods, as well as inhibition of conduction along any bypass tract in both directions. APD prolongation with, possibly, enhanced calcium entry may explain why it causes proarrhythmic after-depolarizations and why the negative inotropic effect is less than expected. It is a noncardioselective, water-soluble (hydrophilic), non–protein-bound agent, excreted solely by the kidneys, with a plasma half-life of 12 hours (US package insert). Dosing every 12 hours gives trough concentrations half of the peak values.

Indications. Because of its combined class II and class III properties, sotalol is active against a wide variety of arrhythmias, including sinus tachycardia, PSVT, WPW arrhythmias with either antegrade or retrograde conduction, recurrence of AF,[18] ischemic ventricular arrhythmias, and recurrent sustained VT or fibrillation. In ventricular arrhythmias, the major outcome study with sotalol was the ESVEM trial[37] in which this drug in a mean dose of approximately 400 mg daily was better at decreasing death and ventricular arrhythmias than any of six class I agents. The major indication was sustained monomorphic VT (or VF) induced in an EP study. Of the wide indications, the major current use is in maintenance of sinus rhythm after cardioversion for AF,[18] for which sotalol is about as effective as flecainide or propafenone, with the advantages that it can be given to patients with structural heart disease and can be given without an additional agent to slow AV-nodal conduction. However, the efficacy of all three is outclassed by amiodarone.[46,47]

Dose. For patients with a history of AF or atrial flutter, and currently in sinus rhythm, the detailed package insert indicates that 320 mg/day (two doses) may give the ideal ratio between therapeutic actions and side effects (especially torsades). The latter risk is 0.3% at 320 mg/day, but goes up to 3.2% at higher doses when used for AF or flutter (US package insert). For ventricular arrhythmias, the dose range is 160 to 640 mg/day given in two divided doses. Keeping the daily dose at 320 mg or lower (as recommended for AF recurrences) lessens side effects, including torsades de pointes. Yet doses of 320 to 480 mg may be needed to prevent recurrent VT or VF. When given in two divided doses, steady-state plasma concentrations are reached in 2 to 3 days. In patients with renal impairment or in older adults, or when there are risk factors for proarrhythmia, the dose should be reduced and the dosing interval increased.

Side effects. Side effects are those of β-blockade, including fatigue (20%) (which appears to be more of a problem in younger patients) and bradycardia (13%), to which is added the risk of torsades de pointes. Being a nonselective β-blocker, bronchospasm may be precipitated. For drug interactions see Tables 8-3 and 8-5.

Precautions and contraindications. For the initial treatment in patients with recurrent AF or flutter, the patient should be hospitalized and monitored for 3 days while the dose is increased (package insert). The drug should be avoided in patients with serious conduction defects, including sick sinus syndrome, second- or third-degree AV block (unless there is a pacemaker), in bronchospastic disease, and when there are evident risks of proarrhythmia. Asthma is a contraindication and bronchospastic disease a strong caution (sotalol is a nonselective β-blocker). The drug is contraindicated in patients with reduced creatinine clearance, below 40 mL/minute (renal excretion). *Torsades de pointes* is more likely when the sotalol dose is high, exceeding 320 mg/day, or when there is bradycardia, when the baseline QT exceeds 450 milliseconds (package insert), in severe LV failure, in women, in patients for whom there are other factors increasing risk (diuretic therapy, other QT-prolonging drugs), or in the congenital long-QT syndrome (LQTS). Co-therapy with class IA drugs, amiodarone, or other drugs prolonging the QT interval should be avoided (Fig. 8-6). In pregnancy, the drug is category B. It is not teratogenic, but does cross the placenta and may depress fetal vital functions. Sotalol is also excreted in mother's milk.

Dronedarone

Dronedarone increases serum digoxin concentrations, and should be used very cautiously in patients taking digitalis.[69,70] Unlike amiodarone, thyroid adverse effects are not an appreciable risk. The European Medicines Agency's Committee has recommended[71] new restrictions (http://www.ema.europa.eu/ema/index.jsp?curl5pages/medicines/human/public_health_alerts/2011/09/human_pha_detail_000038.jsp&murl5menus/medicines/medicines.jsp&mid5WC0b01ac058001d126) on the use of dronedarone that are consistent with the consensus recommendations of the Canadian Cardiovascular Society.[72] This antiarrhythmic medicine should only be prescribed for maintaining sinus rhythm in patients with paroxysmal AF or persistent AF after successful cardioversion. Because of an increased risk of cardiovascular and possibly liver adverse events, dronedarone should only be prescribed to patients without a history of heart failure and with good ventricular function,

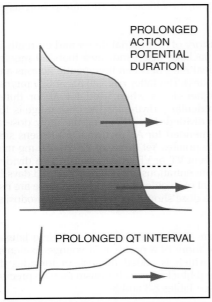

LONG QT WITH RISK OF TORSADE
Opie 2012

PROLONGED ACTION POTENTIAL DURATION

PROLONGED QT INTERVAL

- *DISOPYRAMIDE*
  QUINIDINE
- *IBUTILIDE*
  DOFETILIDE
- *SOTALOL*
  (AMIODARONE)
- *TRICYCLICS*
  HALOPERIDOL
- *ANTIPSYCHOTICS*
- *PHENOTHIAZINES*
- *IV ERYTHROMYCIN*
  QUINOLONES (SOME)
- *ANTIHISTAMINICS*
  - *astemizole*
  - *terfenadine*
- *KETOCONAZOLE*
- *Prolonged QTU:*
  Low K⁺ , Mg²⁺
  (THIAZIDES)

Figure 8-6   Therapeutic agents, including antiarrhythmics that may cause QT prolongation. Hypokalemia causes QTU, not QT, prolongation. Some antiarrhythmic agents act at least in part chiefly by prolonging the action potential duration, such as amiodarone and sotalol. QT prolongation is therefore an integral part of their therapeutic benefit. On the other hand, QT or QTU prolongation, especially in the presence of hypokalemia or hypomagnesemia or when there is co-therapy with one of the other agents prolonging the QT interval, may precipitate torsades de pointes. *IV,* Intravenous. (Figure © L.H. Opie, 2012.)

after alternative treatment options have been considered. Torsades de pointes has not been reported with any frequency.

Pure Class III Agents: Ibutilide, Dofetilide, and Azimilide

The effectiveness of class III antiarrhythmic drugs such as amiodarone and sotalol has prompted the development of purer class III agents. Two such drugs, ibutilide and dofetilide, are presently in clinical practice. The efficacy of ibutilide and dofetilide in the conversion of atrial flutter is noteworthy because, prior to their introduction, drugs have not been found to be efficacious in the cardioversion of atrial flutter.

Ibutilide

Ibutilide (Corvert) is a methanesulfonamide derivative, which prolongs repolarization primarily by inhibition of the delayed rectifier potassium current (I_{Kr}). Ibutilide has no known negative inotropic effects.

Pharmacokinetics. Ibutilide is available only as an intravenous preparation because it undergoes extensive first-pass metabolism when administered orally. The pharmacokinetics of ibutilide are linear and are independent of dose, age, sex, and LV function. Its extracellular distribution is extensive, and its systemic clearance is high. The elimination half-life is variable, 2 to 12 hours (mean of 6), reflecting considerable individual variation.[73]

Efficacy of Ibutilide. This drug is efficacious in the termination of atrial flutter and, to a lesser extent, AF.[73] It is as effective as amiodarone in cardioversion of AF.[18,74] In patients who had persistent AF or atrial flutter, ibutilide had a conversion efficacy of 44% for a single dose and 49% for a second dose.[75] The mean termination time was 27 minutes after the start of the infusion. The efficacy of ibutilide in the cardioversion of atrial flutter is related to an effect on the variability of the cycle length of the tachycardia.[76] Like sotalol, ibutilide exhibits the phenomenon of reverse use dependence in that prolongation of refractoriness becomes less pronounced at higher tachycardia rates. *After cardiac surgery* ibutilide has a dose-dependent effect in conversion of atrial arrhythmias with 57% conversion at a dose of 10 mg.[77] Ibutilide pretreatment facilitates direct-current (DC) cardioversion of AF, but must be followed with 3 to 4 hours of ECG monitoring to exclude torsades.[78]

Adverse effects. QT- and QT$_c$-interval prolongation is a consistent feature in patients treated with ibutilide. QT prolongation is dose-dependent, maximal at the end of the infusion, and returns to baseline within 2 to 4 hours following infusion.[73] *Torsades de pointes* (polymorphic VT with QT prolongation) occurs in approximately 4.3%,[79] and may require cardioversion (in almost 2% of patients).[79] Torsades tends to occur during or shortly after the infusion period (within 1 hour).[79] Patients should be continuously monitored for at least 4 hours after the start of the ibutilide infusion. To avoid proarrhythmia, higher doses of ibutilide and rapid infusion are avoided, the drug is not given to those with preexisting QT prolongation or advanced or unstable heart disease, and the serum K must be greater than 4 mmol/L. Theoretically, other cardiac and noncardiac drugs, which prolong the QT interval, may increase the likelihood of torsades. However, in one study, prior therapy with sotalol or amiodarone did not appear to provoke torsades.[78]

Dose. The recommended dose is 1 mg by intravenous infusion over 10 minutes. If the arrhythmia is not terminated within 10 minutes, the dose may be repeated. For patients who weigh less than 60 kg, the dose should be 0.01 mg/kg.

Drug interactions. Apart from the proposed interaction with sotalol, amiodarone, and other drugs prolonging the QT interval, there are no known drug interactions.

Dofetilide

Like ibutilide, dofetilide (Tikosyn) is a methanesulfonamide drug. Dofetilide prolongs the APD and QT$_c$ in a concentration-related manner. Dofetilide exerts its effect solely by inhibition of the rapid component of the delayed rectifier potassium current I_{Kr}. Like ibutilide and sotalol, dofetilide exhibits the phenomenon of reverse use dependence. Dofetilide has mild negative chronotropic effects, is devoid of negative inotropic activity, and may be mildly positively inotropic. Whereas ibutilide is given only intravenously, dofetilide is given only orally.

Pharmacokinetics. After oral administration, dofetilide is almost completely (92% to 96%) absorbed, and mean maximal plasma concentrations are achieved roughly 2.5 hours after administration. Twice-daily administration of oral dofetilide results in steady state within 48 hours. Fifty percent of the drug is excreted through the kidneys unchanged and there are no active metabolites.

Efficacy. Dofetilide has good efficacy in the cardioversion of AF[18] and is even more effective in the cardioversion of atrial flutter. In addition, dofetilide may also be active against ventricular arrhythmias (not licensed). Dofetilide decreases the VF threshold in patients undergoing defibrillation testing prior to ICD implantation, and suppresses the inducibility of VT. Dofetilide is as effective as sotalol against inducible VT, with fewer side effects.[80] In patients with depressed LV function both with and without a history of MI,[81] dofetilide has a neutral effect on mortality. However, dofetilide reduced the development of new AF, increased the conversion of preexisting AF to sinus rhythm, and improved the maintenance of sinus rhythm in these patients with significant structural heart disease. In this study dofetilide also reduced hospitalization.

Indications. Indications include (1) cardioversion of persistent AF or atrial flutter to normal sinus rhythm in patients in whom cardioversion by electrical means is not appropriate and in whom the duration of the arrhythmic episode is less than 6 months, and (2) maintenance of sinus rhythm (after conversion) in patients with persistent AF or atrial flutter. Because dofetilide can cause ventricular arrhythmias, it should be reserved for patients in whom AF and atrial flutter is highly symptomatic and in whom other antiarrhythmic therapy is not appropriate. Dofetilide has stronger evidence in its favor for acute cardioversion of AF than for maintenance thereafter, according to a metaanalysis.[18] An important point in its favor is that it can be given to those with a depressed EF.

Dose of dofetilide. The package insert *warns in bold* that the dose must be individualized by the calculated creatinine clearance and the QT_c. There must be continuous ECG monitoring to detect and manage any serious ventricular arrhythmias. For the complex six-step dosing instructions, see the package insert. The calculated dose could be 125-500 mcg twice daily. Those with a creatinine clearance of less than 20 mL/minute should not be given dofetilide. If the increase in the QT_c is more than 15%, or if the QT_c is more than 500 milliseconds, the dose of dofetilide should be reduced. If at any time after the second dose the QT_c is greater than 500 milliseconds, dofetilide should be discontinued.

Adverse effects. The major significant adverse effect is torsades de pointes in 3% of patients.[81] The risk of torsades de pointes (80% of events within the first 3 days of therapy) can be reduced by normal serum potassium and magnesium levels, and by avoiding the drug (or reducing its dosage according to the manufacturer's algorithm) in patients with abnormal renal function, or with bradycardia, or with baseline QT prolongation (QT_c should be less than 429 milliseconds).[82] To detect early torsades, patients need continuous ECG monitoring in hospital for the first 3 days of dofetilide therapy.

Drug interactions. Drugs that increase levels of dofetilide should not be co-administered. These include ketoconazole and other inhibitors of cytochrome CYP 3A4, including macrolide antibiotics and protease inhibitors such as the antiviral agent ritonavir, verapamil, and cimetidine. Check for QT_c prolongation (hypokalemia), especially with diuretics or chronic diarrhea and the co-administration of drugs that increase the QT_c (see Fig. 8-6).

Class IV and Class IV-Like Agents

Verapamil and diltiazem. Calcium channel blockade slows conduction through the AV node, and increases the refractory period of AV nodal tissue. Because of vascular selectivity, *dihydropyridine* compounds do not have significant EP effects (see Table 3-3). The nondihydropyridine agents *verapamil* and *diltiazem* are similar in their EP properties. They slow the ventricular response rate in atrial arrhythmias, particularly AF. They can also terminate or prevent reentrant arrhythmias in which the circuit involves the AV node. For the termination of AV nodal dependent supraventricular tachycardias, verapamil and diltiazem are alternatives to adenosine.

ADENOSINE INHIBITION OF AV NODE
Opie 2012

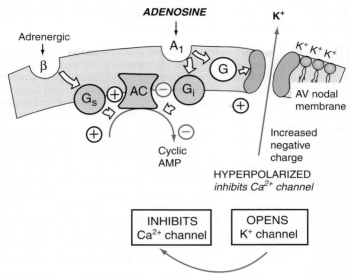

Figure 8-7 Adenosine inhibits the atrioventricular (AV) node by effects on ion channels. Adenosine acting on the adenosine 1 (A_1) surface receptor opens the adenosine-sensitive potassium channel to hyperpolarize and inhibit the AV node and also indirectly to inhibit calcium channel opening. *AC,* Adenylate cyclase; *AMP,* adenosine monophosphate; *β,* β-adrenoreceptor; *G,* G protein, nonspecific; G_i, inhibitory G protein; G_s, stimulatory G protein. (Figure © L.H. Opie, 2012.)

Rare use in ventricular tachycardia. A few unusual forms of VT respond to verapamil or diltiazem. In idiopathic right ventricular outflow tract (RVOT) tachycardia, verapamil is chosen after β-blockade. Fascicular tachycardias often respond to verapamil and torsades de pointes may terminate following verapamil. In all other ventricular arrhythmias, *these agents are contraindicated* because of their hemodynamic effects and inefficacy. Verapamil must be administered cautiously in patients who have received either oral or recent intravenous β-blockade. Severe and irreversible electromechanical dissociation may occur.

Intravenous magnesium. Intravenous magnesium weakly blocks the calcium channel, as well as inhibiting sodium and potassium channels. The relative importance of these mechanisms is unknown. It can be used to slow the ventricular rate in AF but is poor at terminating PSVTs. It may be the agent of choice in torsades de pointes.[83] It has an additional use in refractory VF.

Adenosine

Adenosine (Adenocard) has multiple cellular effects mediated by opening of the adenosine-sensitive inward rectifier potassium channel, with inhibition of the sinus and especially the AV node (Fig. 8-7). It is a first-line agent for terminating narrow complex PSVTs.[84] It is also used in the diagnosis of wide-complex tachycardia of uncertain origin.

Dose. Adenosine is given as an initial rapid intravenous bolus of 6 mg followed by a saline flush to obtain high concentrations in the heart.[84] If it does not work within 1 to 2 minutes, a 12-mg bolus is given that may be repeated once. At the appropriate dose, the antiarrhythmic effect occurs as soon as the drug reaches the AV node, usually within

15 to 30 seconds. The initial dose needs to be reduced to 3 mg or less in patients taking verapamil, diltiazem, or β-blockers or dipyridamole (see drug interactions in "Side Effects and Contraindications" later in this section), or in older adults at risk of sick sinus syndrome. Note the extremely short half-life of less than 10 seconds.

Indications. The chief indication is for *paroxysmal narrow complex SVT* (usually AV nodal reentry or AV reentry such as in the WPW syndrome or in patients with a concealed accessory pathway). In *wide-complex tachycardia* of uncertain origin, adenosine can help the management by differentiating between VT or SVT (with aberrant conduction). In the latter case, adenosine is likely to stop the tachycardia, whereas in the case of VT there is unlikely to be any major adverse hemodynamic effect and the tachycardia continues. It may be particularly helpful in VT with retrograde conduction to block the P wave and to show the diagnosis. Finally, intravenous adenosine may be used to reveal *latent preexcitation* in patients suspected of having the WPW syndrome.[85] When used for this indication adenosine is administered during sinus rhythm while a multichannel ECG rhythm strip is recorded (ideally all 12 leads) and a normal response occurs if transient high-grade AV block is observed. On the other hand, following adenosine the presence of an anterograde conduction accessory pathway is inferred if there is PR interval shortening–QRS widening without interruption in AV conduction.

Side effects and contraindications. Side effects ascribed to the effect of adenosine on the potassium channel are short lived, such as headache (via vasodilation), chest discomfort, flushing, nausea, and excess sinus or AV nodal inhibition. The precipitation of bronchoconstriction in asthmatic patients is of unknown mechanism and can last for 30 minutes. *Transient new arrhythmias* can occur at the time of chemical cardioversion. Because of abbreviating effects on atrial and ventricular refractoriness, adenosine may cause a range of *proarrhythmic consequences,* including atrial and ventricular ectopy, and degeneration of atrial flutter or PSVT into AF.[86] Contraindications are as follows: asthma or history of asthma, second- or third-degree AV block, sick sinus syndrome. Atrial flutter is a relative contraindication, because of the risk of 1:1 conduction and serious tachycardia. *Drug interactions* are as follows: Dipyridamole inhibits the breakdown of adenosine and therefore the dose of adenosine must be markedly reduced in patients receiving dipyridamole. Methylxanthines (caffeine, theophylline) competitively antagonize the interaction of adenosine with its receptors, so that it becomes less effective.

Adenosine versus verapamil or diltiazem. Adenosine is as effective as intravenous verapamil or diltiazem for the rapid termination of narrow QRS complex SVT. It needs to be reemphasized that verapamil or diltiazem, by myocardial depression and peripheral vasodilation, can be fatal when given to patients with VT, whereas adenosine with its very transient effects leaves true VT virtually unchanged. The transience of adenosine's effects is an advantage; on the other hand, adenosine very commonly produces brief but severe systemic discomfort that does not occur with verapamil or diltiazem.

Proarrhythmia, QT Prolongation, and Torsades de Pointes

Proarrhythmic Effects of Antiarrhythmics

Proarrhythmia can offset the potential benefits of an antiarrhythmic agent.[2] There are two basic mechanisms for proarrhythmia: first, prolongation of the APD and QT interval (see Fig. 8-6), and, second, incessant wide-complex tachycardia often terminating in VF (Fig. 8-8). The former

CLASS IA and III AGENTS: TORSADES DE POINTES
Opie 2012

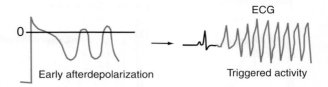

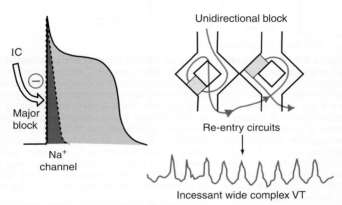

Figure 8-8   Major proarrhythmic mechanisms. *Top:* Class IA and class III agents widen the action potential duration and in the presence of an early after-depolarization can give rise to triggered activity known as *torsades de pointes.* Note major role of QT prolongation (see Fig. 8-6). *Bottom:* Class IC agents have as their major proarrhythmic mechanism a powerful inhibition of the sodium channel, particularly in conduction tissue. Increasing heterogeneity together with unidirectional block sets the stage for reentry circuits and monomorphic wide-complex ventricular tachycardia (VT). *ECG,* Electrocardiogram. (Figure © L.H. Opie, 2012.)

typically occurs with class IA and class III agents, the latter with class IC agents. In addition, incessant VT can complicate therapy with any class I agent when conduction is sufficiently severely depressed. A third type of proarrhythmia is when the patient's own tachycardia, previously paroxysmal, becomes incessant—the result of either class IA or IC agents. Not only is early vigilance required with the institution of therapy with antiarrhythmics of the class IA, IC, and III types, but continuous vigilance is required throughout therapy. Furthermore, the CAST study shows that proarrhythmic sudden death can occur even when ventricular premature complexes are apparently eliminated. Solutions to this problem include (1) avoiding the use of class I, and especially class IC agents, in patients with structural heart disease; (2) not treating unless the overall effect will clearly be beneficial; and (3) ultimately defining better those subjects at high risk for proarrhythmia and arrhythmic death. The latter would now often be treated by an ICD.

Long-QT Syndrome and Torsades de Pointes

The LQTS with delayed repolarization is clinically recognized by a prolonged QT or QT$_c$ (corrected for heart rate exceeding 440 milliseconds) or QTU interval. LQTS may be either an acquired or a congenital

REPOLARIZATION RESERVE

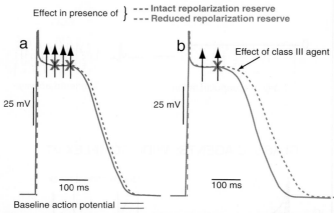

Effect in presence of } --- Intact repolarization reserve
                        --- Reduced repolarization reserve

a

b   Effect of class III agent

25 mV

25 mV

100 ms

100 ms

Baseline action potential ====

Figure 8-9   Repolarization reserve as a determinant of action potential and QT prolongation. The idea of "repolarization reserve," as illustrated in this schematic, has emerged as an important notion in understanding the risk of arrhythmias associated with delayed repolarization. In the normal heart (*Panel a*), there are substantial repolarizing currents (*black arrows*) flowing during the action potential plateau. When one outward current is reduced (e.g., by a class III antiarrhythmic drug), the others increase, so that action potential prolongation (*dashed lines*) is minimized. However, when baseline currents are reduced (e.g., by a congenital gene variant decreasing a potassium current, by hypokalemia, etc.), as in *Panel b,* the reserve currents are reduced and the same class III drug will produce substantial prolongation of the action potential (and QT interval), with an increased risk of proarrhythmia. (Figure © S. Nattel, 2012.)

abnormality. The realization that quinidine, disopyramide, procainamide, and related class IA agents, class III agents, and others (see Fig. 8-6) can all prolong the QT interval has led to a reassessment of the mode of use of such agents in antiarrhythmic therapy. The concept of "repolarisation reserve" is an important idea in the understanding of the risk of long-QT arrhythmias.[87] Cardiac cells have several repolarizing currents, so that if one is blocked, the others increase to compensate (Fig. 8-9). Consequently, in a person with normal repolarisation reserve, drug-induced reduction in potassium current will produce little or no effect on the QT interval or APD (Fig. 8-9, *dashed blue line*). However, when repolarization reserve is already reduced, the same drug will produce marked QT/APD prolongation in the presence of reduced repolarisation reserve (Fig. 8-9, *dashed red line*). Repolarisation reserve is decreased by genetic abnormalities in ion channel subunits, by electrolyte disturbances (e.g., hypokalemia, hypocalcemia, hypomagnesemia), by drugs that block potassium channels, and even as a function of gender in normal women.[87]

The risk of torsades de pointes is determined not only by the QT interval, but also by other channels that are involved in generating the arrhythmia, such as inward sodium and calcium channels.[87] For example, amiodarone is relatively safe for a given degree of QT prolongation, because of concomitant effects on sodium and calcium channels that limit the risk of torsades. Serious problems may arise when QT prolongation by sotalol or class 1A drugs or even amiodarone is combined with any other factor increasing the QT interval or QTU, such as bradycardia, hypokalemia, hypomagnesemia, hypocalcemia, intense or prolonged use of potassium-wasting diuretic therapy, or combined class IA and class III therapy. A number of noncardiac drugs prolong the QT interval by blocking I_{Kr} potassium channels (see Fig. 8-6), including tricyclic antidepressants, phenothiazines, erythromycin, and some antihistamines, such as terfenadine and astemizole. Note that a drug concentration that might slightly prolong the action potential plateau in some patients might in others produce excessive prolongation because of differences in repolarisation reserve and drug pharmacokinetics.

Treatment. The management of patients with drug-induced torsades includes identifying and withdrawing the offending drugs, replenishing the potassium level to 4.5 to 5 mmol/L, and infusing intravenous magnesium (1 to 2 g). An interesting preventative approach is by chronic therapy with the potassium-retaining aldosterone blocker, spironolactone.[88] In resistant cases, isoproterenol or temporary cardiac pacing may be needed to increase the heart rate and shorten the QT interval. Isoproterenol is contraindicated in ischemic heart disease and the congenital LQTS.

Congenital long-QT syndrome. The congenital LQTS is typically caused by genetically based "channelopathies," which are congenital disorders of the cardiac ion channels predisposing to lethal cardiac arrhythmias. The three most common involve loss-of-function mutations in the genes encoding proteins responsible for the slow (LQT1) and rapid (LQT2) components of the repolarising potassium current, and mutations impairing inactivation of the inward sodium current, producing an increased "late" component that retards repolarisation (LQT3). LQT3 is logically treated by sodium channel inhibitors (class I drugs), of which mexiletine and flecainide have been documented to be effective.[89,90] In patients with LQT1, the defect is in the slow delayed-rectifier potassium channel I_{Ks}, which is adrenergic-dependent. I_{Ks} enhancement normally offsets the calcium-current increase caused by adrenergic activation, thus preventing excess APD prolongation in response to adrenergic drive. LQT1 patients have a defective I_{Ks} response that allows unopposed calcium current enhancement to induce excess QT prolongation and torsades de pointes: appropriate treatment is therefore to block β-adrenergic effects with a β-adrenoceptor antagonist.

Which β-blocker? For all forms of symptomatic LQTS patients, β-blockers are the agents of choice. The risk of recurrences is markedly higher with metoprolol than with either propranolol or nadolol.[90A] The underlying reason might be, in part, on the differential effect on the sodium current (peak and delayed) of propranolol, nadolol, and metoprolol (in descending order).[90B] Other drugs that should not be used are flecainide and mexilitine.[90C]

Which Antiarrhythmic Drug or Device?

Paroxysmal Supraventricular Tachycardia

Acute therapy. Understanding the mechanism responsible for this arrhythmia (see Fig. 8-9) is the key to appropriate therapy for PSVT.[91,92] Atrioventricular nodal reentrant tachycardia (AVNRT) and atrioventricular reentrant tachycardia (AVRT) are the forms most frequently seen in patients without structural heart disease (see Fig. 8-14) and maintenance of both arrhythmias depends on intact 1:1 AV nodal conduction. Many patients learn on their own to abort episodes soon after initiation with vagal maneuvers such as gagging, Valsalva, or carotid massage. In infants, facial immersion is effective. If the arrhythmia persists, sympathetic tone increases and these maneuvers then become less effective.

Parenteral therapy. During PSVT, bioavailability of orally administered drugs is delayed, so parenteral drug administration is usually required.[93] One report described oral self-administration of crushed diltiazem and propranolol, but this is not frequently recommended.[94] Adenosine and a nondihydropyridine calcium channel blocker (CCB; verapamil or diltiazem) are the intravenous drugs of choice.[91,92]

Adenosine. After intravenous administration, adenosine is cleared from the circulation within seconds by cellular uptake and metabolism.[84] Administration of an intravenous bolus results in transient AV nodal block when the bolus reaches the heart, usually within 15 to 30 seconds. Central administration results in a more rapid onset of effect, and dosage reduction is required. The recommended adult dosage for peripheral intravenous infusion is 6 mg followed by a second dose of 12 mg if necessary. Higher doses may be required in selected patients. Because adenosine is cleared so rapidly, sequential doses do not result in a cumulative effect. Most patients report transient dyspnea or chest pain after receiving a bolus of adenosine. Sinus bradycardia with or without accompanying AV block is also common after PSVT termination. However, the bradycardia typically resolves within seconds and is replaced with a mild sinus tachycardia. Atrial and ventricular premature beats may occur and can reinitiate PSVT or AF. (For further details and drug interactions of adenosine, see this chapter, p. 299).

Verapamil and diltiazem. Verapamil and diltiazem administered intravenously are alternates to adenosine.[84,91] Both of these drugs affect the calcium-dependent AV nodal action potential and can produce transient AV nodal block, which terminates the intranodal reentry and stops the tachycardia. The recommended initial dose of verapamil is 5 mg intravenously infused over 2 minutes. A second dose of 5 to 7.5 mg may be given 5 to 10 minutes later, if necessary. Diltiazem, 20 mg initially, followed by a second dose of 25 to 35 mg, is equally effective.[95] PSVT termination within 5 minutes of the end of the first or second infusion is expected in more than 90% of patients with AV nodal reentrant tachycardia or AV reentrant tachycardia. Verapamil and diltiazem are vasodilators and may produce hypotension if the PSVT does not terminate. Atrial arrhythmias and bradycardia may also be seen. CCBs should not be used to treat preexcitation arrhythmias (WPW syndrome) or wide-complex tachycardias unless the mechanism of the arrhythmia is known to be AV nodal dependent. Drug-induced hypotension with persistent arrhythmia may lead to cardiovascular collapse and VF in these settings, as in neonates.[96]

Adenosine versus CCBs. In most patients with PSVT caused by an AV node–dependent mechanism, either adenosine or a CCB can be selected.[91,97] Adenosine is preferred in infants and neonates, patients with severe hypotension, if intravenous β-blockers have been recently administered, and in those with a history of heart failure and poor LV function. CCBs are preferred in patients with venous access unsuitable for delivering a rapid bolus infusion, in patients with acute bronchospasm, and in the presence of agents that interfere with adenosine's actions or its metabolism.[92]

Atrial tachycardias. Atrial tachycardias may be due to a number of possible mechanisms, and few data about acute pharmacologic termination of atrial tachycardias are available.[91,94] CCBs or β-blockers may be effective when there is sinus node reentry or in some automatic atrial tachycardias. Atrial tachycardias related to reentry around atriotomy scars are often drug resistant, and their management should resemble that of atrial flutter (see earlier in this chapter, p. 300).

Chronic therapy of PSVT. Many patients with recurrent PSVT do not require chronic therapy. If episodes produce only minor symptoms and can be broken easily by the patient, chronic drug therapy may be avoided. In cases in which recurrent episodes produce significant symptoms or require outside intervention for termination, either pharmacologic therapy or catheter ablation is appropriate. In AV node–dependent PSVT, CCBs and β-blockers are the first-line choices if chronic drug therapy is necessary. Flecainide and propafenone also are effective and are frequently used in combination with a β-adrenergic

SITES AMENABLE TO CATHETER ABLATION
Possible indications
Opie 2012

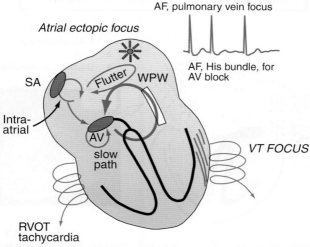

Figure 8-10   Possible sites for intervention by catheter ablation techniques.
AF, Atrial fibrillation; AV, atrioventricular node; flutter, atrial flutter; RVOT, right ventricular outflow tract; SA, sinoatrial node; VT, ventricular tachycardia; WPW, Wolff-Parkinson-White preexcitation syndrome. (Figure © L.H. Opie, 2012.)

blocker.[20,98,99] Sotalol, dofetilide, azimilide, and amiodarone may be effective but are second- or third-line agents. Because of very high efficacy and acceptable safety, ablation procedures directed to a portion of the reentry circuit (either one of two AV-nodal pathways in AVNRT and or the accessory pathway in AVRT) are often the treatment of choice for recurrent PSVTs. Chronic drug therapy of atrial tachycardias (as opposed to AV nodal–dependent tachycardias) has not been extensively studied in clinical trials. Empiric testing of β-blockers, CCBs, and either class I or class III antiarrhythmics may be appropriate.[91,92] Ablation is also often successfully used for atrial tachycardias.

Radiofrequency catheter ablation. Although antiarrhythmic drug therapy is usually efficacious in 70% to 90% of PSVT patients, up to half of these patients will have unwanted side effects and daily therapy is often undesirable. Catheter ablation is an attractive alternative for AV nodal reentrant tachycardias and AV reentrant tachycardias with or without manifest preexcitation that is highly effective, produces a lifelong "cure," and in experienced centers, is a low-risk procedure.[91,100] In AV nodal reentry, the slow AV nodal pathway is the usual target. For AV reentry, the accessory pathway is mapped and ablated. Radiofrequency energy is the most frequent ablation technique but cryoablation may be useful, particularly if the ablation target is close to the normal AV conduction system. Most atrial tachycardias can also be approached with catheter ablation but more complex three-dimensional mapping procedures may be required and the success rate is lower than observed with AV nodal or AV reentry. Patients with extensive atrial scarring, especially those with postoperative congenital heart disease, may have multiple atrial arrhythmias and total elimination of tachycardia in such patients remains challenging. Given the excellent results of catheter ablation in most patients with PSVT, current guidelines allow catheter ablation to be offered to patients as either a first option before any chronic drug trials or if drug treatment has been unsuccessful (Fig. 8-10).[91,92,94]

PATHOPHYSIOLOGY OF ATRIAL FIBRILLATION   Opie 2012

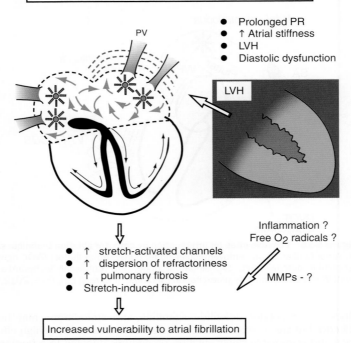

> *"Lone" atrial fibrillation?* - P vein and L atrial triggers?
> *Endurance athletes?*   - role of ↑ vagal tone

PV

- ● Prolonged PR
- ● ↑ Atrial stiffness
- ● LVH
- ● Diastolic dysfunction

LVH

Inflammation ?
Free O_2 radicals ?

- ● ↑   stretch-activated channels
- ● ↑   dispersion of refractoriness
- ● ↑   pulmonary fibrosis
- ● Stretch-induced fibrosis

MMPs - ?

Increased vulnerability to atrial fibrillation

Figure 8-11 Pathophysiologic characteristics of atrial fibrillation, with emphasis on multiple contributory or perpetuating factors. Note role of atrial triggers, increased vagal tone, left ventricular hypertrophy (LVH), atrial stretch, and fibrosis. Inflammatory mediators may also play a role. *L,* left; *MMP,* Metalloproteinases; *P,* pulmonary; *PR,* as measured by the electrocardiogram. (Figure © B.J. Gersh, 2012.)

Atrial Fibrillation

AF is an old disease, first described in 1903, with a "new look" given by the significance of the adverse predisposing factors of left atrial structural and ionic remodeling (Fig. 8-11),[101-103] which have led to the current interest in the initiation and perpetuation of this very common arrhythmia.[104,105] In the United States, approximately 20% of all hospital admissions have AF as either a primary or secondary diagnosis.[106] The ECG in AF is characterized by an undulating baseline without discrete atrial activity, which often has its origin in the pulmonary veins as they enter the atria, to provide sites for therapeutic ablation (Fig. 8-12). The rapid and mostly disorganized atrial rates averaging more than 350 per minute bombard the AV node during all phases of its refractory period. Some impulses that do not conduct to the ventricle will reset the refractory period of the AV node and thereby delay or prevent conduction of subsequent impulses, a phenomenon called *concealed conduction.*

Symptoms of atrial fibrillation. Patients with AF may present with a variety of symptoms, including palpitations, exercise intolerance, dyspnea, heart failure, chest pain, syncope, dizziness, and stroke. Some patients, however, are asymptomatic during some, or even all, episodes. AF is also frequently associated with sinus node dysfunction

MECHANISMS OF ATRIAL FIBRILLATION

Nattel, 2006

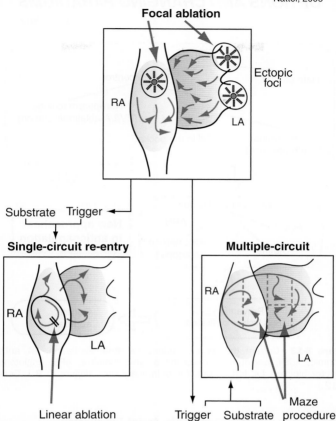

Figure 8-12 Mechanisms of atrial fibrillation, with sites of possible intervention by ablation. Maze procedure (*bottom right panel*) involves multiple incisions of which only two are shown. *LA,* Left atrium; *RA,* right atrium. (Modified from Nattel S, et al., *Lancet* 2006;367:262.)

or AV conduction disease, and patients may experience severe symptoms as a result of bradycardia. Loss of atrial contraction, disturbed atrial endothelial function, and activation of coagulation factor all predispose toward clot formation in the atria.[105] Therapy of AF, therefore, may involve measures to control ventricular rates, to restore and maintain sinus rhythm, and to prevent thromboembolic complications (Fig. 8-13)

Presentation of atrial fibrillation. AF may present in a number of ways, and a classification based on its temporal pattern is often used.[107,108] At the time of first presentation of an acute episode of AF, the future temporal pattern may be difficult to predict so first episodes are often classified separately. If episodes are self-terminating within less than 7 days (usually less than 1 day), they are classified as *paroxysmal*. When episodes require drug or electrical therapy for termination, they are classified as *persistent*. Persistent AF that is resistant to cardioversion or in which cardioversion is not attempted is classified as *permanent*. Unfortunately, individual patients may experience both paroxysmal and persistent episodes in an unpredictable pattern; yet the terms are helpful in analyzing trials dealing with drug therapy for AF.

ATRIAL FIBRILLATION - THERAPEUTIC OPTIONS AND CHANGING PARADIGMS

Gersh 2012

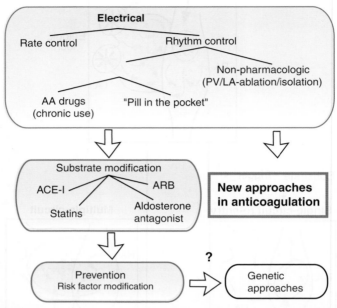

Figure 8-13 Current therapeutic options for atrial fibrillation. *AA,* antiarrhythmic; *ACE-I,* angiotensin-converting enzyme inhibitor; *ARB,* angiotensin receptor blocker; *LA,* left atrium; *PV,* pulmonary vein. (Figure © B.J. Gersh, 2012.)

Rate versus Rhythm Control in Atrial Fibrillation

Is it better to control rate or rhythm in AF? In five randomized trials on chronic AF, there were no differences between these strategies.[102,107] The major risk remains that of thromboembolic stroke, often requiring chronic anticoagulation. Nonetheless, controlling abnormal ventricular rates mostly improves symptoms and exercise capacity. *How strict should rate control be?* Optimal criteria for rate control are presently unknown. Excess bradycardia may lead to syncope or fatigue, whereas consistently faster rates may result in a tachycardia-induced cardiomyopathy. Strict rate control is a resting heart rate less than 80 beats per minute (bpm) and less than 110 bpm with minor exercise.[109,110] The Rate Control Versus Electrical Cardioversion for Persistent Atrial Fibrillation (RACE 2) trial[109,110] showed that strict rate control is not essential, and that in selected patients a target heart rate of less than 100 bpm may suffice.[111]

Although some guidelines[112] recommend that rate control and anticoagulation be the preferred strategy in patients with AF, this may not always be appropriate. The patients who were enrolled in the rate-control versus rhythm-control strategy trials cited previously were considered candidates for either strategy. Patients who were highly symptomatic despite good rate control and those who had failed numerous drug trials to maintain sinus rhythm could not be randomized. Physicians managing patients with AF must base individual therapy on the patient's symptoms, quality of life, and tolerance for procedures. Importantly, it has not been demonstrated that even an apparently successful rhythm control strategy eliminates a need for anticoagulation in patients with risk factors for stroke because there are still frequent episodes of subjectively undetected episodes of AF.[113]

Rate control in heart failure. In those with CHF, rate control is simpler with less cardioversion and fewer hospitalizations. The large, randomized AF-CHF trial showed no advantage to a rhythm control strategy in terms of LV function, exercise tolerance, or mortality.[114] At present, the only indications for trying to maintain sinus rhythm in patients with CHF are persistent symptoms, a clear correlation between the development of AF, and deterioration in CHF status or failure to achieve rate control.[115] The combination of digoxin with carvedilol is logical and effective in reducing the ventricular rate and increasing the EF.[116] It has been suggested that ablation therapy for sinus-rhythm maintenance may improve the cardiac function and prognosis in CHF patients.[117] A small randomized study that was underpowered showed no improvement with an AF-ablation approach.[118] Larger studies are ongoing.

Combinations of two AV-nodal blocking agents. Combinations of two AV-nodal blocking agents may be more effective than higher-dose therapy with a single drug and are required for optimal rate control in many patients, always excluding those with accessory paths (WPW). CCBs should be avoided in patients with CHF resulting from systolic dysfunction, but may add benefit in patients with hypertension and good systolic function. Adding digoxin may also allow lower doses of other AV nodal inhibitors.

Pacemakers. In some patients, it is not possible to achieve effective rate control during AF. Excess bradycardia or prolonged pauses causing syncope may prevent administration of therapy that would be effective for preventing or controlling rates during AF. Bradycardia during sleep or rest may limit control of rates during exercise or stress. Implantation of a permanent pacemaker may be required in such patients. Ablation of AV conduction and insertion of an adaptive rate pacemaker constitutes an effective strategy in patients in whom control of inappropriately rapid rates cannot be achieved with pharmacologic therapy alone. A dual-chamber pacemaker with mode switching during periods of AF may be used in patients with paroxysmal AF. A single-chamber pacemaker is used in patients with permanent AF. Thus *ablate and pace* is a useful alternative for rate control. In patients with baseline LV dysfunction that is not solely due to inadequate rate control, use of a resynchronization device can minimize the deleterious effects of right ventricular apical pacing.[119]

Ventricular preexcitation with atrial fibrillation. The combination of ventricular preexcitation with AF presents a unique problem (see *WPW*, Fig. 8-14). Agents acting primarily on the AV node may paradoxically increase ventricular rates either by shortening the effective refractory period of the accessory pathway or by eliminating concealed conduction into the accessory pathway. Agents that prolong the anterograde refractory period of the accessory pathway (e.g., procainamide, flecainide, and amiodarone) should be used both for rate control and to achieve conversion, but urgent electrical cardioversion is often necessary.

Therapy for acute rate control. Intravenous therapy is usually employed in patients who present acutely with severe symptoms. In this situation, rapid relief of these symptoms is important. Except in patients with preexcitation WPW, rate control is usually achieved with drugs that act primarily on the AV node (Table 8-7). *Digoxin* has historically been the drug of choice for rate control in AF, but its onset of rate-slowing action is delayed and it is ineffective for pharmacologic cardioversion.[107,120,121] *β-blockers* will all slow ventricular rates in AF, and many are available as intravenous, oral short-acting, or oral long-acting preparations (see Table 1-3). Sotalol, a β-blocker with a class III activity, should not be given acutely because of risk of torsades. The

AV NODAL RE-ENTRY VERSUS WPW

Opie 2012

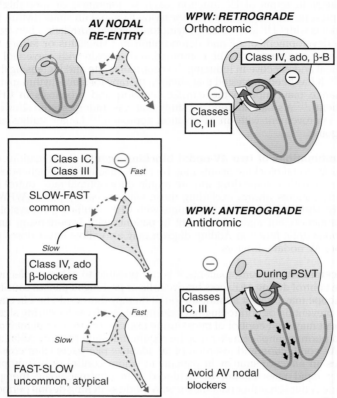

Figure 8-14 Atrioventricular (AV) nodal reentry and Wolff-Parkinson-White (WPW) or preexcitation syndrome. The *top left panel* shows AV nodal reentry without WPW. The common pattern is slow-fast (*middle panel*), whereas fast-slow conduction (*bottom left panel*) is uncommon. The slow and fast fibers of the AV node are artificially separated for diagrammatic purposes. The right panel shows WPW with the bypass tract as a white band. During paroxysmal supraventricular tachycardia (PSVT), when anterograde conduction occurs over the AV node and retrograde conduction most commonly through the accessory pathway, the QRS pattern should be normal (orthodromic supraventricular tachycardia [SVT], *top right panel*). Less commonly, the accessory pathway is used as the anterograde limb and the AV node (or a second accessory pathway) is the retrograde limb (antidromic SVT, *bottom right panel*). The QRS pattern shows the pattern of full preexcitation. In such preexcited atrial tachycardias, agents that block the AV node may enhance conduction over the accessory pathway to the ventricles (*red downward arrows*), leading to rapid ventricular rates that predispose to ventricular fibrillation. Sites of action of various classes of antiarrhythmics are indicated. *Ado,* Adenosine; *β-B,* β-blocker. (Figure © L.H. Opie, 2012.)

nondihydropyridine CCBs, verapamil and diltiazem, reduce heart rates in AF during both rest and exercise. For patients with severe heart failure or marked hemodynamic instability, electrical cardioversion may be required. Intravenous amiodarone is also a pharmacologic option for rate control,[122] with the added advantage that it may facilitate rhythm reversion.

Restoration and maintenance of sinus rhythm. Restoration and maintenance of sinus rhythm is the alternate management strategy in patients with AF. Intuitively, patients feel better when in sinus rhythm, as

Table 8-7

Drug Loading and Maintenance Regimens for Control of Ventricular Rate in Atrial Fibrillation			
		Acute Intravenous Therapy	**Chronic Oral Therapy**
β-blockers	Metoprolol	2.5-5 mg every 5 min up to 15 mg	50-200 mg/day
	Propranolol	0.15 mg/kg (1 mg every 2 min)	40-240 mg/day
	Esmolol	0.5 mg bolus, then 0.05-0.2 mg/kg per min	NA
	Pindolol	NA	7.5-30 mg/day
	Atenolol	5 mg over 5 min, repeat in 10 min	25-100 mg/day
	Nadolol	NA	20-80 mg/day
Calcium-channel blockers	Verapamil	0.075-0.15 mg/kg over 2 min; 0.005 mg/kg per min	120-360 mg/day
	Diltiazem	0.25-0.35 mg/kg followed by 5-15 mg/hour	120-360 mg/day

NA, Not available.

Other β-blockers in addition to those listed may also be useful.

found in a nonrandomized observational study.[123] The agents used for conversion of acute episodes and for long-term prevention of recurrence of AF are listed in Table 8-8. Although early cardioversion can experimentally prevent tachycardia-driven atrial remodeling, such remodeling is only one component of the pathophysiologic characteristics of AF and *should not be an important consideration in decisions regarding the timing of cardioversion.*[102]

DC conversion for distressing acute-onset atrial fibrillation. DC electrical cardioversion is generally the procedure of choice for distressing acute-onset AF. Pharmacologic conversion is useful when DC

Table 8-8

Recommended Antiarrhythmic Drug Doses for Pharmacologic Cardioversion and Prevention of Recurrences of Atrial Fibrillation			
		IV or Oral Therapy for Rapid Conversion	**Chronic Oral Drug Therapy to Prevent Recurrence***
Class IA	Procainamide	500-1200 mg IV over 30-60 min	2000-4000 mg/day
Class IC	Flecainide	1.5-3.0 mg/kg IV over 10 min†; 200-400 mg orally	150-300 mg/day
	Propafenone	1.5-2 mg/kg IV over 10-20 min†	400-600 mg/day
Class III	Ibutilide	1 mg IV over 10 min, repeat once	Not available
	Sotalol	Not recommended	160-320 mg/day
	Amiodarone	5-7 mg/kg IV over 30 min, then 1.2-1.8 g/day	400-1200 mg/day for 7 days, then taper to 100-300 mg/day
	Dofetilide	Insufficient data	125-500 mcg every 12 hours

IV, Intravenous.

*Initiation of oral therapy without loading may also result in conversion.

†Not available in North America.

cardioversion is not possible or has to be delayed. DC cardioversion stops AF in more than 90% of cases.[102] Potential complications include burns, iatrogenic VF (if shocks are not QRS synchronized), and the need for general anesthesia (in North America, or in some other countries if the patient is neuroleptic). Current guidelines give a class I recommendation for DC cardioversion for (1) a rapid ventricular response and ongoing myocardial ischemia, symptomatic hypotension, angina, or heart failure and no prompt response to pharmacologic agents (level of evidence: C); (2) AF involving preexcitation (WPW) with very rapid tachycardia or hemodynamic instability (level of evidence: B); and (3) symptoms unacceptable to the patient.[107]

Pharmacologic facilitation of DC cardioversion. Guidelines also suggest that pretreatment with amiodarone, flecainide, ibutilide, propafenone, or sotalol can facilitate DC cardioversion and prevent recurrent AF (evidence: class IIA, benefit is much decreased risk). In relapses to AF after successful cardioversion, repeating DC cardioversion after prophylactic drugs may be more successful (level of evidence: C).[107]

Pharmacologic conversion of AF. The drugs under consideration are summarized in Table 8-8. They may be used alone or with DC shocks to restore sinus rhythm. Drug therapy is superior to placebo in patients with AF of recent onset, but many episodes will terminate spontaneously without specific therapy within the initial 24 to 48 hours. Most studies suggest higher pharmacologic conversion rates in atrial flutter than in AF. The combined American and European guidelines (see their Table 13[107]) recommend four drugs: dofetilide, flecainide, ibutilide, and propafenone with a class IA recommendation for conversion of AF with a duration of 7 days or less.[107] Of these, dofetilide is only given orally and ibutilide only intravenously. Amiodarone was given a class IIA recommendation because of its delayed onset of action, but amiodarone may be useful in many patients because it also slows ventricular rates and, unlike the others, has no risk of postconversion ventricular arrhythmias. Quinidine was considered effective, but received a lower rating because of potential toxicity. All drugs are less effective in AF of more than 7 days in duration when oral dofetilide, requiring hospitalization, was the only agent given a class I recommendation. Vernakalant (see later) is a mixed channel blocker that has been developed for intravenous AF cardioversion.[124] It is highly effective, generally well tolerated, and available in more than 30 countries (many in Europe), but not yet in the United States.[125]

"Pill-in-the-pocket." Intermittent oral administration of single doses of flecainide (200 to 300 mg) or propafenone (450 to 600 mg) when an episode begins—the "pill-in-the-pocket technique"—may be effective in selected patients with AF and no structural heart disease.[22,126] The major potential complication of this approach is the possibility for organization and slowing of the arrhythmia to atrial flutter, which may then conduct with a 1:1 AV ratio at a very high ventricular rate. Intermittent drug self-administration should be used cautiously and only in patients likely to tolerate this potential proarrhythmic effect. The efficacy of this approach is often tested in a monitored setting before being used on an outpatient basis.

Maintenance of sinus rhythm after cardioversion. In most patients, AF proves to be a recurrent disorder. Unfortunately, the effectiveness of available antiarrhythmic agents is quite limited.[18,61,107] In patients with paroxysmal AF, reduction in the frequency and severity of episodes is the usual goal of therapy. In patients with persistent AF, prolongation of the interval between cardioversions is a reasonable target. Drugs from classes IA, IC, and III are more effective than placebo for maintaining sinus rhythm in patients with AF.[18,107] Only limited data are available comparing two or more agents in similar populations. In the Canadian Trial of Atrial Fibrillation (CTAF),[47] amiodarone was superior to sotalol or propafenone. In a substudy of the Atrial Fibrillation Follow-up Investigation of Rhythm Management (AFFIRM) trial, amiodarone was superior to both sotalol and a mixture of class I drugs.[46] In the Sotalol-Amiodarone Atrial Fibrillation Efficacy Trial (SAFE-T), amiodarone was superior to sotalol in the entire group, but the drugs had similar efficacy in the subgroup of patients with ischemic heart disease.[54]

Algorithm for drug choice for repeat or persistent atrial fibrillation. In patients with no or minimal structural heart disease, the first-line agents are flecainide, propafenone, or sotalol (see Fig. 8-14). Amiodarone or dofetilide are secondary options. In patients with CHF, only amiodarone and dofetilide are thought to be safe and effective. In patients with coronary artery disease, class IC agents are associated with increased mortality, so dofetilide or sotalol followed by amiodarone should be selected. In hypertensive patients without significant LV hypertrophy, flecainide, propafenone, or sotalol may be safely used as first-line agents followed by sotalol or dofetilide. In patients with significant LV hypertrophy, only amiodarone is recommended. By employing several drugs in sequence along with selective use of electrical cardioversion, 75% to 80% of patients with recent AF can maintain sinus rhythm for up to one year.[46]

Newer antiarrhythmic drugs for atrial fibrillation. *Vernakalant* (Kynapid, injectable) is a mixed potassium and sodium ion channel blocker now approved in Europe for acute conversion of AF to sinus rhythm. Contraindications are recent MI, advanced CHF, and obstructive heart disease. Hypotension is another risk. In a phase 3 trial, 336 patients with AF were given an infusion of vernakalant (3 mg/kg over 10 min, followed by a second infusion 15 min later if the arrhythmia had not terminated) resulting in a 52% conversion rate, versus 4% with placebo, in those with short duration of AF (3 hours to 7 days).[114] In patients with longer arrhythmia duration (8 to 45 days), vernakalant was much less successful (8% converted versus zero in the placebo group). A rare possible side effect was transient hypotension. There is no head-to-head comparison with DC cardioversion, which is now standard practice for acute onset AF, with some risks and discomforts, nor with dofetilide and ibutilide, which are the only other currently used drugs with Food and Drug Administration (FDA) approval for the conversion of AF, yet with risk of ventricular arrhythmias.

Dronedarone. Dronedarone (see previous) has structural similarities to amiodarone and a similar antiarrhythmic profile. Without containing iodine and with reduced lipophilicity, dronedarone has fewer adverse effects than amiodarone but is less effective for rhythm control in AF patients.[127] Dronedarone is widely available and is a useful addition to the clinical armamentarium for AF therapy, specifically after conversion to sinus rhythm, but major caution is required because of adverse effects in patients with heart failure and in those with permanent AF,[72] and because of toxic side effects.[71]

Proarrhythmia risk. This drug selection algorithm is heavily influenced by the potential for each drug to cause proarrhythmia in susceptible individuals. All agents, with the possible exception of dofetilide, may cause sinus node dysfunction or AV block. Atrial flutter with 1:1 conduction is a risk with flecainide, propafenone, and quinidine unless other agents are also used to block AV nodal conduction. Flecainide increased mortality in patients with ischemic heart disease and propafenone probably has a similar effect. Agents in classes IA and III prolong the QT interval and may result in polymorphic VT. Patients with LV hypertrophy and CHF are particularly susceptible to proarrhythmia during attempts at therapy for AF.

Postoperative atrial fibrillation. AF in the early postoperative period after cardiac surgery is often self-limited and may not require long-term therapy.[128] In untreated patients, the incidence may be 30% to 40% after coronary revascularization and is even higher in patients undergoing valve surgery. Based on data from randomized trials, short-term therapy with β-blockers and amiodarone, amiodarone alone, or CCBs decreases the incidence of AF.[56,128-130]

Invasive approaches to the maintenance of sinus rhythm. Given the disappointing results of pharmacologic therapy in the maintenance of sinus rhythm after cardioversion, there is growing interest in non-pharmacologic approaches. The initial surgical experience with the "corridor" and "maze" procedures[131] plus the observation that ectopic beats originating from a muscular sleeve surrounding the pulmonary vein orifices can initiate AF, paved the way for radiofrequency catheter-based ablation of AF.[132-136] Focal pulmonary vein stenosis was initially a major complication when lesions were placed within the veins themselves but newer techniques in which the pulmonary veins are circumferentially isolated, in conjunction with the placement of additional left atrial ablation lines, have resulted in a major improvement both in terms of procedural success and complication rates. The ideal candidates are younger patients with paroxysmal AF and without structural heart disease. However, with increased experience, radiofrequency ablation for AF may now be considered in older patients and in those with underlying structural heart disease.[132] There are now detailed recommendations for AF ablation therapy.[137] *Radiofrequency ablation* and antiarrhythmic drug therapy as first-line treatment for patients with paroxysmal atrial fibrillation were compared in a 2-year study. The two modalities were equally effective.[137A]

Predisposing causes. Left atrial size increases with LV hypertrophy and diastolic dysfunction, thereby predisposing to AF (see Fig. 8-11). Thus hypertension is an indirect but common predisposing cause of AF. These conditions should be sought and treated.

Renin-angiotensin inhibition. There is a lower prevalence of AF among patients treated with ACE inhibitors or angiotensin receptor blockers,[138] the proposed mechanisms being reversal of left atrial remodeling,[101] reduced atrial stretch, and lessened atrial fibrosis. To translate this into clinical practice requires results of prospective double-blind trials, one of which is testing the effects of telmisartan. Studies are also underway to determine if antiinflammatory agents will decrease the incidence or prevalence of AF.

Anticoagulation for atrial fibrillation. Nonvalvular AF is associated with an increased risk for stroke. Loss of atrial systolic function results in sluggish blood flow in the atrium. Atrial distention disturbs the atrial endothelium and activates hemostatic factors leading to a hypercoagulable state.[18,107,139] Several factors increase the risk for stroke in patients with AF. The primary risk factors are increased age, history of stroke or transient ischemic attack, hypertension, left atrial enlargement, diabetes, and CHF. The CHADS$_2$ scoring system[140] is now widely used and forms the basis for current guidelines.[107] In CHADS$_2$, one point is given for the following risk factors: recent CHF, hypertension, age older than 75, and diabetes; two points are given for a prior stroke. Patients with a CHADS$_2$ score of 0 should not require antithrombotic therapy. Considering conventional treatment by warfarin, patients with a score of 1 may be treated with either aspirin or warfarin. Patients with a CHADS$_2$ score of 2 or more should be treated with warfarin with a target INR of 2-3. Regarding patients more than 75 years old, the Birmingham Atrial Fibrillation Treatment of the Aged Study supported the use of warfarin, unless there are contraindications or the patient decides that the benefits are not worth the inconvenience.[141]

BRAIN PROTECTION IN ATRIAL FIBRILLATION

Opie 2012

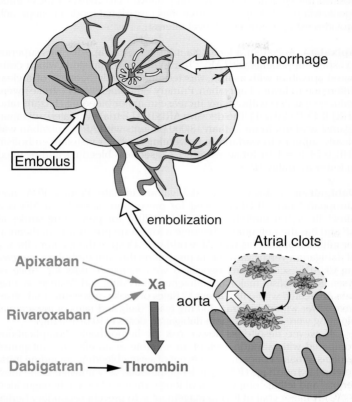

Figure 8-15   Brain protection in atrial fibrillation. Protection of the brain has become the focus of better control of embolization by the newer anti-thrombin and anti-Xa agents. (Figure © L.H. Opie 2012.)

New antithrombotics. In general, antithrombotics (see Fig. 9-10) have either been approved or are likely to be approved by the FDA and European authorities for stroke prevention in nonvalvular AF. The Canadian Cardiovascular Society Recommendations are that when oral anticoagulant therapy is indicated, the new anticoagulants are preferable to warfarin for most patients.[72] Three agents are listed alphabetically. The major problem with all three drugs is the risk of rare but potentially fatal uncontrollable bleeding. No studies in patients have yet assessed the ability of prohemostatic drugs to antagonize excess anticoagulant effects. Regardless of the relatively short half-life of these agents, immediate reversal of the anticoagulant effect may be needed in case of major bleeding or emergency surgery. The major positive aspects of these agents include the following: (1) no need for monitoring of INR, as required for warfarin; (2) reduced risk of adverse interactions following a change in diet or concomitant drugs; and (3) an enhanced ability to prevent strokes (Fig. 8-15).

Using early outcome data with the new agents, and drawing on data with nonvalvular AF from the Danish National Patient Registry, the *net clinical benefit* estimates the benefit of reducing ischemic stroke versus the risk of intracranial hemorrhage.[142] For patients at high risk as assessed by a modified $CHADS_2$ score, all three novel agents can be expected to provide at least as much benefit as warfarin in terms of stroke prevention and have less risk of intracranial hemorrhage by this model. In those at intermediate risk, the net clinical benefit is particularly favorable with apixaban and both doses of dabigatran (110 mg and 150 mg twice daily). For those at low risk, apixaban and dabigatran 110 mg twice daily had a positive net clinical benefit. As comparative trials between these three agents will probably never be done, this provisional modeling approach provides extrapolations of clinical interest.

Apixaban. Apixaban, a factor Xa inhibitor (see Fig. 9-10) was superior to aspirin in patients with AF.[143] The AVERROES trial study, which compared apixaban with aspirin, was terminated early because of a clear difference in favor of apixaban. Primary outcome events (stroke) were reduced (stroke) without any increase in major bleeding (hazard ratio [HR] 0.45; P < 0.001). The decisive ARISTOTLE trial evaluated apixaban against warfarin in more than 18,000 patients with AF.[144] Apixaban was clearly superior to warfarin in preventing stroke or systemic embolism (HR, 0.79; P = 0.01 for superiority), caused less bleeding, and resulted in lower mortality (P = 0.047).

Dabigatran. Dabigatran (as dabigatran-etexilate, Pradax, FDA- and European Union [EU]-approved for prevention of stroke in AF) is a direct thrombin inhibitor approved in 2010 for preventing stroke in AF and has the potential to become a long-term preventive medication for millions of patients with AF worldwide. Despite the greater efficacy of dabigatran versus warfarin in preventing thromboembolism, increasing $CHADS_2$ scores were associated with increased risks for stroke or systemic embolism, major and intracranial bleeding, and death in patients with AF treated with either agent.[145] Rates of stroke or systemic embolism were lower with dabigatran, 150 mg twice daily, and rates of intracranial bleeding were lower with both dabigatran doses (110 or 150 mg).

However, despite its lower risk of hemorrhagic complications compared with warfarin, lack of an antidote or an effective antagonist remains a major concern in the event of severe bleeding, including intracerebral hemorrhage (ICH). The latter, although very unusual, is the most serious and lethal complication of long-term use of oral anticoagulation (OAC). A major goal of ICH management is to prevent secondary hematoma growth because hematoma size substantially affects outcome after ICH. In a murine model of OAC-ICH, hematoma expansion was limited by prothrombin complex concentrate (PCC).[146] The efficacy and safety of this strategy must be further evaluated in appropriate clinical studies.

Rivaroxaban. Rivaroxaban (FDA- and EU-approved for prevention of stroke in AF), an inhibitor of activated Xa (see Fig. 9-10), was an effective anticoagulant in 14,264 patients with nonvalvular AF, adjudged to be at increased risk of stroke in the ROCKET AF trial.[147] Rivaroxaban was noninferior to warfarin for the prevention of stroke or systemic embolism. The rivaroxaban group showed no difference from warfarin-treated patients in the risk of major bleeding, but intracranial hemorrhage (0.5% versus 0.7%, P = 0.02) and fatal bleeding (0.2% verus 0.5%, P = 0.003) were reduced.

Regarding the risk of unexpected bleeding, PCC could overcome the anticoagulant effect induced by thrombin and factor Xa inhibitors because PCC-4 contains the coagulation factors II, VII, IX, and X in a high concentration and in general enhances thrombin generation. In a randomized, double-blind, placebo-controlled study, 12 healthy male volunteers received rivaroxaban 20 mg twice daily (n = 6) or dabigatran 150 mg twice daily (n = 6) for 2½ days, followed by either a single bolus of 50 IU/kg PCC (Cofact) or a similar volume of saline. PCC immediately and completely reversed the anticoagulant effect of rivaroxaban in healthy subjects,[148] but had no influence on the anticoagulant action of dabigatran at the PCC dose used in this human study. However, there are no formal trials on patients with excess bleeding.

Practical considerations with warfarin. Separate guidelines for warfarin anticoagulation around the time of cardioversion have been published.[107,149] For cardioversion of acute episodes of less than 48 hours duration, warfarin anticoagulation is not required. For episodes of greater than 48 hours duration or when the duration is uncertain, 3 to 4 weeks of anticoagulation with warfarin (INR between 2 and 3) before cardioversion is recommended. Alternatively, a transesophageal ECG during anticoagulation can be used to exclude the presence of a left atrial thrombus. If none is found, cardioversion may be performed while anticoagulation is continued. Even in patients without risk factors for stroke, anticoagulation is maintained for at least 4 weeks after conversion. In the AFFIRM trial, the majority of strokes occurred in patients with either subtherapeutic INRs or those who were not on warfarin.[150] Furthermore, many brief recurrences of AF may be asymptomatic. Hence the current trend is for lifelong anticoagulation unless there is unequivocal proof that recurrences are not occurring. Randomized trials show the benefit of anticoagulation with warfarin in patients with nonvalvular AF; yet because warfarin therapy is fraught with potential complications, it is often difficult to judge when a patient's risk for stroke is high enough to warrant long-term warfarin therapy.[107,149,151] The availability of the new anticoagulants may alter risk/benefit ratios for anticoagulation and modify the indications compared with those established with warfarin; however, much more work needs to be done before this issue can be clarified.

Atrial Flutter

Traditionally, atrial flutter has been defined as a regular atrial rhythm with a rate between 250 and 350 bpm in the absence of antiarrhythmic drugs. Several EP mechanisms are responsible. The most common form, typical or classical atrial flutter, involves a macroreentrant circuit with a counterclockwise rotation in the right atrium.[152] This circuit passes through the isthmus between the inferior vena cava and the tricuspid valve. Atrial activity is seen on the ECG as negative flutter waves in the inferior leads II, III, and aVF. Less commonly, a reverse circuit involving a clockwise rotation occurs. These two forms are also called *isthmus-dependent flutters*. Other atrial rhythms at similar rates that do not require conduction through the isthmus are referred to as *atypical flutters*. Most clinical reports on the acute management of atrial flutter have included all types of flutter. Atrial flutter is also commonly associated with AF. There is an extensive literature concerning ablation therapy of atrial flutter and some studies on acute conversion rates, but most studies of long-term pharmacologic therapy have combined atrial flutter patients with those with AF.

Acute therapy. Patients with new-onset atrial flutter commonly are usually highly symptomatic. In the absence of antiarrhythmic drug therapy or disease in the AV conduction system, there is typically 2:1 AV conduction, because alternating atrial impulses either conduct normally or encounter the absolute refractory period of the AV node. There is therefore little concealed conduction in the AV node, and it is difficult to achieve stable control of ventricular rates by the modest increases in AV nodal refractory periods produced with AV nodal blocking agents. AV nodal blocking agents are, however, important adjuncts to protect against 1:1 AV conduction should drug therapy slow the atrial rate.[152]

Acute cardioversion. As with all reentrant arrhythmias, patients with severe symptoms or hemodynamic collapse during atrial flutter should be electrically cardioverted as soon as possible. Atrial flutter is associated with a significant thromboembolic risk, so the same concerns for precardioversion anticoagulation or the exclusion of atrial thrombus with transesophageal echocardiography applies as for AF in the absence of urgent hemodynamic indications.[153] Most patients can tolerate rates of 150 bpm or less during 2:1 or higher AV block. In such patients, either electrical or pharmacologic conversion may be chosen. Both synchronized DC shocks and overdrive atrial pacing are effective techniques for electrical conversion. Intravenous *ibutilide* (1 to 2 mg IV) is reported to correct 38% to 78% of episodes of atrial flutter.[75,78,107] Ibutilide should not be administered to patients with long QT interval or with significant hypokalemia or hypomagnesemia. The major complication of intravenous ibutilide is polymorphic VT with a long QT interval, in approximately 2% of individual trials. Patients with severe LV dysfunction (EF less than 0.21), LV hypertrophy, bradycardia, electrolyte imbalance, and prolonged QT intervals at baseline are at increased risk for developing polymorphic VT. Women are more susceptible than men.

Drug choice. Randomized, double-blind studies show that intravenous ibutilide is more effective than intravenous procainamide or sotalol.[18,75,78] Conversion to sinus rhythm, when it occurs, is seen within 60 minutes, and most commonly within 30 minutes, of the end of the infusion. Polymorphic VT also is seen principally during this interval; therefore monitoring for at least 4 hours is recommended. Class IC drugs and amiodarone, either intravenously or orally, are less effective than ibutilide. Dofetilide is also effective for converting atrial flutter, but an intravenous preparation is not currently available for clinical use.[154] If long-term antiarrhythmic therapy is not planned and there are no contraindications, intravenous ibutilide and electrical therapy are appropriate first-line choices. If long-term antiarrhythmic therapy is planned, it may be preferable to begin therapy with amiodarone, sotalol, dofetilide, or a class IC agent, often with an AV nodal blocking agent, with electrical cardioversion after 24 to 48 hours of therapy if a pharmacologic conversion does not occur.

Chronic therapy. There are insufficient data on chronic drug therapy of atrial flutter on which to base firm clinical recommendations. For patients with normal atrial anatomy and no history of AF, ablation to produce conduction block in the cavotricuspid isthmus is often preferable to drug therapy. In patients with a history of AF, flutter ablation may eliminate the flutter, but AF is likely to recur in the future.[155] Some patients who present with AF and then develop atrial flutter while on an antiarrhythmic drug will do well on drug therapy after flutter ablation. In patients with concomitant AF or abnormal atrial anatomy, chronic drug therapy as discussed previously, either alone or in combination with ablation therapy, is the best approach.

Anticoagulation for Atrial Flutter. Patients with atrial flutter are at risk for cardioembolic stroke and systemic embolism. Guidelines for anticoagulation during acute and chronic management are the same as those for patients with AF.[107,149]

Ventricular Arrhythmias

Acute management. VT with a stable uniform QRS morphologic structure is often referred to as *monomorphic VT.* Monomorphic VT can present in a variety of cardiac conditions and may be caused by several distinct EP mechanisms. Reentry related to scars (MI, surgical incisions, and fibrosis) is the most common mechanism seen clinically. Guidelines for pharmacologic management of sustained monomorphic VT are based almost exclusively on experience treating scar- or fibrosis-related arrhythmias.[156,157] Unless there is specific clinical information available to suggest another mechanism, therapy for patients with sustained monomorphic VT should be based on a presumed reentrant mechanism.

Hemodynamic status. The patient's hemodynamic status should determine the initial therapy used to terminate an episode of sustained monomorphic VT.[156] Patients who are unconscious, severely hypotensive, or highly symptomatic should be treated with synchronized DC shocks. Preadministration of an intravenous anesthetic agent or sedative should be used, if possible. Antiarrhythmic drug therapy, if used at all, in this situation is used to prevent recurrences. In patients with stable hemodynamics during sustained VT, pharmacologic termination may be considered. There are only a few randomized trials published dealing with VT termination. Griffith and colleagues[158] evaluated intravenous lidocaine (1.5 mg/kg), disopyramide (2 mg/kg, ≤ 150 mg), flecainide (2 mg/kg), and sotalol (1 mg/kg) in patients with sustained VT induced during EP studies. Of the 24 patients in the trial, 20 had coronary artery disease with a history of MI. Flecainide and disopyramide were the most effective agents for terminating VT, but especially flecainide was associated with significant side effects and neither would be appropriate chronic therapy in a patient with VT after MI. All drugs worked best in patients without prior infarctions. They recommended lidocaine as a first-line and disopyramide as a second-line drug.

Procainamide (see Table 8-3). Even though procainamide may be useful for terminating an acute episode of sustained VT, it is now almost never used as a single agent for chronic therapy.

Intravenous amiodarone. Intravenous amiodarone has been recommended for patients who present with sustained monomorphic VT.[156,157] Current guidelines suggest it should be preferred over procainamide in patients with severe LV dysfunction,[158] but published data concerning the efficacy of amiodarone for quickly terminating an episode of VT are limited. In one recent survey of the use of intravenous amiodarone in sustained monomorphic VT,[159] termination was seen in only 8 of 28 (29%) patients. The most common use of intravenous amiodarone is in patients with either incessant VT or frequent VT episodes.[160-162] In these patients, an initial intravenous bolus of 150 mg over 10 minutes is followed by an infusion of 360 mg (1 mg/minute) over the next 6 hours and 540 mg (0.5 mg/minute) over the remaining 18 hours. If given during incessant VT, the expected response will be gradual slowing of the VT cycle length with eventual termination. Transition to oral therapy can be made at any time.

Cardiac arrest and amiodarone. In patients with cardiac arrest caused by VF, amiodarone can be an *adjunct to defibrillation*. Two randomized controlled trials have addressed this issue. In the ARREST study,[60] intravenous amiodarone (300 mg) was given to patients not resuscitated after three or more precordial shocks, rather late in the resuscitation attempts (mean time, over 40 min). Patients who received amiodarone were more likely to survive to hospital admission (44% versus 34% with placebo, $P = 0.03$), but survival to hospital discharge was not significantly improved (13.4% versus 13.2%). The ALIVE study compared amiodarone (5 mg/kg estimated body weight) and lidocaine (1.5 mg/kg) in patients with out-of-hospital VF.[52] The mean interval from paramedic dispatch to drug administration was 25 ± 8 minutes. Amiodarone gave better survival to hospital admission (22.8% amiodarone versus 12% lidocaine). Survival to hospital discharge (5% amiodarone, 3% lidocaine) was not significantly improved. These two studies indicate that amiodarone may be useful for resuscitating some cardiac arrest victims. Antiarrhythmic therapy in this setting is an adjunct to defibrillation. Prevention of recurrent episodes of VT or VF after electrical termination is the primary reason for drug administration during resuscitation.

Chronic therapy of VT. Antiarrhythmic drugs can be used in patients with a history of sustained VT and cardiac arrest to decrease the probability of recurrence or to improve symptoms during a recurrence. However, in randomized trials, antiarrhythmic drug therapy has consistently proven inferior to ICDs as initial therapy.[41,163-166] In patients with life-threatening arrhythmias, antiarrhythmic drugs (particularly amiodarone) are often used in conjunction with ICDs to reduce the risk of ICD shocks (see section on ICDs, below).

Ventricular tachycardia in the absence of structural heart disease. In patients without structural heart disease, treatment of VT requires a different approach. The two most common types of monomorphic sustained VT in patients without structural heart disease arise in the RVOT or in the inferior LV septum and have characteristic ECG patterns and mechanisms.[167] When VT starts in the RVOT, the ECG will show a predominant left bundle block pattern with an inferior axis. This arrhythmia presents with both nonsustained bursts and, less commonly, sustained episodes that are often provoked by stress or exercise. The postulated mechanism is cAMP-mediated activity. Acutely, this arrhythmia responds to *intravenous β-blockers or verapamil*. Chronic oral therapy with agents like verapamil, β-blockers, flecainide, or propafenone can be effective, although ablation of the arrhythmogenic region is often preferred. In idiopathic left VT, calcium channel–dependent reentry occurs in or near the left posterior fascicle. The ECG shows a left-axis deviation and a right bundle branch block pattern. This arrhythmia terminates with verapamil administration, and *verapamil* is also the preferred choice for chronic therapy. Both these forms of VT are susceptible to catheter ablation (see Fig. 8-10) and many individuals prefer to undergo ablation as opposed to lifelong drug therapy, particularly because many of these patients are young.

Inherited long-QT syndrome and other channelopathies. There is a rapidly expanding fount of knowledge about arrhythmias caused by genetic mutations in ion channels.[168] For patients with an inherited LQTS, long-acting β-blockers (e.g., nadolol) are often effective, particularly in type 1 and also to some extent in type 2 LQTS.[169] Genotyping of individual patients is still not commonly available, but mutation-specific therapy for patients with LQTS and other genetically determined arrhythmias may be possible in the future.

ICDs for Prevention of Sudden Cardiac Death

Secondary Prevention

In patients with serious symptomatic postinfarct ventricular arrhythmias, trial data conclusively demonstrated the superiority of the ICD over drugs, primarily amiodarone.[170] However, ICD shocks are painful and best avoided. Hence antiarrhythmic drugs (particularly amiodarone) are often used in conjunction with an ICD in many patients, to decrease the need for shocks or to allow termination by antitachycardia pacing.[33] In the OPTIC Trial, amiodarone plus a β-blocker was better than a β-blocker or sotalol alone without major adverse effects on defibrillation threshold.[59,171] In practice β-blockade plus amiodarone is standard therapy for recurrent VT in ICD patients. Catheter ablation of the arrhythmogenic substrate is an effective approach[172] that is being increasingly applied.

Primary Prevention: Post–Myocardial Infarction

In the *primary* prevention of SCD in patients without symptomatic arrhythmias, five trials of patients with underlying coronary artery disease, almost all including patients with a prior history of MI (months to years previously) and low EFs, have provided guidelines. These are MADIT I,[173,174] MUSTT,[42] MADIT II,[175] SCD-HeFT[58] and DINAMIT.[176] What has been problematic and has led to a degree of inconsistency between guidelines has been the relatively wide range of EFs chosen for enrollment into different trials. Nonetheless, a consensus has emerged as reflected in current ICD guidelines.[177]

1. In patients with coronary artery disease and a documented prior MI (>40 days), New York Heart Association (NYHA) Class 2-3 CHF, ICD implantation is indicated in patients with an EF of 35% or less, irrespective of QRS width. This also applies to patients with inducible sustained arrhythmias on EP testing, approximately 4 weeks or more following MI. In patients with NYHA Class 1 symptoms, the evidence is less conclusive and a more stringent EF cut-off of 30% or less is recommended. In patients with an EF of 35% to 40%, invasive EP testing to assess inducibility remains an option although the use of the EP study is declining.

2. In patients with an EF of more than 40%, there is no need for further arrhythmia evaluation unless the patient is experiencing symptomatic palpitations, near syncope, or syncope. The problem arises in the extrapolation of these trials to predischarge survivors of an AMI, because the DINAMIT trial of patients 8-40 days post-MI was neutral.[176] The decision is further complicated by changes in the EF during the first 4 weeks after infarction, especially in patients receiving reperfusion therapy. This underlies current recommendations to wait at least 40 days before deciding whether to implant an ICD for primary prevention of SCD post-MI. The role of the ambulatory external defibrillator during the "waiting period" is currently the subject of an ongoing trial.

ICDs in Dilated Cardiomyopathy

The majority of prior trials were confined to patients with ischemic cardiomyopathy, but recent trials demonstrate that the results appear to apply equally to patients with nonischemic dilated cardiomyopathy although the results of the initial smaller trials were inconclusive.[44,178]

In the DEFINITE multicenter study on 458 patients with a mean EF of 21% and almost all on modern medical therapy including β-blockers and ACE inhibitors, the ICD substantially reduced arrhythmic but not all-cause mortality.[179] A large multicenter trial on approximately 2500 patients with heart failure, the Sudden Cardiac Death-Heart Failure Trial (SCD-HEFT), showed a 23% fall in mortality compared with placebo with ICD therapy but no difference with amiodarone treatment.[58] Results were equally impressive whether or not the origin of the heart failure was ischemic or nonischemic, which is the first time this has been shown. The consensus is that recommendations should be the same for patients with ischemic or nonischemic cardiomyopathy. Thus patients with NYHA Class 2-3 CHF, EFs lower than 35%, and nonischemic dilated cardiomyopathy are candidates for ICD implantation. In patients with Class 1 symptoms this remains a zone of some uncertainty because of a lack of data, and the EF cut-off is 30% or less. Class 4 CHF is a contraindication to ICD use unless the patient has met the requirements for CRT therapy.

In the future, more exact risk stratification will probably help guide the decision of whether to use an ICD. In the meantime, a practical point also discerned in SCD-HEFT[58] is that lack of β-blocker use is an important risk predictor of arrhythmia.[180] Of note, in those with severe LV dysfunction (mean EF only 21%) plus an arrhythmia marker, optimal medical therapy including β-blockade and ACE inhibition reduced the annual mortality to only 6% to 7%, and standard heart failure medications[179,180] are an essential adjunct to ICD implantation. In addition, in two post-MI trials in which there was no ICD aldosterone blockade reduced SCD (EPHESUS and RALES). Co-morbidities play an important role in deciding whether an ICD will improve survival.[181]

ICD Plus Cardiac Resynchronization Therapy

The previous arguments for ICD placement in selected patients with severe heart failure lead to a further question: Can added CRT by biventricular pacing do even better? This issue arises especially in those with a prolonged QRS interval, who in their own right are candidates for resynchronization. In the large COMPANION study this combination of devices reduced all-cause mortality in those with class III or IV chronic heart failure (QRS interval ≥120 milliseconds) by 36% (Fig. 8-16).[182] Unfortunately, the effect of an ICD alone was not assessed, so that this combined approach is not yet firmly established. CRT acts in complex ways to achieve some remodeling of the failing left ventricle, which in itself may reduce the incidence of SCD.[183] Although CRT gave benefit in some studies even with a "narrow" QRS, a wide QRS means a greater likelihood of mechanical delay and thus a greater potential for success.[184,185]

ICD Shocks: Antiarrhythmic Drug Prophylaxis

ICDs deliver high-voltage shocks to terminate potentially fatal ventricular arrhythmias. Shocks may also be caused by atrial arrhythmias. Modern dual-chamber ICDs are able to terminate some ventricular arrhythmias, thereby reducing but not eliminating shocks, which still occur especially in the first year after ICDS implant.[59] Although β-blockade is standard therapy, the combination with amiodarone is much better.[59]

ICD PREVENTION OF SUDDEN DEATH

Opie 2012

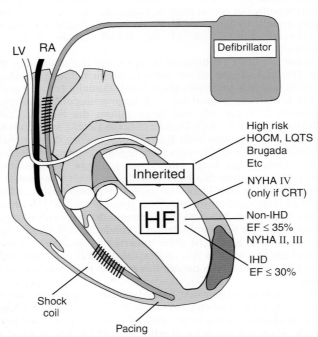

Figure 8-16 Suggested policy for use of implantable cardioverter defibrillator to prevent sudden cardiac death, including patients with ischemic heart disease (IHD) and heart failure (HF). The implantable automatic defibrillator is an electronic device designed to detect and treat life-threatening tachyarrhythmias. The device consists of a pulse generator and electrodes for sensing and defibrillating. *CRT,* cardiac resynchronization therapy; *EF,* ejection fraction; *HOCM,* hypertrophic obstructive cardiomyopathy; *LQTS,* long-QT syndrome; *LV,* left ventricular; *NYHA,* New York Heart Association; *R,* Right atrial. For further details see Epstein A et al., 2008. (Figure © L.H. Opie, 2012.)

SUMMARY

1. *Antiarrhythmic drug classification.* These are grouped into four classes: class I, sodium channel blockers; class II, β-adrenergic blockers; class III, repolarization blockers; and class IV, those agents that block the calcium current in the AV node, such as some CCBs (verapamil and diltiazem) and adenosine. Class I agents are used less and less because of adverse long-term effects, except for the acute use of intravenous lidocaine or procainamide, and agents that are safe only in the absence of structural heart disease (flecainide and propafenone). Class II, the β-blockers, are especially effective in hyperadrenergic states such as chronic heart failure, some repetitive tachycardias, and ischemic arrhythmias. Among class III agents, amiodarone is a powerful antiarrhythmic agent, acting on both supraventricular and ventricular arrhythmias, but potentially toxic, sometimes even when used in a very low dose, and therefore often not regarded as a first-line agent except when intravenously given as in cardiac arrest. Class IV agents are excellent in arresting acute supraventricular tachycardias (adenosine is preferred), and also reduce ventricular rates in chronic AF (verapamil and diltiazem).

2. *Current trends in arrhythmia therapy.* The complexity of the numerous agents available and the ever-increasing problems with side effects and proarrhythmic events have promoted a strong trend toward intervention by ablation or devices. For example, an ICD is now increasingly used in the presence of severe heart failure.

3. *Supraventricular arrhythmias.* In terms of drug effects, the acute therapy of supraventricular arrhythmias is assuming an increasingly rational basis with a prominent role for adenosine, verapamil, or diltiazem in inhibition of supraventricular tachycardias involving conduction through the AV node. Sodium blockers can inhibit the bypass tract or retrograde fast AV nodal conduction, as can class III agents, such as sotalol or amiodarone. Ablation is increasingly used for long-term management of most symptomatic cases of SVT.

4. *Atrial flutter.* Ibutilide, given intravenously, or dofetilide, given orally, are effective for drug-induced reversion of atrial flutter. These should not be given to patients at risk of torsades de pointes (check QT interval, electrolyte status, and other drugs taken). Cardioversion is often the treatment of choice. Ibutilide sensitizes the flutter to the effects of cardioversion. Ablation is often chosen for chronic therapy.

5. *Acute-onset AF.* For acute-onset AF, control of the ventricular rate can be achieved by AV nodal inhibitors, such as verapamil or diltiazem, or intravenous β-blockade by esmolol, metoprolol, or propranolol, or by combinations. Pharmacologic conversion can usually be achieved by intravenous ibutilide or, if there is no structural heart disease, flecainide or propafenone. Note the risk of postconversion ventricular arrhythmias. Amiodarone has a slower onset of action, but also slows the heart rate and has no postconversion ventricular arrhythmias. If drugs fail to restore sinus rhythm, DC defibrillation given externally or (even better) transvenously has a very high success rate.

6. *Recurrent AF: rate control.* For patients with recurrent forms of AF, the choice between rate and rhythm control is never easy. With either policy, optimal anticoagulation should be continued indefinitely because many episodes of AF are asymptomatic and unsuspected. The AFFIRM and smaller European trials have, however, changed practice by showing that rate control has similar outcomes to rhythm control. *One practical policy* is to attempt cardioversion for the first episode of AF. Then if this arrhythmia returns and is asymptomatic, rate control is in order. In the absence of heart failure, the drugs of choice are β-blockers, rate-lowering CCBs (verapamil and diltiazem), or combination therapy, with digoxin for selected patients. In those with heart failure, the rate-lowering CCBs are omitted, leaving β-blockers with or without digoxin. In those with coronary artery disease, β-blockers and rate-lowering CCBs are preferred because of their concomitant antianginal actions. Radiofrequency ablation of the AV node (followed by pacing) is increasingly selected for patients who find drugs difficult or who are refractory to their effects.

7. *Algorithm for rhythm control for recurrent or persistent AF.* In patients with normal systolic function and no history of heart failure, the first-line agents are flecainide, propafenone, or sotalol. Thereafter, amiodarone becomes a secondary option, in view of its potentially serious side effects. Use of dronedarone is now more limited because of recent warnings about the risk of serious organ side effects, although it can nevertheless be quite useful in selected patients.

8. *Rhythm control for patients with a history of heart failure or with LV systolic dysfunction.* If the EF is more than 35%, then amiodarone or sotalol are the choices. If the EF is 35% or less, amiodarone is chosen. Repeated cardioversion may also be required. There may be a rapidly firing pulmonary vein focus that responds to ablation.

9. *Chronic AF.* Here again the choice is between rate and rhythm control with careful anticoagulation. However, defibrillation is less likely when AF is more than 7 days in duration when dofetilide is chosen.

10. *New anticoagulant agents for chronic AF.* The major recent advance has been the introduction of the new specific anticoagulants, dabigatran as an antithrombin agent and the antifactor Xa agents apixaban and rivaroxaban. These drugs have simple fixed doses that do not require monitoring. They reduce the risk of intracranial strokes or bleeding when compared with warfarin. Rarely, they may give rise to excess bleeding for which there is no clinically established therapeutic antidote. PCC may be tried without, however, any solid positive clinical evidence as yet.

11. *Ventricular arrhythmias.* Ventricular arrhythmias and their therapy remain controversial and constantly evolving. Antiarrhythmic drug therapy is only one avenue of overall management, as ICDs are increasingly used in severe ventricular arrhythmias, especially when the EF is low. Moreover, antiarrhythmic drugs have been disappointing in preventing SCD, other than β-blockers and other antifailure drugs. A distinction must be made between suppression of premature ventricular complexes, which is useless (unless causing persistent symptoms) and the control of VT and VF, which can prolong life. In acute AMI, lidocaine is no longer given prophylactically. In postinfarct patients, β-blockers remain the drugs of choice, although amiodarone has good evidence in its favor. ICDs are now the standard of choice in selected patients.

12. *ICDs.* In CHF, optimal management of the hemodynamic and neurohumoral status, including the use of ACE inhibitors and β-blockade, must be instituted before the prophylactic use of antiarrhythmic drugs or an ICD. In severe heart failure, ICD therapy is probably the single most important aspect of antiarrhythmic therapy. The combination of ICD and cardiac resynchronization by biventricular pacing is increasingly considered, especially when there is QRS prolongation.

13. *Hybrid pharmacologic drugs and device or ablation therapy.* Hybrid pharmacologic drugs and device or ablation therapy are options increasingly used for disabling AF or for severe and serious ventricular arrhythmias. Thus β-blockade and amiodarone may be combined with ICDs to give optimal results.

14. *New antiarrhythmic agents.* New agents have been investigated in recent years. Most have been variations of the class IC or class III drugs that are already available. In many instances the assessment of these drugs has revealed a negative benefit-risk ratio. Only ibutilide and dofetilide have so far been approved for clinical use. Ibutilide is given intravenously and dofetilide orally. Both benefit atrial tachyarrhythmias, yet both have prominent warnings regarding torsades. Dronedarone has proven value in preventing hospitalizations and reducing cardiovascular death rates in patients with paroxysmal and persistent cardioverted AF, but concerns have been raised by risk profiles in permanent-AF patients and those with a history of heart failure.

References

1. Curtis AB, et al. Arrhythmias in women. *Clin Cardiol* 2012;35:166–171.
2. CAST Investigators. Preliminary report: effect of encainide and flecainide on mortality in randomized trial of arrhythmia suppression after myocardial infarction. The Cardiac Arrhythmia Suppression Trial (CAST) Investigators. *N Engl J Med* 1989;321:406–412.
3. Teo KK, et al. Effects of prophylactic antiarrhythmic drug therapy in acute myocardial infarction. An overview of results from randomized controlled trials. *JAMA* 1993;270:1589–1595.
4. Arshad A, et al. New antiarrhythmic drugs for treatment of atrial fibrillation. *Lancet* 2010;375:1212–1223.
5. Nattel S, et al. What is an antiarrhythmic drug? From clinical trials to fundamental concepts. *Am J Cardiol* 1990;66:96–99.
6. Das MK, et al. Antiarrhythmic and nonantiarrhythmic drugs for sudden cardiac death prevention. *J Cardiovasc Pharmacol* 2010;55:438–449.
7. Sheldon R, et al. On behalf of the CIDS Investigators. Identification of patients most likely to benefit from implantable cardioverter-defibrillator therapy. The Canadian Implantable Defibrillator Study. *Circulation* 2000;101:1660–1664.
8. Task Force of the Working Group on Arrhythmias of the European Society of Cardiology. The Sicilian Gambit. A new approach to the classification of antiarrhythmic drugs based on their actions on arrhythmogenic mechanisms. *Circulation* 1991;84:1831–1851.
9. Parmley W, et al. Attenuation of the circadian patterns of myocardial ischemia with nifedipine GITS in patients with chronic stable angina. *J Am Coll Cardiol* 1992; 19:1380–1389.
10. Sadowski ZP, et al. Multicenter randomized trial and systemic overview of lidocaine in acute myocardial infarction. *Am Heart J* 1999;137:792–798.
11. ACC/AHA Guidelines, Ryan TK, et al. ACC/AHA guidelines for the management of patients with acute myocardial infarction: Executive summary. *Circulation* 1996; 94: 2341–2350.
12. Piccini JP, et al. Antiarrhythmic drug therapy for sustained ventricular arrhythmias complicating acute myocardial infarction. *Crit Care Med* 2011;39:78–83.
13. CASH Study, Siebels J, et al. Preliminary results of the Cardiac Arrest Study Hamburg (CASH). *Am J Cardiol* 1993;72:109–113.
14. Reiffel JA, et al. The actions of ibutilide and class Ic drugs on the slow sodium channel: new insights regarding individual pharmacologic effects elucidated through combination therapies. *J Cardiovasc Pharmacol Ther* 2000;5:177–181.
15. Cahill SA, et al. Propafenone and its metabolites preferentially inhibit I_{Kr} in rabbit ventricular myocytes. *J Pharmacol Exp Ther* 2004;308:59–65.
16. Hwang HS, et al. Inhibition of cardiac Ca2+ release channels (RyR2) determines efficacy of class I antiarrhythmic drugs in catecholaminergic polymorphic ventricular tachycardia. *Circ Arrhythm Electrophysiol* 2011;4:128–135.
17. Reiffel JA, et al. Sotalol for ventricular tachyarrhythmias; beta blocking and class III contributions, and relative efficacy versus class 1 drugs after prior drug failure. *Am J Cardiol* 1997;79:1048–1053.
18. McNamara RL, et al. Management of atrial fibrillation: review of the evidence for the role of pharmacologic therapy, electrical cardioversion, and echocardiography. *Ann Intern Med* 2003;139:1018–1033.
19. Ruffy R. Flecainide. *Electrophysiol Rev* 1998;2:191–193.

20. UK Propafenone PSVT Study Group. A randomized, placebo-controlled trial of propafenone in the prophylaxis of paroxysmal supraventricular tachycardia and paroxysmal atrial fibrillation. *Circulation* 1995;92:2550–2557.
21. Kochiadakis GE, et al. Amiodarone versus propafenone for conversion of chronic atrial fibrillation: results of a randomized, controlled study. *J Am Coll Cardiol* 1999;33:966–971.
22. Boriani G, et al. Oral propafenone to convert recent-onset atrial fibrillation in patients with and without underlying heart disease. A randomized, controlled trial. *Ann Intern Med* 1997;126:621–625.
23. Joglar JA, et al. Propafenone. *Cardiac Electrophysiol Rev* 1998;28:204–206.
24. Ellison KE, et al. Effect of beta-blocking therapy on outcome in the Multicenter UnSustained Tachycardia Trial (MUSTT). *Circulation* 2002;106:2694–2699.
25. Dargie HJ. Beta blockers in heart failure. *Lancet* 2003;362:2–3.
26. CIBIS II Study. The Cardiac Insufficiency Bisoprolol Study II (CIBIS-II): a randomised trial. *Lancet* 1999; 353:9–13.
27. MERIT-HF Study Group. Effect of metoprolol CR/XL in chronic heart failure: Metoprolol CR/XL Randomized Trial in Congestive Heart Failure (MERIT-HF). *Lancet* 1999;353: 2001–2007.
28. Exner DV, et al. Beta-blocker use and survival in patients with ventricular fibrillation or symptomatic ventricular tachycardia: The Antiarrhythmics Versus Implantable Defibrillators (AVID) Trial. *J Am Coll Cardiol* 1999;34:325–333.
29. Boutitie F, et al. Amiodarone interactions with beta-blockers. Analysis of the merged EMIAT (European Myocardial Infarct Trial) and CAMIAT (Canadian Amiodarone Myocardial Infarct Trial) databases. *Circulation* 1999;99:2268–2275.
30. Nademanee K, et al. Treating electrical storm: sympathetic blockade versus advanced cardiac life support-guided therapy. *Circulation* 2000;102:742–747.
31. Wiest D. Esmolol. A review of its therapeutic efficacy and pharmacokinetic characteristics. *Clin Pharmacokinet* 1995;28:190–202.
32. Manz M, et al. Interactions between drugs and devices: experimental and clinical studies. *Am Heart J* 1994;127:978–984.
33. Pacifico A, et al. Prevention of implantable-defibrillator shocks by treatment with sotalol. d,l-Sotalol Implantable Cardioverter-Defibrillator Study Group. *N Engl J Med* 1999;340: 1855–1862.
34. Gottlieb SS, et al. Effect of beta-blockade on mortality among high-risk and low-risk patients after myocardial infarction. *N Engl J Med* 1998;339:489–497.
35. ESVEM Investigators. Electrophysiologic Study Versus Electrocardiographic Monitoring for selection of antiarrhythmic therapy of ventricular tachycardia. *Circulation* 1989;70: 1354–1360.
36. Steinbeck G, et al. A comparison of electrophysiologically guided antiarrhythmic drug therapy with beta-blocker therapy in patients with symptomatic, sustained ventricular tachyarrhythmias. *N Engl J Med* 1992;327:987–992.
37. ESVEM Investigators, Mason JW. For the Electrophyisiologic Study Versus Electrocardiographic Monitoring Investigators. A comparison of seven antiarrhythmic drugs in patients with ventricular tachyarrhythmias. *N Engl J Med* 1993;329:452–458.
38. Julian DG, et al. Randomized trial of effect of amiodarone on mortality in patients with left ventricular dysfunction after recent myocardial infarction. EMIAT. *Lancet* 1997;347: 667–674.
39. Cairns JA, et al. Randomised trial of outcome after myocardial infarction in patients with frequent or repetitive ventricular premature depolarisations: CAMIAT. Canadian Amiodarone Myocardial Infarction Arrhythmia Trial Investigators. *Lancet* 1997;349:675–682.
40. Moss AJ, et al. For the Multicenter Automatic Defibrillator Implantation Trial (MADITT) Investigators. Improved survival with an implanted defibrillator in patients with coronary artery disease at high risk for ventricular arrhythmia. *N Engl J Med* 1996;335: 1933–1940.
41. AVID Investigators. A comparison of antiarrhythmic-drug therapy with implantable defibrillators in patients resuscitated from near-fatal ventricular arrhythmias. *N Engl J Med* 1997;337:1576–1583.
42. MUSTT Investigators, Buxton AE, et al. For the Multicenter Unsustained Tachycardia Trial (MUSTT) Investigators. A randomized study of the prevention of sudden death in patients with coronary artery disease. *N Engl J Med* 1999;341:1882–1890.
43. Moss AJ, et al. Prophylactic implantation of a defibrillator in patients with myocardial infarction and reduced ejection fraction. *N Engl J Med* 2002;346:877–883.
44. Strickberger SA, et al. Amiodarone versus implantable cardioverter-defibrillator: randomized trial in patients with nonischemic dilated cardiomyopathy and asymptomatic nonsustained ventricular tachycardia—AMIOVIRT. *J Am Coll Cardiol* 2003;41:1707–1712.
45. Connolly SJ. Evidence-based analysis of amiodarone efficacy and safety. *Circulation* 1999;100:2025–2034.
46. AFFIRM Investigators. First Antiarrhythmic Drug Substudy. Maintenance of sinus rhythm in patients with atrial fibrillation. *J Am Coll Cardiol* 2003;42:20–29.
47. Roy D, et al. Amiodarone to prevent recurrence of atrial fibrillation. Canadian Trial of Atrial Fibrillation Investigators. *N Engl J Med* 2000;342:913–920.
48. Sicouri S, et al. Potent antiarrhythmic effects of chronic amiodarone in canine pulmonary vein sleeve preparations. *J Cardiovasc Electrophysiol* 2009;20:803–810.
49. Shinagawa K, et al. Effects of antiarrhythmic drugs on fibrillation in the remodeled atrium: insights into the mechanism of the superior efficacy of amiodarone. *Circulation* 2003;107:1440–1446.
50. Nattel S. Pharmacodynamic studies of amiodarone and its active N-desethyl metabolite. *J Cardiovasc Pharmacol* 1986;8:771–777.
51. Zimetbaum P. Amiodarone for atrial fibrillation. *N Engl J Med* 2007;356:935–941.

52. Nademanee K, et al. Amiodarone and post-MI patients. *Circulation* 1993;88:764–774.
53. Dorian P, et al. Amiodarone as compared with lidocaine for shock-resistant ventricular fibrillation. *N Engl J Med* 2002;346:884–890.
54. Singh BN, et al. Amiodarone versus sotalol for atrial fibrillation. *N Engl J Med* 2005; 352:1861–1872.
55. Jong GP, et al. Long-term efficacy and safety of very-low-dose amiodarone treatment for the maintenance of sinus rhythm in patients with chronic atrial fibrillation after successful direct-current cardioversion. *Chin Med J* (Engl) 2006;119:2030–2035.
56. Crystal E, et al. Atrial fibrillation after cardiac surgery: update on the evidence on the available prophylactic interventions. *Card Electrophysiol Rev* 2003;7:189–192.
57. Amiodarone Trials-Meta-Analysis Investigators (ATMAI). Effect of prophylactic amiodarone on mortality after acute myocardial infarction and in congestive heart failure; meta-analysis of individual data from 6500 patients in randomized trials. *Lancet* 1997; 350:1417–1424.
58. Bardy GH, et al. Amiodarone or an implantable cardioverter-defibrillator for congestive heart failure. *N Engl J Med* 2005;352:225–237.
59. Connolly SJ, et al. Comparison of beta-blockers, amiodarone plus beta-blockers, or sotalol for prevention of shocks from implantable cardioverter defibrillators: the OPTIC Study: a randomized trial. *JAMA* 2006;295:165–171.
60. Kudenchuk PJ, et al. Amiodarone for resuscitation after out-of-hospital cardiac arrest due to ventricular fibrillation. *N Engl J Med* 1999;341:871–878.
61. Lafuente-Lafuente C, et al. Antiarrhythmic drugs for maintaining sinus rhythm after cardioversion of atrial fibrillation: a systematic review of randomized controlled trials. *Arch Intern Med* 2006;166:719–728.
62. Vassallo P, et al. Prescribing amiodarone: an evidence-based review of clinical indications. *JAMA* 2007;298:1312–1322.
63. Conen D, et al. Amiodarone-induced thyrotoxicosis: clinical course and predictors of outcome. *J Am Coll Cardiol* 2007;49:2350–2355.
64. Batcher EL, et al. Thyroid function abnormalities during amiodarone therapy for persistent atrial fibrillation. *Am J Med* 2007;120:880–885.
65. Vorperian VR, et al. Adverse effects of low dose amiodarone: a meta-analysis. *J Am Coll Cardiol* 1997;30:791–798.
66. Doval HC, et al. Randomised trial of low-dose amiodarone in severe congestive heart failure. Grupo de Estudio de la Sobrevida en la Insuficiencia Cardiaca en Argentina (GESICA). *Lancet* 1994;344:493–498.
67. Kato R, et al. Electrophysiologic effects of the levo- and dextrorotatory isomers of sotalol in isolated cardiac muscle and their in vivo pharmacokinetics. *JACC* 1986;7:116–125.
68. SWORD Investigators, Waldo AL, et al. Prevention of sudden death in patients with LV dysfunction after myocardial infarction. The SWORD trial. *Lancet* 1996;348:7–12.
69. Connolly SJ, for the PALLAS Investigators. Dronedarone in high-risk permanent atrial fibrillation. *N Engl J Med* 2011;365(24):2268–2276.
70. Opie LH. Dronedarone in high-risk permanent atrial fibrillation. *N Engl J Med* 2012; 366(12):1159.
71. Elgazaverly AN, et al. Dronedarone in high-risk permanent atrial fibrillation. *N Engl J Med* 2012;366:1160–1161.
72. Skanes AC, et al. Focused 2012 update of the Canadian Cardiovascular Society atrial fibrillation guidelines: recommendations for stroke prevention and rate/rhythm control. *Can J Cardiol* 2012;28:125–136.
73. Murray KT. Ibutilide. *Circulation* 1998;97:493–497.
74. Bernard EO, et al. Ibutilide versus amiodarone in atrial fibrillation: a double-blinded, randomized study. *Crit Care Med* 2003;31:1031–1034.
75. Stambler BS, et al. Efficacy and safety of repeated doses of ibutilide for rapid conversion of atrial flutter or fibrillation. *Circulation* 1996;94:1613–1621.
76. Guo GB, et al. Conversion of atrial flutter by ibutilide is associated with increased atrial cycle length variability. *J Am Coll Cardiol* 1996;27:1083–1089.
77. VanderLugt J, et al. Efficacy and safety of ibutilide fumarate for the conversion of atrial arrhythmias after cardiac surgery. *Circulation* 1999;100:369–375.
78. Oral H, et al. Facilitating transthoracic cardioversion of atrial fibrillation with ibutilide pretreatment. *N Engl J Med* 1999;340:1849–1854.
79. Kowey PR, et al. Safety and risk/benefit analysis of ibutilide for acute conversion of atrial fibrillation/flutter. *Am J Cardiol* 1996;78 (Suppl. 8A):46–52.
80. Boriani G, et al. A multicentre, double-blind randomized crossover comparative study on the efficacy and safety of dofetilide vs sotalol in patients with inducible sustained ventricular tachycardia and ischaemic heart disease. *Eur Heart J* 2001;22:2180–2191.
81. Torp-Pedersen C, et al. Dofetilide in patients with congestive heart failure and left ventricular dysfunction. Danish Investigations of Arrhythmia and Mortality on Dofetilide Study Group. *N Engl J Med* 1999;341:857–865.
82. Brendorp B, et al. Survival after withdrawal of dofetilide in patients with congestive heart failure and a short baseline QTc interval; a follow-up on the Diamond-CHF QT substudy. *Eur Heart J* 2003;24:274–279.
83. Tzivoni D, et al. Treatment of torsade de pointes with magnesium sulfate. *Circulation* 1988;77:392–397.
84. DiMarco JP. Adenosine and digoxin. In Zipes DP, Jalife J, editors. *Cardiac electrophysiology: from cell to bedside.* 3rd ed. Philadelphia: Saunders; 2000. pp. 933–938.
85. Garratt CJ, et al. Use of intravenous adenosine in sinus rhythm as a diagnostic test for latent pre-exitation. *Am J Cardiol* 1990;65:868–873.
86. Jaeggi E, et al. Adenosine-induced atrial pro-arrhythmia in children. *Can J Cardiol* 1999;15:169–172.

87. Farkas AS, et al. Minimizing repolarization-related proarrhythmic risk in drug development and clinical practice. *Drugs* 2010;70:573–603.
88. Etheridge SP, et al. A new oral therapy for long QT syndrome: long-term oral potassium improves repolarization in patients with HERG mutations. *J Am Coll Cardiol* 2003;42: 1777–1782.
89. Priori SG, et al. Molecular biology of the long QT syndrome: impact on management. *Pacing Clin Electrophysiol* 1997;20:2052–2057.
90. Windle JR, et al. Normalization of ventricular repolarization with flecainide in long QT syndrome patients with SCN5A:DeltaKPQ mutation. *Ann Noninvasive Electrocardiol* 2001;6:153–158.
90A. Chockalingham P, et al. Not all beta-blockers are equal in the management of Long QT Syndrome Types 1 and 2: Higher recurrence of events under metoprolol. *J Am Coll Cardiol*, 2012, in press.
90B. Besana A, et al. Nadolol block of *Nav 1.5* does not explain its efficacy in the long QT syndrome. *J Cardiovasc Pharmacol* 2012;59:249.
90C. Priori SG, et al. The elusive link between LQT3 and Brugada syndrome: the role of flecainide challenge. *Circulation* 2000;102:945–947.
91. Blomstrom-Lundqvist C, et al. ACC/AHA/ESC guidelines for the management of patients with supraventricular arrhythmias—executive summary: a report of the American College of Cardiology/American Heart Association Task Force on Practice Guidelines and the European Society of Cardiology Committee for Practice Guidelines (Writing Committee to Develop Guidelines for the Management of Patients With Supraventricular Arrhythmias). *Circulation* 2003;108:1871–1909.
92. Ferguson JD, et al. Contemporary management of paroxysmal supraventricular tachycardia. *Circulation* 2003;107:1096–1099.
93. Hamer AW, et al. Failure of episodic high-dose oral verapamil therapy to convert supraventricular tachycardia: a study of plasma verapamil levels and gastric motility. *Am Heart J* 1987;114:334–342.
94. Alboni P, et al. Efficacy and safety of out-of-hospital self-administered single-dose oral drug treatment in the management of infrequent, well-tolerated paroxysmal supraventricular tachycardia. *J Am Coll Cardiol* 2001;37:548–553.
95. Dougherty AH, et al. Acute conversion of paroxysmal supraventricular tachycardia with intravenous diltiazem. IV Diltiazem Study Group. *Am J Cardiol* 1992;70:587–592.
96. Epstein ML, et al. Cardiac decompensation following verapamil therapy in infants with supraventricular tachycardia. *Pediatrics* 1985;75:737–740.
97. DiMarco JP, et al. Adenosine for paroxysmal supraventricular tachycardia: dose ranging and comparison with verapamil. Assessment in placebo-controlled, multicenter trials. The Adenosine for PSVT Study Group. *Ann Intern Med* 1990;113:104–110.
98. Akhtar M, et al. Role of adrenergic stimulation by isoproterenol in reversal of effects of encainide in supraventricular tachycardia. *Am J Cardiol* 1988;62:45L–49L.
99. Dorian P, et al. A randomized comparison of flecainide versus verapamil in paroxysmal supraventricular tachycardia. The Flecainide Multicenter Investigators Group. *Am J Cardiol* 1996;77:89A–95A.
100. Scheinman M, et al. The 1998 NASPE prospective catheter ablation registry. *Pacing Clin Electrophysiol* 2000;23:1020–1028.
101. Casaclang-Verzosa G, et al. Structural and functional remodeling of the left atrium: clinical and therapeutic implications for atrial fibrillation. *J Am Coll Cardiol* 2008;51:1–11.
102. Nattel S, et al. Controversies in atrial fibrillation. *Lancet* 2006;367:262–272.
103. Spach MS. Mounting evidence that fibrosis generates a major mechanism for atrial fibrillation. *Circ Res* 2007;101:743–745.
104. Lip G, et al. Atrial fibrillation. In: Crawford M, DiMarco J, Paulus W, editors. *Cardiology*, 2nd ed. London: Elsevier; 2004. pp. 699–716.
105. Lip GY, et al. Management of atrial fibrillation. *Lancet* 2007;370:604–618.
106. Wattigney WA, et al. Increasing trends in hospitalization for atrial fibrillation in the United States, 1985 through 1999: implications for primary prevention. *Circulation* 2003;108:711–716.
107. Fuster V, et al. ACC/AHA/ESC 2006 guidelines for the management of patients with atrial fibrillation—executive summary: a report of the American College of Cardiology/ American Heart Association Task Force on Practice Guidelines and the European Society of Cardiology Committee for Practice Guidelines (Writing Committee to Revise the 2001 Guidelines for the Management of Patients With Atrial Fibrillation). *J Am Coll Cardiol* 2006;48:854–906.
108. Gallagher MM, et al. Classification of atrial fibrillation. *Am J Cardiol* 1998;82: 18N–28N.
109. Van Gelder IC, et al. Rate control efficacy in permanent atrial fibrillation: a comparison between lenient versus strict rate control in patients with and without heart failure. Background, aims, and design of RACE II. *Am Heart J* 2006;152:420–426.
110. Van Gelder IC, et al. Does intensity of rate-control influence outcome in atrial fibrillation? An analysis of pooled data from the RACE and AFFIRM studies. *Europace* 2006;8:935–942.
111. Van Gelder IC. For the RACE II Investigators. Lenient versus strict rate control in patients with atrial fibrillation. *N Engl J Med* 2010;362:1363–1373.
112. Snow V, et al. Management of newly detected atrial fibrillation: a clinical practice guideline from the American Academy of Family Physicians and the American College of Physicians. *Ann Intern Med* 2003;139:1009–1017.
113. Israel CW, et al. Long-term risk of recurrent atrial fibrillation as documented by an implantable monitoring device: implications for optimal patient care. *J Am Coll Cardiol* 2004;43:47–52.

114. Roy D, et al. A multicenter randomized trial of rhythm-control versus rate-control in patients with atrial fibrillation and congestive heart failure. *N Engl J Med* 2008;358: 2667–2677.

115. Roy D, et al. For the Atrial Arrhythmia Conversion Trial Investigators. Vernakalant hydrochloride for rapid conversion of atrial fibrillation: a phase 3, randomized, placebo-controlled trial. *Circulation* 2008;117:1518–1525.

116. Khand AU, et al. Carvedilol alone or in combination with digoxin for the management of atrial fibrillation in patients with heart failure? *J Am Coll Cardiol* 2003;42:1944–1951.

117. Hsu LF, et al. Catheter ablation for atrial fibrillation in congestive heart failure. *N Engl J Med* 2004;351:2373–2383.

118. MacDonald MR, et al. Radiofrequency ablation for persistent atrial fibrillation in patients with advanced heart failure and severe left ventricular systolic dysfunction: a randomised controlled trial. *Heart* 2011;97:740–747.

119. Doshi RN, et al. Left ventricular-based cardiac stimulation post AV nodal ablation evaluation (the PAVE study). *J Cardiovasc Electrophysiol* 2005;16:1160–1165.

120. Sarter BH,. Redefining the role of digoxin in the treatment of atrial fibrillation. *Am J Cardiol* 1992;69:71G–78G; discussion 78G–81G.

121. The Digitalis in Acute Atrial Fibrillation (DAAF) Trial Group. Intravenous digoxin in acute atrial fibrillation. Results in a randomized, placebo-controlled multicentre trial in 239 patients. *Eur Heart J* 1997;18:649–654.

122. Deedwania PC, et al. Spontaneous conversion and maintenance of sinus rhythm by amiodarone in patients with heart failure and atrial fibrillation: observations from the veterans affairs congestive heart failure survival trial of antiarrhythmic therapy (CHF-STAT). The Department of Veterans Affairs CHF-STAT Investigators. *Circulation* 1998;98:2574–2579.

123. Singh SN, et al. Quality of life and exercise performance in patients in sinus rhythm versus persistent atrial fibrillation: a Veterans Affairs Cooperative Studies Program Substudy. *J Am Coll Cardiol* 2006;48:721–730.

124. Pratt CM, et al. for the Atrial Arrhythmia Conversion Trial (ACT-III) Investigators. Usefulness of vernakalant hydrochloride injection for rapid conversion of atrial fibrillation. *Am J Cardiol* 2010;106:1277–1283.

125. Buccelletti F, et al. Efficacy and safety of vernakalant in recent-onset atrial fibrillation after the European Medicines Agency Approval: Systematic review and meta-analysis. *J Clin Pharmacol* 2011. [Epub ahead of print] PMID: 22167572.

126. Capucci A, et al. Effectiveness of loading oral flecainide for converting recent-onset atrial fibrillation to sinus rhythm in patients without organic heart disease or with only systemic hypertension. *Am J Cardiol* 1992;70:69–72.

127. Le Heuzey JY, et al. A short-term, randomized, double-blind, parallel-group study to evaluate the efficacy and safety of dronedarone versus amiodarone in patients with persistent atrial fibrillation: the DIONYSOS study. *J Cardiovasc Electrophysiol* 2010;21: 597–605.

128. Crystal E, et al. Interventions on prevention of postoperative atrial fibrillation in patients undergoing heart surgery. A meta-analysis. *Circulation* 2002;106:75–80.

129. Barucha D, et al. Management and prevention of atrial fibrillation after cardiovascular surgery. *Am J Cardiol* 2000;85:20D–24D.

130. Mahoney EM, et al. Cost-effectiveness of targeting patients undergoing cardiac surgery for therapy with intravenous amiodarone to prevent atrial fibrillation. *J Am Coll Cardiol* 2002;40:737–745.

131. Reston JT, et al. Meta-analysis of clinical outcomes of maze-related surgical procedures for medically refractory atrial fibrillation. *Eur J Cardiothorac Surg* 2005;28:724–730.

132. Calkins H, et al. HRS/EHRA/ECAS expert consensus statement on catheter ablation of atrial fibrillation. Recommendations for personnel policy, procedures and follow-up. *Heart Rhythm* 2007;6:1–46.

133. Hissaguerre M, et al. Spontaneous initiation of atrial fibrillation by ectopic beats originating in the pulmonary veins. *N Engl J Med* 1999;339:659–665.

134. Marine JE, et al. Catheter ablation therapy for atrial fibrillation. *Prog Cardiovasc Dis* 2005;48:178–192.

135. Oral H, et al. Catheter ablation for paroxysmal atrial fibrillation: segmental pulmonary vein ostial ablation versus left atrial ablation. *Circulation* 2003;108:2355–2360.

136. Pappone C, et al. Mortality, morbidity, and quality of life after circumferential pulmonary vein ablation for atrial fibrillation: outcomes from a controlled nonrandomized long-term study. *J Am Coll Cardiol* 2003;42:185–197.

137. Calkins H, et al. 2012 HRS/EHRA/ECAS expert consensus statement on catheter and surgical ablation of atrial fibrillation: recommendations for patient selection, procedural techniques, patient management and follow-up, definitions, endpoints, and research trial design. *J Interv Card Electrophysiol* 2012;33:171–257.

137A. Nielsen JC, et al. Radiofrequency ablation as initial therapy in paroxysmal atrial fibrillation. *N Engl J Med* 2012; 367:1587–1595.

138. Ehrlich JR, et al. Role of angiotensin system and effects of its inhibition in atrial fibrillation: clinical and experimental evidence. *Eur Heart J* 2006;27:512–518.

139. Wang TJ, et al. A risk score for predicting stroke or death in individuals with new-onset atrial fibrillation in the community: the Framingham Heart Study. *JAMA* 2003;290: 1049–1056.

140. van Walraven C, et al. A clinical prediction rule to identify patients with atrial fibrillation and a low risk for stroke while taking aspirin. *Arch Intern Med* 2003;163:936–943.

141. Mant J, et al. Warfarin versus aspirin for stroke prevention in an elderly community population with atrial fibrillation (the Birmingham Atrial Fibrillation Treatment of the Aged Study, BAFTA): a randomised controlled trial. *Lancet* 2007;370:493–503.

142. Banerjee A, et al. Net clinical benefit of new oral anticoagulants (dabigatran, rivaroxaban, apixaban) versus no treatment in a "real world" atrial fibrillation population: a modelling analysis based on a nationwide cohort study. *J Thromb Haemost* 2012; 107:584–589.

143. Connolly SJ, et al. for the AVERROES Steering Committee and Investigators. Apixaban in patients with atrial fibrillation. *N Engl J Med* 2011;364:806–817.

144. Granger CB, et al. for the ARISTOTLE Committees and Investigators. Apixaban versus warfarin in patients with atrial fibrillation. *N Engl J Med* 2011;365:981–992.

145. Oldgren J, et al. on behalf of the RE-LY Investigators. Risks for stroke, bleeding, and death in patients with atrial fibrillation receiving Dabigatran or Warfarin in relation to the CHADS2 score: a subgroup analysis of the RE-LY trial. *Ann Intern Med* 2011;155:660–667.

146. Zhou W, et al. Hemostatic therapy in experimental intracerebral hemorrhage associated with the direct thrombin inhibitor dabigatran. *Stroke* 2011;42:3594–3599.

147. Patel MR, et al., ROCKET AF Investigators. Rivaroxaban versus warfarin in nonvalvular atrial fibrillation. *N Engl J Med* 2011;365:883–891.

148. Eerenberg ES, et al. Reversal of rivaroxaban and dabigatran by prothrombin complex concentrate: a randomized, placebo-controlled, crossover study in healthy subjects. *Circulation* 2011;124:1573–1579.

149. Singer I, et al. Azimilide decreases recurrent ventricular tachyarrhythmias in patients with implantable cardioverter defibrillators. *J Am Coll Cardiol* 2004;43:39–43.

150. AFFIRM Investigators. The Atrial Fibrillation Follow-up Investigation of Rhythm Management. A comparison of rate control and rhythm control in patients with atrial fibrillation. *N Engl J Med* 2002;347:1825–1833.

151. Hylek EM, et al. Major hemorrhage and tolerability of warfarin in the first year of therapy among elderly patients with atrial fibrillation. *Circulation* 2007;115:2689–2696.

152. Murgatroyd F. Atrial tachycardias and atrial flutter. In: Crawford M, DiMarco J, Paulus W, editors. *Cardiology.* 2nd ed. London: Elsevier; 2004. pp. 717–728.

153. Stiell IG, et al, CCS Atrial Fibrillation Guidelines Committee. Canadian Cardiovascular Society atrial fibrillation guidelines 2010: management of recent-onset atrial fibrillation and flutter in the emergency department. *Can J Cardiol* 2011;27:38–46.

154. Falk RH, et al. Intravenous dofetilide, a class III antiarrhythmic agent, for the termination of sustained atrial fibrillation or flutter. Intravenous Dofetilide Investigators. *J Am Coll Cardiol* 1997;29:385–390.

155. Gilligan DM, et al. Long-term outcome of patients after successful radiofrequency ablation for typical atrial flutter. *Pacing Clin Electrophysiol* 2003;26:53–58.

156. American Heart Association Guidelines for Cardiopulmonary Resuscitation and Emergency Cardiovascular Care. Part 7.3: management of symptomatic bradycardia and tachycardia. *Circulation* 2005;112:IV-68–IV-77.

157. Zipes DP, et al. ACC/AHA/ESC 2006 guidelines for management of patients with ventricular arrhythmias and the prevention of sudden cardiac death—executive summary: a report of the American College of Cardiology/American Heart Association Task Force and the European Society of Cardiology Committee for Practice Guidelines (Writing Committee to Develop Guidelines for Management of Patients with Ventricular Arrhythmias and the Prevention of Sudden Cardiac Death) developed in collaboration with the European Heart Rhythm Association and the Heart Rhythm Society. *Eur Heart J* 2006;27:2099–2140.

158. Griffith MJ, et al. Relative efficacy and safety of intravenous drugs for termination of sustained ventricular tachycardia. *Lancet* 1990;336:670–673.

159. Marill KA, et al. Amiodarone is poorly effective for the acute termination of ventricular tachycardia. *Ann Emerg Med* 2006;47:217–224.

160. Kowey PR, et al. Randomized double-blind comparison of intravenous amiodarone and bretylium in the treatment of patients with recurrent, hemodynamically destabilizing ventricular tachycardia or fibrillation. The Intravenous Amiodarone Multicenter Investigators Group. *Circulation* 1995;92:3255–3263.

161. Levine JH, et al. Intravenous amiodarone for recurrent sustained hypotensive ventricular tachyarrhythmias. Intravenous Amiodarone Multicenter Trial Group. *J Am Coll Cardiol* 1996;27:67–75.

162. Scheinman MM, et al. Dose-ranging study of intravenous amiodarone in patients with life-threatening ventricular tachyarrhythmias. The Intravenous Amiodarone Multicenter Investigators Group. *Circulation* 1995;92:3264–3272.

163. Connolly SJ, et al. Canadian implantable defibrillator study (CIDS): a randomized trial of the implantable cardioverter defibrillator against amiodarone. *Circulation* 2000;101: 1297–1302.

164. Connolly SJ, et al. Meta-analysis of the implantable cardioverter defibrillator secondary prevention trials. AVID, CASH and CIDS studies. Antiarrhythmics vs Implantable Defibrillator study. Cardiac Arrest Study Hamburg . Canadian Implantable Defibrillator Study. *Eur Heart J* 2000;21:2071–2078.

165. DiMarco JP. Implantable cardioverter-defibrillators. *N Engl J Med* 2003;349:1836–1847.

166. Kuck KH, et al. Randomized comparison of antiarrhythmic drug therapy with implantable defibrillators in patients resuscitated from cardiac arrest: the Cardiac Arrest Study Hamburg (CASH). *Circulation* 2000;102:748–754.

167. Borggrefe M, et al. Ventricular tachycardia. In: Crawford M, DiMarco J, Paulus W, editors. *Cardiology.* 2nd ed. London: Elsevier; 2004. pp. 753–764.

168. Priori SG, et al. Task Force on Sudden Cardiac Death of the European Society of Cardiology. *Eur Heart J* 2001;22:1374–1450.

169. Roden DM. Clinical practice. Long-QT syndrome. *N Engl J Med* 2008;358:169–176.

170. Bokhari F, et al. Long-term comparison of the implantable cardioverter defibrillator versus amiodarone: eleven-year follow-up of a subset of patients in the Canadian Implantable Defibrillator Study (CIDS). *Circulation* 2004;110:112–116.

171. Hohnloser SH, et al. Effect of amiodarone and sotalol on ventricular defibrillation threshold: the optimal pharmacological therapy in cardioverter defibrillator patients (OPTIC) trial. *Circulation* 2006;114:104–109.

172. Reddy VY, et al. Prophylactic catheter ablation for the prevention of defibrillator therapy. *N Engl J Med* 2007;357:2657–2665.

173. Mason JW. A comparison of electrophysiologic testing with Holter monitoring to predict antiarrhythmic-drug efficacy for ventricular tachyarrhythmias. Electrophysiologic Study versus Electrocardiographic Monitoring Investigators. *N Engl J Med* 1993;329:445–451.

174. Mason JW. A comparison of seven antiarrhythmic drugs in patients with ventricular tachyarrhythmias. Electrophysiologic Study versus Electrocardiographic Monitoring Investigators. *N Engl J Med* 1993;329:452–458.

175. For the Multicenter Automatic Defibrillator Implantation Trial II Investigators, Moss AJ, et al. Prophylactic implantation of a defibrillator in patients with myocardial infarction and reduced ejection fraction. *N Engl J Med* 2002;346:877–883.

176. Hohnloser SH, et al. Prophylactic use of an implantable cardioverter-defibrillator after acute myocardial infarction. *N Engl J Med* 2004;351:2481–2488.

177. Foley PW, et al. Implantable cardioverter defibrillator therapy for primary prevention of sudden cardiac death after myocardial infarction: implications of international guidelines. *Pacing Clin Electrophysiol* 2009;32(Suppl. 1):S131–134.

178. Bänsch D, et al. Primary prevention of sudden cardiac death in idiopathic dilated cardiomyopathy: the Cardiomyopathy Trial (CAT). *Circulation* 2002;105:1453–1458.

179. Kadish A, et al. Prophylactic defibrillator implantation in patients with nonischemic dilated cardiomyopathy. *N Engl J Med* 2004;350:2151–2158.

180. Grimm W, et al. Noninvasive arrhythmia risk stratification in idiopathic dilated cardiomyopathy: results of the Marburg Cardiomyopathy Study. *Circulation* 2003;108:2883–2891.

181. Lee DS, et al. Effect of cardiac and noncardiac conditions on survival after defibrillator implantation. *J Am Coll Cardiol* 2007;49:2408–2415.

182. Bristow MR, et al. Cardiac-resynchronization therapy with or without an implantable defibrillator in advanced chronic heart failure. *N Engl J Med* 2004;350:2140–2150.

183. Cleland JG, et al. Longer-term effects of cardiac resynchronization-Heart Failure on mortality in heart failure [the CArdiac REsynchronization-Heart Failure (CARE-HF) trial extension phase]. *Eur Heart J* 2006;27:1928–1932.

184. Beshai JF, et al. Cardiac-resynchronization therapy in heart failure with narrow QRS complexes. *N Engl J Med* 2007;357:2461–2471.

185. Kass DA. Predicting cardiac resynchronization response by QRS duration: the long and short of it. *J Am Coll Cardiol* 2003;42:2125–2127.

9

Antithrombotic Agents: Platelet Inhibitors, Acute Anticoagulants, Fibrinolytics, and Chronic Anticoagulants

KEITH A.A. FOX · HARVEY D. WHITE ·
BERNARD J. GERSH · LIONEL H. OPIE

The Emperor said: "I wonder whether breathlessness results in death or life?"

Chi'i P answered: "When there are blockages in the circulation between the viscera, then death follows."

The Emperor said: "What can be done with regard to treatment?"

Chi'i P replied: "The method of curing is to establish communication between the viscera and the vascular system."

The Yellow Emperor's Classic of Internal Medicine (circa 2000 BC)

Mechanisms of Thrombosis

The proaggregatory and antiaggregatory factors of the hemostatic system are normally finely balanced, opposing mechanisms. To protect against vascular damage and the risk of bleeding too strong, the proaggregatory system is poised to rapidly form a thrombus to limit any potential hemorrhage. As coronary endothelial damage is a prominent feature of ischemic heart disease, there is a constant risk that antiaggregatory forces will be overcome by the proaggregatory forces, with the risk of further vascular damage and, potentially, thrombosis.

The three main types of agent discussed in this chapter act at different stages of the thrombotic process. First, *platelet inhibitors* act on arterial thrombogenesis and help prevent consequences such as myocardial infarction (MI) and transient ischemic attacks (TIAs). Second, *anticoagulants* given acutely (e.g., heparin) limit the further formation of thrombus, and, when given chronically (e.g., warfarin), help prevent thromboembolism from a dilated left atrium or from the venous system. Both antiplatelet and antithrombotic agents are required to inhibit thrombotic complications of percutaneous coronary intervention (PCI) with revascularization. Third, *fibrinolytic agents* are most useful in the setting of acute arterial thrombosis and occlusion, such as ST-elevation myocardial infarction (STEMI) and peripheral arterial thrombosis, especially when prompt mechanical revascularization (primary PCI) is not feasible. The different sites of action of these three types of agent mean that combination therapy can be beneficial. For example, fibrinolytic agents are used together with antiplatelet agents and anticoagulants in the management of acute myocardial infarction (AMI), but the greater efficacy of combinations is offset by the increased incidence of bleeding.

The *formation of thrombus* (clot in Fig. 9-1) occurs in four steps according to the cell-based concept that stresses the initial role of tissue factor:[1-3] (1) *Subendothelial tissue factor is exposed* to circulating blood as when vascular endothelium is damaged as by atherosclerotic plaque rupture. (2) *Coagulation factors are rapidly activated* by tissue factor to generate thrombin, thus converting fibrinogen into fibrin, which is an essential step to thrombus –formation. (3) *Platelet adhesion, activation, and aggregation* occur almost simultaneously as thrombin acts on the platelets already adhering to the site of injury (Fig. 9-1). During platelet activation there are shape and conformational changes. Activated platelet receptors promote aggregation by cross-links that result in the formation of the *primary platelet plug*. Thrombin, generated both by coagulation factors and platelets (next section), is a very powerful stimulator of platelet adhesion and aggregation. Thrombin forms fibrin, which stabilizes the inherently weak primary platelet plug. Thus platelet adhesion, activation, and aggregation are overlapping processes, with the platelets releasing substances that further promote

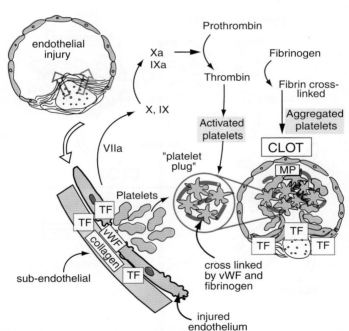

FROM PLAQUE TO THROMBOSIS

Opie 2012

Figure 9-1 From unstable plaque to thrombus. As the plaque becomes unstable with endothelial damage, platelets become exposed to tissue factor (TF) found in either the damaged dysfunctional endothelium or in the subendothelial tissue. TF, acting via factor VIIa (and IXa), activates factor X to Xa, which then converts prothrombin to thrombin. Thrombin converts fibrinogen to fibrin and activates platelets. Platelets then change shape and readily aggregate under the influence of fibrin and other cross-linking molecules (see Fig. 9-2) that bind the platelets together to form the stable fibrin-linked clot (thrombus). Further activation of the coagulation system occurs via TF conveyed in microparticles (MP) to the developing thrombus (TF in lumen of the artery, *bottom left*). There are several paths for rapid self-amplification of these complex platelet changes, including those shown in Figure 9-2. *vWF,* von Willebrand factor. (Figure © L.H. Opie, J.J.S Opie, 2012.)

aggregation and cause vasoconstriction. (4) *Thrombus forms* as fibrin forms polymer cross-links and aggregated platelets tightly combine. The thrombus is not free floating, but adheres to the damaged vessel wall by platelet adhesion.[4] However, fragments of thrombus and platelet aggregates may embolize, stimulating changes in vascular tone and potentially causing microinfarcts in the distal territory. The typical arterial thrombus at the site of a coronary stenosis has a white head caused by platelet aggregation, and a red friable clot forming distally in continuity to the thrombus, caused by stasis beyond the lesion.

Tissue factor and thrombin. Tissue factor and thrombin warrant more detailed consideration. Tissue factor is a cell surface glycoprotein (Gp) abundantly expressed in damaged endothelial and exposed subendothelial cells, and in the atherosclerotic plaque (Fig. 9-2). Tissue factor is also derived from circulating *microparticles* released during plaque rupture.[3] Tissue factor forms a complex with and activates coagulation factor VII. Factor VIIa activates factor X to Xa (first step of the final common coagulation pathway), both directly and indirectly by also activating factor IX (part of the intrinsic pathway, next section).

PLATELET ADHESION AND ACTIVATION

Opie 2012

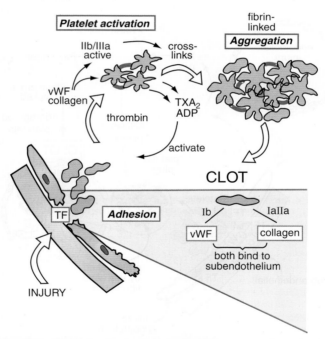

Figure 9-2   Platelet adhesion and activation. Injury to the endothelium exposes the subendothelial receptors for von Willebrand Factor (vWF) and collagen that promotes adhesion of platelets at the site of injury. Platelet activation then occurs under the influence of thrombin, rapidly formed by the effects of subendothelial tissue factor (TF), also exposed by the injury. Thus the glycoprotein IIb/IIIa receptor is now activated, allowing the vWF and fibrinogen to form strong cross-links between them. Platelet activation also liberates thromboxane A_2 (TXA$_2$) and adenosine diphosphate (ADP), which further promotes platelet activation (self-amplification; see Fig. 9-3). The overlapping third stage of aggregation occurs as fibrin, also rapidly formed by the activation of the extrinsic and intrinsic pathways, binds the platelets even more tightly together. The result is the formation of the thrombus (clot). (Figure © L.H. Opie, J.J.S Opie, 2012.)

Factor Xa converts prothrombin to thrombin. Although thrombin is the end-product of the coagulation process, it also activates two platelet receptors (protease-activated receptors [PARs], Table 9-1).[5] Signals from both receptors lead by different routes to rapid platelet activation (Figs. 9-3, 9-4).[6] Thrombin also positively feeds back on the coagulation pathway activating factors including V, VIII, XI, and XIII (these are shown in Fig. 9-5). XIIIa is necessary for full stabilization of the fibrin clot. *Thrombin is thus the lynchpin of the coagulation process.*

Does the intrinsic pathway have a role? Traditionally, the extrinsic and intrinsic pathways are distinguished. The intrinsic coagulation pathway involves a series of interactions starting with activation of factors XII to XIIa, XI to XIa, IX to IXa, and X to Xa, which acts on prothrombin to form thrombin. The activation of X to Xa is where the traditional extrinsic and intrinsic pathways converge (Fig. 9-5), and marks the start of the "common pathway." Although the extrinsic coagulation pathway takes the lead in vivo,[2] there is interpathway interaction,[7] and the traditional model helps in interpretation of in vitro coagulation tests.

Von Willebrand factor and collagen platelet receptors. Superficial platelet injury activates many platelet receptors, which are membrane Gps.[5] Since our last edition in 2005, more receptors have been identified (see Table 9-1), all basically promoting platelet participation in clotting, but without new clinically available antiplatelet agents. At medium and high shear rates, activated platelet receptors bind more

Table 9-1

Platelet Receptors and Their Function				
Receptor	**Alternate or Related Name**	**Function**	**Therapeutic Inhibitor**	**Reference**
GpIb-IX-V (receptor complex)	GpIbα	Adhesion receptor; tethers platelets to tissue-bound vWF	None	9
GPVI/FcR-γ	GpIa	Binds collagen to platelets; generates inside-out integrin activation	None	4,8
αIIbβ3	GpIIbIIIa (integrin)	Binds fibrinogen and vWF to form platelet crosslinks and platelet plug	Abciximab Tirofiban Eptifibatide	4
α2β1	GpIaIIa (integrin)	Collagen receptor	None	4,8
P2Y$_1$ P2Y$_{12}$	ADP receptors (G-protein linked)	Platelet activation; Ca ↑ by IP$_3$ ↑ (P2Y$_1$) or cAMP ↓ (Y$_{12}$)	P2Y$_{12}$ receptor: Clopidogrel Ticlopidine Prasugrel AZD6140 Cangrelor	5,10
PAR	Thrombin, TXA$_2$ (G-protein linked receptors)	Respond to thrombin and TXA$_2$ to activate platelets	Aspirin, indirectly (blocks TXA$_2$ synthesis)	5

ADP, Adenosine diphosphate; *Ca,* calcium; *cAMP,* cyclic adenosine monophosphate; *PAR,* protease activated receptors; *TXA$_2$,* thromboxane A$_2$; *vWF,* von Willebrand factor.

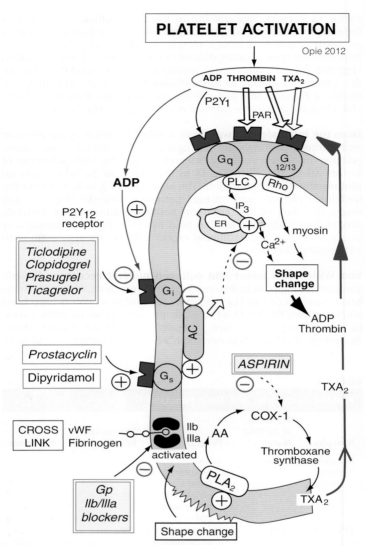

Figure 9-3 Platelet activation and receptors involved. Different platelet inhibitors act at different sites and on different mechanisms, ultimately to inhibit the calcium-dependent pathways of platelet activation. Note the self-amplification platelet activation cycle on the *right side* of the figure, initiated by platelet membrane damage that "exposes" and alters membrane configuration, and activates crucial receptors (thrombin, thromboxane A$_2$ [TXA$_2$], glycoprotein (Gp) IIb/IIIa, and others). *AC,* Adenyl cyclase; *ADP,* adenosine diphosphate; *Ca^{2+},* calcium; *ER,* endoplasmic reticulum; *G$_i$,* G protein, inhibitory form; *G$_s$,* G protein, stimulatory form; *PAR,* protease-activated receptors; *PLC,* phospholipase c; *Rho,* Rho kinase; *vWF,* von Willebrand factor. (Figure © L.H. Opie, J.J.S Opie, 2012.)

readily to the subendothelial matrix, exposed by plaque rupture or tissue trauma, containing *von Willebrand factor* (vWF) and collagen. A large multimeric protein, vWF is normally present in high levels but inactive in the plasma. At the site of vessel injury, vWF becomes immobilized and activated. The vWF interacts with its platelet receptor glycoprotein Ib-alpha (GpIbα) to tether the platelets to the site of injury. The vWF platelet receptors also help to activate platelets by releasing calcium from the endoplasmic reticulum (not shown in Fig. 9-3). Collagen interacts with the platelet *collagen receptor,* GpVI (not shown in

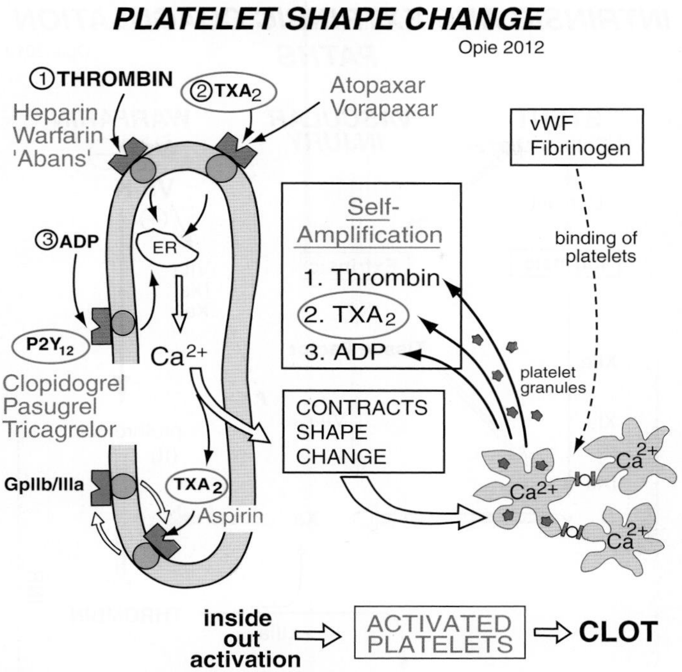

PLATELET SHAPE CHANGE

Opie 2012

Figure 9-4　Platelet shape change. Note the process of self-amplification. '*Abans,*' dabigatran, rivaroxaban, apixaban; *ADP,* adenosine diphosphate; *Ca²⁺*, calcium; *ER,* endoplasmic reticulum; *Gp,* glycoprotein; *TXA₂*, thromboxane A₂; *vWF,* von Willebrand factor. (Figure © L.H. Opie, 2012.)

Fig. 9-3), which powerfully induces platelet activation,[8] thereby liberating more vWF from platelet granules.

Platelet activation and receptor self-amplification. Platelets play a pivotal role in the pathophysiologic findings of AMI. They are involved not only in the initiation of clot formation after plaque fissuring or rupture, but also in the propagation of clot, the secretion of plasminogen activator inhibitor (PAI)–1, which causes clots to become resistant to lysis, and the secretion of thromboxane A_2 (TXA_2), which causes vasoconstriction. They may also embolize to cause plugging of the microvasculature. Platelet aggregates are resistant to fibrinolytic therapy

A critical aspect of platelet activation is the transition from the low- to high-affinity binding state of the platelet receptors,[9] sometimes called "inside-outside" activation (see Table 9-1). Thrombin, readily generated at the site of plaque rupture (see Fig. 9-2), is a potent activator, which leads to release of more thrombin from platelets, followed by release of adenosine diphosphate (ADP) and TXA_2. These three bind to their respective platelet receptors and promote further activation (see Fig. 9-3), a process called *self-amplification.*[9] Activated receptors bind more readily to vWF factor, subendothelial collagen, and fibrinogen. These macromolecules bind platelets to each other (platelet aggregation) and to the platelets already adhering to the vessel wall.

Platelet shape change. Activated platelets have activated contractile proteins. New actin filaments are formed, and myosin light chain kinase responds to signals from the TXA_2 and thrombin receptors (see Fig. 9-3) to promote platelet shape change (see Figs. 9-2 and 9-4). The shape change results in increased surface membrane available for platelet activation and promotion of receptor conformational changes to further activate

INTRINSIC AND EXTRINSIC COAGULATION PATHS

Opie 2012

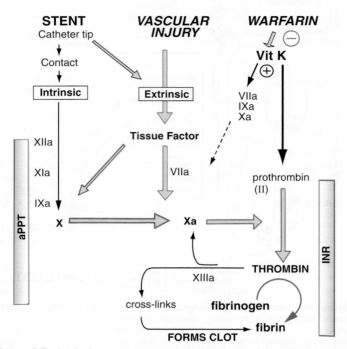

Figure 9-5   Intrinsic contact and extrinsic coagulation pathways. Note major sites of action of heparin and low-molecular-weight heparin. Note which processes are measured by activated partial prothrombin time (aPPT) and by international normalized ratio (INR). (Figure © L.H. Opie, 2012.)

platelets. The shape change also releases platelet ADP, TXA$_2$, and thrombin, which in turn activate other platelets,[10] like a whirlwind effect.

Platelet calcium. A critical event during platelet activation is the rise in the intracellular platelet calcium level. Several mediators (including collagen from endothelial injury, thrombin, ADP released from injured platelets) mobilize calcium from the endoplasmic reticulum (see Fig. 9-3). Enhanced platelet calcium has several consequences, including (1) stimulation of formation of TXA$_2$ (see Figs. 9-3 and 9-4), (2) activation of platelet contraction and shape change to promote the conformational activation of GpIIb/IIIa so that fibrinogen and other adhesive proteins can interlink platelets, and (3) enhanced release of ADP from platelet granules to act on their receptors further to promote platelet activation.[11]

Platelet rapid propagation. The adherent, activated, and aggregated platelets continue to stimulate further thrombus formation. The large concentration of local thrombin, derived both from platelet release and both coagulation pathways, produces local fibrin that polymerizes in "end-to-end" and "side-to-side" reactions to form a fibrin clot. Thrombin also changes circulating factor XIII to active XIIIa, which cross-links the fibrin units. The cross-linked polymers and entrapped platelets make up the thrombus (clot).

Drugs inhibiting platelets. Only some of the many platelet receptors can be blocked by aspirin, clopidogrel, the GpIIb/IIIa antagonists, and the blockers of the platelet P2Y$_{12}$ and PAR receptors

(see Figs. 9-3 and 9-4; Table 9-1). Antagonists to several major receptors such as those to which collagen, the vWF, thrombin, and TXA_2
bind, have yet to be developed. Indirectly many of these receptors
could be inhibited by blocking tissue factor, so new agents are in
development.

Therapeutic activation of coagulation. When urgent activation of the clotting mechanism is essential (for example, traumatic
hemorrhage with life-threatening bleeding), then powerful activation of thrombosis can be attempted by giving recombinant factor
(rF) VIIa. Its only approved use is for hemophiliacs with inhibitors to
factors VIII and IX (licensed in the United States as *Novoseven*). rF
VIIa is increasingly used for off-label indications. Limited available
evidence from 28 studies for five off-label indications suggests no
mortality reduction with rFVIIa use.[12] Rather, there is risk of increased thromboembolism. For factor Xa–induced bleeding, prothrombin complex concentrate (PCC) immediately and completely
reverses the anticoagulant effect of *rivaroxaban* but not dabigatran
in healthy human subjects.[13] For dabigatran, PCC slows hematoma
expansion in experimental brain hematoma in murine intracerebral
hemorrhage.[14]

Tranexamic acid. Tranexamic acid inhibits plasmin. Recent
large-scale trial evidence has shown reduced bleeding when administered after trauma and especially in the first 3 hours after trauma.[15,16]
Importantly, deaths and cardiovascular deaths were reduced without
an increase in MI, venous thrombosis, or pulmonary embolism. This
inexpensive one-time treatment has the potential to reduce bleeding
and mortality. However, there was a trend to increased mortality when
given more than 3 hours after the onset of the trauma.

Antiplatelet Agents: Aspirin and Cardiovascular Protection

Platelet inhibition. Acetylsalicylic acid (aspirin) irreversibly acety-
lates cyclooxygenase (COX; see Fig. 9-3), and activity is not restored
until new platelets are formed. The COX isoform is COX-1, the inhibition
of which gives both the cardiovascular therapeutic benefit and the
toxic gastric side effects. In contrast, aspirin does not strongly inhibit
COX-2; this pathway produces the prostaglandins (PGs), including PGE_2,
that contribute to the inflammatory response. By inhibiting COX-1, aspirin interferes with the synthesis of prothrombotic TXA_2, important in the
platelet activation cycle (see Fig. 9-3) and at a low dose permits the
continued secretion of PGI_2 (prostacyclin).[17] Being very primitive cells,
platelets cannot synthesize new proteins, hence aspirin prevents all
platelet COX-1 activity for the lifespan of the platelet, which is 8-10 days.
Aspirin also has important nonplatelet effects. In the vascular endothelium it inactivates COX, which may diminish the formation of antiaggregatory prostacyclin as well as TXA_2.

Despite these potentially conflicting effects of aspirin, the overwhelming clinical effect is antithrombotic. Also note that vascular COX
can be resynthesized within hours, whereas platelet COX can only re-
form with the birth of new platelets in the absence of aspirin. On the
negative side, aspirin can cause gastric irritation, and gastrointestinal
(GI) bleeding requiring hospitalization occurs in 2 per 1000 patients
treated per year,[18] with a small increase in risk of hemorrhagic stroke.[19,20]
However, in the secondary prevention of MI, aspirin is approximately
100 times more effective in preventing cardiovascular events than in
provoking major bleeding[21] although aspirin resistance may limit the
response (see later). Bleeding is related to the dose of aspirin, with
major bleeding doubling as the dose is increased from less than 100 mg
to less than 200 mg/day.[22] (See "Low-Dose Aspirin and Efficacy" later in
this chapter for discussion of ideal doses.)

Additional effects. Aspirin blocks aggregation only in response to stimulation by thromboxane. Its effects can be overcome by other stimuli, particularly thrombin, which is the most powerful stimulus of platelet aggregation.[23] However, aspirin may have important additional effects on platelet-neutrophil interactions,[24] and on inflammation, but many of these effects require concentrations much higher than currently used for secondary prevention.[25]

Aspirin nonresponsiveness ("resistance"). *Resistance* is a commonly used but loosely defined and controversial term. Of patients with arterial thrombosis, 5% to 20% or more experience a recurrent vascular event during long-term follow-up despite an apparently adequate therapeutic dose.[26] Nonadherence must first be eliminated.[27] "Resistance" may occur in 16% of patients with prior MI, and was associated a fourfold risk of death, reinfarction, or rehospitalization over 12 months.[28] Antiplatelet responsiveness (to aspirin or thienopyridines) is not an "all or nothing" phenomenon. Rather, there is a continuous spectrum. In addition, the clinical response depends on the potency of the thrombogenic stimulus. When aspirin resistance is defined as failure of suppression of thromboxane generation with high urinary concentrations of a metabolite of TXA_2, then the risk of MI is doubled.[26] When defined by platelet function tests and presumed clinical unresponsiveness to aspirin, there is a long-term trebling of the risk of death, myocardial infarct, or stroke.[29] The diverse mechanisms of aspirin resistance include platelet Gp polymorphisms, activation of platelets by pathways other than the COX pathway, and enhanced inflammatory activity with increased expression of COX-2 that is not strongly inhibited by aspirin.[26] Laboratory diagnosis is not easy, as there is no accepted definition, so that clinical suspicion usually provides the cue. Clopidogrel, as an add-on or replacement, may help,[10] but aspirin-resistant patients may also have a reduced response to clopidogrel.[30]

Clinical Use of Aspirin

Because platelets play such an important role in vascular disease of all kinds, there are many clinical indications for aspirin. A meta-analysis of 135,000 patients in 287 studies confirmed its prophylactic effects after a previous MI, in effort and unstable angina, after a stroke, and after coronary artery bypass surgery, while establishing its efficacy in women as well as in men.[21] The major problem is balancing the benefits of aspirin versus the risks, the chief being major GI bleeding and a smaller risk of hemorrhagic stroke. When aspirin is used for secondary prevention, the balance strongly favors benefit. In primary prevention assessing potential risk versus overall benefit (including cancer prevention) is the key.

Secondary prevention by aspirin. All patients with a prior cardiovascular event should be considered for aspirin therapy, which on average reduces the risk of any further vascular event by approximately one-quarter. *In stable angina* in β-blocked patients, aspirin 75 mg daily reduced AMI or sudden death by 34% compared with placebo.[31] The risk reductions extend to those with unstable angina (46%), coronary angioplasty (53%), prior MI (25%), prior stroke or TIA (22%), and peripheral arterial disease (23%).[21]

Primary prevention by aspirin: only for those at high risk? Our previous recommendation, supported by a metaanalysis on more than 30,000 subjects, was that aspirin is indicated only in high-risk populations.[21] In a small but well-designed trial on 1276 diabetic persons with peripheral vascular disease followed for up to 8 years, and judged to have higher cardiovascular risk, aspirin, disappointingly, failed in the primary prevention of cardiovascular events including deaths from heart disease or stroke.[32] The largest study on aspirin and bleeding comes from the Italian National Health System on new users of low-dose aspirin (≤300 mg) from 2003 to 2008.[33] The study authors selected 186,425 patient's using propensity-score matching and compared them with an equal number not currently taking low-dose aspirin. During a median follow-up of 5.7 years, there were 1.6 million person-years of observation. For those currently taking aspirin, the rate of total hemorrhagic events per 1000 person-years was 5.58, whereas the rate was 3.60 per 1000 person-years in those not taking aspirin, with an incidence rate ratio (IRR) of 1.55 (confidence interval [CI], 1.48-1.63). The excess aspirin-induced bleeding was similar in numbers to the expected aspirin-induced reduction of major cardiovascular events for those with a 10-year risk of between 10% and 20%. Of note, an increased intake of proton pump inhibitors (PPIs) was associated with reduced major bleeding. A major problem with this study is that "low dose" could be 300 mg daily, much higher than our recommendation.[34]

Aspirin to prevent cancer. In a series of papers Rothwell's group at Oxford has shown a remarkable effect of aspirin in lessening the development of cancer, including early metastases. In eight primary and secondary prevention trials allocation to aspirin reduced death resulting from cancer by 21% (CI 0.68-0.92, p = 0.003).[35] Even though this study is a retrospective analysis, in three large UK trials long-term posttrial follow-up was obtained from death certificates and cancer registries. Strong support for the inhibitory effect of aspirin on colorectal cancer comes from a prospective randomized study in which aspirin 600 mg daily (a dose normally not used because of the bleeding risk) for a mean of 25 months substantially reduced cancer incidence in carriers of hereditary colorectal cancer.[36]

Furthermore, in an analysis of 51 trials with 77,549 participants, allocation to aspirin gave fewer nonvascular deaths overall (p = 0.003;) and decreased cancer deaths (odds ratio [OR] 0.85, p = 0.008; 34 trials, 69,224 participants).[37] The lower risks were initially offset by increased major bleeding, but both effects decreased with increasing follow-up, leaving only the reduced risk of cancer (absolute reduction 3.13 per 1000 patients per year) from 3 years onward. As the effect of both low and high doses of aspirin in decreasing cancer metastases convincingly (all P values <0.005) started at approximately 4-5 years after initiation of aspirin, the proposal is that aspirin inhibits the growth of metastases.[38]

What should we recommend to our patients? From the earlier studies, we calculate that there is a strong case for prevention of GI cancers that vastly outweigh the risks of major bleeds in those at low cardiovascular risk.[39] In the light of the recent Rothwell analysis on 51 trials, we agree with the editorialists in the *Lancet* that the case for prolonged aspirin use is now very convincing.[40] Benefit exceeds harm (Fig. 9-6). Without clear data for guidance, aspirin could be started at a low dose of 75 mg perhaps in the patient's early 50s to allow for both the early and the delayed anticancer benefit shown in this study.

Thus we change our previous opinion that prophylactic aspirin for the general apparently healthy population should not be encouraged. We remain concerned about starting aspirin in older adults in whom decreased renal function is a possible side effect. Nonetheless, in the absence of data for aspirin use for primary prevention at different severities of chronic kidney disease (CKD), in practice low-dose aspirin less than 100 mg is often used even in the presence of severe CKD.[41]

Aspirin for cardiovascular indications. *In acute coronary syndromes* (ACS), including AMI with fibrinolytic therapy or primary PCI, and unstable angina with either conservative or invasive strategies,

ASPIRIN BENEFITS VERSUS HARM
Opie 2012

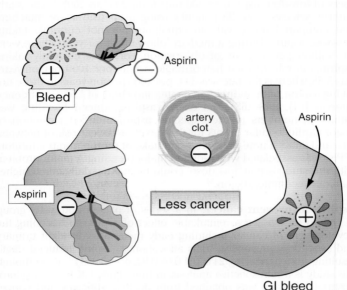

Figure 9-6   Aspirin benefit exceeds harm. Besides the well-known arterio-protective effects of aspirin on heart and brain, balanced to some extent by increased cerebral bleeding, the newly reported decreased risk of cancer argues for its use in primary prevention. *GI,* Gastrointestinal. (Figure © L.H. Opie, 2012.)

aspirin should be given in both the acute and follow-up phases, and is part of triple antiplatelet blockade. A large trial comparing 300-325 mg daily doses with lower-dose aspirin (75-100 mg daily) showed no outcome differences and no differences in bleeding.[42] Aspirin 160 mg was the dose used in the first large AMI trial in 1988[43] and was also favored by a retrospective analysis.[44]

Aspirin as an antiinflammatory drug. Although the Framingham-based risk factor calculation is an excellent guide, it does not factor in the role of the inflammatory response in the genesis of vascular disease. In the Physicians' Health Study, the benefit of aspirin in primary prevention was largely localized to men with high blood levels of C-reactive protein.[25] Logically, but without prospective trial support, aspirin by its antiinflammatory effect should be more effective than expected from current risk factor calculations, and might be considered for primary prevention in those with high C-reactive protein levels. However, the benefits of this approach remain to be proven.

Other indications for aspirin. (1) *In postcoronary bypass surgery,* aspirin should be started within 48 hours of surgery, which reduces total mortality by about two-thirds,[45] and continued indefinitely. (2) Use for *prevention of stroke in atrial fibrillation (AF),* when warfarin is contraindicated or the patient has a CHADS-VASc score of less than 2 (congestive heart failure; hypertension; age 75 years or older [2 points]; diabetes mellitus; stroke, TIA, or thromboembolism [2 points]; vascular disease; age 65-74 years; sex category; graded 0–9)[46] and thus is not at modest risk of stroke (6%-10% 10-year risk).[34] (3) For *arteriovenous shunts,* aspirin decreases thrombosis. (4) For *stroke prevention* in intracranial arterial stenosis, high-dose aspirin (325-1300 mg daily) was better than warfarin (see "Possible Indications for Warfarin").

(5) For urgent therapy in *TIAs and minor stroke,* aspirin is part of a comprehensive strategy (with clopidogrel, a statin, blood pressure lowering, and anticoagulation if indicated).[46] (For dual therapy with clopidogrel, see p. 348.)

Low-dose aspirin and efficacy. Low doses theoretically retain efficacy yet limit GI side effects and bleeding. Metaanalysis suggests that the dose range should be 75-150 mg daily for a wide range of indications.[21] In a follow-up study of patients with non–ST-elevation (NSTE) ACSs the optimal dose of aspirin was 75 to 100 mg.[22] Aspirin 80 mg/day completely blocks platelet aggregation induced by COX.[47] Doses of only 30 mg daily were as effective as higher doses in preventing TIAs,[48] but other endpoints were not tested. The problem with very low doses is that the full antithrombotic effect takes up to 2 days to manifest, explaining why higher dose aspirin (approximately 160 mg) should be given urgently at the onset of symptoms of AMI or unstable angina. Much higher dose aspirin, formerly used to prevent recurrences of stroke or TIAs, is seldom appropriate.[18,48,49]

Bleeding, gastrointestinal, and renal side effects of aspirin. Whereas bleeding is the most serious side effect, GI side effects are much more common. Dyspepsia, nausea, or vomiting may be dose-limiting in approximately 10%-20% of patients. Such side effects may be reduced by buffered or enteric-coated aspirin, or by taking aspirin with food. Low-dose enteric coated aspirin (Ecotrin 81 mg in the United States) is often prescribed to avoid GI side effects, yet by delivering aspirin to the small intestine rather than the stomach, bioavailability is reduced with risk of suboptimal clinical response.[27] Standard "low"-dose aspirin (75-300 mg daily) more than doubles the risk of major GI bleeding (relative risk, 2.07; CI 1.61-2.66) and increases intracranial bleeds by 65%.[50] In absolute terms, however, the risk is low: 769 patients must be treated for 1 year to cause one major bleed.[50] *Impaired renal function and decreased excretion of uric acid* with risk of gout are less commonly emphasized, but are frequent in older adults even with low-dose aspirin.[51]

Contraindications to aspirin. The major contraindications are aspirin intolerance, history of GI bleeding, and peptic ulcer or other potential sources of GI or genitourinary bleeding. Hemophilia is not an absolute contraindication to aspirin when there are strong cardiovascular indications. Because it retards the urinary excretion of uric acid and creatinine, blood uric acid, and creatinine should be monitored, especially in older adults.[52] Relative contraindications include gout, dyspepsia, iron-deficiency anemia, and the possibility of increased perioperative bleeding.

Drug interactions with aspirin. Concurrent warfarin and aspirin therapy increases the risk of bleeding, especially if aspirin doses are high. Aspirin inhibits COX-1 activity approximately 170 times more than COX-2[53] so that interaction with COX-2 inhibitors is unlikely. Among nonsteroidal antiinflammatory drugs (NSAIDs), those with dominant COX-1 activity (ibuprofen and naproxen) but not those with dominant COX-2 activity (diclofenac [Voltaren]) interfere with the cardioprotective effects of aspirin.[27,54] Angiotensin-converting enzyme (ACE) inhibitors and aspirin have potentially opposing effects on renal hemodynamics, with aspirin inhibiting and ACE inhibitors promoting the formation of vasodilatory PGs.

When ACE inhibitors are chronically used for heart failure, postinfarct protection, or high-risk prevention, they are still beneficial even when aspirin is added. Two metaanalyses have addressed this issue. Aspirin did reduce but not eliminate the ACE inhibitor's beneficial effect on major clinical events. The risk reduction in those also receiving aspirin at baseline was an OR of 0.80 versus 0.71 in those given an

ACE –inhibitor only.[55] In 96,712 patients with AMI, there was no interaction over 30 days.[56] A practical policy is to keep the aspirin dose low, especially in those with hemodynamic problems such as heart failure.[57] The risk of aspirin-induced GI bleeding is increased by alcohol, corticosteroid therapy, and NSAIDs. Phenobarbital, phenytoin, and rifampin decrease the efficacy of aspirin through induction of the hepatic enzymes metabolizing aspirin. The effect of oral hypoglycemic agents and insulin may be enhanced by aspirin. Aspirin may reduce the efficacy of uricosuric drugs such as sulfinpyrazone and probenecid. Both thiazides and aspirin retard the urinary excretion of uric acid, increasing the risk of gout.

Treatment of aspirin-induced gastrointestinal bleeding. In those with healed ulcers, aspirin plus a PPI reduces recurrent bleeding more effectively than a change to clopidogrel.[58] Could primary use of clopidogrel avoid or lessen the incidence of GI bleeding that occurs with aspirin? Indirect evidence suggests that almost 1000 patients would have to be treated for 1 year with clopidogrel instead of aspirin to avoid one major bleed at the cost of more than $1 million.[50]

Other Antiplatelets: Clopidogrel and Dipyridamole (Used as Single Antiplatelet Therapy)

ADP is released from platelets during platelet activation and, when externalized, interacts with two G protein–coupled platelet receptors ($P2Y_1$, $P2Y_{12}$), which act through different intracellular signals (see Fig. 9-3). $P2Y_1$ activation induces platelet shape change and initiates GpIIb/IIIa activation, whereas $P2Y_{12}$ perpetuates GpIIb/IIIa activation and critically stabilizes platelet aggregation.[27] $P2Y_{12}$ antagonism may not only prevent platelet aggregation but also promote disaggregation.[27] Another indirect effect of ADP is to rapidly activate intravascular tissue factor. Therefore ADP antagonists may not only decrease platelet thrombosis, but may directly affect coagulation.[27] Clopidogrel is the most widely used agent of this group, with the more recent agents being prasurgel and ticagrelor (see Fig. 9-3). Ticlopidine was the first agent of this group, yet now is seldom used because of potentially serious side effects. First, we present a brief review of ticlopidine.

Ticlopidine

Ticlid and clopidogrel are both thienopyridine derivatives that irreversibly inhibit the binding of ADP to the $P2Y_{12}$ receptor (see Fig. 9-7). Ticlopidine can cause neutropenia, liver abnormalities, and thrombotic thrombocytopenic purpura (TTP), making it much less safe than clopidogrel. Both agents when added to aspirin give added antiaggregatory effects and improve clinical outcomes.[21] The neutropenia associated with ticlopidine occurs within the first 3 months of treatment. It is therefore essential that a complete blood cell count and white cell differential be performed before starting treatment, and every 2 weeks until the end of the third month, according to the manufacturer's information. Ticlopidine has two licensed indications in the United States, to prevent repeat stroke or TIA in those intolerant of or resistant to aspirin and for coronary artery stenting for up to 30 days with aspirin. In practice, ticlopidine is rarely used in countries where clopidogrel is available except in cases of clopidogrel resistance or allergy.

Pharmacokinetics of ticlopidine. The kinetics of ticlopidine tablets are nonlinear, with a markedly decreased clearance on repeated dosing.

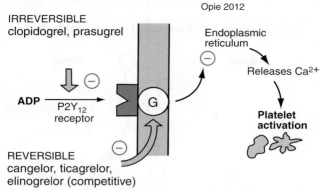

Figure 9-7   Sites of adenosine diphosphate (ADP)–receptor (P2Y$_{12}$) block, either irreversible (e.g., by clopidogrel) or reversible (e.g., by ticagrelor). G$_i$ protein, inhibitory form. For role of P2Y$_{12}$ also see Figure 9-3. Ca^{2+}, Calcium. (Figure © L.H. Opie, 2012.)

Thus it takes 4-7 days to achieve maximum inhibition of platelet aggregation when given with aspirin.[59] However, a quicker response can be achieved by oral loading. Ticlopidine is largely metabolized by the liver, followed by renal excretion. The plasma half-life during constant dosing is 4-5 days.

Clopidogrel

Clopidogrel is a widely used inhibitor of the platelet ADP receptor P2Y$_{12}$.[7] It is substantially safer than ticlopidine with a low rate of myelotoxicity (0.8%, package insert). There is no study that compares the rate of GI bleeding to that with placebo, but there is less major GI bleeding than with aspirin.[50] Clopidogrel acts at a different site from aspirin by *irreversibly* inhibiting the binding of ADP to the P2Y$_{12}$ receptor, thereby preventing the transformation and activation of the GpIIb/IIIa receptor (Figs. 9-3 and 9-7). Thus clopidogrel has gained considerable importance in the treatment of ACS. Compared with ticlopidine, metaanalysis suggests a superior reduction of major adverse cardiac events[60] to which may be added better tolerability (fewer GI and allergic side effects). As with aspirin, clopidogrel resistance also occurs.

Pharmacokinetics and dosage. Clopidogrel is an inactive prodrug that requires in vivo oxidation by the hepatic or intestinal cytochrome CYP3A4 and 2C19 isoenzymes (Fig. 9-8).[61] The onset of action on platelets is within hours of a single oral dose,[62] but steady state inhibition requires between 3 and 7 days (package insert).[63] When given upstream before PCI, a 600-mg oral *loading dose* of clopidogrel achieves maximal inhibition of platelets after 2 hours,[64] compared with 24-48 hours with a 300-mg loading dose, both doses achieving greater inhibition than ticlopidine.[64] In a prospective trial, in a secondary analysis double-dose clopidogrel (a loading dose of 600 mg and then150 mg for 7 days) was superior to standard-dose prior (a loading dose of 300 mg and then 75 mg/day) for PCI for ACS at 30 days.[65] Kinetics of clopidogrel are nonlinear and variable, with a markedly decreased clearance on repeated dosing. When dosing is stopped, it takes approximately 5 days for the generation of new platelets and the bleeding to be reduced, so that cessation for 5 days is recommended before coronary artery bypass grafting (CABG) to avoid major bleeding that may require 30 transfusions per 1000 patients.[63] No dose

ACTIVATION OF ANTI-PLATELET AGENTS
Opie 2012

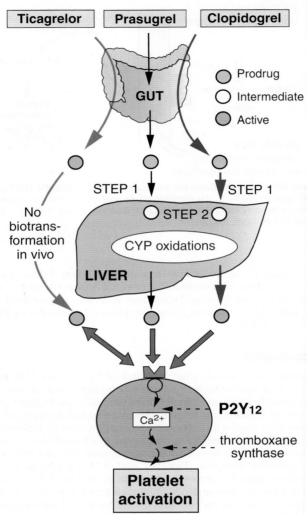

Figure 9-8 Activation of antiplatelet agents. Note that both prasurgel and clopidogrel require hepatic activation with risk of interactions with other drugs at that site. Ticagrelor requires no hepatic step and was superior to clopidogrel in the PLATO trial.[61] Ca^{2+}, Calcium; *CYP,* cytochrome P-450. (Figure © L.H. Opie, 2012.)

adjustment of clopidogrel is needed for older adults or for patients with renal impairment (package insert).

Major side effects. Neutropenia occurs in 0.02% versus 2.4% for ticlopidine (package inserts). The major side effect of clopidogrel is increased major bleeds (approximately 1% excess), without an increase in intracranial bleeds.[21] A *contraindication* is active bleeding.

Clopidogrel genetic testing. Clopidogrel is a prodrug that requires metabolic activation by hepatic cytochrome P450 (see Fig. 9-8). The CYP2C19*2 allele is a common genetic variant and is associated with increased rates of ischemic events and stent thrombosis after PCI. This and other genetic variants are carried by nearly 30% of individuals of western European ancestry and approximately 40% of those of Asian descent and of blacks. On-site genetic testing completed within 1 hour can now identify those with specific genetic variants.[66] Prasugrel or ticagrelor can be given instead of clopidogrel in those individuals. Although this is a promising approach, prospective genetic-based trials are now needed to determine whether clinical outcome benefit of such rapid genetic testing is achieved. A recent *Lancet* editorial concludes, "Funders await evidence establishing the value of genetic testing–guided antiplatelet treatment before making reimbursement decisions."[66] Of note, the US Food and Drug Administration (FDA) has controversially stated that CYP2C19 genotyping be considered prior to prescribing clopidogrel.

Drug interactions. Atorvastatin and omeprazole competitively inhibit hepatic activation of clopidogrel, reducing clopidogrel responsiveness.[67] Despite such theoretical concerns and ex vivo testing suggesting a potential negative interaction with concomitant clopidogrel and CYP3A4-metabolized statins (atorvastatin, simvastatin, pravastatin), there was no evidence of a clinical interaction in a large placebo-controlled trial with long-term follow-up.[68] Nonetheless, higher doses of clopidogrel (600 mg) and atorvastatin (40-80 mg as currently used) may interact, as is being tested in the prospective SPICE trial.[67]

PPIs, and particularly the ones that effect the cytochrome P450 pathway, may decrease the efficacy of clopidogrel.[69] Reassuringly, in a randomized trial that stopped early because of lack of funding, in 3761 patients given clopidogrel with or without omeprazole, there was a reduction in upper GI tract bleeding with omeprazole (hazard ratio [HR]: 0.13; CI: 0.03-0.56; p = 0.0001) with no apparent interaction with cardiovascular events (HR: 0.99; CI: 0.68-1.44).[70]

Reduced response to clopidogrel resistance and effects of platelet reactivity. According to the test used, the incidence varies. There is no simple classification into responders and nonresponders, but rather a gradation of responses. Increased on-treatment platelet reactivity, as measured by a direct sensitive $P2Y_{12}$ assay, is related to serious clinical outcomes. There were increased long-term cardiovascular events after PCI, including death, MI, and stent thrombosis. These events were all increased in half of 3000 patients who had increased platelet reactivity, as shown by metaanalysis.[71] When giving a loading dose of 600-mg at the time of PCI, followed by 150 mg/day versus 75 mg/day of clopidogrel over 6 months, there is modest 22% reduction in the rate of high platelet reactivity at 30 days, but that did not translate into any change in the primary endpoint nor in the incidence of death from cardiovascular causes at 6 months.[72] There are no data on appropriate therapy of such increased platelet reactivity, but the current European Society of Cardiology (ESC) guidelines prefer other $P2Y_{12}$ blockers.[73]

Preferred use of other $P2Y_{12}$ blockers. Of $P2Y_{12}$ blockers, ticagrelor has some advantages over prasugrel, which requires hepatic activation (see Fig. 9-8), so that the issue of the effects of hepatic genetic variations does not arise. In case of excess bleeding, ticagrelor may be more readily reversible with a shorter duration of action of 3-4 days versus 5-10 days for prasugrel. Furthermore, ticagrelor has strong trial data with mortality reduction in ACS in PLATO.[74] Prasugrel gives more effective platelet inhibition than does clopidogrel in patients with high residual platelet reactivity, but without change in outcome events, a trial stopped early because of low event rates.[75] This was a trial with high residual platelet reactivity and low event rates e.g.: 1 vs 0.

Indications, dose, and use. Clopidogrel is licensed in the United States for (1) *reduction of atherosclerotic events* (MI, stroke, vascular death) in patients with recent stroke, recent MI, or with established peripheral arterial disease; and (2) for *ACS* whether or not PCI (with or without stent) or CABG is performed. For loading, 600 mg is better.[65] For *prevention of late poststent thrombosis* after drug-eluting stent (DES), clopidogrel should be used for at least 12 months post-DES insertion,[76] and aspirin must be kept on indefinitely. *For aspirin resistance,* clopidogrel often replaces aspirin; however, there is no outcome study.

How long to keep on after PCI? The standard recommendation is to use clopidogrel for 1 year with DES and 1 month with bare metal stents. However, there are no definitive data. An observational study suggests an increased risk of an adverse cardiovascular event when stopping after a mean of 278 days.[77]

Aspirin intolerance. Clopidogrel can be used in place of aspirin and has modest superiority in a chronic population at broad vascular risk (9% relative risk reduction versus aspirin).[78]

Summary. Clopidogrel is an effective agent, but with variable metabolism and a relatively high rate of in vitro platelet resistance. The precise frequency of clinical resistance is unknown, but greater variation in platelet reactivity is seen with clopidogrel than with newer platelet antagonists (see "Prasugrel" and "Ticagrelor," both later in this chapter). In acute vascular injury it should be added to aspirin to obtain better platelet inhibition and clinical results but not routinely for stable coronary disease; it can replace aspirin in cases of intolerance. Upstream clopidogrel has replaced routine administration of GpIIb/IIIa blockers for high-risk patients with NSTE ACS. The ESC guidelines recommend the use of ticagrelor with discontinuation of clopidogrel if already used for pretreatment.[73]

Dipyridamole and Sulfinpyrazone

In general, platelet inhibition by dipyridamole (site of action the same as prostacyclin, see Fig. 9-3) with or without aspirin or sulfinpyrazone, produces results very similar to those seen with aspirin alone.[21] By contrast, clopidogrel or ticlopidine added to the effects of aspirin, reducing vascular events by approximately 20%.[21] Therefore *dipyridamole* is no longer the nonaspirin antiplatelet agent of choice even in the cerebrovascular circulation for which data are stronger. Dipyridamole helps to reduce recurrent stroke when given with aspirin as in the ESPRIT trial, and when combined with earlier studies the overall risk ratio of vascular death, stroke, or MI was 0.82 (CI: 0.74-0.91).[79] The only cardiovascular-licensed indication of dipyridamole is for prosthetic mechanical valves, in combination with anticoagulation by warfarin.[80] Note the dangerous drug interaction of dipyridamole with the antiarrhythmic adenosine (see Fig. 8-7). *Sulfinpyrazone* inhibits COX, with effects similar to those of aspirin, yet is more expensive. It requires multiple daily doses and has no benefit in patients already on aspirin. However, in contrast to aspirin it is also a uricosuric agent. In the United States, the only licensed indication is chronic or intermittent gouty arthritis.

Dual Antiplatelet Therapy

Aspirin-clopidogrel combined. As aspirin and clopidogrel act differently (see Fig. 9-3), better results should logically be obtained by using the combination in higher-risk patients. The general principle is as follows. Substantial data shows that adding clopidogrel to aspirin is beneficial in the setting of acute vascular injury, whether procedure-induced as in stenting, or spontaneous as in ACS,[81] including AMI.[82] In

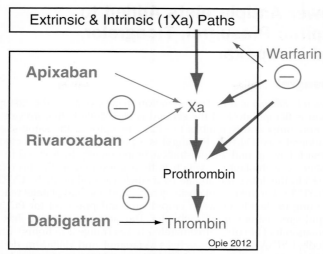

Figure 9-9   Extrinsic and intrinsic paths (see Fig. 9-10) showing sites of action of various indirect and direct thrombin inhibitors. (Figure © L.H. Opie, 2012.)

high-risk subgroups of CHARISMA, dual antiplatelet therapy appeared protective.[83]

For STEMI or unstable angina and non–ST-elevated myocardial infarction (NSTEMI) *with intended invasive therapy* by PCI, the revised American College of Cardiology (ACC)–American Heart Association (AHA) 2011 guidelines[84] advise clopidogrel 300-600 mg given as soon as possible as a loading dose, then 75 mg daily for at least 1 year.[84] In the large OASIS-7 trial that randomized 17,263 patients who had PCI to a 7-day double-dose clopidogrel regimen (600 mg on day 1; 150 mg on days 2-7, then 75 mg daily) reduced cardiovascular events and stent thrombosis compared with standard doses at 30 days (300 mg on day 1 then 75 mg daily).[42] Efficacy and safety did not differ between high-dose and low-dose aspirin.[65]

Clopidogrel added to aspirin reduced the composite of combined death, MI, and stroke at 1 year by 27% ($p < 0.02$).[85] Dual antiplatelet resistance has been reported but optimal therapies have not been defined.[30] *Drug interaction:* PPIs, advised in guidelines to prevent GI bleeding especially when clopidogrel is given with aspirin, may counteract platelet inhibition, but the evidence is not robust.[86]

In atrial fibrillation at high risk of stroke. In patients with AF at high risk of stroke, maximal benefits are found with the new direct thrombin or factor Xa inhibitors (Fig. 9-9). For those with *prior TIAs or minor stroke,* aspirin added to clopidogrel (both 75 mg daily over 18 months in the MATCH trial) increased life-threatening bleeds from 1% to 3% ($p < 0.0001$) without improving cardiovascular outcomes,[87] thus making the case for only one antiplatelet agent in these patients.

Clinical summary. In *NSTE ACS,* regardless of whether management is conservative or invasive, clopidogrel provides benefit (combined with aspirin). In the CURE trial of 12,562 patients, clopidogrel added to aspirin reduced the combined incidence of death, nonfatal MI, and stroke by 20% versus aspirin alone ($p < 0.001$) over an average 9-month period.[88] Clopidogrel increased major bleeding (3.7% versus 2.7%, $P = 0.003$). Loading with upstream clopidogrel is used for PCI for ACS at moderate to high risk,[89,90] as now recommended by ESC guidelines.[73]

Newer Antiplatelets Added to Aspirin: Prasugrel, Ticagrelor, and Vorapaxar

Prasugrel

Prasugrel (Effient) is a newer-generation thienopyridine (the first generation is ticlopidine and the second is clopidogrel) that irreversibly and noncompetitively inhibits the $P2Y_{12}$ receptor at the same site as clopidogrel (see Fig. 9-7). Prasugrel is a prodrug. It is not detected in plasma following oral administration, being rapidly hydrolyzed in the intestine to a thiolactone, which is then converted in the liver (see Fig. 9-8) to the active metabolite by a single step, primarily by CYP3A4 and CYP2B6. For the role of onsite genetic and residual platelet reactivity testing to decide between clopidogrel and prasugrel for PCI, see "Clopidogrel" earlier in this chapter. The active metabolite has an elimination half-life of approximately 7 hours (range 2-15 hours). Unexpectedly, CYP3A inhibitors such as verapamil and diltiazem do not appear to alter prasugrel activity, but may decrease the maximum concentration (Cmax) by 34% to 46%. Prasugrel-mediated inhibition of platelet aggregation is approximately five to nine times more potent than that of clopidogrel,[91] achieving greater platelet inhibition than 600 mg of clopidogrel with an onset of action within 1 hour.[92]

Major clinical trial. In the TRITON-TIMI 38 Trial[92] prasugrel (60 mg loading dose, then 10 mg daily) was compared with clopidogrel (300 mg loading dose followed by 75 mg daily) in patients undergoing PCI and followed for 6-15 months. Prasugrel reduced the primary endpoint of cardiovascular death, MI, and stroke from 12% to 9.9% (p < 0.001). Stent thrombosis fell from 2.4% to 1.1% (p < 0.001). Forty-six patients would have to be treated for 5 months to avoid one primary endpoint, compared with 167 treated to result in one major hemorrhage (not CABG related). Overall, greater efficacy came at the price of greater bleeding. The FDA and the European Medicines Agency (EMA) have both approved prasugrel with warnings about the bleeding risk. The EMA also warns of hypersensitivity reactions with prasugrel, affecting anywhere from 0.1% to 1% of patients.

FDA-approved indications. Prasugrel is indicated for the reduction of thrombotic cardiovascular events (including stent thrombosis) in patients with ACS who are to be managed with PCI for unstable angina or NSTEMI, or STEMI when managed with either primary or delayed PCI. Note, however, that the approval did not include superiority to clopidogrel. The FDA states that prasugrel's greater treatment effect and greater bleeding rate in TRITON might in part be explained by the decreased conversion of clopidogrel to active metabolites in approximately 30% of white patients, and also because the concurrent use of PPIs in an unspecified number of the subjects in the trial might have led to a genetically based interaction that also decreased clopidogrel's effective activity. Another factor is that clopidogrel was intentionally given at the same time as prasugrel in TRITON, whereas ideally it should have been given earlier for an optimal effect.[93]

Bleeding risk. The black box FDA warning on the label states that prasugrel can cause serious bleeding and occasionally TTP. Bleeding should, if possible, be managed without stopping prasugrel, particularly in the first few weeks after ACS, which would increase the risk of subsequent cardiovascular events. Further analysis of the TRITON-38 reveals that the major predictors of serious bleeding were a combination of the patient and procedural characteristics and antiplatelet therapies.[94] Although serious bleeding was strongly associated with mortality within the first month of the bleeding event, this association was not significant beyond 40 days (HR for mortality 1.38; 95% CI 0.72 to 2.66; P = 0.33). Factors increasing the risk were (1) the use of a GPIIb/IIIa inhibitor which, when given even only for a short period, showed a stronger association with serious bleeding than did assignment to prasugrel (HR 1.59; p < 0.001); (2) a history of stroke or TIA (HR 1.58; P = 0.01); (3) age 75 years or older (HR 2.58; P < 0.001); (4) female gender (HR 1.77; p < 0.0001); (5) body weight of less than 60 kg (HR 2.30; P < 0.001); and (6) femoral access (HR 1.60; P = 0.02). Patients with a history of stroke or TIA or low body weight (<60 kg) should not receive prasugrel.

Ticagrelor

Ticagrelor belongs to a novel chemical class, cyclopentyl-triazolopyrimidine, and is an oral reversibly binding noncompetitive inhibitor of the $P2Y_{12}$ receptor with a plasma half-life of approximately 12 hours.[73] The level of $P2Y_{12}$ inhibition is determined by the plasma ticagrelor level and, to a lesser extent, an active metabolite. Like prasugrel, it has a more rapid and consistent onset of action than clopidogrel, but additionally it has a quicker offset of action so that recovery of platelet function is faster. Unlike prasugrel, it requires no hepatic activation (see Fig. 9-8).

Drug interactions. Ticagrelor inhibits hepatic CYP3A to increase blood levels of drugs metabolized through CYP3A, such as amlodipine and two commonly used statins (simvastatin and atorvastatin), whereas moderate CYP3A inhibitors such as diltiazem, verapamil, and amlodipine increase the levels of ticagrelor and reduce the speed of its offset. (For a proposed interaction with high dose aspirin, see "Approval Status" later in this chapter.)

Clinical studies. In the PLATO trial, patients with either moderate to high risk NSTE-ACS (planned for either conservative or invasive management) or STEMI planned for primary PCI were randomized to either clopidogrel 75 mg daily, with a loading dose of 300 mg, or ticagrelor 180 mg loading dose followed by 90 mg twice daily.[74] In this trial over 12 months ticagrelor given to 9333 patients reduced deaths compared with clopidogrel given to 9291 patients (4.5% versus 5.9%, p < 0.0001). In the overall cohort, in which 61% of patients came to PCI either early or within 24 hours the primary composite endpoint (death from vascular causes, MI, or stroke) was reduced from 11.7% in the clopidogrel group to 9.8% in the ticagrelor group (HR 0.84; CI 0.77-0.92; P < 0.001). The primary endpoint in patients undergoing a planned invasive strategy, the primary composite endpoint occurred in 9% of patients in the ticagrelor group, versus 10.7% in the clopidogrel group (P = 0.0025)[95] of the benefit in terms of reduced MI and death accrued progressively with continued separation of event curves at 12 months

Adverse effects of ticagrelor. Adverse effects are reviewed in Hamm et al.[73] In addition to increased rates of minor or non–CABG-related major bleeding with ticagrelor, adverse effects include dyspnea, increased frequency of ventricular pauses, and asymptomatic increases in uric acid. Dyspnea occurs most frequently (up to 14%) within the first week of treatment and may be transient or persist until cessation of treatment, but is usually not severe enough to stop treatment. The dyspnea does not seem to be linked to deterioration in cardiac or pulmonary function. Ventricular pauses of 3 seconds or more occurred more frequently (but not significant for ≥5 second pauses) and were mostly asymptomatic nocturnal sinoatrial pauses occurring in the first week. Caution is required in advanced sinoatrial disease or second- or third-degree atrioventricular block, unless already treated by a permanent pacemaker. The mechanisms of the dyspnea and ventricular pauses remain uncertain.

Approval status. Health Canada and the European Union have granted approval to ticagrelor for the secondary prevention of atherothrombotic events in patients with ACS. The FDA approval is to reduce the risk of cardiovascular death and MI in patients with ACS, but with a boxed warning stating that use of ticagrelor with aspirin in doses exceeding 100 mg/day decreases the effectiveness of the medication. This dose limitation might be explained by a drug-drug interaction with high-dose aspirin such as 300-mg daily that is thought to account for the lesser effectiveness of ticagrelor in the North American component of the PLATO trial.

Cangrelor

Cangrelor is a rapid-acting, reversible, potent, competitive inhibitor of the $P2Y_{12}$ receptor (see Fig. 9-7). Given intravenously, it acts within 20 minutes to achieve 85% inhibition of ADP-induced platelet aggregation. In a pooled analysis of the two large phase 3 CHAMPION trials, with the use of the universal definition of MI, cangrelor was associated with a significant reduction in early ischemic events when compared with clopidogrel in patients with NSTE ACS undergoing PCI.[96] A third phase 3 trial, the PHOENIX trial, is underway. In a small trial, when added to clopidogrel, cangrelor decreased platelet reactivity but did not alter cardiac surgery–related bleeding.[97]

Vorapaxar and Atopaxar

Vorapaxar. *Vorapaxar* is a potent, competitive PAR-1 antagonist (see Fig. 9-3) that was tested in two large outcome trials. In 12,944 patients with ACS (NSTE),[98] vorapaxar did not significantly reduce the primary endpoint of a composite of major cardiovascular events (P = 0.07), although it did reduce the secondary endpoint of cardiovascular death, MI, or stroke (P = 0.02). Unfortunately, it significantly increased the risk of major bleeding, including intracranial hemorrhage (P < 0.0001), so that the trial was terminated early after a safety review.[98] In the second study, a secondary-prevention study in 26,449 patients with MI, ischemic stroke, or peripheral vascular disease,[99] vorapaxar reduced by 12% (p = 0001) the protocol-specified primary endpoint of the composite of cardiovascular death, MI, stroke, or urgent coronary revascularization compared with standard of care, but again at the cost of increased bleeding (4.2% versus 2.5%, P < 0.001), including intracranial hemorrhage (ICH). However, there was a lower risk of ICH in patients without a history of stroke.

Atopaxar. *Atopaxar* is still under evaluation. In one phase 2 trial on patients with ACS (NSTE), no major cardiovascular benefits were detected, hepatic enzymes rose, and QTc was prolonged.[100] However, Holter-detected ischemia decreased 48 hours following dosing.

Glycoprotein IIb/IIIa Receptor Antagonists

GpIIb/IIIa blockers inhibit one of the platelet integrin adhesion receptors known as the $\alpha IIb\beta3$ receptor (see Fig. 9-3 and Table 9-1).[10] Thereby they block final platelet activation and cross-linking by fibrinogen and vWF. Importantly, the trials of GpIIb/IIIa antagonists were conducted before the advent of dual antiplatelet therapy so that recent guidelines have given them less strong recommendation. Thus according to current ESC guidelines it is reasonable to withhold GpIIb/IIIa receptor inhibitors until after angiography.[73] Maximum platelet inhibition should logically consist of three types of agents acting at three different sites: aspirin, $P2Y_{12}$ blockers, and GpIIb/IIIa inhibitors (see Fig. 9-3). However, high doses of all three combined with anticoagulant therapy should only be reserved for ACS with continuing ischemia while awaiting PCI because of the increased risk of bleeding.[73]

Risk of thrombocytopenia and bleeding. The three commonly used GpIIb/IIIa antagonists are abciximab, tirofiban, and eptifibatide, each with somewhat different approved indications in the United States (Table 9-2).

Table 9-2

GpIIb/IIIa Receptor Antagonists: Key Properties

Compound and US Licensed Indications	Supporting Trials	Pharmacokinetics	Doses (all with aspirin and heparin)*	Special Points	Side Effects and Contraindications
Abciximab 1. PCI 2. Unstable angina requiring PCI within 24 h	CAPTURE, EPIC, EPILOG, EPISTENT, TARGET	Monoclonal antibody High affinity to platelet receptor (low K_D); 67% bound to receptor; plasma $t_{1/2}$ 10-30 min; remains platelet-bound in circulation up to 15 days with some residual activity	0.25 mg/kg bolus 10-60 before PCI, then 0.125 mcg/kg/min up to max of 10 mcg over 12 h, up to 24 h if ACS with planned PCI	Keep vials cold (not frozen); filter bolus injection before use, use in-line filter for infusion; discard vial after use.	Bleeding—most contraindications relate to risk of bleeding. Use extra care at puncture sites. Thrombocytopenia—Caution: obtain platelet count before starting, 2-4 h after bolus and 24 h before discharge of patient Hypersensitivity—rare.
Eptifibatide 1. PCI 2. Non-ST elevation ACS	IMPACT-II, PURSUIT, ESPIRIT	Cyclic heptapeptide Lower receptor affinity than others; plasma $t_{1/2}$ 2-3 h; renal clearance 50%	180 mcg/kg bolus, then 2 mcg/kg/min up to 72 h Reduce dose to 0.5 mcg/kg/min at time of PCI, then for 20-24 h post-PCI. If no prior ACS but PCI, 135 mcg/kg bolus then 0.5 mcg/kg/min	Store vials at 2-8° but can keep at room temperature up to 2 months.	Bleeding, as for abciximab. Renal disease: C/I if serum creatinine > 4 mg/dL (350 µmol/L). If serum creatinine 2-4 mg/dL (175-350 µmol/L) reduce dose to 135 mcg/kg bolus then 0.5 mcg/kg/min. Thrombocytopenia: no excess is claimed in package insert, but real risk probably similar to other agents (see text).
Tirofiban 1. Non-ST elevation ACS 2. ST-elevation MI	PRISM, PRISM-Plus RESTORE On-TIME 2	Peptidomimetic nonpeptide Intermediate affinity for receptor, closer to abciximab; hence 35% unbound in circulation, renal (65%) and fecal (25%) clearance	1. Non-STEMI, Two stage infusion: 0.4 mcg/kg/min for 30 min, then 0.1 mcg/kg/min up to 48 min 2. STEMI, 25-mcg/kg bolus and 0.15-mcg/kg/min maintenance infusion	Store vials at room temperature, 25 °C or 77 °C protected from light (easiest to store)	Bleeding, as for abciximab. Renal disease: ↓ dose if creatinine clearance <30 mL/min. Thrombocytopenia: 1.5% vs 0.6% heparin alone. Do platelet count before (C/I if count < 150,000/µL, 6 h after initial dose, then daily, stop if platelets <90,000//µL.

ACS, Acute coronary syndrome; C/I, contraindications; MI, myocardial infarction; PCI, percutaneous intervention; STEMI, ST-elevation myocardial infarction; $t_{1/2}$, half-time.

*For heparin doses, see text.

Berg JM, et al. J Am Coll Cardiol 2010;55:2446.

They have all been studied on a background of aspirin and antithrombotic therapy, but the main trials were conducted prior to the use of thienopyridines and the current $P2Y_{12}$ blockers. The major problem with these agents is acute thrombocytopenia at rates ranging from 0.3% to 6%[101] with added risk of delayed thrombocytopenia after 5-11 days; both acute types are thought to be caused by drug-dependent antibodies. Abciximab more than doubles the incidence of severe thrombocytopenia, which can rarely be fatal, with much lower risks for eptifibatide or tirofiban.[73] Thus all three are contraindicated in the presence of a bleeding site or increased bleeding potential, or preexisting thrombocytopenia. All are administered with either low-molecular-weight heparin (LMWH) or low-dose intravenous unfractionated heparin (UFH). All are given intravenously and only for a limited time, to cover the intervention.[73] For patients who are not at high risk and in the absence of PCI, their effect is modest or neutral and no current guidelines recommend their use in such settings.

Combination with unfractionated or LMWHs or other anticoagulants. The GpIIb/IIIa blockers must be combined with aspirin and anticoagulant therapy, the latter being UFH in most major trials. This in turn calls for constant monitoring of the heparin dose by activated clotting time (ACT) testing. However, current practice usually prefers LMWH to UFH. Based on the results of the ACUITY trial, bivalirudin may be used in place of GpIIb/IIIa inhibition plus UFH and LMWH.[63,102] Fondaparinux is recommended by the ESC in nonurgent situations,[63] although there has been no formal test of its combination with GpIIb/IIIa inhibitors.

Intracoronary administration. Compared with intravenous administration, intracoronary administration of GpIs has favorable effects on thrombolysis in myocardial infarction (TIMI) flow, target vessel revascularization, and short-term mortality after PCI, with similar rates of bleeding. Data regarding mid- and long-term outcomes are inconclusive. Large trials with longer follow-up are required to determine long-term safety and efficacy.[103]

Abciximab

Abciximab *(ReoPro)* is a monoclonal antibody against the platelet GpIIb/IIIa receptor. It consists of a murine variable portion of the Fab fragment combined with the human constant region. Abciximab also blocks the binding of vitronectin to its receptor ($\alpha_v\beta_3$) on endothelial cells, but it is not known whether this has any therapeutic advantage. Inhibition of platelet aggregation is maximal at 2 hours after a bolus injection, and returns to almost normal at 12 hours. However, the antibody is transmitted to new platelets and can be detected 14 days after administration. Its action can be reversed by platelet transfusions. Abciximab is very effective in patients undergoing PCI,[90] which is currently its only license in the United States, unless dealing with NSTE ACS with known angiographic findings and requiring PCI within 24 hours (see Table 9-2). When given very early, in the ambulance, to those with STEMI it only decreased distal embolization during PCI.[104]

Dose, side effects, and contraindications. An initial bolus is followed by an infusion to a maximum of 24 hours (see Table 9-2). High-risk patients are pretreated with clopidogrel (see previous paragraph). Careful control of heparin is important to lessen bleeding, using a reduced dose as with all GpIIb/IIIa inhibitors. In EPILOG[105] heparin was given as an initial bolus of 70 U/kg, or less according to the initial ACT (maximum initial bolus, 7000 units), followed by 20 U/kg boluses as needed to keep the ACT at 200 seconds (see package insert). Acute severe *thrombocytopenia* (platelet count of <20,000), occurs in approximately 0.5% to 1% of patients.[106] Therefore platelet counts are

required in the first few hours after beginning the infusion. Readministration of abciximab may provoke antibodies to cause severe thrombocytopenia in approximately 2.4%.[107] Thus previous thrombocytopenia
is a clear *contraindication* to readministration; use alternative IIb/IIIa
blockers. It can be given intracoronary.

Tirofiban

Tirofiban *(Aggrastat)* is a highly specific nonpeptide peptidomimetic
GpIIb/IIIa inhibitor, which is inherently less likely to cause hypersensitivity than a monoclonal antibody. Nonetheless, the end result of both
methods of blockade is inhibition of binding of fibrinogen and vWF to
the GpIIb/IIIa receptor (see Fig. 9-3). It has an acute onset and a half-life
of approximately 2 hours. Indications, dosage, side effects, and contraindications are in Table 9-2. In the TACTICS trial on patients with unstable
angina, tirofiban with PCI was compared with tirofiban alone, and the
combination was better except for the low-risk group of patients, arguing for the value of risk assessment in ACS (see Fig. 12-3). Tirofiban is
only licensed for unstable angina and NSTEMI, but is the easiest of the
three agents to store (vials at room temperature). The European approval is for unstable angina or non–Q-wave MI with the last episode of
chest pain occurring within 12 hours and with electrocardiogram
(ECG) changes or elevated cardiac enzymes. Increased bleeding is
given in the tirofiban package insert as the most common adverse
event. In those who received heparin and tirofiban, the incidence of
thrombocytopenia (defined as $<50,000/mm^3$) was 0.3% versus 0.1%
for those who received heparin alone (package insert).

Comparison with abciximab. In the TARGET trial of patients receiving triple antiplatelet therapy (aspirin, clopidogrel, and a GpIIb/IIIb
inhibitor) plus heparin, tirofiban was compared with abciximab in
4809 patients undergoing PCI for an ACS or for stable angina.[108] Both
drugs were given according to the package inserts. By 30 days, MI had
occurred in 6.9% of tirofiban patients versus 5.4% of abciximab patients
(p = 0.04). Minor bleeding was more frequent with abciximab. At
12-month follow-up there was no difference in the composite endpoint
of death, MI, or urgent revascularization.[109] Thus, overall, at these doses
used and long-term the agents were equal although very different in
price.

Use of tirofiban in STEMI. The new higher doses (25 mcg/kg bolus and
0.15 mcg/kg/min maintenance infusion)[110] were given to patients with
STEMI in the ambulance or referral center in the On-TIME 2 Study.[111] All
patients also received an intravenous bolus of UFH (5000 IU), together
with intravenous aspirin 500 mg and an oral 600-mg loading dose
of clopidogrel. Then, before primary PCI, an additional 2500 IE UFH was
administered only if the ACT was less than 200. Major adverse cardiac
events at 30 days were significantly reduced (5.8% versus 8.6%, p = 0.043).
There was a strong trend toward a decrease in mortality (2.2% versus 4.1%,
p = 0.051) in patients who were randomized to tirofiban pretreatment,
which was maintained during the 1-year follow-up (3.7% versus 5.8%,
p = 0.08). Tirofiban pretreatment reduced major adverse cardiac events
at 30 days (5.8% versus 8.6%, p = 0.043), with a strong trend toward a
decrease in mortality.[111]

Summary. For STEMI tirofiban pretreatment reduced major adverse
cardiac events at 30 days.

Eptifibatide

Eptifibatide *(Integrilin)* is a synthetic cyclic heptapeptide. Structural differences from tirofiban mean that they bind at different sites on
the GpIIb/IIIa receptor, yet with the same end result. The affinity for the

receptor is, however, lower than with the other GpIIb/IIIa blockers, which explains the higher dose in absolute terms. Indications, dosage, side effects, and contraindications are in Table 9-2. UFH was given with eptifibatide in the PURSUIT trial as a bolus of 5000 units (weight adjusted), and then infused at 1000 U/hour to keep the activated partial prothrombin time (aPPT) at between 50 and 70.[112] As for all GpIIb/IIIa blockers, the major problem is increased bleeding. Although the package insert claims that thrombocytopenia (<100,000/mm³) is not augmented, in PURSUIT[112] profound platelet depression (<20,000/mm³) occurred within 0.3% eptifibatide versus 0.1 % in controls, both groups receiving aspirin and heparin. Thus thrombocytopenia is a risk as with other GpIIb/IIIa blockers. Eptifibatide is currently the only GpIIb/IIIa blocker that is licensed for both ACS and for PCI. It can be given by the intracoronary route.

Oral Anticoagulants: Warfarin, Antithrombin, and Anti-Xa Agents (Dabigatran, Rivaroxaban, Apixaban)

Oral Anticoagulation by Warfarin

Warfarin (Coumarin, Coumadin, Panwarfin) is the most commonly used oral anticoagulant. Warfarin also has few side effects, except for the major complication associated with over-anticoagulation, which is bleeding including serious risk of intracranial hemorrhage. The metabolism of warfarin is influenced by many other drugs. In general, when comparing warfarin with aspirin, higher-intensity warfarin (international normalized ratio [INR] 3-4) is more effective, but associated with more bleeding that may be unacceptable. Moderate-intensity warfarin (INR 2-3) still has the risk of bleeding but protects better than aspirin from stroke prevention in AF.[113] Currently there is a strong trend away from warfarin toward the new antithrombin agents (dabigatran, rivaroxaban, apixaban). Yet in carefully managed situations as in Finland,[114] the risk of intracranial hemorrhage with warfarin is declining. Patients currently already stabilized on warfarin with INR 2-3 are currently best left on warfarin.

Cost-effective considerations. Thus an important contemporary question is whether a new candidate for anticoagulant therapy for nonvalvular AF should receive one of the newer antithrombin agents or warfarin. One of the deciding factors may be cost effectiveness, suggesting that dabigatran is superior to warfarin. Dabigatran was associated with 4.27 quality-adjusted life-years compared with 3.91 quality-adjusted life-years with warfarin.[115] Dabigatran provided 0.36 additional quality-adjusted life-years at a cost of $9000, yielding an incremental cost-effectiveness ratio of $25,000. This conclusion is, however, limited as it is based on a substudy of a single randomized trial. Furthermore, these results may not apply to good stabilized INR control using warfarin.

Mechanism of action. As a group, the warfarin-like oral anticoagulants inactivate vitamin K in the hepatic microsomes, thereby interfering with the formation of vitamin K–dependent clotting factors such as prothrombin (see Fig. 9-5). In addition, factor X may be reduced.[113] The onset of therapeutic levels of anticoagulation is delayed by 2-7 days.

Pharmacokinetics. After rapid and complete absorption, oral warfarin is almost totally bound to plasma albumin, with a half-life of 37 hours. It is metabolized in the hepatic microsomes by the enzymes cytochrome P450(CYP)2C9 and vitamin K epoxide reductase (VKORC1) to produce inactive metabolites excreted in the urine and stools. *Genetic variation* in these enzymes probably account for much of the variability of the warfarin dose from patient to patient.[116] For pharmacogenetic testing, see below.

Dose. A standard procedure is to give warfarin 5 mg/day for 5 days, checking the INR daily until it is in the therapeutic range, and then to check it three times weekly for up to 2 weeks. *Lower starting doses* should be given to older adults and to those with increased risk of bleeding (including prior aspirin use). Genetic variations in hepatic enzymes explain lower doses for persons of Asian descent[117] and higher doses for black and some Jewish populations.[117,118] In those transitioning from parenteral anticoagulation, warfarin should be commenced at least 4 days before heparin is discontinued to allow for the inactivation of circulating vitamin K–dependent coagulation factors; the heparin can be discontinued once the INR (next section) has been in the therapeutic range for 2 days.[113] Avoiding a large primary dose helps prevent an excessively high INR. Patients with heart failure or liver disease require lower doses. The usual dose maintenance is 4-5 mg daily, but may vary from 1 mg to 20 mg daily. Warfarin resistance is largely genetic in origin.[118] This wide range means that doses must be individualized according to the INR. In the United States, genetic-based testing is available to identify those with very low warfarin requirements.[116] In the first trial of warfarin dosing guided by genetic testing, more accurate early control of anticoagulation was achieved. However, the primary endpoint of reduced out-of-range INRs was not achieved.[119]

INR range. The effect of warfarin is monitored by reporting the INR (see Fig. 9-5), which represents the prothrombin time according to international reference thromboplastin, as approved by the World Health Organization. In general clinical practice, the aim is moderate intensity of inhibition with an INR of 2-3. Thus an INR of 2-3 is also appropriate for patients who have deep vein thrombosis (DVT) with pulmonary embolism, those at risk of thromboembolism, and for AF. Patients with *prosthetic heart valves* require the greatest intensity of safe anticoagulation, and the recommended INR range is variable, from 2 to 4.5, with lower values for those with bioprosthetic valves and mechanical aortic rather than mitral valves.[113] A metaanalysis on 23,145 patients recommended a target of more than 3.[120] As Asian populations have a higher rate of intracranial hemorrhage, a lower INR target may be needed.[117] Once the steady-state warfarin requirement is known, the INR need only be checked once every 4-6 weeks. Importantly, variation in INR control and variation in warfarin requirements may be influenced in individual patients by dietary changes and alcohol intake (modifying metabolism) and by drug interactions (see p. 358).

Self-monitoring and self-guided warfarin therapy. Selected patients who can both self-monitor and self-guide have less thromboembolic events and lower mortality than those who only self-monitor.[121] Thus with computer-guided dose adjustment the educated patient may achieve control superior to that achieved even by the experienced physician.

Pharmogenetic-guided dosing. Bleeding risks are highest within the first 1-3 months of starting warfarin, up to 10 times more than later risk. In the CoumaGen-II study of VKORC genotype-guided warfarin dosing, the prior analysis of VKORC gave the genetically appropriate first dose. The result was 10% absolute reduction in the out-of-range INRs, 66% lower rate of DVT, and a reduction in serious adverse events at 90 days from 9.4% in controls to 4.5%. These data argue for the pharmacogenetic approach, if available and if rapid and affordable, prior to the initiation of warfarin.[122]

Dose reduction. The dose should be reduced in the presence of congestive heart failure; liver damage from any source, including alcohol; renal impairment (which increases the fraction of free drug in the plasma); and malnutrition (which leads to vitamin K deficiency). Thyrotoxicosis enhances the catabolism of vitamin K, reducing the dose of warfarin needed, whereas myxedema has the opposite effect. In older adults, the dose should be reduced because the response to warfarin increases with age. A high intake of dietary vitamin K (e.g., green vegetables such as broccoli) reduces the efficacy of warfarin. Some fad diets alternate high and low salad periods, which causes INR control to fluctuate.

Drug interactions with warfarin. Warfarin interacts with approximately 80 other drugs. It is inhibited by drugs such as barbiturates or phenytoin that accelerate warfarin degradation in the liver. Potentiating drugs include the cardiovascular agents allopurinol and amiodarone, and cephalosporins that inhibit the generation of Vitamin K.[113] Drugs that decrease warfarin degradation and increase the anticoagulant effect include a variety of antibiotics such as metronidazole *(Flagyl)* and co-trimoxazole *(Bactrim)*.

Antiplatelet drugs such as aspirin, clopidogrel, and NSAIDs may potentiate the risk of bleeding, but this varies considerably. Sulfinpyrazone powerfully displaces warfarin from blood proteins, reducing the required dose of warfarin down to 1 mg in some patients. The safest rule is to tell patients on oral anticoagulation not to take any over-the-counter nor any new drugs without consultation, and for the physician to checklist any new drug that is used. If in doubt, the INR should be monitored more frequently. This is also necessary when dietary changes are anticipated, as during travel.

Contraindications. Contraindications include recent stroke; uncontrolled hypertension; hepatic cirrhosis; and potential GI and genitourinary bleeding points such as hiatus hernia, peptic ulcer, gastritis, gastroesophageal reflux, colitis, proctitis, and cystitis. If anticoagulation is deemed essential, the risk-benefit ratio must be evaluated carefully. Old age is not in itself a contraindication against anticoagulation, although older adults are more likely to bleed, particularly if prone to falls.

Renal impairment. The warfarin doses for moderate reduction in renal function may need reduction (approximately 25% in a small study for a mean creatinine clearance [CrCl] of 47 mL/min) while watching for increased warfarin instability.[113]

Pregnancy and warfarin. Warfarin is contraindicated in the first trimester because of its teratogenicity, and 2 weeks before birth because of the risk of fetal bleeding. The alternative, UFH, may be less effective than warfarin and the FDA has issued a warning against LMWH. One approach is to use heparin or LMWH in the first trimester; warfarin in the second trimester until about 38 weeks; and changing to heparin or LMWH, which is discontinued 12 hours before labor induction, restarted postpartum, and overlapped with warfarin for 4-5 days. Heparin should be regularly monitored by aPPT and LMWH by anti-Xa levels. Heparin requirements increase in the third trimester because heparin-binding proteins increase.

Complications and cautions. The most common complication is bleeding with increased risk of intracranial hemorrhage, especially in older adults.[123,124] This finding has accelerated the trend toward replacement of warfarin by direct thrombin inhibitors; yet they, too, are relatively contradicted in much older adults. Although rare, a very serious complication is *warfarin-associated skin necrosis*. The cause is not well understood; it may possibly be acute depletion in protein C, a natural anticoagulant. The skin necrosis may occur between the third and the eighth day of therapy, especially when high-dose warfarin is initiated after cardiopulmonary bypass. The best protection is to start with lower doses under the cover of heparin. If it is necessary to carry on with warfarin despite the necrosis, the dose should be reduced to approximately 2 mg daily, covered by heparin, and gradually increased over several weeks.[113] Long-term use of warfarin (>1 year) may be complicated by osteoporotic fracture, which is more marked in men.[125]

Warfarin overdose and bleeding. Bleeding is more common in older adult patients soon after starting therapy, which is a high danger period.[126] During chronic therapy, the risk of bleeding can be reduced dramatically by lowering the intended INR from 3-4.5 down to 2-3.[113] Even high INR values up to 9 may (in the absence of bleeding) be managed by dose omission and then reinstating warfarin at a lower dose. If bleeding becomes significant, or if the INR is more than 9, 3-5 mg of oral vitamin K_1 should be given to reduce the INR within 24-48 hours. The subcutaneous route gives variable results and should be avoided, rather than using the slow intravenous route (5-10 mg over 30 min) for an emergency.[113] In patients with *prosthetic valves,* vitamin K should be avoided because of the risk of valve thrombosis, unless there is a life-threatening intracranial bleed. A comparison between fresh frozen plasma (FFP) and vitamin K in patients with mechanical heart valves and mild to moderate over-anticoagulation showed quicker response within 6 hours to FFP.[127] In patients unresponsive to vitamin K or with life-threatening bleeding, the intravenous treatment could be (1) a concentrate of the prothrombin group of coagulation factors including II, IX, and X; or (2) FFP (15 mL/kg).

Indications for Warfarin

Acute myocardial infarction. We maintain the viewpoint expressed in our previous editions that we do not advise using oral anticoagulants routinely after infarction; rather, there should be a careful evaluation of the needs of each individual patient, with a preference for aspirin started as soon as possible after the onset of myocardial ischemia and continued indefinitely unless there are clear contraindications. We also recommend a $P2Y_{12}$ blocker for 12 months. The downside is the risk of increased bleeding with warfarin[128] and with triple therapy.

In chronic heart failure post-MI (mean ejection fraction, 25%) in sinus rhythm, there was no significant overall difference in the primary outcome between treatment with warfarin and treatment with aspirin.[129] In this 6-year study of 2305 patients, 48% with previous MI with low and in sinus rhythm, there was no difference in the composite of death, ischemic stroke, or intracranial bleed. The reduced rate of ischemic stroke with warfarin was offset by an increased risk of major hemorrhage. The authors concluded that choice between warfarin and aspirin should be individualized. Because aspirin is cheap and requires no monitoring, it wins the day in most instances. Aspirin was provided by Bayer HealthCare; thus the likely dose was 100 mg daily.

Venous thromboembolism. In patients with DVT, warfarin should be initiated concurrently with intravenous heparin or LMWH. Thereafter, oral anticoagulation alone should be continued for at least 3 months. A less intensive regimen (INR 2-3) is effective and safer than a more intensive regimen (INR 3-4.5).[113] Long-term follow-up by low-intensity warfarin (INR 1.5 to 2) reduces repeat events.[130] Indefinite treatment should be considered in patients with recurrent venous thrombosis, or with risk factors such as antithrombin-III deficiency, protein-C or protein-S deficiency, persistent antiphospholipid antibodies, or malignancy. For documented *pulmonary embolism,* either LMWH or UFH should be given, followed by oral warfarin continued for approximately

6 months in the absence of recurrences. However, should there be a recurrence, indefinite therapy should be considered.

Atrial fibrillation. AF is strongly associated with thromboembolism and the risk rises additively in those with congestive heart failure, left ventricular (LV) dysfunction, hypertension, older age, diabetes, TIA, previous thromboembolism, prior MI, peripheral atrial disease, the presence of aortic plaques, and especially stroke. Treatment should be guided by the use of the European guidelines[46] taking into account the CHADS$_2$ score[131] and the CHADS-VASC or CHA$_2$DS$_2$-VASc scores.[132] (For assessment of these scoring systems, seeChapter 12, p. 498.) The benefits of warfarin far exceed the risk of hemorrhage. The only clear indications for withholding warfarin are (1) lone AF in younger patients (aged <65 years) without risk factors; (2) bleeding diathesis; and (3) older adult patients with high risk of bleeding, which can be quantified by the HAS-BLED[133] or ATRIA bleeding risk scores.[134] Cardioversion increases the risk of an embolus in patients with AF. After 48 hours of AF, anticoagulation for 3 weeks is strongly recommended (if feasible) prior to elective cardioversion. Transesophageal echo may be used to look for atrial thrombus with the aim of proceeding to cardioversion in the absence of thrombus, and where the duration is uncertain. In most patients the duration of anticoagulation even after resumption of sinus rhythm should be lifelong.[135] Patients with paroxysmal AF have increased risk of stroke, the same as persistent AF.[136]

Paroxysmal atrial fibrillation. The choices vary from no treatment in "lone" AF to warfarin in those older adult patients at higher risk of stroke.[137] For the latter, one of the newer antithrombins would be preferred because of their lower risk of stroke (see later, Table 9-6). Treatment should again be guided by the use of the European guidelines,[46] taking into account the CHADS$_2$ score[131] or the CHADS-VASC or CHA$_2$DS$_2$-VASc scores.[132] (For assessment of these scoring systems and the HAS-Bled indexes, see Chapter 12, p. 499.) We recommend the CHA$_2$DS$_2$-VASc scores.

Atrial fibrillation presenting with acute embolic stroke. Although anticoagulation is required, cerebral hemorrhage must first be excluded by computed tomography or magnetic resonance imaging. In the case of large strokes, warfarin should be delayed for approximately 1 week to allow full evolution to occur.

Atrial fibrillation: proposals. There is strong evidence for the use of moderate-intensity anticoagulation (INR target 2-3) in "high-risk" patients, in whom warfarin is much more effective than aspirin in preventing stroke (CHADS$_2$ >1).[46,137] Patients should be risk-stratified CHA$_2$DS$_2$-VASc scores, and aspirin (or no antithrombotic) should only be used in those at low stroke risk (score of 0 or 1). The clinical assessment required to assess the need for warfarin is shown in Table 7 of the European recommendations on anticoagulation.[138] The major risk factors are age older than 65 years, a history of hypertension, diabetes, congestive heart failure, and a history of stroke or TIA. Increased left atrial (LA) dimension, a mitral valve gradient, or regurgitation indicate higher risk.[138] Patients with a recent TIA or minor stroke are at particularly high risk of a recurrence.[139]

Atrial fibrillation in older adults. This common combination requires careful balancing of the advantages of reduced thromboembolism versus the risk of serious hemorrhage, especially in those with increased risk of hemorrhage and those with an inadvertent INR of 4 or more.[126]

Mitral stenosis or regurgitation. In patients with mitral valve disease, the risk of thromboembolism is greatest in those with AF, marked

LA enlargement, or previous embolic episodes; anticoagulation is strongly indicated in patients with any of these features. In contrast, anticoagulation is not indicated in patients with mitral stenosis with sinus rhythm. *Percutaneous mechanical LA appendage closure* with the Watchman device is a new approach. In a comparison of such closure against warfarin in AF patients with CHADS$_2$ of 1 or more,[140] the procedure was noninferior to warfarin therapy for the prevention of stroke, systemic embolism, and cardiovascular death. Yet there was a significantly higher risk of complications, predominantly pericardial effusion and procedural stroke related to air embolism. These complications could be decreased by meticulous care and increased operator experience.[140] Peri-device flow occurred in 32% of implanted patients at 12 months but was not associated with an increased risk of thromboembolism.[141]

Dilated cardiomyopathy. There is a substantial risk of systemic embolism, particularly if there is AF. Although anticoagulants are effective in reducing thromboembolism, the risk versus benefit is the subject of ongoing trials. In heart failure, aspirin is as protective as warfarin.[129] Thus we do not recommend routine anticoagulation in the absence of additional thrombotic risk or evidence of mural thrombus.

The tachycardia-bradycardia syndrome. Tachycardia-bradycardia syndrome may be complicated by AF and thromboembolism. Anticoagulation should be considered, especially if there is underlying organic heart disease, such as ischemic heart disease, hypertension, or cardiomyopathy.

Atrial septal defects. In older patients with atrial septal defects and pulmonary hypertension, anticoagulation is strongly recommended as prophylaxis against in situ pulmonary arterial thromboses or, rarely, paradoxical emboli. Anticoagulation is also required for patients with repaired septal defects who subsequently develop AF.

Warfarin for prosthetic heart valves. Warfarin is recommended in patients with mechanical prosthetic heart valves, usually at a level of 2.5 to 3.5.[113] However, a metaanalysis proposed a relatively high target INR of 3 to 4.5, with aortic mechanical valves at the lower end and mitral valves at the higher end of the INR range.[120] In patients with bioprosthetic mitral valves, the risk of thromboembolism is highest in the first 6-12 weeks, when warfarin is mandatory. Thereafter, aspirin may be given or antithrombotic therapy may be discontinued if there are no other indications. There is strong evidence supporting the continuation of warfarin when mitral bioprosthetic valves are combined with AF, a large left atrium, or LV failure. In patients with bioprosthetic aortic valves the risk is low, and aspirin for 6-12 weeks is appropriate.[142]

Warfarin for moderate chronic kidney disease: warfarin-related nephropathy. CKD is associated with both a lower warfarin maintenance dose and decreased stability of anticoagulation, requiring tighter anticoagulation management.[142A] In those with stage 3 CKD, AF is associated with double the rate of adverse events,[143] including increased bleeding.[41] Adjusted-dose warfarin compared with aspirin and very-low-dose warfarin reduced ischemic stroke and systemic embolism by 76% (P < 0.001), yet without increased major hemorrhage.[143] However, note that for this degree of stage 3 renal impairment, dabigatran or rivaroxaban can also be used, whereas apixaban also seems safer, although without comparative trials (see later, Table 9-6).

Warfarin-related nephropathy is a newly described entity in those with an acutely increased INR of more than 3 soon after the initiation of warfarin.[144] This, if confirmed, is especially serious in patients with CKD in whom it is more often associated with an unexplained acute increase in serum creatinine and an accelerated progression of CKD. In 4006 patients with CKD and an INR exceeding 3, the 1-year mortality was 31.1% compared with 18.9% without warfarin-related nephropathy.[144] The *bottom line* is that INR should be kept below 3 in all patients soon after starting warfarin, but especially in those with CKD or who use antithrombin inhibitors (see later, Table 9-6).

Possible indications for warfarin.
Cerebrovascular accidents and transient ischemic attacks. There is no evidence to support anticoagulation in patients who have had a completed stroke (in the absence of AF). When patients present with an acute stroke and AF, warfarin is indicated providing cerebral hemorrhage is excluded by computed tomography. In patients with recent TIAs, warfarin is only recommended when symptoms persist despite aspirin or clopidogrel therapy, or when there is a major cardiac source of embolism. In symptomatic intracranial arterial stenosis, high-dose aspirin is better than warfarin (same stroke outcomes, less bleeding and death).[145]

Mitral valve prolapse. In patients with definite echocardiographic documentation of mitral valve prolapse and evidence suggestive of thrombotic or thromboembolic events, warfarin or platelet inhibitors may be indicated.

Low-dose warfarin: is it indicated to prevent thromboembolism? As reviewed in the seventh edition of this book, low-dose warfarin is theoretically attractive for a variety of thromboembolic conditions, yet not supported by trial data. In secondary prevention after venous thromboembolism (VTE), low-intensity warfarin (INR 1.5-1.9) was better than placebo[130] but inferior to the conventional intensity (INR 2-3).[146] For patients with unprovoked VTE, a low level of anticoagulation with *rivaroxaban* was noninferior to warfarin for the primary efficacy outcome (symptomatic recurrent VTE) and reduced major bleeding from 2.2 to 1.1% (HR, 0.49; 0.31 to 0.79; P = 0.003). Rates of other adverse events were similar.[147]

Oral anticoagulation by warfarin: summary. Oral anticoagulants are indicated in many *patients with AF and in those with prosthetic heart valves.* They are used in both the treatment and prevention of venous thrombosis and pulmonary embolism. *A small minority of patients with AMI qualify for limited anticoagulation with warfarin for 3-6 months.* Very few require prolonged anticoagulation. Long-term anticoagulation requires careful consideration of the risk-benefit ratio (bleeding versus decreased thromboembolism) for each individual patient. There is the increasingly recognized risk of increased intracranial bleeding with warfarin. For example, although a patient with chronic AF may benefit from meticulous anticoagulation, aspirin may be a safer choice for a relatively noncompliant or frail older adult patient. The major problem with warfarin is the large variation in the doses needed to achieve and maintain the required INR. Genetic-based dosing is gaining ground but is costly and not straightforward.

Anticoagulation with Direct Thrombin Inhibitors and Anti-Xa Agents

As noted in Chapter 7, with the recognition of the importance of stroke as the principal clinically significant complication of AF, stroke prevention by new oral anticoagulants has moved to the fore. These agents are at least as effective as warfarin in preventing embolic stroke among patients with AF and are safer with less intracranial bleeding or complicating hemorrhagic strokes.[148] There may be a small increase in the incidence of MI with dabigatran, with an HR of 1.27 versus warfarin; the mechanism is unknown.[149] On offer are more convenient and potentially safer ways of maintaining optimal anticoagulation, which should encourage physicians to use these agents more widely for patients with AF. These agents are discussed here. The major remaining issues are cost effectiveness versus warfarin and the lack of any clinically established antidotes to inadvertent uncontrolled bleeding. However, the risk of bleeding may have been over emphasized (see discussion of the EMA under "Doses and Approval" in "Dabigatran"), the exception being in the much older adults.

Dabigatran

Dabigatran etexilate (Pradaxa) is a new direct thrombin inhibitor.[150] Dabigatran and its acyl glucuronides are competitive, direct thrombin inhibitors (see Fig. 9-9). Because thrombin enables the conversion of fibrinogen into fibrin during the coagulation cascade, its inhibition prevents thrombosis. Both free and clot-bound thrombin as well as thrombin-induced platelet aggregation are inhibited by the active moieties. Dabigatran etexilate mesylate is absorbed as the ester, which is then hydrolyzed, forming dabigatran, the active moiety. Dabigatran is metabolized to four different acyl glucuronides, which have similar pharmacokinetics and activity to dabigatran. These have similar dose-proportional pharmacokinetics in healthy subjects and patients in the range of doses from 10 to 400 mg. Dabigatran etexilate is a substrate of the efflux transporter P-Gp. However, there appear to be no significant drug interactions with P-Gp inducers or inhibitors. After oral administration of dabigatran etexilate in healthy volunteers, Cmax occurs at 1 hour postadministration in the fasted state. The half-life of dabigatran in healthy subjects is 12 to 17 hours; its bioavailability is 6.5%, and 80% of the drug is excreted by the kidneys. Gastric discomfort is a potential side effect.

Clinical studies. In the RE-LY study dabigatran 150 mg twice daily reduced the combined endpoint of stroke and systemic embolism in patients with AF when compared with warfarin, yet with approximately similar rates of bleeding and four fewer intracranial hemorrhages per 1000 patients.[151] With dabigatran there was a trend toward increased MI, more than balanced by the major finding that stroke or systemic embolism was reduced compared with warfarin.[152] At a dose of 110 mg twice daily dabigatran gave similar rates of stroke and systemic embolism as warfarin, yet with 30% lower rates of major hemorrhage and five fewer intracranial hemorrhages per 1000 patients.[153] A major advantage over warfarin is that dabigatran reduces stroke or systemic embolism more effectively than warfarin. A broader composite that included "net clinical benefit" of all major events (all strokes, systemic embolism, MI, pulmonary embolism, major bleeding, and all-cause death) occurred at annual rates of 4.76% with dabigatran 110 mg, 4.47% with dabigatran 150 mg, and 5.10% with warfarin. The HRs versus warfarin were 0.93 ($P = 0.24$) for dabigatran 110 mg and 0.88 (95%, CI 0.78-0.98, $P = 0.03$) for dabigatran 150 mg. Thus the higher dose was better than warfarin at reducing all adverse cardiovascular events.[154]

Coadministration. Coadministration of aspirin and dabigatran increased the risk of major bleeding compared with dabigatran alone (HR 1.91; $P < 0.001$) without any evidence of benefit in reducing stroke and other serious vascular events.

Risks in older adults. Impaired renal function and low body weight are hazards. There must be a careful evaluation of the risks and possible benefits of treatment before starting dabigatran. In RE-LY, dabigatran at the higher dose of 150 mg twice daily was superior to adjusted-dose warfarin in reducing ischemic and hemorrhagic stroke. The risk for major bleeds was similar across subgroups.

Doses and approvals. Doses and approvals are complex. The FDA has licensed the higher dose (150 mg twice daily) for prevention of stroke in patients with AF and the lower dose of 110 mg twice daily is also licensed in Europe. In May 2012 the FDA-approved new label stated that the 150-mg twice-daily dose is superior to warfarin in preventing ischemic and hemorrhagic stroke in nonvalvular AF.[155] The FDA also approved the 75 mg twice-daily dose for severe renal impairment. The Canadian Health authority approved dabigatran for the prevention of stroke and systemic embolism in patients with AF in whom anticoagulation is appropriate. The 150-mg twice-daily dose was recommended and the 110-mg twice-daily dose was specifically for patients more than 80 years of age and for patients at high risk of bleeding. Dabigatran 150 and 110 mg are both approved by the EMA for prevention of stroke or embolism in patients with nonvalvular AF and one or more risk factors, as well as the prevention of venous thromboembolic events in total hip- and knee-replacement surgery. In patients older than 75 or with renal impairment, renal function should be assessed after 1-3 months and then at least annually, and the drug should not be given to patients with CrCl less than 30 mL/min. Although more expensive than warfarin, the great cost of having a stroke often followed by lifelong physical impairment must be taken into account in financial analyses.

In renal impairment. In the presence of renal impairment, the dose must be reduced because dabigatran and its moieties are renally excreted (80%) and should not be given to those with CrCl of less than 30 mL/min. However, these populations were excluded in RE-LY. Thus the FDA recommends a 75-mg dose[156] and the EMA suggests the 110-mg dose available in Europe.[41] Note that with time renal function may deteriorate, leading to increased plasma concentrations of dabigatran.[150]

Risk of bleeding. Dabigatran increases the risk of bleeding and can cause significant and sometimes fatal bleeding. In January 2012, in response to the reports of bleeding, the FDA revised the dabigatran label, stressing the need to monitor renal function and adjusting the dabigatran dose if necessary. In May 2012, the EMA noted that the incidence of bleeding with dabigatran had significantly fallen during postregistration use.[157] More information will be available from RELY-ABLE, a long-term safety study, the results of which will soon be available and from GLORIA-AF, a patient registry, the second phase of which was recently launched.

Risk factors and contraindications for bleeding include much advanced age and the use of drugs that increase the risk of bleeding in general (e.g., antiplatelet agents, heparin, and chronic use of NSAIDs). Overall in the RE-LY study there was similar risk of major bleeds during dabigatran as with warfarin use, with a higher rate of major GI bleeds with dabigatran 150 mg than with warfarin (1.85% versus 1.25%, respectively),[153] and a higher rate of any GI bleeds (6.1% versus 4%, respectively) but lower rates of intracranial bleeding.

Active therapy for major bleeds. With a short half-life, minor bleeds are treated by dose reduction or omission. Dabigatran etexilate is a lipophilic molecule successfully adsorbed in vitro by activated charcoal therapy. Although not clinically tested, it is reasonable to administer charcoal within 1 to 2 hours of overdose before dabigatran etexilate is absorbed from the GI tract.[150] In experimental brain hematoma in a murine intracranial hematoma model associated with dabigatran, PCC and, less consistently, FFP prevented excess hematoma expansion.[14] PCC was not effective in reversing anticoagulation with dabigatran in a small clinical trial.[13]

Dabigatran versus warfarin. Hankey and Eikelboom[150] argue as follows. Warfarin will probably remain the treatment of choice for compliant patients well stabilized on warfarin, in those with a CrCl less than 30 mL/min, those who cannot afford dabigatran, those suffering from gastric discomfort, and when there are concerns about compliance with the twice-daily dose of dabigatran. In addition, even patients taking warfarin and achieving good INR control may prefer dabigatran because dabigatran 150 mg twice daily reduces stroke and intracranial bleeding compared with warfarin. *Switching* from warfarin to dabigatran requires warfarin to be stopped and the INR to be monitored daily. When the INR falls below 2, usually 2 to 3 days later, dabigatran can be started.

Dabigatran: Summary. Dabigatran, a direct thrombin inhibitor, is the first of the oral antithrombin agents; hence it has the largest and longest experience. The advantages of dabigatran versus warfarin are that it is rapidly effective, does not interact with foods nor with most medications (which are particularly problematic for patients taking warfarin), does not require monitoring, and is associated with a lower risk of ischemic stroke and intracranial bleeding than warfarin. It is more expensive than warfarin, but is more cost effective.

Rivaroxaban

Rivaroxaban (Xarelto) is an oral inhibitor of factor Xa (10a) and, like dabigatran and apixaban, it does not require monitoring. Unlike dabigatran or apixiban, it is given only once daily in AF. It is well tested in chronic nonvalvular AF.[158]

Pharmacokinetics. Unchanged rivaroxaban is the most important compound in human plasma, with no major or active circulating metabolites present. The absolute bioavailability of rivaroxaban is approximately 100% for the 10-mg dose. Rivaroxaban is rapidly absorbed with Cmax appearing 2-4 hours after tablet intake. Rivaroxaban has a half-life of approximately 5 to 13 hours. Plasma protein binding in humans is high at approximately 92% to 95%. Approximately two thirds of rivaroxaban is cleared by the liver and the other one third is cleared by direct renal excretion of unchanged compound. Hepatic metabolism is mediated by cytochromes P450-(CYP3A4, CYP2J2). Renal excretion of the unchanged drug involves the P-Gp–breast cancer resistance protein transporter systems. Rivaroxaban does not induce nor inhibit CYP3A4. In cirrhotic patients with moderate hepatic impairment, rivaroxaban clearance is impaired so that inhibition of Factor Xa is increased by a factor of 2.6. Thus the dose needs reduction. For renal impairment see next section.

Drug interactions. Rivaroxaban must be used with caution in patients receiving concomitant systemic treatment with azole antimycotics (e.g., ketoconazole) or human immunodeficiency virus (HIV) protease inhibitors (e.g., ritonavir) or rifampin (rifampicin). These drugs are strong inhibitors of both CYP3A4 and P-Gp. Co-administration of rivaroxaban with the strong CYP3A4 and P-Gp inducers (e.g., phenytoin, carbamazepine, phenobarbitone, or St. John's Wort) may also lead to a decreased rivaroxaban plasma concentration.

Use in nonvalvular atrial fibrillation. To prevent stroke or systemic embolism in patients with a $CHADs_2$ score of 2 or more the dose was 20 mg once daily,[158] reduced to 15 mg daily in those with moderate to severe renal impairment.[159] In the ROCKET-AF study rivaroxaban was at least noninferior to warfarin (superior while on treatment).[158] There was no difference between groups in the risk of major bleeding, yet intracranial and fatal bleeding occurred less frequently in the rivaroxaban group.

Use in recent acute coronary syndrome. Because factor 10a (Xa) plays a central role in thrombosis, the inhibition of factor Xa by low-dose rivaroxaban was tested with the aim of showing improved cardiovascular outcomes in patients with a recent ACS.[160] In the ATLAS

ACS 2–TIMI 51 trial 15,526 patients with a recent ACS received low-dose aspirin and a thienopyridine (almost all clopidogrel) plus 2.5-mg rivaroxaban twice daily (one fourth of the daily dose used in AF). Results were better than with 5 mg twice daily, with reduced rates of cardiovascular death (2.7% versus 4.1%, P = 0.002) and all-cause deaths (2.9% versus 4.5%, P = 0.002). The same dose reduced the risk of the composite endpoint of death from cardiovascular causes, MI, or stroke. Rivaroxaban, however, increased the risk of major bleeding (2.1% versus 0.6%, P < 0.001) and intracranial hemorrhage (0.6% versus 0.2%, P = 0.009), but not the risk of fatal bleeding. There were no hepatic side effects. The problem with this otherwise impressive trial is that FDA approval for patients with ACS was declined in May 2012 because of imperfect follow-up of a small number of trial patients. Nonetheless, this study shows that a much lower dose than before could be used and that rivaroxaban has the potential to improve outcome in those with recent ACS.

Prevention of pulmonary embolism. In 4832 patients who had acute symptomatic pulmonary embolism with or without deep vein thrombosis, rivaroxaban (15 mg twice daily for 3 weeks, followed by 20 mg once daily) equaled standard therapy.[147] Rivaroxaban was noninferior to warfarin for the primary efficacy outcome (symptomatic recurrent VTE), and reduced major bleeding from 2.2% to 1.1% (HR, 0.49; 0.31 to 0.79; P = 0.003). Rates of other adverse events were similar.

Renal disease. In the ROCKET-AF trial, the reduced dose of 15 mg once daily was given to those with moderate to severe renal impairment and a CrCl of 30-49 mL/min.[159] The outcomes in this cohort were similar to those with warfarin, as were rates of major and nonmajor bleeding.

Bleeding as a side effect. Should bleeding occur, delay the next dose or discontinue. For serious bleeding, consider procoagulant PCC as tested on human volunteers.[13] If not available, resort to activated prothrombin complex concentrate (rF VIIa).

FDA and European Union approvals. The FDA approved rivaroxaban in standard doses for the prevention of stroke and systemic embolism in nonvalvular AF and to reduce the risk of blood clots, DVT, and pulmonary embolism following knee- or hip-replacement surgery. Rivaroxaban is approved in the European Union for the prevention of nonvalvular-related AF, stroke, and systemic embolism, and for the treatment of DVT.

Rivaroxaban: Summary. The major advantage compared with other agents is the once-daily dose, whereas the major problem is that such a wide range of doses from 20 mg once daily to 2.5-mg twice daily appears to have clinical activity.

Apixaban

Apixaban (Eliquis), a direct factor Xa inhibitor, is a relatively new drug and is still being assessed by regulatory agencies. Apixaban has one high-grade study, ARISTOTLE,[161] so that it may become among the first choices for anticoagulation in patients with AF.

Pharmacokinetics. Maximum plasma concentrations are 3 to 4 hours after an oral dose. The bioavailability of the drug is approximately 50% for a 10-mg dose. The half-life is 8-15 hours (see later, Table 9-6). It is given twice daily for all indications. Liver metabolism is by CYP3A4-dependent and CYP3A4-independent mechanisms, with approximately 25% of the dose excreted unchanged in the urine. For *drug interactions*, see Table 9-6, later. Apixaban is not recommended in patients receiving concomitant treatment with strong inhibitors of both CYP3A4 and P-Gp, such as azole antimycotics and HIV virus protease inhibitors.

Dosage. For stroke prevention in AF, 5 mg twice daily is standard, with a recommended 2.5-mg twice-daily dose for patients with two or more of the following criteria: age 80 years and older, body weight less than 60 kg, or a serum creatinine level of 1.5 mg/dL (133 micromol/l) or more.

Outcome studies. This oral direct factor Xa inhibitor, given 5 mg twice daily, was clearly better than warfarin in 18,201 patients with AF and at least one additional risk factor for stroke (CHADS$_2$ score mean of 2.1).[161] It does not require anticoagulant monitoring. Apixaban was superior to warfarin in preventing stroke or systemic embolism, caused less bleeding, and resulted in lower mortality (see Chapter 8, p. 316). In a separate study of those with AF at increased risk of stroke (CHADS$_2$ score mean 2.1), but considered unsuitable for warfarin, apixaban was clearly superior to aspirin without increased bleeding.[162] However, in thromboprophylaxis, as for DVT, a prolonged course of apixaban was inferior to a short course of enoxaparin and gave more bleeding.[163] Apixaban is *contraindicated* in high-risk patients after an ACS. When added at a dose of 5 mg twice daily to standard antiplatelet therapy, major bleeding events increased without reduction in recurrent ischemic events.[164]

Severe renal impairment. There are limited clinical data in patients with a CrCl of 15 to 29 mL/min; thus only use with caution in such patients.

Overdose or excess bleeding. There is currently no specific reversal agent or antidote for apixaban. The same considerations as for rivaroxaban apply.

Apixaban: Summary. As this agent in still being assessed for registration by the FDA and European authorities, widespread clinical experience is still to come. Yet it has attractive properties such as the low rate of renal elimination, and, of note, reduced mortality in a major trial in patients with nonvalvular AF.

Novel Anticoagulants (NOACs). These have ben summarized in the current European Society of Cardiology –Europace Guidelines as follows (Camm et al., 2012). The NOACs offer better efficacy, safety, and convenience compared with OAC with VKAs. Thus, where an OAC is recommended, one of the NOACs—either a direct thrombin inhibitor (dabigatran) or an oral factor Xa inhibitor (e.g. rivaroxaban, apixaban)—should be considered instead of adjusted-dose vitamin K antagonists such as warfarin (with INR 2–3) for most patients with AF.

There is insufficient evidence to recommend one NOAC over another, although some patient characteristics, drug compliance and tolerability, and cost may be important considerations in the choice of agent.[164A]

Acute Anticoagulation: Heparin

Mechanism of action and use. Heparin, traditionally the backbone of antithrombotic therapy, is a heterogeneous mucopolysaccharide with extremely complex effects on the coagulation mechanism and on blood vessels. The major effect of UFH is on the interaction of antithrombin and thrombin (factor IIa) to inhibit the thrombin-induced platelet aggregation that initiates ACS and venous thrombosis (see Fig. 9-6).

Mode of action: comparison with LMWH. Inhibition of thrombin by heparin requires (1) binding of heparin to antithrombin by a unique pentasaccharide segment of the heparin molecule, and (2) simultaneous binding of heparin to thrombin by 13 additional saccharide units (see Fig. 9-6).[165] Heparin-antithrombin also inhibits factor Xa, to a lesser extent Xia, and others in the contact "intrinsic" path. Antithrombin contains an active center (arginine) that inhibits the active center serine not only in thrombin but also in several of the coagulation proteases, so the name *antithrombin* means more than a specific interaction only with thrombin. The dose-effect relationship is difficult to predict because heparin is a heterogeneous group of molecules extracted by a variety of procedures, and its strength varies from batch to batch. Heparin also binds variably to plasma proteins, endothelial cells, and macrophages. Such binding inactivates some of the heparin. Furthermore, there is the risk of heparin-induced thrombocytopenia (HIT; see section following). These complexities, added to the difficulty of controlling the dose and the need for monitoring, mean that heparin is far from ideal as an intravenous anticoagulant. However, its advantages compared with LMWH are that the anticoagulant effects can be promptly discontinued by stopping the intravenous infusion and it is completely and readily reversed by protamine. Also, in clinical doses it is not cleared by the kidneys; hence it is safer in renal failure.[165] Furthermore, it has a wider spectrum of antithrombotic activity (see Fig. 9-6).[165]

Controlling the dose of intravenous heparin. When heparin is administered after fibrinolytic therapy to patients with ACS, meticulous laboratory control of the heparin dose is required. The heparin may be diluted in either isotonic saline or dextrose water. European dosage recommendations are an intravenous bolus of 60-70 IU/kg up to 5000 IU, followed by an infusion of 12-15 IU/kg/hour (maximum 1000 IU/hour).[63] The dose should be adjusted to an aPPT of 1.5-2.5 times the upper limit of normal, or 50-75 seconds with monitoring at 6, 12, and 24 hours. The AHA-ACC more cautiously recommend lower doses: an initial bolus of 60 U/kg (maximum 4000 U), with an initial infusion rate of 12 U/kg/hour (maximum 1000), aiming at aPPT levels of 60-80 seconds.[166]

Higher aPPTs increase the risk of cerebral bleeding without conferring any survival advantage. The use of nomograms results in fewer subtherapeutic aPPTs, and there may also be less bleeding. If the aPPT is three times the control value, the infusion rate should be decreased by 50%; if 2-3 times the control value, the infusion rate should be decreased by 25%; if 1.5-2 times the control value, there should be no change. If the aPPT is less than 1.5 times the control value, the infusion should be increased by 25% to a maximum rate of 2500 IU/hour. At the same time, overheparinization should be guarded against to avoid cerebral bleeding. The inherent limitation of the aPPT is that different commercial reagents and laboratory instruments give different aPPT values. The ACT is preferred in the catheterization laboratory (see p. 369).

Heparin: precautions and side effects. To reduce the risk of HIT (next section) current guidelines stress that intravenous heparin should not be given for longer than 48 hours.[167] There is an increased risk of heparin-induced hemorrhage in patients with subacute bacterial endocarditis or hematologic disorders such as hemophilia, hepatic disease, or GI or genitourinary ulcerative lesions. There is a narrow therapeutic window for the use of heparin in conjunction with fibrinolytic therapy. To avoid intracerebral hemorrhage, the recommended doses of heparin should not be exceeded. Some patients are *resistant to heparin*, and in these patients administration of high-dose heparin with aPPT monitoring every 4 hours is advised. Heparin is derived from animal tissue, and occasionally causes allergy. *Heparin overdosage* is treated by stopping the drug and, if clinically required, giving protamine sulfate (checking first for salmon allergy) as a very slow infusion of a 1% solution, no more than 50 mg in any 10-minute period.

Heparin-induced thrombocytopenia and thrombosis syndrome. HIT and heparin-induced thrombocytopenia-thrombosis syndrome

(HITTS) occurs in approximately 3%-5% of patients during or after UFH treatment for 5 days or more. The incidence is much lower, less than 1% during and after LMWH therapy (see later, Table 9-4). A subset of these patients develop venous or arterial thrombosis (HITTS).[168] A retest clinical scoring system (the *"4 Ts"*) is used to assess the likelihood of this syndrome: the platelet count drops by 50% or more (thrombocytopenia), 5-10 days after commencing UFH (timing), there is new thrombosis, and other causes of thrombocytopenia have been excluded.[169] HIT is an immune-mediated potentially fatal syndrome in which the heparin-induced immunoglobulins bridge platelets causing both thrombocytopenia and thrombosis. In most patients the onset occurs during heparin therapy; however, in less than 5% onset is after discontinuation of heparin therapy (delayed-onset HIT).[86] Heparin or LMWH must be discontinued on suspicion. Laboratory tests are available to support the diagnosis. As the condition is prothrombotic, these patients require alternative anticoagulation, and most patients are treated with direct thrombin inhibitors or heparinoid and later commenced on warfarin when the platelet count has recovered.

HIT therapy. In the United States, *lepirudin, argatroban, and bivalirudin,* are licensed for HIT therapy (see later, Table 9-4). In patients with suspected or proven HIT who need PCI for ACS, argatroban (direct thrombin inhibitor, 240 mcg/kg bolus followed by 20 mcg/kg/min infusion, doses rounded) can cover the intervention, even without added GpIIb/IIIa blockade.[170] Valid alternatives in ACS are fondaparinux, an indirect antithrombin (see later),[171,172] or bivalirudin, a direct thrombin inhibitor[173] that is licensed for use when HIT or HITTS complicates PCI (see later, Table 9-4). The heparinoid danaparoid is also used elsewhere but has molecular overlap with heparin. Of note, the British Society of Haematology advises that *all patients receiving prolonged heparin of any sort should have platelet counts on day 1 and every 2-4 days.*[174]

Indications for Heparin

In acute myocardial infarction. In AMI heparin is given together with thrombolysis or primary percutaneous coronary intervention. *In ACS,* UFH was the reference standard,[165] but this is no longer the case now that LMWH, fondaparinux, and bivalirudin are available. Reinfarction may occur following the cessation of intravenous heparin usually as a result of "heparin rebound" and the procoagulant state that ensues. *In elective PCI,* no placebo-controlled trials have been performed with UFH; the standard regimen is 70-100 IU/kg, with additional weight-adjusted boluses to achieve and maintain an ACT of 250-300 seconds.[106] If a GpIIb/IIIa antagonist is co-administered, the initial heparin dosage is reduced to 70 IU/kg (bolus) followed by 100 U/kg infused to maintain an ACT of at least 250-300 seconds.[106] In Europe and other countries, bolus-reduced heparin doses may be used (e.g., 70-100 IU/kg without monitoring of the ACT[175] and no additional heparin is given during the procedure[106]). Heparin should be discontinued immediately after the interventional procedure. In the *prevention and treatment of DVT,* subcutaneous heparin has been replaced by LMWH or fondaparinux.

Anticoagulation in pregnant women. UFH may be used (Category C, see Table 12-10), but can cause osteoporosis if given in doses of more than 20,000 IU daily for more than 5 months.[142,176] Alternatives are fondaparinux or LMWH (Category B) (also see p. 374).

Low-Molecular-Weight Heparins

LMWHs are approximately one third of the molecular weight of heparin, and are also heterogeneous in size. LMWHs have greater bioavailability and a longer plasma half-life than standard heparin (see later, Table 9-4). They bind to antithrombin, effectively to inhibit factor Xa with also some direct inhibition of thrombin (see Fig. 9-6). Approximately 25%-30% of the molecules of various preparations contain the crucial 18 or more saccharide units needed to bind to both antithrombin III and thrombin; hence inhibition of thrombin is less powerful than that of heparin. The ratio of LMWHs binding to antithrombin III and inhibition of factor Xa:IIa (where IIa is thrombin) varies with each agent, for example, 2:1 with dalteparin and 3:1 with enoxaparin. The bleeding side effects of LMWHs can be reduced but not completely reversed by protamine (residual anti-Xa activity remains). LMWHs given subcutaneously in a fixed dose are much easier to use than standard UFH, and risk of HIT is less (see Table 9-2). Regular platelet counts are required, and the LMWH should be stopped if the count falls to less than $100,000/mm^2$.

LMWH for acute coronary syndromes. Several trials show the superiority or equivalence of LMWH to UFH. A meta-analysis on more than 49,000 patients in 12 trials showed superiority of enoxaparin as adjunct therapy in those with STEMI. For every 1000 patients treated, 21 deaths or MI events were prevented at the cost of four nonfatal major bleeds, thus showing net clinical benefit.[177] In NSTEMI, nine death or MI events were prevented for every 1000 patients treated by enoxaparin, at the cost of eight nonfatal major bleeds, showing a net neutral clinical effect.[177]

   In elective PCI, in the STEEPLE trial, intravenous doses of enoxaparin 0.5-0.75 mg/kilo gave less major bleeding than UFH.[178] Furthermore, 0.75 mg/kg achieved better target anti-factor Xa levels (92%) than did the lower dose (79%), both much better than with UFH (20%). Concurrent GpIIb/IIIa use increased bleeding substantially (OR 2.28, p < 0.001). Sheath removal occurred 4-6 hours after the end of PCI with 0.75 mg/kg and immediately at the end of PCI with the lower dose. This trial was not powered for outcome events, which were similar in UFH- and enoxaparin-treated patients. No adjustment is needed for *renal dysfunction* if only a single bolus is given for elective PCI (for other situations, see Table 9-4).[179] SYNERGY demonstrated that switching between UFH and LMWH increases bleeding risks.[179]

Dalteparin. *Dalteparin (Fragmin)* comes in a single-dose prefilled syringe or as multidose vials. Each syringe contains 2500 to 10,000 international units antifactor Xa (see Fig. 9-6) equal to 16-64 mg of dalteparin. It is given as a deep subcutaneous injection and NOT intramuscularly. In the FRISC study the dose was 120 IU twice daily plus aspirin for 6 days, then 7500 IU for 35-45 days, starting after admission for unstable angina. At 6 days the composite endpoint of death or MI was reduced from 4.8% with aspirin to 1.8% with dalteparin plus aspirin (p = 0.001),[180] but by 6 months these differences were no longer apparent. In the United States, dalteparin is licensed for prevention of ischemic complications in unstable angina and non–Q wave MI, and for prevention of DVT. It is contraindicated by major bleeding or thrombocytopenia or past HITTS (Heparin-induced thrombocytopenia and thrombosis syndrome). There is a boxed warning against its use with spinal anesthesia and pregnancy, category B (see Table 12-10).

Choice of LMWH or UFH. LMWH is in general preferred to UFH because it is convenient, overall less expensive, eliminates the need for aPPT monitoring, avoids the problem of intravenous site infections, and gives superior results.[177,181] The inability to monitor the degree of anticoagulation with LMWH in contrast to UFH, and the lack of a complete antidote are potential disadvantages, especially when urgent PCI is undertaken in high-risk ACS.[90]

Bivalirudin

Bivalirudin (Angiomax) is the only intravenous anticoagulant that reduces ischemia similarly to UFH, yet with a consistent reduction in bleeding complications associated with PCI. Bivalirudin binds directly to thrombin (factor IIa) and thereby inhibits the thrombin-induced conversion of fibrinogen to fibrin (Fig. 9-10). It inactivates fibrin-bound as well as fluid-phase thrombin.

Pharmacokinetics. Bivalirudin is easy to use, has linear kinetics, and, because it is not protein-bound, has few drug interactions. It inhibits both soluble and clot-bound thrombin and blocks thrombin-mediated platelet activation and aggregation.[182] Elimination is predominantly achieved by proteolytic cleavage and, to a lesser extent, by renal excretion so that clearance is reduced by only approximately 20% in moderate and severe renal impairment (FDA information). This may be particularly advantageous in *CKD* as the risk of bleeding is approximately doubled.[183] Coagulation tests (activated partial thromboplastin time and ACT) correlate well with plasma concentrations.

Nonurgent PCI. In nonurgent PCI and almost half for ACS, the long-term outcome events with bivalirudin and selective adjunctive GpIIb/IIIa blockade (7.2%), was similar to that of UFH plus planned GpIIb/IIIa blockade.[184] In the acute phase, major bleeding was less common with bivalirudin (2.4% versus 4.1%, p < 0.001). The bivalirudin dose was 0.75 mg/kg prior to the intervention followed by an infusion of 1.75 mg/hour for the duration of the procedure.

ACS with planned PCI. In ACS with planned PCI, the ACUITY trial showed that bivalirudin alone gave similar outcome rates to heparin plus GpIIb/IIIa inhibition with less bleeding.[102,185,186]

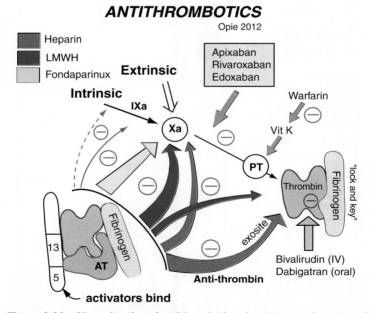

Figure 9-10   Sites of action of antithrombotics. Crucial to the formation of the clot is the interaction between thrombin and fibrinogen to form fibrin (see Fig. 9-5) that cross-links the platelets (see Fig. 9-1). The thickness of the arrows indicates the strength of the binding of the antithrombotics to various molecular sites. *AT,* antithrombin; *IV,* intravenous; *LMWH,* low-molecular-weight heparin; *PT,* prothrombin. (Figure © L.H. Opie, 2012.)

Urgent PCI in high-risk non–ST elevation ACS. For urgent PCI in non-STE ACS, bivalirudin is a cost-effective alternative to UFH plus GpIIb/IIIa blockade and gives less bleeding.[186] In this trial (ACUITY), GpIIb/IIIa antagonists added to bivalirudin increased bleeding but gave no outcome benefit.[102] Despite absence of firm data,[187] the AHA-ACC guidelines suggest that bivalirudin should be combined with clopidogrel to optimize outcomes.[166] Given the adverse relationship of bleeding[185,188] to long-term mortality, bivalirudin is a reasonable alternative to UFH or LMWH with added GpIIb/IIIa antagonists. The current preferred approach for *non-STE ACS* is to use bivalirudin in patients at high risk of bleeding (Fig. 12-3).

Primary PCI in STEMI. For primary PCI in STEMI, in the HORIZONS study on 3602 patients bivalirudin reduced major bleeding by 40% (4.9 versus 8.3%, p < 0.001) and also reduced 30-day mortality (1.8% verus 2.9%, p = 0.035) as compared with UFH and a GpIIb/IIIa receptor antagonist.[189] Thus this agent is an attractive antithrombotic

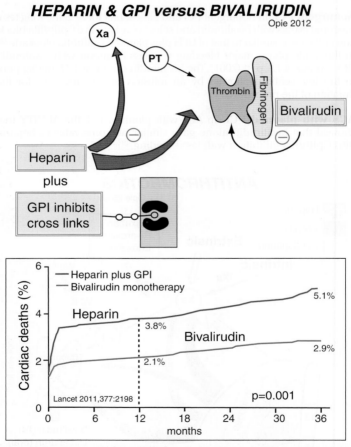

Figure 9-11   Comparison of effects of heparin plus glycoprotein IIb/IIIa inhibitor (GPI) versus bivalirudin. *Upper panel* shows mechanisms of action. *Lower panel* shows superior effects of bivalirudin in decreasing deaths in acute myocardial infarction. *PT,* Prothrombin. (Figure modified from Stone GW, et al. HORIZONS-AMI Trial Investigators. Heparin plus a glycoprotein IIb/IIIa inhibitor versus bivalirudin monotherapy and paclitaxel-eluting stents versus bare-metal stents in acute myocardial infarction (HORIZONS-AMI): final 3-year results from a multicentre, randomised controlled trial. *Lancet* 2011;377:2193-2204; © L.H. Opie, 2012.)

option for primary PCI compared with UFH plus GpIIb/IIIa antagonists and can be given to all those with ACS, but trial data in those whom PCI is not planned are not superior to heparin.[190] Long-term final 3-year results of the primary PCI trial HORIZONS-AMI show continued mortality benefit of bivalirudin and also suggest possible late benefits on stent thrombosis and repeat MI (Fig. 9-11).[191]

Less bleeding vs. heparin. At similar ACTs in patients undergoing PCI, bivalirudin had consistently less bleeding than did heparin or heparin plus a Gp inhibitor.[192]

Chromic kidney disease. The ESC recommends an infusion rate of 1.75 mg/kg/hour for moderate renal impairment (CrCl, 30-59 mL/min); if the clearance is less than 30 mL/min, reduce to 1 mg mg/kg/hour.[73]

Bivalirudin, licensed use. The FDA license is for use with aspirin for patients with unstable angina undergoing percutaneous transluminal coronary angioplasty. Bivalirudin is also licensed for patients with or at risk of HIT or HITTS who are undergoing PCI.[173]

Bivalirudin evaluation. Bivalirudin is a valuable agent to replace heparin or UFH during PCI. An important outcome study shows mortality reduction versus heparin and a GpIIb/IIIa antagonist when used for acute STEMI. It causes relatively less bleeding than does heparin in unselected patients undergoing PCI.

Enoxaparin

Enoxaparin (Lovenox, Clexane) is the most used and most tested LMWH. It predominantly inhibits factor Xa but also inhibits thrombin to some degree. It is given by subcutaneous injection, and comes in concentrations of 100 or 150 mg/mL, in prefilled single-dose syringes or as ampules. Indications are similar to dalteparin, including treatment of acute DVT. Warnings are similar to dalteparin plus warning against use with prosthetic valves, especially in pregnant women (pregnancy category B) risk of thrombocytopenia, although this is rare. This drug has been well studied in several major trials. It is excreted renally.

Use in AMI. Enoxaparin was superior to UFH in STEMI as shown in a metaanalysis on more than 49 000 patients.[177] Although bleeding was increased with enoxaparin, this increase was offset by a reduction in death or MI. In the NSTEMI patients, the comparison was neutral. In a current metaanalysis, 23 trials representing 30,966 patients were selected, including 10,243 patients (33.1%) undergoing PCI for STEMI and 8750 (28.2%) undergoing secondary PCI after fibrinolysis.[193] Enoxaparin was superior to UFH in reducing mortality and bleeding outcomes during PCI and particularly in patients undergoing PCI for STEMI.

Comparisons with oral thrombin inhibitors. Compared with apixaban in patients undergoing hip replacement, enoxaparin was associated with higher rates of VTE, without differences in bleeding rates.[194] In this study, apixaban compared with enoxaparin reduced all VTE and death from any cause (P < 0.001). Regarding rivaroxaban, also for prevention of VTE, it gave better protection than enoxaparin at similar rates of bleeding.[194] Dabigatran in a similar setting and given at a high dose (220 mg daily) reduced the primary efficacy outcome (p < 0.0001) as also major VTE plus VTE-related death (<0.03) when compared with subcutaneous enoxaparin 40 mg once daily.[195] On the positive side, enoxaparin was superior to apixaban for medically ill patients requiring prophylaxis for VTE in that outcomes were similar but enoxaparin had fewer major bleeding events than apixaban (P = 0.04).[163]

Dosage. The standard dose for ACS is 1 mg/kg subcutaneously every 12 hours with aspirin and clopidogrel and, sometimes, a GpIIb/IIIa inhibitor. For thromboprophylaxis, the standard dose is 40 mg subcutaneously daily. Enoxaparin is given until PCI or throughout hospitalization or for 8 days. In older adult patients the dose should be reduced (e.g., omit the intravenous bolus and give 0.75 mg/kg twice daily[179]). In CKD with a CrCl less than 30 mL/min, the ESC recommendation is that the dose be reduced to 1 mg/kg once daily.[73]

Summary: Enoxaparin. Enoxaparin given subcutaneously is the standard LMWH, predominantly inhibiting factor Xa. It is superior to UFH for AMI (specifically STE) and superior to apixaban for prophylaxis against thromboembolism for medical patients. In patients undergoing major hip or knee operations, enoxaparin is being displaced by the new oral thrombin inhibitors (apixaban, dabigatran, rivaroxaban).

Fondaparinux

Fondaparinux (Arixtra) is the only selective activated factor X (factor Xa) inhibitor available for clinical use in ACS.

Pharmacokinetics. It is a synthetic pentasaccharide structurally similar to the antithrombin-binding sequence found in heparin. It inhibits the coagulation factor Xa (see Fig. 9-10) by binding with a high affinity and reversibly and noncovalently to antithrombin, thereby catalyzing and promoting antithrombin-mediated inhibition of factor Xa. It increases the ability of antithrombin to inhibit factor Xa 300-fold. The specific anti-Xa activity is approximately sevenfold higher that of LMWH.[138] Fondaparinux has 100% bioavailability after subcutaneous injection, with an elimination half-life of 17 hours, and can therefore be given once daily. For use in PCI it needs no monitoring. The risk of hemorrhage increases with impaired hepatic or renal function (contraindicated if CrCl less than 30 mL/min), in patients with very low body weight, or in for older adult patients for whom the dose must be reduced according to the FDA-approved package insert. Thrombocytopenia can occur but HIT has not yet been reported (see Table 9-2); thus monitoring of platelet count is unnecessary.[63]

License in the United States. In the United States fondaparinux is licensed only for prevention of DVT and (with warfarin) for acute pulmonary embolism, although the large trials in ACS[196] suggest that additional off-license use could be appropriate. A boxed warning introduced in 2010 warns of the risks of epidural or spinal hematomas in patients given neuraxial anesthesia or undergoing spinal punctures.

Non-STE ACS. In non-STE ACE, in 20,078 patients in OASIS-5, fondaparinux was similar to enoxaparin, both usually given with clopidogrel, in reducing death or MI at 9 days (the primary endpoint), but also reduced deaths at 30 days and 6 months.[197] Major bleeding was much less (approximately halved) with fondaparinux (dose 2.5 mg subcutaneously once daily, extra 2.5 or 5 mg intravenously before PCI). In a subgroup of those who underwent PCI,[196] death, MI, and stroke as separate endpoints were not reduced at any time. Rather, it was when major bleeding was added to the rates of death, MI, and stroke that fondaparinux was superior to enoxaparin at 9 days, 30 days, and 6 months of follow-up. For PCI, European guidelines suggest the addition of UFH to fondaparinux initiated prior to the procedure.[63] Specifically, catheter thrombosis[196] can be thereby avoided.[196] *In the conservative management of ACS,* fondaparinux is superior to heparin.[190]

STEMI. In STEMI in OASIS-6, fondaparinux was compared in a large complex trial conducted in 41 countries in 12,092 patients with either no anticoagulation or UFH who may or may not have received a fibrinolytic agent.[197] The most commonly used fibrinolytic agent was streptokinase (without UFH).[197] In patients undergoing primary PCI, there was no advantage of fondaparinux given as an intravenous bolus (2.5 or 5 mg, the latter if no GpIIb/IIIa) followed by subcutaneous dosing up to 8 days, but there was an excess of catheter thrombosis and coronary complications. (By extrapolation from OASIS-5, added UFH at the time of PCI might have avoided the thrombosis).[196] In others without PCI but receiving thrombolysis, subcutaneous fondaparinux was superior to UFH for reducing death or reinfarction at 90-180 days by 23% (p = 0.008). Of note, fondaparinux was given for approximately 8 days, whereas UFH was given for approximately 2 days. Fondaparinux was also superior to placebo in patients that received no reperfusion therapy. Thus the benefit of fondaparinux over UFH in STEMI is less clear and the longer duration of therapy could have accounted for part of the benefit. However, fondaparinux is clearly easier to administer than UFH.

Catheter thrombosis. A problem with fondaparinux is the low albeit real risk of catheter thrombosis at the time of PCI. This risk is countered by a covering bolus injection of UFH given at PCI,[73] as studied in the FUTURA/OASIS-8 trial.[198] The standard-dose UFH, namely 85 IU/kg (reduced to 60 IU/kg in the case of the use of GP IIb/IIIa receptor inhibitors) was better than a lower bolus (50 IU/kg), because there was more favorable net clinical benefit and lower risk of catheter thrombosis compared with low-dose UFH.[198]

Chronic renal disease. For chronic renal disease, fondaparinux is the drug of choice in moderately reduced renal function (CrCl 30-60 mL/min) but contraindicated in severe renal failure (CrCl <20 mL/min).[73]

Summary: Fondaparinux. Fondaparinux is superior to placebo (but not to UFH) in STEMI (treated with thrombolytic agent or without reperfusion). Fondaparinux is superior to LMWH in non-STE ACS (lower bleeding and fewer deaths). The ESC guidelines favor fondaparinux in non-STE ACS unless the patient is planned for early intervention.[63] The ACC-AHA guidelines recommend either UFH or enoxaparin.[166]

Lepirudin. *Lepirudin (Refludan)* is a recombinant hirudin licensed only for HIT and the associated thromboembolic disorder to prevent further thromboembolism. It is contraindicated in pregnancy (category B) and in breast feeding, with a warning against use with thrombolytic agents or in bleeding disorders. The infusion dose (0.15 mg/kg after an initial bolus of 0.4 mg/kg) is adjusted by the aPPT (1.5 to 2.5). It is almost exclusively cleared in the kidneys, so that renal impairment requires lower doses (see package insert for table).

Which regimen is better? There are several approved options (UFH versus LMWH versus bivalirudin versus fondaparinux). The chosen regimen may differ between interventional and noninterventional centres. When intervention is likely, bivalirudin has excellent data, whereas if a conservative strategy is employed, fondaparinux is well tested. If bleeding is a concern, bivalirudin and fondaparinux (if PCI is unlikely) are good choices. Some factors guiding choice are shown in Tables 9-2, 9-3, 9-4, and 9-5.

Table 9-3

Antiplatelets, Antithrombotics, and Fibrinolytics in Acute Coronary Syndromes and in Percutaneous Coronary Intervention			
Condition	**Antiplatelet Agents**	**Antithrombotics**	**Fibrinolytics**
ACS, low-risk or conservative strategy	Aspirin, clopidogrel (if no CABG)	Heparin/LMWH or fondaparinux or bivalirudin	None
ACS, high-risk* invasive strategy	Previous, plus GpIIb/IIIa (Eptifibatide/tirofiban/if continuing ischaemia; abciximab if anatomy known)	Heparin/LMWH; bivalirudin may replace both IIb/IIIa and heparin/LMWH	None
ACS, ST-elevation MI, PCI not available	Aspirin plus clopidogrel[†]	Heparin/LMWH or fondaparinux (OASIS-6)	TNK/tPA/rPA/ streptokinase
Primary PCI	Aspirin, clopidogrel ± abciximab (may consider selective IC abciximab or eptifibatide)	Bivalirudin/UFH	
Elective PCI, low risk	Aspirin, clopidogrel	Heparin/LMWH/ bivalirudin	None
Elective PCI, high risk	Above, plus abciximab or eptifibatide	Heparin/LMWH/ bivalirudin	None

ACS, Acute coronary syndrome; CABG, coronary artery bypass graft; IIb/IIIa, glycoprotein IIb/IIIa inhibitor; LMWH, low-molecular-weight heparin; MI, myocardial infarction; PCI, percutaneous coronary intervention; rPA, reteplase; TNK, tenecteplase; tPA, tissue plasminogen activator; UFH, unfractionated heparin.

*Elevated troponins, ischemic ST-depression or similar ongoing ischemia.
†Aspirin 162 mg, clopidogrel 75 mg in COMMIT trial.[82,236]

Table 9-4

Aspirin, Clopidogrel, and Warfarin for Secondary Prevention and Risk Reduction for Coronary and Vascular Disease: Class I Recommendations from the AHA and ACC Foundation

1. Aspirin 75-162 mg daily recommended in all patients with CAD unless contraindicated. **(Level of Evidence: A)**
   Clopidogrel 75 mg daily if intolerant or allergic to aspirin. **(Level: B)**
2. A P2Y12 receptor antagonist in combination with aspirin is indicated for patients after ACS or PCI with stent placement. **(Level: A)**
   Give clopidogrel 75 mg daily, prasugrel 10 mg daily, or ticagrelor* 90 mg twice daily for at least 12 months. **(Level: A)**
3. For patients undergoing CABG, give aspirin within 6 hours after surgery, 100-325 mg daily for 1 year. **(Level: A)**
4. For patients with atherosclerosis, use antiplatelet therapy rather than warfarin. **(Level: A)**
5. Compelling indications for anticoagulant therapy: atrial fibrillation, prosthetic heart valve, LV thrombus, or concomitant venous thromboembolic disease; add warfarin to the low-dose aspirin (75-81 mg daily). **(Level: A)**
6. Warfarin with aspirin and/or clopidogrel: increased risk of bleeding. Monitor closely. **(Level: A)**

ACC, American College of Cardiology; ACS, acute coronary syndrome; AHA, American Heart Association; CABG, coronary artery bypass grafting; CAD, coronary artery disease; LV, left ventricular; PCI, percutaneous coronary intervention.

*We prefer ticagrelor as in the PLATO trial (Wallentin et al., New Engl J Med 2009;361:1045).[61] Ticagrelor has proven outcome benefit including mortality reduction in ACS, which remains a repeat risk despite secondary prevention.

From Smith SC Jr, et al. World Heart Federation and the Preventive Cardiovascular Nurses Association. AHA/ACCF secondary prevention and risk reduction therapy for patients with coronary and other atherosclerotic vascular disease: 2011 update: a guideline from the American Heart Association and American College of Cardiology Foundation. Circulation 2011;124:2458–73.

Table 9-5

Unfractionated Heparin Versus Low-Molecular-Weight Heparin, Fondaparinux, and Bivalirudin

	UFH	LMWH	Fondaparinux*	Bivalirudin (Hirulog)
Molecular weight	5000-30,000 Da	Mean 5000 Da	1728 Da	2180
Mechanism of action	Major antithrombin (IIa) activity, less on Xa and on Xia[165]	Greater anti Xa activity: also antithrombin (IIa) activity	Specific conformational change in antithrombin, factor Xa strongly inhibited	Inhibits both soluble and clot-bound thrombin[237]
Mode of administration	IV infusion or SC 2-3 times daily	SC only, 1-2 times daily	SC daily; added IV bolus for PCI in ACS	IV infusion
Therapeutic dose	Bolus, then IV infusion with monitoring of aPTT	Fixed dose by body weight for creatinine clearance <60-30 mL/min 1 mg/kg daily; if <30 mL/min avoid unless single-bolus dosing for elective PCI Age ≥75 yr reduced dosing; no bolus and 0.75 mg/kg b.i.d. with fibrinolysis	2.5 mg; reduce dose in older adults or renal impairment; C/I creatinine clearance <30 ml/min; body wt <50 kg	FDA: IV bolus 0.75 mg/kg; infuse 1.75 mg/kg/h for PCI duration[†] Reduce in renal disease
Bioavailable half-life	≈1.5 h	≈4 h	≈17 h	25 min
Monitoring of anticoagulant activity	aPTT	Usually not necessary Anti-Xa levels advised in renal failure, severe obesity, pregnancy	Usually none needed, anti-Xa possible	aPTT; ACT (not usually done)
Reversal	Reversed with IV injection protamine sulphate	Only partially reversible with protamine	rVIIa potential partial antagonist	Baseline coagulation times within 1 h of drug cessation; no single reversal agent; combinations may work
HIT; of these, 20%-50% develop HITTS	HIT incidence in those receiving therapy for ≥5 days 3%-5%	HIT incidence in those receiving therapy for ≥5 days <1%	Very low cross-reactivity with HIT antibodies; thrombotic HIT not yet found, package insert warns severe thrombocytopenia in 0.2%	FDA: indicated to treat HIT/HITTS or risk thereof during PCI; IV bolus 0.75 mg/kg; infuse 1.75 mg/kg/h

ACS, Acute coronary syndrome; ACT, activated clotting time; aPTT, activated partial thromboplastin time; b.i.d., twice daily; C/I, contraindicated; FDA, Food and Drug Administration; HIT, heparin-induced thrombocytopenia; HITTS, heparin-induced thrombocytopenia thrombosis syndrome; IV, intravenous; LMWH, low-molecular-weight heparin; PCI, percutaneous coronary intervention; SC, subcutaneous; UFH, unfractionated heparin.

*Fondaparinux: package insert; Wester, 2007.[172]

[†]Alternate dosage: bolus 0.1 mg/kg, then infused at 0.25 mg/kg/h; before PCI added bolus 0.5 mg/kg, infusion increased to 1.75 mg/kg/h.[102]

Fibrinolytic (Thrombolytic) Therapy

Although primary PCI is superior to thrombolytic therapy for STEMI, there are many regions where this is not feasible (especially within 3 hours of presentation). Hence, internationally, fibrinolysis remains the most commonly used reperfusion therapy.

Role of plasmin. Thrombolytic agents have a common goal: the generation of plasmin that lyses the clot (Fig. 9-12). Physiologically, the plasminogen activator system forms plasminogen that binds to the clot surface to lyse the clot,[199] opposing thrombus formation. PAI-1, made by adipose tissue, inhibits the formation of plasmin. Chronic inhibition of fibrinolysis by PAI-1 can promote accumulation of intravascular fibrin, which may be invaded by proliferating vascular smooth muscle cells and circulating progenitor cells gradually to form a cellular neointima (see Fig. 9-8). These effects may be important in provoking a thrombotic response in the presence of minor endothelial damage.[199] Future inhibitors of PAI-1 may help to control slow thrombus formation, which could be effective as long-term preventative therapy[200] as opposed to the rapid therapeutic effects of current agents such as tissue plasminogen activator (tPA), and tenecteplase (TNK) or reteplase (rPA) used to achieve clot lysis in acute thrombotic conditions (Fig. 9-13).

Goals of fibrinolysis. The goals of reperfusion therapy are early patency, increased myocardial salvage, preservation of LV function, and lower mortality.[201,202] The major aim is to achieve early reperfusion with short "symptom-to-needle'" and "door-to-needle" times in patients with suspected AMI and STE or new-onset left bundle branch block. Early reperfusion can be achieved by either fibrinolysis or by PCI. Primary PCI is established as providing better reperfusion than lysis, but for patients within the first 3 hours of symptom onset more prompt reperfusion with lysis may balance the delayed but more complete and sustained reperfusion with PCI.[203] Symptom-to-balloon time and door-to-balloon times are crucial. The principle of modern fibrinolytic therapy is the use of agents such as alteplase (tPA), rPA,

THROMBOSIS AND LYSIS

Opie 2012

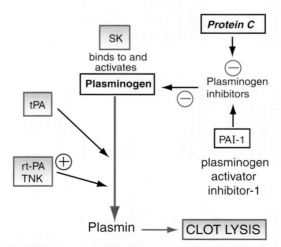

Figure 9-12   Sites of action of thrombolytic agents. *PAI,* Plasminogen activator inhibitor; *rt-PA,* reteplase; *SK,* streptokinase; *tPA,* tissue-type plasminogen activator; *TNK,* tenecteplase. (Figure © L.H. Opie, 2012.)

NOVEL THROMBOTIC RESPONSE

Opie 2012

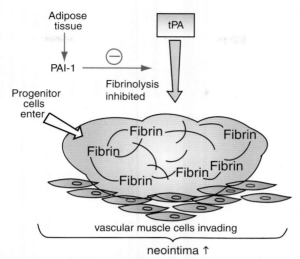

Figure 9-13   Novel thrombotic mechanisms. Plasminogen activator inhibitor-1 (PAI-1), made by adipose tissue, inhibits fibrinolysis and thus the formation of plasmin from tissue plasminogen activator (tPA). This process, when chronic, can promote accumulation of intravascular fibrin, which may then be invaded by proliferating vascular smooth muscle cells and circulating progenitor cells gradually to form a cellular neointima in the fibrin-rich clot. These effects could provoke a delayed thrombotic response in the presence of minor endothelial damage. (Figure © L.H. Opie, 2012.)

TNK, and streptokinase (Table 9-6), which convert plasminogen into active plasmin. Because fibrinolytic agents simultaneously exert clot-dissolving and procoagulant actions and have significant serious side effects, *they must not be used in non-STE ACS (unstable angina and non-STEMI)* where they have no benefit and increase risks of bleeding.

Early reperfusion: the golden hours. Dramatic reductions in mortality can be achieved if treatment is obtained during the "golden" first hour. STE can resolve without the development of Q waves, and with very prompt reperfusion (usually within the first hour) there may be no elevation in biomarkers of necrosis ("aborted MI"). In the MITI trial, alteplase and aspirin were started as soon as possible either at home or in hospital.[204] Thrombolytic perfusion within 70 minutes reduced the early death rate from 8.7% to 1.2%, and infarct size fell from 11.2% to 4.9% when compared with a longer delay of up to 180 minutes. Among patients undergoing early primary PCI, the relationship between symptom-to-balloon time and mortality is less striking, but this may relate in part to the relative lack of data as few patients achieve very early primary PCI.[205]

The window of opportunity. In the FTT Collaborative Overview of 58,000 randomized patients in fibrinolytic trials,[206] mortality was reduced by 25% in patients randomized to fibrinolysis between 2 and 3 hours after symptom onset and by 18% in patients randomized to fibrinolysis between 4 and 6 hours. MI may also be "aborted."[207] Patients randomized between 7 and 12 hours still had a 14% reduction in mortality, the later improvement perhaps related more to the benefits of a patent infarct-related artery that to myocardial salvage.[208,209] Gersh

Table 9-6

New Oral Anticoagulants: Pharmacologic Features and Major Trials

	Dabigatran	Rivaroxaban	Apixaban	Edoxaban
Mechanism of action	Selective direct thrombin inhibitor	Selective direct Xa inhibitor	Selective direct Xa inhibitor	Selective direct Xa inhibitor
Doses, daily	110 or 150 mg b.i.d or 75 g b.i.d.	20 mg with evening meal (FDA)	5 mg b.i.d.	60 mg
Doses, renal impairment	CrCl <30 mL/min excluded	CrCl 30-49 mL/min, 15 mg	Half dose for increased serum creatinine; <80 yr; low BMI	Half dose for renal impairment
Renal eliminated	85%	66%	27%	50%*
Oral availability	6.5%	80%-100%	50%	62%
Half-life, h	12-17	5-13	8-15	6-11
Renal eliminated	85%	66%	27%	50%
Max inhibition, h	0.5-2	1-4	1-4	1-2
Drug interactions	Reduce dose: verapamil, dronedarone, amiodarone Avoid antifungals and protease inhibitors	Avoid verapamil, dronedarone, amiodarone Caution: antifungals and protease inhibitors	Avoid verapamil, dronedarone, amiodarone Caution antifungals and protease inhibitors	Reduce dose: verapamil, dronedarone, amiodarone Avoid antifungals and protease inhibitors
Major phase III trial	RELY	ROCKETT (ATLAS ACS2†)	ARISTOTLE	ENGAGE AF (under way)
CHAD$_2$ score mean in trial	2.1	3.5	2.1	2 or more

Primary endpoint result	150 mg HR 0.65, P < 0.001; 100 mg, NS	Noninferior to warfarin in high-risk patients with atrial fibrillation	HR 0.79; p = 0.01 Stroke/systemic emboli; 0.81 mortality, p < 0.05	Aim: Noninferior to warfarin for stroke and systemic emboli
Safety	Intracranial bleeds less than warfarin; more GI bleeds (150 mg)	Intracranial bleeds less than warfarin; more GI bleeds	Less major bleeds and hemorrhagic stroke than warfarin; also in HF†	
FDA approval	Stroke prevention in nonvalvular AF; DVT prevention after hip or knee replacement	Stroke prevention in nonvalvular AF; DVT prevention after hip or knee replacement; not FDA approved for ACS†, DVT		Not yet known

ACS, Acute coronary syndrome; AF, atrial fibrillation; b.i.d., twice daily; BMI, body mass index; CrCl, creatinine clearance; CHAD, congestive heart failure, hypertension, age, diabetes mellitus; DVT, deep-vein thrombosis; FDA, Food and Drug Administration; GI, gastrointestinal; HF, heart failure; NS, not significant.

*Of the absorbed drug.

†ATLAS-ACS TIMI 46 trial, theheart.org, May 23, 2012.

Modified from De Caterina R, et al. Coordinating Committee. New oral anticoagulants in atrial fibrillation and acute coronary syndromes: ESC Working Group on Thrombosis–Task Force on Anticoagulants in Heart Disease position paper. *J Am Coll Cardiol* 2012;59:1413–1425.

Also see Lip GY, et al. Indirect comparisons of new oral anticoagulant drugs for efficacy and safety when used for stroke prevention in atrial fibrillation. *J Am Coll Cardiol* 2012; 60:738-746.

and colleagues describe the relationship between mortality reduction and the extent of myocardial salvage.[210] Within the first 60-90 minutes, mortality with reperfusion by fibrinolytic therapy can be reduced by 50%[203]; during the first 2-3 hours a striking but rapidly declining benefit of reperfusion is present; from 6-12 hours gains achieved by reperfusion are only modest as the curve flattens, so that there is almost no added benefit thereafter (see Fig. 12-5). Overall, during the first 1-3 hours of symptoms, the time to treatment is critical, whereas later when the patient is on the "flat" part of the curve time is less of a factor and opening the infarct-related artery is the priority. In this later time, a mechanical approach is superior to fibrinolytic agents that have lesser effectiveness on more mature coronary artery clots.

Alteplase (tPA)

Tissue plasminogen activator *(Activase in the United States, Actilyse in Europe)* is a naturally occurring enzyme that binds to fibrin with a greater affinity than streptokinase or urokinase; once bound, it starts to convert plasminogen to plasmin on the fibrin surface. Hence it is relatively "clot selective," although in clinical doses some systemic effects do occur. The very short half-life of alteplase mandates co-therapy with intravenous heparin to avoid reocclusion. In the GUSTO trial[211] mortality was 14% lower (1% absolute decrease) with tPA compared with streptokinase.

Dose of alteplase. The US package insert states that alteplase is infused as 100 mg over 3 hours, with 60 mg in the first hour (of which 6-10 mg is given as a bolus), 20 mg over the second hour, and 20 mg over the third hour. For smaller patients (<65 kg), a dose of 1.25 mg/kg is administered. As with the other fibrinolytics (see later), aspirin 300 mg should be given as soon as possible. Any aspirin can be given, but if enteric should be chewed. Clopidogrel 300 mg followed by 75 mg per day (no loading dose in patients 75 years old or older) should also be commenced. An initial heparin bolus of 4000 IU is standard, although lower doses should be considered in older adults and in patients of low body weight. Intravenous heparin should be continued for at least 48 hours, adjusted to an aPPT of 50-75 seconds.

Use in stroke. Intravenous alteplase is the only US-approved treatment for acute ischemic stroke. Alteplase was tested in doses of 0.9 mg/kg versus TNK, the first 10% administered as an initial bolus and the remainder over a 1-hour period, with a maximum dose of 90 mg. In a small trial high-dose TNK was better than alteplase (see TNK).[212]

Side effects and contraindications. Side effects and hence contraindications relate chiefly to hemorrhage, for example, risk of hemorrhage or hemorrhagic stroke (Table 9-7). (For a full list of contraindications see *Drugs for the Heart,* sixth edition, Table 9-5). Gentamicin sensitivity is a specific exclusion for alteplase therapy because gentamicin is used in the preparation of alteplase.

Cost effectiveness of alteplase. An important disadvantage of alteplase is its cost, which is approximately five times that of streptokinase.

Tenecteplase

TNK is a genetically engineered mutant of native tPA with amino acid substitutions at three sites. These properties result in decreased plasma clearance, a longer half life (Table 9-8), increased fibrin specificity, and resistance to the PAI-1. In the ASSENT-2 trial, a single bolus of TNK (in a weight-adjusted dose of 0.5 mg/kg) was compared with accelerated alteplase. At 30 days, mortality was the same with both agents (6.18% with TNK versus 6.15% with alteplase), as was the stroke rate.[213]

Table 9-7

Clinical Factors in Choosing an Antithrombotic Agent				
Condition	**UFH**	**LMWH**	**Fonda**	**Bival**
Severe renal impairment	Caution	Avoid	Avoid	Caution
↑ bleeding risk	Neutral	Selective use	Good*	Good*
Thrombocytopenia	Worst risk for HIT	Better: lower risk for HIT	Better, but some thrombocytopenia	Best
Early invasive strategy	Good*	Selective use†	Avoid†	Good*

Bival, Bivalirudin; *Fonda,* fondaparinux; *HIT,* heparin-induced thrombocytopenia; *LMWH,* low-molecular-weight heparin; *UFH,* unfractionated heparin.
*Can use; positive data.
†Missed primary endpoint, positive data for fibrinolysis and rescue PCI.[177]
†Positive data for fibrinolysis, not for primary percutaneous coronary intervention.[188]

Table 9-8

Characteristics of Fibrinolytic Agents				
	Streptokinase	**Alteplase (tPA)**	**Reteplase (rPA)**	**Tenecteplase (TNK)**
Fibrin selective	No	Yes	Yes	Yes > tPA
Plasminogen binding	Indirect	Direct	Direct	Direct
Duration of infusion (min)	60	90	10 + 10	5-10 sec
Half-life (min)	23	<5	13-16	20
Fibrinogen breakdown	4+	1-2+	Not known	>tPA
Early heparin	Probably yes	Yes	Yes	Yes
Hypotension	Yes	No	No	No
Allergic reactions	Yes	No	No	No
Approximate current cost/dose	$750* per 1.5 MU	$5863 per 100 mg	$5212 per 20-u kit	$3848 per 50-mg kit
TIMI flow grade 3, 90 min	32%	45%-54%	60%	≈tPA
TIMI flow grade 2-3 at 90 minutes	53%	81%-88%	83%	No data
at 2-3 hours	70%-73%	73%-80%	No data	No data
at 24 hours	81%-88%	78%-89%	No data	No data

MU, Million units; *rPA,* reteplase; *TIMI,* thrombolysis in myocardial infarction; *TNK,* tenecteplase; *tPA,* tissue plasminogen activator.
    Dollar prices for Mayo Clinic, 2012; TIMI flow grade 1 = some penetration of contrast material past prior obstruction; grade 2 = perfusion of entire infarct-related artery but delayed perfusion of distal bed; grade 3 = full perfusion, normal flow.
    *Estimate.

However, there was less major bleeding with TNK (4.7% versus 5.9%, p < 0.01). Thus the same or marginally better clinical results can be found with only one bolus of TNK-tPA versus the infusion required for alteplase, so that TNK is now preferred over tPA.

Use in stroke. In a phase 2B trial, 75 patients with early stroke received alteplase or TNK-tPA (0.1 mg/kg, administered as a single bolus, with a maximum dose of 10 mg; or 0.25 mg/kg, administered as a single bolus, with a maximum dose of 25 mg) less than 6 hours after the onset of ischemic stroke.[212] The higher dose of TNK-tPA was superior to the lower dose and to alteplase for all efficacy outcomes, including absence of serious disability at 90 days (in 72% of patients, versus 40% with alteplase; P = 0.02). Together, the two TNK-tPA groups had greater reperfusion (P = 0.004) and clinical improvement (P < 0.001) at 24 hours than the alteplase group.

Reteplase

Reteplase *(Retavase)* is a deletion mutant of alteplase with elimination of the kringle-1, finger, and epidermal growth factor domains, as well as some carbohydrate side chains. This results in prolonged plasma clearance, so that a double-bolus regimen (10 U + 10 U intravenously, each over 10 minutes and 30 minutes apart) can be used. Heparin must not be given through the same intravenous line (physical incompatibility). In large trials, mortality was similar with rPA and streptokinase, and mortality and stroke rates were similar with rPA and alteplase.

Streptokinase

Streptokinase is the original thrombolytic agent (see Fig. 9-13). It has no direct effect on plasminogen, but rather works by binding with plasminogen to form a 1:1 complex that becomes an active enzyme to convert plasminogen to plasmin. In addition, streptokinase may increase circulating levels of activated protein-C, which enhances clot lysis. The second and third generation of thrombolytics are superior drugs, but streptokinase is cheap and still widely used in many parts of the world. The standard rate of infusion is 1.5 million IU of streptokinase in 100 mL of physiologic saline over 30-60 minutes.[214] The major problem with streptokinase is that the majority of generic preparations (13 of 16 tested) are underpowered with activities of 21%-87% of those claimed.[215]

Streptokinase and heparin or bivalirudin. The combination of intravenous heparin with streptokinase remains controversial. We recommend heparin on the basis of the following trials. First, in an analysis of 68,000 patients (all of whom received aspirin, 93% of whom received fibrinolytic therapy and many of whom received streptokinase), the benefits of added heparin translates into a benefit/risk ratio of five deaths and three infarctions prevented at a cost of three transfusions per 1000 patients treated and a nonsignificant increase in stroke.[216] Second, in the 5-year follow-up of US patients in the GUSTO-1 Trial,[217] mortality was similar in the alteplase group and the streptokinase plus intravenous heparin group, but significantly higher in the streptokinase plus subcutaneous heparin group. Regarding streptokinase and bivalirudin in AMI, this combination was superior to streptokinase and UFH in prevention of reinfarction at the cost of modestly more bleeding.[218]

Side effects and contraindications of streptokinase. In the GUSTO-I Trial,[211] there were two more hemorrhagic strokes per 1000 patients treated with alteplase than with streptokinase (p < 0.03; Table 9-9). Allergic reactions and hypotension were more common with streptokinase. The overall incidence of major bleeding was similar with both regimens. Major bleeding requires cessation of the fibrinolytic agent and adjunctive heparin, administration of protamine sulfate to reverse the actions of heparin, and FFP or whole blood. *Contraindications* are similar to those against alteplase, with the exception of gentamicin sensitivity. Additional contraindications are (1) major recent streptococcal infection, because antistreptococcal antibodies cause resistance to streptokinase; and (2) previous treatment by streptokinase, because the antibodies diminish efficacy and there is an increased risk of allergy.

Which fibrinolytic? Several large trials randomizing over 100,000 patients have compared the effects of streptokinase and alteplase. In the GUSTO-I

Table 9-9

	Streptokinase (GUSTO)*	Alteplase (GUSTO)*	Alteplase (ASSENT-2)†	Tenecteplase (ASSENT-2)†
Side Effects of Streptokinase, Alteplase, and Tenecteplase in the GUSTO-I and ASSENT-2 Trials				
Patient number	10,410	10,396	8,461	8,488
Mortality at 30 days	7.4%	6.3%*	6.2%	6.2%
Overall stroke	1.40%	1.55%	1.66%	1.78%
Hemorrhagic stroke†	0.54%	0.72%*	0.93%	0.94%
Major bleeds	6.3%*	5.4%	5.9%	4.7%*
Allergic reactions	5.8%*	1.6%	0.2% (ana)	0.1% (ana)
Hypotension	12.5%	10.1%	16.1%	15.9%

ana, Anaphylaxis.
All three agents were used in conjunction with intravenous heparin.
*Significant difference.
†See Reference 213.
†For risk factors, see Simoons et al.[238] In patients with streptokinase and no risk factors, the probability of stroke is 0.3%. In patients with alteplase and three risk factors, the probability is more than 3%.

Trial, there was a 14% relative and a 1% absolute mortality reduction with alteplase infused over 90 minutes compared with streptokinase,[211] at the cost of two extra strokes per 1000 patients randomized. Thus when stroke reduction is important (as in older adults), streptokinase may be better (and much cheaper). In the GUSTO-III trial, rPA was the equivalent to accelerated alteplase. In the ASSENT-2 trial, TNK was equivalent to alteplase, but with less major bleeding.[213] TNK and rPA have the advantage of bolus administration, TNK being given only once. The bolus agents are more convenient, simpler to use, and help to reduce medication errors. Alteplase, streptokinase, TNK, and rPA are licensed in the United States for mortality reduction in AMI. Of these, TNK is most widely used in the United States. All have similar contraindications.

Current trends. Improvements have occurred with the addition of clopidogrel, enoxaparin, or fondaparinux, and more frequent use of rescue and systematic PCI or the pharmacoinvasive approach. Attention is also switching to improvements that can be achieved by lessening reperfusion injury.[219] Early studies in humans with reperfused AMI suggest that reperfusion injury can cause death of approximately one-third of the reperfused myocytes, and that postconditioning can limit such damage.[220]

Active Intervention: Fibrinolysis or PCI?

The premise that the best form of reperfusion therapy is PCI is established as preferred treatment when door-to-balloon times are more than 90 minutes, but the outcomes depend on the expertise and logistics present in individual institutions. Primary PCI has the distinct advantage of lower bleeding rates than fibrinolytic therapy, and achieves higher TIMI grade 3 flow rates in the infarct-related artery. A metaanalysis of 23 randomized trials documented a benefit from primary PCI on both short- and longer-term mortality and morbidity.[221] However, fibrinolysis is likely to have been improved by the addition of clopidogrel, new antithrombotics and high rates of rescue or systematic PCI.

Goodbye to combined fibrinolysis and PCI? The challenging hypothesis that reduced dose fibrinolytics could be combined with subsequent angioplasty, thereby helping to avoid the adverse effects of long delays to

PCI, has been set aside by the FINESSE[222] and ASSENT-4 studies.[223] However, very early thrombolysis with an average time delay of 100 minutes to the onset of therapy and preceding mandatory invasive study within 24 hours gave results similar to primary PCI in a small study.[224] Pharmacodynamic reperfusion strategy may make a comeback. Half-dose fibrinolysis, clopidogrel and UFH combined with transfer as soon as feasible to the nearest PCI-capable hospital is a practical strategy.[225]

"Rescue" or routine postthrombolytic PCI. Some degree of resistance of thrombi to lysis can be expected in perhaps 10%-15% of patients; the cause may include deep fissuring or rupture of the plaque or platelet-rich thrombus, which is very resistant to lysis. Rescue PCI may be beneficial in patients with continuing pain or hemodynamic instability, or when very early fibrinolysis appears to have failed.[226] Rescue PCI is superior to repeat thrombolysis and to no treatment for failed reperfusion.[227] Following thrombolysis, routine early catheterization and frequent PCI within 24 hours appears to be more beneficial than a conservative strategy.[228] Thus if fibrinolytic agents are given, patients should ideally be rapidly transferred to a PCI-capable center if rescue PCI is required. Further studies are required to define whether all patients following fibrinolysis should undergo angiography and PCI regardless of symptomatic status and whether this should occur within 24 hours of fibrinolysis or at some later stage.

Effect of time delay. PCI and fibrinolysis may be similarly effective in patients presenting within 3 hours, as shown in the PRAGUE-2 study,[229] and the CAPTIM data argue for fibrinolysis within the first 2 hours provided that prompt "rescue PCI" is available for failed reperfusion.[203] Other trials suggest that the advantage of PCI is greater in patients treated late.[230] Fibrinolytic therapy may be the treatment of choice in the first 2 hours, and PCI the treatment of choice both in patients with contraindications against fibrinolytic therapy and in those presenting after 3 hours, provided that the procedure can be performed with less than 60 minutes of PCI-related time delay. Nonetheless, the trend is toward increasing use of primary PCI where facilities are available. Much depends on how soon the patient can reach a center with high-quality emergency primary PCI facilities, and the door-to-balloon delay at those centers should be less than 90 minutes.[205,231] *As the delay increases, the mortality advantage for primary PCI over fibrinolysis decreases.* Primary PCI is now the commonest form of reperfusion therapy in the United Kingdom. Unfortunately, however, less than 30% of patients in the United States and less than 20% in most of Europe have access to primary PCI, and probably even fewer in India or China, meaning that only thrombolytic reperfusion is available. Whenever facilities for primary PCI are available for STEMI, the current emphasis is on minimizing the door-to-balloon time.[231] Most emphasis should be placed on reducing the overall "ischemic time" (symptom onset to reperfusion). Effective and integrated prehospital systems (including paramedic ambulance with telemetry of the ECG and rapid coordination with the PCI center) can substantially reduce prehospital delays.[232,233]

Fibrinolysis versus PCI: Practical Problems in Developing Countries*

Primary PCI ideally within 2-3 hours of presentation of AMI is the most desirable therapy. The Western world has established the necessary network to hasten the procedure with ever-shortening pain-to-balloon times. This policy is difficult to apply in the developing countries because of (1) problems in transportation in the form of well-equipped road or air ambulances; (2) slow traffic in bigger cities; (3) unavailability of PCI

---

*Section by Mardikar HM, et al. Management of AMI in the Indian scenario. In Opie LH, Gersh BJ, editors: *Acute myocardial infarction*, India, 2012, Elsevier.

centers and well-trained operators across the country; (4) failure of insurance system to work efficiently, especially in countries like India where universal health insurance is not available. Within these limits, individual physicians and cardiologists as well as regional centres are putting efforts into optimizing the management of AMI both in urban and periurban areas in the developing countries. The following are important points:

1. Because the availability of catheter laboratory facilities and the finances for primary PCI are scarce, most of the patients in developing countries are treated in the coronary care unit (CCU) of a nearby hospital with thrombolysis. Although thrombolytic therapy remains the cornerstone treatment, 40% of STEMI patients in India did not receive any reperfusion therapy.[234]

2. This is the most important missed opportunity when it comes to improving the outcomes of STEMI. Even though tPA molecules have better evidence, most of the patients receive streptokinase because of its cost effectiveness.[234] Recently biosimilar tenecteplase has become less expensive in India, Asia, and some parts of South America, so that its use is increasing. β-Blockers and ACE inhibitors are also underused in developing countries during hospitalization in CCU.[234]

3. There is also a delay in the diagnosis of AMI when ECG is equivocal as few hospitals can provide troponin assays. "Point-of-care" troponin assays would tremendously enhance the early diagnosis and management of AMI.

4. *The potential for greater improvements in patient outcomes can be achieved with improved delivery of care rather than by the potential gains achieved by switching therapeutic strategies.* The ideal aim in the chain from patient to health care delivery provider is to shorten the time to thrombolysis and reperfusion and early transfer to PCI-available center as soon as possible, preferably within 6 hours.[235]

5. Pharmacodynamic reperfusion strategy: Half-dose fibrinolysis, clopidogrel, and UFH combined with transfer as soon as feasible to the nearest PCI-capable hospital is a practical strategy.[225]

6. Another area of opportunity is the early recognition of symptoms of AMI. Public education is the key to early reporting for chest pain. Physicians also need to be educated and motivated to participate in community activities to educate patients to not waste the "golden hour."

SUMMARY

1. *Adherent, activated and aggregated platelets* (the three As) form the thrombus by a series of events initiated by tissue factor, which becomes exposed when a plaque ruptures or the endothelium is injured. Antiplatelet agents are effective and widely used both prophylactically and in ACS, including STEMI.

2. *Aspirin.* This well-tested, widely used, and cheap antiplatelet agent is beneficial in a wide variety of vascular disorders, including the prevention and treatment of coronary heart disease. It inhibits platelet COX-1 over a wide dose range. Prophylactic aspirin is indicated for all stages of symptomatic ischemic heart disease, including chronic effort angina, unstable angina, AMI, postinfarction management, after CABG, and during PCI. In the past, primary prevention by aspirin was considered only for high-risk patients. In those at moderate risk, there are almost as many disabling side effects. In view of the series of papers by Rothwell's group that have shown a remarkable effect of aspirin in lessening the development of cancer, including early metastases, *we change our previous opinion that prophylactic aspirin for the general apparently healthy population should not be encouraged, but rather that prophylactic use of aspirin can be considered.*

3. *ADP-receptor (P2Y₁₂) antagonists: Clopidogrel, ticlopidine and prasugrel.* These ADP receptor antagonists decrease events in ACS and help to prevent acute thrombotic closure after coronary artery stenting and are used for stroke prevention in patients with aspirin intolerance or resistance. Clopidogrel has fewer serious side effects, especially thrombocytopenia, than ticlopidine. For elective PCI, high-dose clopidogrel is sufficient without GpIIb/IIIa receptor inhibitors. With planned PCI, upstream high-dose clopidogrel (300-600 mg loading) is commonly used without GpIIb/IIIa blockade, with ticagrelor being the preferred alternative. Clopidogrel should be continued together with aspirin for at least 12 months with ACS and following DES implantation.

4. *Other antiplatelet agents.* Other agents such as sulfinpyrazone and dipyridamole are used less. Dipyridamole plus aspirin reduces repeat stroke.

5. *GpIIb/IIIa receptor blockers.* GpIIb/IIIa receptor blockers, including intravenous abciximab, tirofiban, and eptifibatide, act by blocking the final pathway of platelet aggregation. In ACS, in high-risk patients, and in PCI, they give outcome benefit beyond that obtained by aspirin and heparin *or* LMWH. The current policy is to replace heparin plus GpIIb/IIIa antagonists by bivalirudin (see Fig. 12-3). Upstream IIb/IIIa receptor antagonists are no longer recommended except for recurrent ischaemia while awaiting PCI. Intravenous abciximab or eptifibatide may be given prior to primary PCI and are usually reserved for a high thrombus or poor coronary flow when they may be given by the intracoronary route. In STEMI treated by fibrinolytics, the GpIIb/IIIa blockers should not be used.

6. *Intravenous UFH.* Intravenous UFH has a rapid onset of action, and is widely used in acute MI with or without fibrinolysis. LMWH produces less reinfarction (with fibrinolysis) than UFH and is simpler to use. Other indications for heparin (or LMWH) are in ACS, PCIs, and VTE. In all of these situations it is combined with aspirin. The drawbacks of UFH are that (1) anticoagulation is seldom well controlled, so that over-anticoagulation and under-anticoagulation are frequent despite repetitive measurements of aPPT or ACT; and (2) rebound can occur on discontinuation.

7. *LMWH.* LMWH is easier to administer than UFH, being given in standard weight-adjusted doses subcutaneously without the need for aPPT testing. There is no complete antidote for overdosing although protamine reverses the antithrombin effect. Enoxaparin is superior to UFH as adjudicative therapy to fibrinolysis in STE ACS and similar in total outcome (events avoided versus bleeding) in NSTEMI.[177] Further data are required for primary PCI.

8. *Bivalirudin.* In patients with moderate- to high-risk ACS and planned early catheterization, bivalirudin infusion results in similar outcomes to UFH or enoxaparin plus GpIIb/IIIa antagonists, with less bleeding.[185] In primary PCI for STEMI, bivalirudin produces less bleeding (and a modest reduction in mortality) compared with heparin plus GpIIb/IIIa.

9. *Fondaparinux.* For conservative management, fondaparinux is convenient to use (2.5 mg subcutaneously once daily) and represents a preferred anticoagulant strategy in those at higher risk of bleeding, but must be avoided in renal impairment with CrCl less than 30 mL/min.[166] Added UFH appears to reduce catheter thrombosis.

10. *Which regimen provides better therapy for ACS?* There are several approved options (UFH versus LMWH versus bivalirudin versus fondaparinux).The chosen regimen may differ between interventional and noninterventional centers.When intervention is likely, bivalirudin has excellent data, whereas if a conservative strategy is employed, fondaparinux is well tested in combination with fibrinolysis. If bleeding is a concern, bivalirudin and fondaparinux (if PCI is unlikely) are good alternative choices.

11. Oral anticoagulation. *Warfarin* has a slow onset of action over several days. Anticoagulation with warfarin is essential for those with prosthetic mechanical heart valves. For most patients with AF, warfarin is superior to aspirin in stroke prevention. Two major problems with warfarin are, first, the genetically induced large interpatient variation in the dose required, and, second, the serious risk of intracranial hemorrhage as use of warfarin in older adults has increased as world populations age. The risk of brain hemorrhage can be predicted by genetic profiling where available and affordable, and lessened by using the new oral agents. Oral thrombin inhibitors such as *dabigatran, rivaroxaban, and apixaban* compare well with warfarin in large-scale studies, often giving better outcome reduction. Their major advantage is a fixed oral dose that needs no monitoring, and reduced intracranial bleeding versus warfarin. They are already widely used to prevent stroke in nonvalvular AF. Their major disadvantages are cost and renal excretion, requiring dose decrease or even exclusion. Increased bleeding is usually not serious, but if it occurs, there is no tested antidote.

12. Fibrinolytic agents form the basis of therapy in many situations in which primary PCI is not feasible, as in the early stages of STE AMI. They are usually given in combination with UFH or LMWH, together with oral aspirin and clopidogrel. TNK and rPA need only one or two (respectively) bolus injections versus the infusion over 90 min needed for alteplase, which is associated with more systemic bleeding than TNK. For those at high risk of intracranial bleeds, such as older women with hypertension, streptokinase lessens the risk, but the lowest risk of intracranial and other bleeding is achieved with primary PCI. If patients present within 12 hours of onset of AMI, and appropriate facilities are available, the best approach to opening the occluded infarct-related artery is primary PCI. The door-to-balloon time should be 90 minutes or less. Combined fibrinolysis and PCI is harmful and not helpful. The next development could be therapy aimed at reduction of reperfusion injury in the ambulance.

13. Ongoing trials. Ongoing trials are testing newer antiplatelet and antithrombotic agents, with or without PCI. Yet more important than the type of reperfusion regimen used is the urgent need to make the "symptom-to-needle" or the "symptom-to-PCI" time as short as possible and to ensure that all potentially eligible patients receive reperfusion (internationally at least one fourth do not).

14. Future progress. The major yield from a society perspective is to treat all eligible patients with STEMI as quickly as possible. If this is achieved, overall gain is far greater than the difference between reperfusion regimens. Unfortunately, many patients, including those at highest risk, receive no reperfusion therapy at all. It is here that the least amount of effort could provide the highest yield.

Acknowledgment

We gratefully acknowledge the help of Dr. Jessica Opie, Senior Laboratory Haematologist, Groote Schuur Hospital and University of Cape Town, South Africa.

References

1. Hoffman M, et al. A cell-based model of hemostasis. *Thromb Haemost* 2001;85:958–965.
2. Mackman N, et al. Role of the extrinsic pathway of blood coagulation in hemostasis and thrombosis. *Arterioscler Thromb Vasc Biol* 2007;27:1687–1693.
3. Steffel J, et al. Tissue factor in cardiovascular diseases: molecular mechanisms and clinical implications. *Circulation* 2006;113:722–731.
4. Ruggeri ZM, et al. Adhesion mechanisms in platelet function. *Circ Res* 2007;100:1673–1685.
5. Offermanns S. Activation of platelet function through G protein-coupled receptors. *Circ Res* 2006;99:1293–1304.
6. Rao LV, et al. Tissue factor-factor VIIa signaling. *Arterioscler Thromb Vasc Biol* 2005;25: 47–56.
7. Schneider DJ, et al. Conundrums in the combined use of anticoagulants and antiplatelet drugs. *Circulation* 2007;116:305–315.
8. Nieswandt B, et al. Platelet-collagen interaction: is GPVI the central receptor? *Blood* 2003;102:449–461.
9. Denis CV, et al. Platelet adhesion receptors and their ligands in mouse models of thrombosis. *Arterioscler Thromb Vasc Biol* 2007;27:728–739.
10. Meadows TA, et al. Clinical aspects of platelet inhibitors and thrombus formation. *Circ Res* 2007;100:1261–1275.
11. Hankey GJ, et al. Aspirin resistance. *Lancet* 2006;367:606–617.
12. Yank V, et al. Systematic review: benefits and harms of in-hospital use of recombinant factor VIIa for off-label indications. *Ann Intern Med* 2011;154:529–540.
13. Eerenberg ES, et al. Reversal of rivaroxaban and dabigatran by prothrombin complex concentrate: a randomized, placebo-controlled, crossover study in healthy subjects. *Circulation* 2011;124:1573–1579
14. Zhou W, et al. Hemostatic therapy in experimental intracerebral hemorrhage associated with the direct thrombin inhibitor dabigatran. *Stroke* 2011;42:3594–3599.
15. CRASH-2 trial collaborators; Shakur H, et al. Effects of tranexamic acid on death, vascular occlusive events, and blood transfusion in trauma patients with significant haemorrhage (CRASH-2): a randomised, placebo-controlled trial. *Lancet* 2010;376:23–321.
16. Prieto-Merino D, et al. The importance of early treatment with tranexamic acid in bleeding trauma patients: an exploratory analysis of the CRASH-2 randomised controlled trial. *Lancet* 2011;377:1096–1101; 1101.
17. Antman EM, et al. Cyclooxygenase inhibition and cardiovascular risk. *Circulation* 2005;112:759–770.
18. UK-TIA Study Group. The United Kingdom Transient Ischaemic Attack (UK-TIA) Aspirin Trial: final results. *J Neurol Neurosurg Psychiatry* 1991;54:1044–1054.
19. Hayden M, et al. Aspirin for the primary prevention of cardiovascular events: a summary of the evidence for the U.S. Preventive Services Task Force. *Ann Intern Med* 2002;136: 161–172.
20. Ridker PM, et al. Low-dose aspirin therapy for chronic stable angina. A randomized placebo-controlled clinical trial. *Ann Int Med* 1991;114:835–839.
21. Antithrombotic Trialists' Collaboration. Collaborative meta-analysis of randomized trials of antiplatelet therapy for prevention of death, myocardial infarction and stroke in high-risk patients. *Brit Med J* 2002;324:71–86.
22. Peters RJ, et al. Effects of aspirin dose when used alone or in combination with clopidogrel in patients with acute coronary syndromes: observations from the Clopidogrel in Unstable angina to prevent Recurrent Events (CURE) study. *Circulation* 2003; 108:1682–1687.
23. Heras M, et al. Effects of thrombin inhibition on the development of acute platelet-thrombus deposition during angioplasty in pigs. *Circulation* 1989;79:657–665.
24. López-Farré A, et al. Effects of aspirin on platelet-neutrophil interactions. Role of nitric oxide and endothelin-1. *Circulation* 1995;91:2080–2088.
25. Ridker PM, et al. Inflammation, aspirin and the risk of cardiovascular disease in apparently healthy men. *N Engl J Med* 1997;336:973–979.
26. Eikelboom JW, et al. Aspirin-resistant thromboxane biosynthesis and the risk of myocardial infarction, stroke, or cardiovascular death in patients at high risk for cardiovascular events. *Circulation* 2002;105:1650–1655.
27. Maree AO, et al. Variable platelet response to aspirin and clopidogrel in atherothrombotic disease. *Circulation* 2007;115:2196–2207.
28. Cotter G, et al. Lack of aspirin effect: aspirin resistance or resistance to taking aspirin? *Am Heart J* 2004;147:293–300.
29. Gum PA, et al. A prospective, blinded determination of the natural history of aspirin resistance among stable patients with cardiovascular disease. *J Am Coll Cardiol* 2003;41: 961–965.
30. Lev EI, et al. Aspirin and clopidogrel drug response in patients undergoing percutaneous coronary intervention: the role of dual drug resistance. *J Am Coll Cardiol* 2006; 47:27–33.
31. Juul-Möller S, et al. For the Swedish Angina Pectoris Aspirin Trial (SAPAT) Group. Double-blind trial of aspirin in primary prevention of myocardial infarction in patients with stable chronic angina pectoris. *Lancet* 1992;340:1421–1425.
32. Belch J, et al. The prevention of progression of arterial disease and diabetes (POPADAD) trial: factorial randomised placebo controlled trial of aspirin and antioxidants in patients with diabetes and asymptomatic peripheral arterial disease. *Brit Med J* 2008;337:a1840.
33. De Berardis, et al. Association of aspirin use with major bleeding in patients with and without diabetes. *JAMA* 2012;307:2286–2294.

34. Goldstein LB, et al. Guidelines for the primary prevention of stroke: a guideline for healthcare professionals from the American Heart Association/American Stroke Association. *Stroke* 2011;42:517–584. Erratum in *Stroke* 2011;42:e26.
35. Rothwell PM, et al. Effect of daily aspirin on long-term risk of death due to cancer: analysis of individual patient data from randomised trials. *Lancet* 2011;377:31–41.
36. Burn J, et al. for the CAPP2 Investigators. Long-term effect of aspirin on cancer risk in carriers of hereditary colorectal cancer: an analysis from the CAPP2 randomised controlled trial. *Lancet* 2011;378; 2081–2087.
37. Rothwell PM, et al. Short-term effects of daily aspirin on cancer incidence, mortality, and non-vascular death: analysis of the time course of risks and benefits in 51 randomised controlled trials. *Lancet* 2012;379:1602–1612.
38. Rothwell PM, et al. Effect of daily aspirin on risk of cancer metastasis: a study of incident cancers during randomised controlled trials. *Lancet* 2012;379:1591–1601.
39. Opie LH. Aspirin and the prevention of cancer. *Lancet* 2011;377:1651.
40. Chan AT, et al. Editorial comment. Are we ready to recommend aspirin for cancer prevention? *Lancet* 2012; 379:1569–1571.
41. Capodanno D, et al. Antithrombotic therapy in patients with chronic kidney disease. *Circulation* 2012;125:2649–2661.
42. Mehta SR, et al. CURRENT-OASIS 7 Investigators. *N Engl J Med* 2010;363:930–942. Erratum in *N Engl J Med* 2010;363:1585.
43. ISIS-2 (Second International Study of Infarct Survival) Collaborative Group. Randomised trial of intravenous streptokinase, oral aspirin, both, or neither among 17,187 cases of suspected acute myocardial infarction. *Lancet* 1988;2:349–360.
44. Berger JS, et al. Initial aspirin dose and outcome among ST-elevation myocardial infarction patients treated with fibrinolytic therapy. *Circulation* 2008;117:192–199.
45. Mangano DT. Aspirin and mortality from coronary bypass surgery. *N Engl J Med* 2002;347:1309–1317.
46. Rothwell PM, et al. Effect of urgent treatment of transient ischaemic attack and minor stroke on early recurrent stroke (EXPRESS study): a prospective population-based sequential comparison. *Lancet* 2007;370:1432–1442.
47. Fuster V, et al. Aspirin as a therapeutic agent in cardiovascular disease. *Circulation* 1993;87:659–675.
48. Dutch TIA Trial Study Group. A comparison of two doses of aspirin (30 mg vs 283 mg a day) in patients after a transient ischemic attack or minor ischemic stroke. *New Engl J Med* 1991;325:1261–1266.
49. Taylor D, et al. Low-dose and high-dose acetylsalicylic acid for patients undergoing carotid endarterectomy: a randomised controlled trial. *Lancet* 1999;353:2179–2184.
50. McQuaid KR, et al. Systematic review and meta-analysis of adverse events of low-dose aspirin and clopidogrel in randomized controlled trials. *Am J Med* 2006;119:624–638.
51. McNamara RL, et al. Management of atrial fibrillation: review of the evidence for the role of pharmacologic therapy, electrical cardioversion, and echocardiography. *Ann Intern Med* 2003;139:1018–1033.
52. Segal R, et al. Early and late effects of low-dose aspirin on renal function in elderly patients. *Am J Med* 2002;115:462–466.
53. Awtry EH, et al. Aspirin. *Circulation* 2000;101:1206–1218.
54. MacDonald TM, et al. Effect of ibuprofen on cardioprotective effect of aspirin. *Lancet* 2003;361:573–574.
55. Teo KK, et al. Effects of long-term treatment with angiotensin-converting-enzyme inhibitors in the presence or absence of aspirin: a systematic review. *Lancet* 2002;360:1037–1043.
56. Latini R, et al. Clinical effects of early angiotensin-converting enzyme inhibitor treatment for acute myocardial infarction are similar in the presence and absence of aspirin: systematic overview of individual data from 96,712 randomized patients. Angiotensin-converting Enzyme Inhibitor Myocardial Infarction Collaborative Group. *J Am Coll Cardiol* 2000;35:1801–1807.
57. van Wijngaarden, et al. Effects of acetylsalicylic acid on peripheral hemodynamics in patients with chronic heart failure treated with angiotensin-converting enzyme inhibitors. *J Cardiovasc Pharmacol* 1994;23:240–245.
58. Chan FK, et al. Clopidogrel versus aspirin and esomeprazole to prevent recurrent ulcer bleeding. *N Engl J Med* 2005;352:238–244.
59. Steinhubl SR, et al. Ticlopidine pretreatment before coronary stenting is associated with sustained decrease in adverse cardiac events: data from the Evaluation of Platelet IIb/IIIa Inhibitor for Stenting (EPISTENT) Trial. *Circulation* 2001;103:1403–1409.
60. Bhatt DL, et al. Meta-analysis of randomized and registry comparisons of ticlopidine with clopidogrel after stenting. *J Am Coll Cardiol* 2002;39:9–14.
61. Wallentin L, et al. For the PLATO Investigators. Ticagrelor versus clopidogrel in patients with acute coronary syndromes. *N Engl J Med* 2009;361:1045–1057.
62. Hochholzer W, et al. Impact of the degree of peri-interventional platelet inhibition after loading with clopidogrel on early clinical outcome of elective coronary stent placement. *J Am Coll Cardiol* 2006;48:1742–1750.
63. Bassand JP, et al. Guidelines for the diagnosis and treatment of non-ST-segment elevation acute coronary syndromes. The Task Force for the Diagnosis and Treatment of Non-ST-Segment Elevation Acute Coronary Syndromes of the European Society of Cardiology. *Eur Heart J* 2007;28:1598–1660.
64. Müller I, et al. Effect of a high loading dose of clopidogrel on platelet function in patients undergoing coronary stent placement. *Heart* 2001;85:92–93.
65. Mehta SR, et al. CURRENT-OASIS 7 trial investigators. Double-dose versus standard-dose clopidogrel and high-dose versus low-dose aspirin in individuals undergoing percutaneous coronary intervention for acute coronary syndromes (CURRENT-OASIS 7): a randomised factorial trial. *Lancet* 2010;376:1233–1243.

66. Roberts JD, et al. Point-of-care genetic testing for personalisation of antiplatelet treatment (RAPID GENE): a prospective, randomised, proof-of-concept trial. *Lancet* 2012;379:1705–1711.
67. Bates ER, et al. Clopidogrel-drug interactions. *J Am Coll Cardiol* 2011;57:1251–1263.
68. Saw J, et al. CHARISMA Investigators. Lack of evidence of a clopidogrel-statin interaction in the CHARISMA trial. *J Am Coll Cardiol* 2007;50:291–295.
69. Sibbing D, et al. Impact of proton pump inhibitors on the antiplatelet effects of clopidogrel. *Thromb Haemost* 2009;101:714–719.
70. Bhatt DL, et al. Clopidogrel with or without omeprazole in coronary artery disease. *N Engl J Med* 2010;363:1909–1917.
71. Brar SS, et al. Impact of platelet reactivity on clinical outcomes after percutaneous coronary intervention a collaborative meta-analysis of individual participant data. *J Am Coll Cardiol* 2011;58:1945–1954.
72. Price MJ, et al. Standard- vs high-dose clopidogrel based on platelet function testing after percutaneous coronary intervention: the GRAVITAS randomized trial. *JAMA* 2011;305:1097–1105. Erratum *JAMA* 2011;305:2174.
73. Hamm CW, et al. ESC Guidelines for the management of acute coronary syndromes in patients presenting without persistent ST-segment elevation: the Task Force for the management of acute coronary syndromes (ACS) in patients presenting without persistent ST-segment elevation of the European Society of Cardiology (ESC). *Eur Heart J* 2011; 32:2999–3054.
74. Wallentin L, et al. For the PLATO Investigators. Ticagrelor versus clopidogrel in patients with acute coronary syndromes. *N Engl J Med* 2009;361:1045–1057.
75. Trenk D, et al. Results of the TRIGGER-PCI (Testing Platelet Reactivity In Patients Undergoing Elective Stent Placement on Clopidogrel to Guide Alternative Therapy With Prasugrel) Study. *J Am Coll Cardiol* 2012;59:2159–2164.
76. Grines CL, et al. Prevention of premature discontinuation of dual antiplatelet therapy in patients with coronary artery stents: a science advisory from the American Heart Association, American College of Cardiology, Society for Cardiovascular Angiography and Interventions, American College of Surgeons, and American Dental Association, with representation from the American College of Physicians. *Circulation* 2007;115:813–818.
77. Ho PM, et al. Incidence of death and acute myocardial infarction associated with stopping clopidogrel after acute coronary syndrome. *JAMA* 2008;299:532–539.
78. CAPRIE Steering Committee. A randomized, blinded trial of clopidogrel versus aspirin in patients at risk of ischemic events (CAPRIE). *Lancet* 1996;348:1329–1339.
79. ESPIRIT Study Group, Halkes PH, et al. Aspirin plus dipyridamole versus aspirin alone after cerebral ischaemia of arterial origin (ESPRIT): randomised controlled trial. *Lancet* 2006;367:1665–1673.
80. Penny W, et al. Antithrombotic therapy for patients with cardiac disease. *Curr Probl Cardiol* 1988;13:433–513.
81. Pfeffer MA, et al. The charisma of subgroups and the subgroups of CHARISMA. *N Engl J Med* 2006;354:1744–1746.
82. Chen ZM, et al. Addition of clopidogrel to aspirin in 45,852 patients with acute myocardial infarction: randomised placebo-controlled trial. *Lancet* 2005;366:1607–1621.
83. Bhatt DL, et al. Patients with prior myocardial infarction, stroke, or symptomatic peripheral arterial disease in the CHARISMA trial. *J Am Coll Cardiol* 2007;49:1982–1988.
84. Wright RS, et al. 2011 ACCF/AHA Focused update of the guidelines for the management of patients with unstable angina/non-ST-elevation myocardial infarction (updating the 2007 Guideline): a report of the ACC Foundation/AHA Task Force on Practice Guidelines. *Circulation* 2011;123:2022–2060.
85. Steinhubl SR, et al. Early and sustained dual oral antiplatelet therapy following percutaneous coronary intervention: a randomized controlled trial. *JAMA* 2002;288:2411–2420.
86. Gilard M, et al. Influence of omeprazole on the antiplatelet action of clopidogrel associated with aspirin: The Randomized Double-Blind OCLA (Omeprazole CLopidogrel Aspirin) Study. *J Am Col Cardiol* 2008;51:256–260.
87. Diener HC, et al. Aspirin and clopidogrel compared with clopidogrel alone after recent ischaemic stroke or transient ischaemic attack in high-risk patients (MATCH): randomised, double-blind, placebo-controlled trial. *Lancet* 2004;364:331–337.
88. The Clopidogrel in Unstable Angina to Prevent Recurrent Events Trial Investigators. Effects of clopidogrel in addition to aspirin in patients with acute coronary syndromes without ST-segment elevation. *N Engl J Med* 2001;345:494–502.
89. Cuisset T, et al. Benefit of a 600-mg loading dose of clopidogrel on platelet reactivity and clinical outcomes in patients with non-ST-segment elevation acute coronary syndrome undergoing coronary stenting. *J Am Coll Cardiol* 2006;48:1339–1345.
90. Kastrati A, et al. Abciximab in patients with acute coronary syndromes undergoing percutaneous coronary intervention after clopidogrel pretreatment: the ISAR-REACT 2 randomized trial. *JAMA* 2006;295:1531–1538.
91. Wiviott SD, et al. Randomized comparison of prasugrel (CS-747, LY640315), a novel thienopyridine P2Y12 antagonist, with clopidogrel in percutaneous coronary intervention: results of the Joint Utilization of Medications to Block Platelets Optimally (JUMBO)-TIMI 26 trial. *Circulation* 2005;111:3366–3373.
92. Wiviott SD, et al. Prasugrel versus clopidogrel in patients with acute coronary syndromes. *N Engl J Med* 2007;357:2001–2015.
93. Serebruany VL. Timing of thienopyridine loading and outcomes in the TRITON trial: the FDA Prasugrel Action Package outlook. *Cardiovasc Revasc Med* 2011;12:94–98.
94. Hochholzer W, et al. Predictors of bleeding and time dependence of association of bleeding with mortality: insights from the Trial to Assess Improvement in Therapeutic Outcomes by Optimizing Platelet Inhibition With Prasugrel—Thrombolysis in Myocardial Infarction 38 (TRITON-TIMI 38). *Circulation* 2011;123:2681–2689.

95. Cannon C, et al. for the PLATelet inhibition and patient Outcomes (PLATO) investigators. Ticagrelor compared with clopidogrel in acute coronary syndromes patients with a planned invasive strategy (PLATO): a randomized double-blind study. *Lancet* 2010;375:283–293.

96. White HD, et al. Reduced immediate ischemic events with cangrelor in PCI: a post-hoc pooled analysis of the CHAMPION trials using the Universal Definition of Myocardial Infarction. *Am Heart J* 2012;163:182–190.

97. Angiolillo DJ, et al. Bridging antiplatelet therapy with cangrelor in patients undergoing cardiac surgery. A randomized controlled trial. *JAMA* 2012;307:265–274.

98. Tricoci P, et al. for the TRACER Investigators. Thrombin-receptor antagonist vorapaxar in acute coronary syndromes. *N Engl J Med* 2012;366:20–33.

99. Morrow DA, et al, TRA 2P–TIMI 50 Steering Committee and Investigators. Vorapaxar in the secondary prevention of atherothrombotic events. *N Engl J Med* 2012;366:1404–1413.

100. White HD. Oral antiplatelet therapy for atherothrombotic disease: current evidence and new directions. *Am Heart J* 2011;161:450–461. Erratum in *Am Heart J* 2011;162:569.

101. Caixeta A, et al. Incidence and clinical consequences of acquired thrombocytopenia after antithrombotic therapies in patients with acute coronary syndromes: results from the Acute Catheterization and Urgent Intervention Triage Strategy (ACUITY) trial. *Am Heart J* 2011;161:298–306.

102. Stone GW, et al. Routine upstream initiation vs deferred selective use of glycoprotein IIb/IIIa inhibitors in acute coronary syndromes: the ACUITY Timing trial. *JAMA* 2007;297:591–602.

103. Friedland S, et al. Meta-analysis of randomized controlled trials of intracoronary versus intravenous administration of glycoprotein IIb/IIIa inhibitors during percutaneous coronary intervention for acute coronary syndrome. *Am J Cardiol* 2011;108:1244–1251.

104. Ohlmann P, et al. Prehospital Abciximab in ST-Segment Elevation Myocardial Infarction: Results of the Randomized, Double-Blind MISTRAL Study. *Circ Cardiovasc Interv* 2012; 5:69–76.

105. EPILOG Investigators. Platelet glycoprotein IIb-IIIa receptor blockade and low-dose heparin during percutaneous coronary revascularization. *N Engl J Med* 1997;336:1689–1696.

106. Kastrati A, et al. A clinical trial of abciximab in elective percutaneous coronary intervention after pretreatment with clopidogrel. *N Engl J Med* 2004;350:232–238.

107. Tcheng J, et al. Readministration of abciximab is as effective as first time administration with similar risks: results from the ReoPro Readministration Registry (R³) [abstract]. *J Am Coll Cardiol* 1999;33(Suppl. A):14A–15A.

108. Topol EJ, et al. TARGET Investigators. Do Tirofiban and ReoPro Give Similar Efficacy Trial. Comparison of two platelet glycoprotein IIb/IIIa inhibitors, tirofiban and abciximab, for the prevention of ischemic events with percutaneous coronary revascularization. *N Engl J Med* 2001;344:1888–1894.

109. Mukherjee D, et al. Mortality at 1 year for the direct comparison of tirofiban and abciximab during percutaneous coronary revascularization: do tirofiban and ReoPro give similar efficacy outcomes at trial 1-year follow-up. *Eur Heart J* 2005;26:2524–2528.

110. Valgimigli M, et al. Tirofiban as adjunctive therapy for acute coronary syndromes and percutaneous coronary intervention: a meta-analysis of randomized trials. *Eur Heart J* 2010;31:35–49.

111. ten Berg JM, et al. On-TIME 2 Study Group. Effect of early, pre-hospital initiation of high bolus dose tirofiban in patients with ST-segment elevation myocardial infarction on short- and long-term clinical outcome. *J Am Coll Cardiol* 2010;55:2446–2455.

112. PURSUIT Trial Investigators. Inhibition of platelet glycoprotein IIb/IIIa with eptifibatide in patients with acute coronary syndromes. *N Engl J Med* 1998;339:436–443.

113. Hirsh J, et al. American Heart Association/American College of Cardiology Foundation guide to warfarin therapy. *J Am Coll Cardiol* 2003;41:1633–1652.

114. Huhtakangas J, et al. Effect of increased warfarin use on warfarin-related cerebral hemorrhage: a longitudinal population-based study. *Stroke* 2011;42:2431–2435.

115. Kamel H, et al. Cost-effectiveness of dabigatran compared with warfarin for stroke prevention in patients with atrial fibrillation and prior stroke or transient ischemic attack. *Stroke* 2012;43:881–883.

116. Millican EA, et al. Genetic-based dosing in orthopedic patients beginning warfarin therapy. *Blood* 2007;110:1511–1515.

117. Shen AY, et al. Racial/ethnic differences in the risk of intracranial hemorrhage among patients with atrial fibrillation. *J Am Coll Cardiol* 2007;50:309–315.

118. Loebstein R, et al. A coding VKORC1 Asp36Tyr polymorphism predisposes to warfarin resistance. *Blood* 2007;109:2477–2480.

119. Anderson JL, et al. Randomized trial of genotype-guided versus standard warfarin dosing in patients initiating oral anticoagulation. *Circulation* 2007;116:2563–2570.

120. Vink R, et al. The optimal intensity of vitamin K antagonists in patients with mechanical heart valves: a meta-analysis. *J Am Coll Cardiol* 2003;42:2042–2048.

121. Heneghan C, et al. Self-monitoring of oral anticoagulation: a systematic review and meta-analysis. *Lancet* 2006;367:404–411.

122. Johnson JA. Warfarin pharmacogenetics: a rising tide for its clinical value. *Circulation* 2012;125:1964–1966.

123. Flaherty ML, et al. The increasing incidence of anticoagulant-associated intracerebral hemorrhage. *Neurology* 2007;68:116–121.

124. Huhtakangas J, et al. Effect of increased warfarin use on warfarin-related cerebral hemorrhage: a longitudinal population-based study. *Stroke* 2011;42:2431–2435.

125. Gage BF, et al. Risk of osteoporotic fracture in elderly patients taking warfarin: results from the National Registry of Atrial Fibrillation 2. *Arch Intern Med* 2006; 166:241–246.

126. Hylek EM, et al. Major hemorrhage and tolerability of warfarin in the first year of therapy among elderly patients with atrial fibrillation. *Circulation* 2007;115:2689–2696.
127. Yiu KH, et al. Comparison of the efficacy and safety profiles of intravenous vitamin K and fresh frozen plasma as treatment of warfarin-related over-anticoagulation in patients with mechanical heart valves. *Am J Cardiol* 2006;97:409–411.
128. Mohler ER, 3rd. Atherothrombosis—wave goodbye to combined anticoagulation and antiplatelet therapy? *N Engl J Med* 2007;357:293–296.
129. Homma S, et al. WARCEF Investigators. Warfarin and aspirin in patients with heart failure and sinus rhythm. *N Engl J Med* 2012;366:1859–1869.
130. Ridker PM, et al. Long-term, low-intensity warfarin therapy for the prevention of recurrent venous thromboembolism. *N Engl J Med* 2003;348:1425–1434.
131. Gage BF, et al. Validation of clinical classification schemes for predicting stroke: results from the National Registry of Atrial Fibrillation. *JAMA* 2001;285:2864–2870.
132. Lip GY, et al. Refining clinical risk stratification for predicting stroke and thromboembolism in atrial fibrillation using a novel risk factor-based approach: the Euro heart survey on atrial fibrillation. *Chest* 2010;137:263–272.
133. Pisters R, et al. A novel user-friendly score (HAS-BLED) to assess 1-year risk of major bleeding in patients with atrial fibrillation: the Euro Heart Survey. *Chest* 2010;138:1093–1100.
134. Fang MC, et al. A new risk scheme to predict warfarin-associated hemorrhage: The ATRIA (Anticoagulation and Risk Factors in Atrial Fibrillation) Study. *J Am Coll Cardiol* 2011;58:395–401.
135. AFFIRM Investigators. First Antiarrhythmic Drug Substudy. Maintenance of sinus rhythm in patients with atrial fibrillation. *J Am Coll Cardiol* 2003;42:20–29.
136. Hart RG, et al. Stroke with intermittent atrial fibrillation: incidence and predictors during aspirin therapy. Stroke Prevention in Atrial Fibrillation Investigators. *J Am Coll Cardiol* 2000;35:183–187.
137. Mant J, et al. Warfarin versus aspirin for stroke prevention in an elderly community population with atrial fibrillation (the Birmingham Atrial Fibrillation Treatment of the Aged Study, BAFTA): a randomised controlled trial. *Lancet* 2007;370:493–503.
138. De Caterina R, et al. Anticoagulants in heart disease: current status and perspectives. *Eur Heart J* 2007;28:880–913.
139. Kennedy J, et al. Fast assessment of stroke and transient ischaemic attack to prevent early recurrence (FASTER): a randomised controlled pilot trial. *Lancet Neurol* 2007;6:961–969.
140. Reddy VY, et al. Safety of percutaneous left atrial appendage closure: results from the Watchman Left Atrial Appendage System for Embolic Protection in Patients with AF (PROTECT AF) clinical trial and the Continued Access Registry. *Circulation* 2011;123:417–424.
141. Viles-Gonzalez JF, et al. The clinical impact of incomplete left atrial appendage closure with the Watchman Device in patients with atrial fibrillation: a PROTECT AF substudy. *J Am Coll Cardiol* 2012;59:923–929.
142. Hirsh J, et al. Guide to anticoagulant therapy. Part 1: Heparin. *Circulation* 1994;89:1449–1468.
142A. Kleinow ME, et al. Effect of chronic kidney disease on warfarin management in a pharmacist-managed anticoagulation clinic. *J Manag Care Pharm* 2011;17:523–530.
143. Hart RG, et al. Warfarin in atrial fibrillation patients with moderate chronic kidney disease. *Clin J Am Soc Nephrol* 2011;6:2599–2604.
144. Brodsky SV. Warfarin-related nephropathy occurs in patients with and without chronic kidney disease and is associated with an increased mortality rate. *Kidney Int* 2011;80:181–189.
145. Chimowitz MI, et al. Comparison of warfarin and aspirin for symptomatic intracranial arterial stenosis. *N Engl J Med* 2005;352:1305–1316.
146. Kearon C, et al. Comparison of low-intensity warfarin therapy with conventional-intensity warfarin therapy for long-term prevention of recurrent venous thromboembolism. *N Engl J Med* 2003;349:631–639.
147. Büller HR, et al. for the EINSTEIN–PE Investigators. Oral rivaroxaban for the treatment of symptomatic pulmonary embolism. *N Engl J Med* 2012;366:1287–1289.
148. Katsnelson M, et al. Progress for stroke prevention with atrial fibrillation: emergence of alternative oral anticoagulants. *Circulation* 2012;125:1577–1583.
149. Nainggolan L. *New analysis extends dabigatran MI signal to other thrombin inhibitors.* <http://www.theheart.org/article/1380075.do>; [accessed 05.10.2012].
150. Hankey GJ, et al. Dabigatran etexilate: a new oral thrombin inhibitor. *Circulation* 2011;123:1436–1450.
151. Wallentin L, et al. Efficacy and safety of dabigatran compared with warfarin at different levels of international normalised ratio control for stroke prevention in atrial fibrillation: an analysis of the RE-LY trial. *Lancet* 2010;376:975–983.
152. Connolly SJ, et al. Dabigatran versus warfarin in patients with atrial fibrillation. RE-LY Study. *N Engl J Med* 2009;361:1139–1151.
153. Eikelboom JW, et al. Risk of bleeding with 2 doses of dabigatran compared with warfarin in older and younger patients with atrial fibrillation: an analysis of the randomized evaluation of long-term anticoagulant therapy (RE-LY) trial. *Circulation* 2011;123:2363–2372.
154. Hohnloser SH, et al. Myocardial ischemic events in patients with atrial fibrillation treated with dabigatran or warfarin in the RE-LY (Randomized Evaluation of Long-Term Anticoagulation Therapy) trial. *Circulation* 2012;125:669–676.
155. *Label update for dabigatran.* <http://www.theheart.org/article/1411191.do>; [accessed 05.10.12].
156. FDA label, revised November 2001. FDA website, www.fda.gov/ [accessed 07.06.12].
157. *Dabigatran fatal bleeding less than in clinical trials.* <http://www.theheart.org>; [accessed 05.10.12].
158. Patel MR, et al. ROCKET AF Investigators. Rivaroxaban versus warfarin in nonvalvular atrial fibrillation. *N Engl J Med* 2011;365:883–891.

159. Fox KAA, et al. Prevention of stroke and systemic embolism with rivaroxaban compared with warfarin in patients with non-valvular atrial fibrillation and moderate renal impairment. *Eur Heart J* 2011;32:2387–2394.
160. Mega JL, et al. for the ATLAS ACS 2–TIMI 51 Investigators. Rivaroxaban in patients with a recent acute coronary syndrome. *N Engl J Med* 2012;366:9–19.
161. Granger CB, et al. for the ARISTOTLE Committees and Investigators. Apixaban versus warfarin in patients with atrial fibrillation. *N Engl J Med* 2011;365:981–992.
162. Connolly SJ, et al. for the AVERROES Steering Committee and Investigators. Apixaban in patients with atrial fibrillation. *N Engl J Med* 2011;364:806–817.
163. Goldhaber SZ, et al. for the ADOPT Trial Investigators. Apixaban versus enoxaparin for thromboprophylaxis in medically ill patients. *N Engl J Med* 2011;365:2167–2177.
164. Alexander JH, et al. for the APPRAISE-2 Investigators Apixaban with antiplatelet therapy after acute coronary syndrome. *N Engl J Med* 2011;365:699–708.
164A. Camm AJ, et al. HYPERLINK "http://www.ncbi.nlm.nih.gov/pubmed/22923145" 2012 focused update of the ESC Guidelines for the management of atrial fibrillation: An update of the 2010 ESC Guidelines for the management of atrial fibrillation. Europace 2012;14:1385–1413
165. Hirsh J, et al. Beyond unfractionated heparin and warfarin: current and future advances. *Circulation* 2007;116:552–560.
166. Anderson JL, et al. ACC/AHA 2007 guidelines for the management of patients with unstable angina/non-ST-Elevation myocardial infarction: a report of the American College of Cardiology/American Heart Association Task Force on Practice Guidelines (Writing Committee to Revise the 2002 Guidelines for the Management of Patients With Unstable Angina/Non-ST-Elevation Myocardial Infarction) developed in collaboration with the American College of Emergency Physicians, the Society for Cardiovascular Angiography and Interventions, and the Society of Thoracic Surgeons endorsed by the American Association of Cardiovascular and Pulmonary Rehabilitation and the Society for Academic Emergency Medicine. *J Am Coll Cardiol* 2007;50:652–726.
167. Antman EM, et al. 2007 Focused Update of the ACC/AHA 2004 Guidelines for the Management of Patients With ST-Elevation Myocardial Infarction: a report of the American College of Cardiology/American Heart Association Task Force on Practice Guidelines: developed in collaboration With the Canadian Cardiovascular Society endorsed by the American Academy of Family Physicians: 2007 Writing Group to Review New Evidence and Update the ACC/AHA 2004 Guidelines for the Management of Patients With ST-Elevation Myocardial Infarction, Writing on Behalf of the 2004 Writing Committee. *Circulation* 2008;117:296–329.
168. Davoren A, et al. Heparin-induced thrombocytopenia and thrombosis. *Am J Hematol* 2006;81:36–44.
169. Lo GK, et al. Evaluation of the pretest clinical score (4T's) for the diagnosis of heparin-induced thrombocytopenia in two clinical settings. *J Thromb Haem* 2006;4: 759–765.
170. Cruz-Gonzalez I, et al. Efficacy and safety of argatroban with or without glycoprotein IIb/IIIa inhibitor in patients with heparin induced thrombocytopenia undergoing percutaneous coronary intervention for acute coronary syndrome. *J Thromb Thrombolysis* 2007;25:214–218.
171. Spinler SA. New concepts in heparin-induced thrombocytopenia: diagnosis and management. *J Thromb Thrombolysis* 2006;21:17–21.
172. Wester JP, et al. Low-dose fondaparinux in suspected heparin-induced thrombocytopenia in the critically ill. *Neth J Med* 2007;65:101–108.
173. Koster A, et al. Bivalirudin during cardiopulmonary bypass in patients with previous or acute heparin-induced thrombocytopenia and heparin antibodies: results of the CHOOSE-ON trial. *Ann Thorac Surg* 2007;83:572–577.
174. Keeling D, et al. The management of heparin-induced thrombocytopenia. *Br J Haematol* 2006;133:259–269.
175. Schulz S, et al. Intracoronary Stenting and Antithrombotic Regimen: Rapid Early Action for Coronary Treatment (ISAR-REACT) 3A Trial Investigators. ISAR-REACT 3A: a study of reduced dose of unfractionated heparin in biomarker negative patients undergoing percutaneous coronary intervention. *Eur Heart J* 2010;31:2482–2489.
176. Hirsh J, et al. Guide to anticoagulant therapy. Part 2: Oral anticoagulants. *Circulation* 1994;89:1469–1480. Erratum in *Circulation* 1995;91:A55–A56.
177. Murphy SA, et al. Efficacy and safety of the low-molecular weight heparin enoxaparin compared with unfractionated heparin across the acute coronary syndrome spectrum: a meta-analysis. *Eur Heart J* 2007;28:2077–2086.
178. Bhatt DL, et al. Clopidogrel and aspirin versus aspirin alone for the prevention of atherothrombotic events. *N Engl J Med* 2006;354:1706–1717.
179. White H, et al. The use of intravenous enoxaparin in elective percutaneous coronary intervention in patients with renal impairment: results from the STEEPLE trial. *Am Heart J* 2009; 157:125–131.
180. FRISC Study Group. Fragmin During Instability in Coronary Artery Disease (FRISC). Low molecular-weight heparin during instability in coronary artery disease. *Lancet* 1996; 347:561–568.
181. Eikelboom JW, et al. Unfractionated and low-molecular-weight heparin as adjuncts to thrombolysis in aspirin-treated patients with ST-elevation acute myocardial infarction: a meta-analysis of the randomized trials. *Circulation* 2005;112:3855–3867.
182. Reed MD, et al. Clinical pharmacology of bivalirudin. *Pharmacotherapy* 2002;22:105S–111S.
183. Hanna EB, et al. Characteristics and in-hospital outcomes of patients with non-ST-segment elevation myocardial infarction and chronic kidney disease undergoing percutaneous coronary intervention. *JACC Cardiovasc Interv* 2011;4:1002–1008.

184. Lincoff AM, et al. Long-term efficacy of bivalirudin and provisional glycoprotein IIb/IIIa blockade vs heparin and planned glycoprotein IIb/IIIa blockade during percutaneous coronary revascularization: REPLACE-2 randomized trial. *JAMA* 2004;292:696–703.

185. Stone GW, et al. Bivalirudin for patients with acute coronary syndromes. *N Engl J Med* 2006;355:2203–2216.

186. Stone GW, et al. Bivalirudin in patients with acute coronary syndromes undergoing percutaneous coronary intervention: a subgroup analysis from the Acute Catheterization and Urgent Intervention Triage strategy (ACUITY) trial. *Lancet* 2007;369:907–919.

187. Waksman R. ACUITY-PCI: one drug does not fit all. *Lancet* 2007;369:881–882.

188. Yusuf S, et al. Comparison of fondaparinux and enoxaparin in acute coronary syndromes. *N Engl J Med* 2006;354:1464–1476.

189. Mehran R, et al. HORIZONS-AMI Trial Investigators. Bivalirudin in patients undergoing primary angioplasty for acute myocardial infarction (HORIZONS-AMI): 1-year results of a randomised controlled trial. *Lancet* 2009;374:1149–1159.

190. Hanna EB, et al. Antiplatelet and anticoagulant therapies in acute coronary syndromes. *Cardiovasc Drugs Ther* 2010;24:6.

191. Stone GW, et al. HORIZONS-AMI Trial Investigators. Heparin plus a glycoprotein IIb/IIIa inhibitor versus bivalirudin monotherapy and paclitaxel-eluting stents versus bare-metal stents in acute myocardial infarction (HORIZONS-AMI): final 3-year results from a multicentre, randomised controlled trial. *Lancet* 2011;377:2193–2204.

192. Bangalore S, et al. EVENT Registry Investigators. Bleeding risk comparing targeted low-dose heparin with bivalirudin in patients undergoing percutaneous coronary intervention: results from a propensity score-matched analysis of the Evaluation of Drug-Eluting Stents and Ischemic Events (EVENT) registry. *Circ Cardiovasc Interv* 2011;4:463–473.

193. Silvain J, et al. Efficacy and safety of enoxaparin versus unfractionated heparin during percutaneous coronary intervention: systematic review and meta-analysis. *Brit Med J* 2012 Feb 3;344:e553.

194. Lassen MR, et al. RECORD3 Investigators. Rivaroxaban versus enoxaparin for thrombo-prophylaxis after total knee arthroplasty. *N Engl J Med* 2008;358:2776–2786.

195. Eriksson BI, et al. RE-NOVATE II Study Group Oral dabigatran versus enoxaparin for thromboprophylaxis after primary total hip arthroplasty (RE-NOVATE II*). A randomised, double-blind, non-inferiority trial. *Thromb Haemost* 201;105:721–729.

196. Mehta SR, et al. Efficacy and safety of Fondaparinux versus Enoxaparin in patients with acute coronary syndromes undergoing percutaneous coronary intervention. Results from the OASIS-5 Trial. *JACC* 2007;50:1742–1751.

197. Yusuf S, et al. Effects of fondaparinux on mortality and reinfarction in patients with acute ST-segment elevation myocardial infarction: the OASIS-6 randomized trial. *JAMA* 2006;295:1519–1530.

198. Steg PG, et al. FUTURA/OASIS-8 Trial Group. Low-dose vs standard-dose unfractionated heparin for percutaneous coronary intervention in acute coronary syndromes treated with fondaparinux: the FUTURA/OASIS-8 randomized trial. *JAMA* 2010;304:1339–1349.

199. Fay WP, et al. Vascular functions of the plasminogen activation system. *Arterioscler Thromb Vasc Biol* 2007;27:1231–1237.

200. Alessi MC, et al. Plasminogen activator inhibitor-1, adipose tissue and insulin resistance. *Curr Opin Lipidol* 2007;18:240–245.

201. Gersh BJ, et al. Thrombolysis and myocardial salvage: results of clinical trials and the animal paradigm—paradoxic or predictable? *Circulation* 1993;88:296–306.

202. White H, et al. Clinical cardiology: new frontiers: thrombolysis for acute myocardial infarction. *Circulation* 1998;97:1632–1646.

203. Steg PG, et al. Impact of time to treatment on mortality after prehospital fibrinolysis or primary angioplasty: data from the CAPTIM randomized clinical trial. *Circulation* 2003;108:2851–2856.

204. Weaver WD, et al. For the Myocardial Infarction Triage and Intervention Trial. Prehospital-initiated vs hospital-initiated thrombolytic therapy. *J Am Med Assoc* 1993;270:1211–1216.

205. Van de Werf FJ. Fine-tuning the selection of a reperfusion strategy. *Circulation* 2006;114:2002–2003.

206. Fibrinolytic Therapy Trial (FTT) Collaborative Group. Indications for fibrinolytic therapy in suspected acute myocardial infarction; collaborative overview of early mortality and major morbidity results from all randomised trials of more than 1000 patients. *Lancet* 1994;343:311–322.

207. Taher T, et al. Aborted myocardial infarction in patients with ST-segment elevation: insights from the Assessment of the Safety and Efficacy of a New Thrombolytic Regimen-3 Trial Electrocardiographic Substudy. *J Am Coll Cardiol* 2004;44:38–43.

208. Giugliano RP, et al. Selecting the best reperfusion strategy in ST-elevation myocardial infarction: it's all a matter of time. *Circulation* 2003;108:2828–2830.

209. White HD. Optimal treatment of patients with acute coronary syndromes and non-ST-elevation myocardial infarction. *Am Heart J* 1999;138:S105–114.

210. Gersh BJ, et al. Pharmacological facilitation of primary percutaneous coronary intervention for acute myocardial infarction: is the slope of the curve the shape of the future? *JAMA* 2005;293:979–986.

211. GUSTO Investigators. An international randomized trial comparing four thrombolytic strategies for acute myocardial infarction. *New Engl J Med* 1993;329:673–682.

212. Parsons M, et al. A randomized trial of tenecteplase versus alteplase for acute ischemic stroke. *N Engl J Med* 2012;366:1099–1107.

213. ASSENT-2 Investigators. Assessment of the Safety and Efficacy of a New Thrombolytic (ASSENT-2) Investigators. Single-bolus tenecteplase compared with front-loaded alteplase in acute myocardial infarction: the ASSENT-2 double-blinded randomised trial. *Lancet* 1999;354:716–722.

214. ISIS-3 Study Group. (Third International Study of Infarct Survival) Collaborative Group. ISIS-3: a randomised comparison of streptokinase vs tissue plasminogen activator vs anistreplase and of aspirin plus heparin vs aspirin alone among 41,299 cases of suspected acute myocardial infarction. *Lancet* 1992;339:753–770.
215. Hermentin P, et al. Comparative analysis of the activity and content of different streptokinase preparations. *Eur Heart J* 2005;26:933–940.
216. Collins R, et al. Clinical effects of anticoagulant therapy in suspected acute myocardial infarction: systematic overview of randomised trials. *Brit Med J* 1996;313:652–659.
217. Tardiff BE, et al. Long term results from the Global Utilization of Streptokinase and TPA for Occluded Coronary Arteries (GUSTO-I) Trial: sustained benefit of fibrin-specific therapy (Abstract). *Circulation* 1999;100 (18):I-498–I-499.
218. Deswal A, et al. Cytokines and cytokine receptors in advanced heart failure: an analysis of the cytokine database from the Vesnarinone Trial (VEST). *Circulation* 2001;103:2055–2059.
219. Minners J, et al. Diazoxide-induced respiratory inhibition—a putative mitochondrial K(ATP) channel independent mechanism of pharmacological preconditioning. *Mol Cell Biochem* 2007;294:11–18.
220. Staat P, et al. Postconditioning the human heart. *Circulation* 2005;2143–2148.
221. Keeley E, et al. Primary angioplasty versus intravenous thrombolytic therapy for acute myocardial infarction: a quantitative review of 23 randomised trials. *Lancet* 2003;361:13–20.
222. Ellis S. *ESC Congress, Vienna*. <http://www.escardio.org>; [accessed 05.10.12].
223. ASSENT-4 PCI. Primary versus tenecteplase-facilitated percutaneous coronary intervention in patients with ST-segment elevation acute myocardial infarction (ASSENT-4 PCI): randomised trial. *Lancet* 2006;367:569–578.
224. Armstrong PW. A comparison of pharmacologic therapy with/without timely coronary intervention vs. primary percutaneous intervention early after ST-elevation myocardial infarction: the WEST (Which Early ST-elevation myocardial infarction Therapy) study. *Eur Heart J* 2006;27:1530–1538.
225. Larson DM, et al. Safety and efficacy of a pharmaco-invasive reperfusion strategy in rural ST-elevation myocardial infarction patients with expected delays due to long-distance transfers. *Eur Heart J* 2012;33:1232–1240.
226. Bonnefoy E, et al. Primary angioplasty versus prehospital fibrinolysis in acute myocardial infarction: a randomised study. *Lancet* 2002;360:825–829.
227. Gershlick AH, et al. Rescue angioplasty after failed thrombolytic therapy for acute myocardial infarction. *N Engl J Med* 2005;353:2758–2768.
228. Fernandez-Aviles F, et al. Routine invasive strategy within 24 hours of thrombolysis versus ischaemia-guided conservative approach for acute myocardial infarction with ST-segment elevation (GRACIA-1): a randomised controlled trial. *Lancet* 2004; 364:1045–1053.
229. Widimsky P, et al. On behalf of the PRAGUE Study Group Investigators. Long distance support for primary angioplasty vs immediate thombolysis in acute myocardial infarction. *Eur Heart J* 2002;2003:94–104.
230. Schomig A, et al. Therapy-dependent influence of time-to-treatment interval on myocardial salvage in patients with acute myocardial infarction treated with coronary artery stenting or thrombolysis. *Circulation* 2003;108:1084–1088.
231. Nallamothu BK, et al. Time to treatment in primary percutaneous coronary intervention. *N Engl J Med* 2007;357:1631–1638.
232. Kalla K, et al. Implementation of guidelines improves the standard of care: the Viennese registry on reperfusion strategies in ST-elevation myocardial infarction (Vienna STEMI registry). *Circulation* 2006;113:2398–2405.
233. Ting HH, et al. Regional systems of care to optimize timeliness of reperfusion therapy for ST-elevation myocardial infarction: the Mayo Clinic STEMI Protocol. *Circulation* 2007;116:729–736.
234. Xavier D, et al. Treatment and outcomes of acute coronary syndromes in India (CREATE): a prospective analysis of registry data. *Lancet* 2008;371:1435–1442.
235. Cantor WJ, et al. Routine early angioplasty after fibrinolysis for acute myocardial infarction. *N Engl J Med* 2009;360:2705–2718.
236. Chen H, et al. Functional properties of a novel mutant of staphylokinase with platelet-targeted fibrinolysis and antiplatelet aggregation activities. *Eur J Pharmacol* 2007;566: 137–144.
237. Lefkovits J, et al. Direct thrombin inhibitors in cardiovascular medicine. *Circulation* 1994;90:1522–1536.
238. Simoons ML, et al. Individual risk assessment for intracranial haemorrhage during thrombolytic therapy. *Lancet* 1993;342:1523–1528.

10

Lipid-Modifying and Antiatherosclerotic Drugs

ANTONIO M. GOTTO, Jr. · LIONEL H. OPIE

"In the great majority of cases ordinary atheroma (Greek, meal or porridge) is to blame; this consists of softening, the precursor of arteriosclerosis, with yellowish fatty (cholesterol) areas in the endarterium."

Paul Dudley White, 1944[1]

Very large reductions in coronary disease might attend pharmacologic achievement of LDL levels characteristic of "traditional" populations such as hunter-gatherers and Arctic Eskimos.

Modified from Domanski, 2007[2]

Blood lipid assessment forms an essential step in the evaluation of almost every cardiac patient, whether young, middle aged, or older. Physicians may help guide younger patients toward long-term cardiovascular health by addressing early risk factors, whereas middle-aged and older patients may need a more intensive approach because of their near-term risk for coronary disease. The widespread availability, persuasive and substantial clinical database, and relative safety of the statins have established pharmacologic control of blood lipids as an increasingly acceptable strategy. Of the lipid aims, the early reduction of low-density-lipoprotein cholesterol (LDL-C) levels by statins is the current key to lessening clinical cardiovascular disease.[2-4] Since the last edition of this book, results of a major clinical trial in primary prevention have demonstrated the utility of the inflammatory marker C-reactive protein (CRP) in identifying individuals at increased risk despite having low to normal levels of LDL-C.[5] Patients in this trial who attained LDL-C levels less than 50 mg/dL experienced greater reductions in cardiovascular morbidity and mortality than the rest of the study cohort.[6] These findings are indicative of two major trends in current research: (1) the potential benefit of high-intensity therapy to very low LDL-C levels, and (2) the growing recognition of the role of vascular inflammation in the genesis of arterial disease (Fig. 10-1) and the increased integration of inflammatory markers in cardiovascular risk assessment. These developments and their translation into clinical practice hold the potential to improve patient outcomes.

Inflammation and Atherogenesis

Atherosclerotic inflammation is triggered when circulating LDL enters the arterial wall and is retained through interaction with proteoglycans in the extracellular matrix.[7] LDL modification within the arterial

ENDOTHELIUM AND VASCULAR DISEASE

Opie 2012

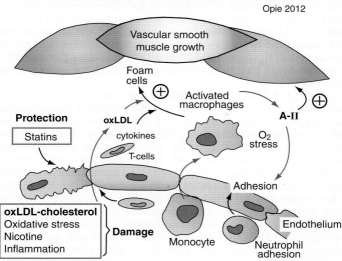

Figure 10-1   From endothelial damage to atheroma: the proposed role of the vascular endothelium in atherogenesis. Note early endothelial damage, prompted by several factors including oxidized low-density lipoprotein (oxLDL) cholesterol, and hypothetically prevented by treatment. Neutrophils roll on and adhere to the damaged endothelium to promote adhesion of macrophages. Vascular cell adhesion molecule (VCAM) promotes the binding of macrophages to the endothelium, after which they penetrate the endothelium to become activated and, by uptake of oxLDL, to become foam cells. Activated macrophages also synthesize angiotensin II (A-II) that in turn promotes oxidative stress that stimulates the formation of VCAM. A-II also promotes growth of vascular smooth muscle cells, an integral part of atherogenesis. O_2, Oxygen. (Figure © L.H. Opie, 2012.)

wall occurs through a series of oxidative steps, which damages the endothelium and stimulates an immune and inflammatory response with increased production of chemoattractant molecules, cytokines, and adhesion molecules.[8] In addition to LDL oxidation, hypertension and cigarette smoking can also cause endothelial dysfunction. Subsequently, the dysfunctional endothelium is more permeable to circulating monocytes and T-cells; both are transported into the intima, where the monocytes are converted into macrophages. Activated macrophages and T-cells release a variety of mediators that collectively exacerbate inflammation and oxidation within the vessel wall.[9,10] Macrophages also synthesize angiotensin II, which further disrupts normal endothelial function. Foam cells are formed when macrophages ingest oxidized LDL through receptors, including CD36. Growth of the atherosclerotic lesion is characterized by smooth muscle cell proliferation and increased production of matrix metalloproteinases, which can cause deterioration of elastin and collagen within the extracellular matrix. Mature plaques typically consist of a lipid-rich necrotic core encased by a weakened fibrous cap. Inflammatory cells may make mature plaques more prone to rupture by promoting the deterioration of fibrous caps.

C-reactive protein. Much interest has centered on CRP, a general measure of inflammation that is produced in the liver in response to interleukin-6. This inflammatory marker is used to assess patients at intermediate risk (10% to 20% 10-year risk) according to traditional risk factor assessment.[11] A high level of CRP is an independent risk factor for atherogenesis and adds to the predictive value of other risk factors. It is unclear whether CRP plays a causal role in atherosclerosis or whether it is simply a marker of the atherosclerotic inflammatory response. Experimental studies have suggested that CRP may contribute to atherogenesis by promoting endothelial dysfunction and altering the behavior of monocytes, macrophages, and smooth muscle cells.[12] However, individuals with genetically determined CRP elevations over a lifetime do not appear to be at increased cardiovascular risk.[13]

The cutoff values are less than 1 mg/L for low risk and greater than 3 mg/L for high risk, the latter tertile indicating an approximate doubling of the relative risk compared with the low-risk tertile. Elevated CRP is associated with obesity and the metabolic syndrome, and levels can be reduced through weight loss, increased physical activity, and smoking cessation. Apparently healthy persons at increased risk because of age, elevated CRP (>2 mg/L), and one additional cardiovascular risk factor should be treated with a statin as in the JUPITER trial with rosuvastatin 20 mg daily (see later).[5] Because statins lower both LDL-C and CRP, it is currently unclear whether reducing CRP, and inflammation more generally, has an independent effect on cardiovascular risk apart from LDL-C reduction. At least two trials with antiinflammatory agents that do not affect lipids are currently planned to begin in the near future.[10]

Prevention and Risk Factors

Primary prevention. Primary prevention in patients without evident coronary disease remains a highly desirable aim. Lifestyle interventions (diet, smoking cessation, and physical activity) are the first line of treatment and may achieve cholesterol reduction in many patients. The national American campaign, promoting dietary management and other lifestyle measures, has resulted in a reduction of mean blood cholesterol levels and a fall in coronary heart disease (CHD) mortality rates. Clinical trials of statins in the past decade have demonstrated safety and clinical event reduction across the spectrum of cardiovascular risk, even in populations with low baseline risk such as the Japanese.[14] Still debated, however, are the fiscal and ethical issues related to the cost-effectiveness of lipid drug therapy in lower-risk primary prevention.[15]

Global risk evaluation: Adult Treatment Panel III. Rather than assign patients to primary or secondary prevention, the 2004 U.S. Adult Treatment Panel III (ATP III) argued for three risk categories that use the concept of global risk (Table 10-1): high (CHD or equivalent); medium (two or more risk factors, 10-year risk of 20% or less); and low (zero to one major risk factor, 10-year risk 10% or less). LDL-C values form the primary basis for treatment decisions (Table 10-2). In the updated ATP III guidelines, the patient's absolute risk for developing CHD in the next 10 years determines the aggressiveness of lipid intervention.[16] This global risk is calculated using an algorithm based on the Framingham Heart Study that considers not only total cholesterol, but also high-density-lipoprotein cholesterol (HDL-C), smoking, age, hypertension, and sex. Also featured in ATP III is the concept of the *CHD equivalent*, a risk factor that identifies a patient who should receive treatment as aggressively as someone with a history of heart attack, angina, or revascularization. Included in this category of risk factors are diabetes, noncoronary atherosclerosis (peripheral vascular disease or stroke), and aortic aneurysm.

   Other algorithms. Besides the ATP III model, a number of other algorithms are available for estimating absolute risk, including guidelines of the Joint Task Force of the European Society of Cardiology and Other Societies on Cardiovascular Disease Prevention in Clinical Practice,[17] the PROCAM risk calculators of the International

Table 10-1

LDL-C Goals Based on Global Risk in Latest American and European Guidelines	
	LDL-C Goal
ATP III Risk Categories and LDL-C Goals (Highest to Lowest)	
CHD	<100 mg/dL (2.6 mmol/L)
CHD Risk Equivalents	(for <70 mg/dL or 1.8 mmol/L;
Other cardiovascular disease *or*	see Table 10-2)
Diabetes mellitus *or*	
Aortic aneurysm *or*	
10-year risk greater than 20%	
Multiple (2+) Risk Factors	<130 mg/dL (3.4 mmol/L)
0—1 Risk Factors	<160 mg/dL (4.1 mmol/L)
European Guidelines Risk Priorities (Highest to Lowest)	
Patients with **established CVD**	<96 mg/dL (2.5 mmol/L)
Asymptomatic patients who have	<115 mg/dL (3 mmol/L)
Multiple risk factors *or*	
Markedly raised levels of single risk	
factors *or*	
Type 2 diabetes *or* **type 1 diabetes**	
with microalbuminuria	
Close relatives of	<115 mg/dL (3 mmol/L)
Patients with early-onset CVD *or*	
Asymptomatic, high-risk patients	
Other individuals encountered in routine	<115 mg/dL (3 mmol/L)
practice	

ATP III, U.S. Adult Treatment Panel III; *CHD*, coronary heart disease; *CVD*, cardiovascular disease; *LDL-C*, low-density-lipoprotein cholesterol.
ATP III and joint European guidelines.[16,17,18]

Table 10-2

LDL-C Treatment Thresholds for Diet and for Drugs			
Risk Category	**LDL-C Goal**	**Diet, Lifestyle Initiation Level**	**Drug Treatment Initiation Level**
0-1 Other risk factors*	<160 mg/dL (4.14 mmol/L)	≥160 mg/dL	≥190 mg/dL (4.91 mmol/L) (160-189 mg/dL; LDL-C–lowering drug optional)
2+ Other risk factors (10-year risk ≤20%)	<130 mg/dL (3.36 mmol/L)	≥130 mg/dL	10-year risk 10%-20%: ≥130 mg/dL 10-year risk <10%: ≥160 mg/dL
CHD or CHD risk equivalents (10-year risk >20%)	<100 mg/dL *or* <70 mg/dL (1.8 mmol/L)†	≥100 mg/dL	≥100 mg/dL†

CHD, Coronary heart disease; *LDL-C*, low-density-lipoprotein cholesterol.
  *Almost all people with 0 to 1 other risk factors have a 10-year risk less than 10%: thus 10-year risk assessment in people with 0 to 1 risk factor is not necessary.
  †Revised to lower levels in light of the PROVE-IT and REVERSAL trials.[22,23] Clinical judgment may call for deferring drug therapy in this subcategory.
Adapted from Expert Panel on Detection, Evaluation, and Treatment of High Blood Cholesterol in Adults.[3]

Task Force (see http://www.chd-taskforce.com), and the Reynolds Risk Score incorporating CRP (see http://www.reynoldsriskscore. org). Differences in the data sets used and the methods for calculation may yield different risk predictions, but these schemas share a common intention: to facilitate the discrimination of higher-risk patients from lower-risk ones. Both U.S. and European guidelines prioritize categories of patients and modify the LDL-C goal accordingly (see Table 10-1).

Secondary prevention. The latest guidelines from the American Heart Association (AHA) and American College of Cardiology (ACC) on secondary prevention support aggressive risk reduction therapies for patients with established coronary and other atherosclerotic vascular disease (Table 10-3).[18] For patients at very high risk for future CHD, results from two clinical trials demonstrated the cardiovascular benefit of lipid lowering to levels significantly less than those prescribed by ATP III.[19,20] Thus the updated 2011 AHA-ACC guidelines support the recommended LDL-C goal of less than 100 mg/dL (2.6 mmol/L) for all patients with CHD and other clinical forms of atherosclerotic disease, but allow for an optional goal of less than 70 mg/dL (1.8 mmol/L) in such patients. These guidelines do not modify the ATP III recommendations for patients without atherosclerotic disease who have diabetes or multiple risk factors and a 10-year risk level for CHD greater than 20% (LDL-C < 100 mg/dL). Although *drug-induced LDL-C reduction remains an essential component* of cardiovascular risk factor management, total risk can also be modified through blood pressure (BP) control, dietary changes, increased exercise, weight loss, and strictly no smoking.

Table 10-3

Lipid Management in Secondary Prevention

Lifestyle and Diet

1. Daily exercise and weight control. *(Evidence: B)*
2. Reduce saturated fats, avoid trans fatty acids, limit cholesterol. *(Evidence: B)*
3. Omega-3 fatty acids from fish* or fish oil capsules (1 g/day). *(Evidence: B)*

Lipids and Statins

1. Statins. Aim: LDL-C of <100 mg/dL (2.6 mmol/L). *(Evidence: A)*
2. Lipid profile, all patients. *(Evidence: B)*
3. Statins for triglycerides ≥200 mg/dL (2.26 mmol/L); aim to lower non–HDL-C to <130 mg/dL (3.4 mmol/L). *(Evidence: B)*
4. Statins plus fibrates for triglycerides >500 mg/dL (5.65 mmol/L), to prevent acute pancreatitis. *(Evidence: C)*
5. Statins dosed to reduce LDL-C to <100 mg/dL (2.6 mmol /L), AND by ≥30%. *(Evidence: C)*

Beyond Statins

1. Cholestyramine[†] and/or niacin for statin intolerance, or for statin failure despite higher-dose and higher-potency. *(Evidence: B)*
2. Niacin or fibrate therapy for elevated non–HDL-C despite statin therapy: *(Evidence: B)* or fish oil. *(Evidence: C)*
3. Ezetimibe: consider if above fail. *(Evidence: C)*

For Very High-Risk Patients

1. If triglycerides ≥200 mg/dL (2.26 mmol/L), non–HDL-C goal is <100 mg/dL (2.6 mmol/L). *(Evidence: B)*
2. Statin aim is LDL-C to <70 mg/dL (1.8 mmol/L). *(Evidence: C)*

HDL-C, High-density-lipoprotein cholesterol; *LDL-C,* low-density-lipoprotein cholesterol. *Evidence levels:* A: Data from multiple randomized clinical trials or metaanalyses. B: Data from single randomized trial or nonrandomized trials. C: Only consensus opinion of experts, case studies, or standard of care.
    *Not for pregnant or lactating women because of mercury risk.
    [†]Or colesevelam, colestipol.
Very high risk:[18]- Established cardiovascular disease plus (1) multiple major risk factors (especially diabetes), (2) severe and poorly controlled risk factors (especially continued cigarette smoking), (3) multiple risk factors of the metabolic syndrome (especially high triglycerides ≥ 200 mg/dL (2.26 mmol/L) plus non–HDL-C ≥ 130 mg/dL (3.4 mmol/L) with low HDL-C <40 mg/dL (1.03 mmol/L), and (4) patients with acute coronary syndrome. Modified from Smith et al.[18]

Blood Lipid Profile

Total blood cholesterol and LDL-C. Optimal total blood cholesterol levels are less than 200 mg/dL (5.2 mmol/L)[3,16] or even much lower at 150 mg/dL (3.9 mmol/L), but it bears reemphasizing that cholesterol level is only part of the patient's absolute global risk. Furthermore, the LDL-C level is the real goal of therapy. Both European and American guidelines emphasize a low LDL-C (<100 mg/dL) as the prime aim of therapy in patients with established coronary disease or equivalent risks. In other patients, higher values of up to 115 mg/dL (3 mmol/L) are acceptable according to the European guidelines, with the Americans being somewhat more tolerant, going up to 130 or even 160 mg/dL as the risk level falls (see Table 10-1). Every reduction in LDL-C of 40 mg/dL (1 mmol/L) is accompanied by a 22% reduction in vascular events.[21]

It has been unclear whether there is a lower limit of LDL-C beyond which no further benefit occurs or whether *"lower is better."* This argument is now largely settled in patients with recent acute coronary syndrome (ACS) because LDL-C values of only 62 mg/dL (1.60 mmol/L) gave convincingly better clinical outcomes than levels of 95 mg/dL (2.46 mmol/L).[22] An alternate interpretation of this study is that high-dose atorvastatin was better at reducing the increased levels of CRP (see previous discussion) found in recovering ACS patients than was low-dose pravastatin. However, in a companion study involving patients with stable coronary disease and much lower values of CRP, high-dose atorvastatin reduced atheroma volume at an LDL-C of 79 mg/dL.[23] In a third series, an LDL-C value of approximately 75 mg/dL (2 mmol/L) marked the point at which progression and regression of the atheroma volume were in balance.[24] The primary prevention JUPITER study (see later) suggests that even lower LDL-C levels may be ideal: a subgroup of patients achieving LDL-C levels less than 50 mg/dL experienced a 65% reduction in cardiovascular events compared with placebo, whereas risk reduction was 44% in the study overall.[6] Thus a provisional conclusion, subject to further verification, is that an LDL-C level between 50-70 mg/dL (2 mmol/L) may be a desirable aim with statin therapy.[25]

High-density lipoproteins. HDLs are a new focus of interest. In vitro, HDL aids in clearing cholesterol from the foam cells that develop in diseased arteries (Fig. 10-2), either by returning cholesteryl ester directly to the liver through the SR-BI receptor or through transfer to the apolipoprotein (apo) B–containing lipoproteins in exchange for triglycerides (reverse cholesterol transport mediated by cholesteryl ester transfer protein [CETP], see later). HDL is also hypothesized to exert antiinflammatory and antioxidant effects.[26]

A low HDL-C is an independent risk factor that is strongly and inversely associated with risk for CHD.[3] In the CARE study, every 10-mg/dL decrease in HDL-C led to a similar 10% increase in risk.[27] Because this is a continuously variable relation, and because a low HDL-C is often associated with other lipid abnormalities such as high triglycerides, an HDL-C of less than 40 mg/dL (<1.03 mmol/L) is seen in ATP III in part as a marker for other risk factors, as in the metabolic syndrome (see later). A value of 60 mg/dL (1.6 mmol/L) or more is a negative (protective) risk factor, although it remains to be proven that raising HDL-C is in itself cardioprotective.[3] Even minor elevations of HDL-C to only 42 mg/dL (1.1 mmol/L) are associated with protection in some large studies.[28] Overall, normalization of HDL-C is desirable, but not as essential as reduction of LDL-C (to <100 mg/dL). Evidence is mixed regarding the potential benefit of increasing HDL-C even when LDL-C levels are very low (<70 mg/dL), with some studies showing that HDL-C levels remain predictive of risk and others showing that it is not.[29,30] The combination of low HDL-C and high triglycerides is believed to play a contributory role in increasing cardiovascular risk, although there is insufficient evidence to make the same claim about each of these lipid components separately.[31] The AIM-HIGH study[32] (see later), which

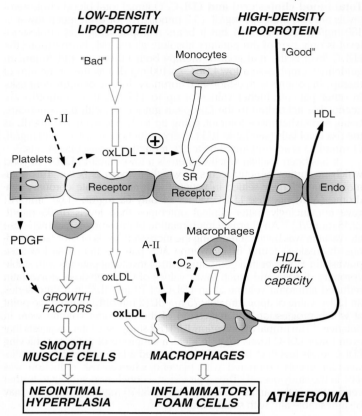

Figure 10-2   Proposed round trip of cholesterol through the vascular endo-thelium and intima. Oxidized low-density lipoprotein (oxLDL) promotes the formation of foam cells. LDL that remains unoxidized can potentially be reex-ported. High-density lipoprotein (HDL) acts hypothetically to help export lipid from the foam cells; free radicals form either in the endothelium (endo) or in foam cells. *A-II,* Angiotensin II; *O₂,* oxygen; *PDGF,* platelet-derived growth factor; *receptor,* receptor for oxLDL; *SR,* scavenger receptor. (Figure © L.H. Opie, 2012.)

investigated the effect of raising HDL-C with niacin, did not show cardiovascular benefit in CHD patients who were already treated with a statin to a baseline mean LDL-C of 71 mg/dL. Although ATP III and European guidelines do not propose a target value for HDL-C, they do recommend correction when possible by lifestyle modification (exercise, modest alcohol intake, loss of weight, nonsmoking). A low HDL-C is often part of a lipid triad known as *atherogenic dyslipidemia,* with the other two components being elevated triglycerides and small, dense LDL particles. The lipid triad is a risk factor in its own right[33] and is commonly found in patients with the metabolic syndrome, type 2 diabetes, and premature CHD.[3] Lifestyle modification, combined with nicotinic acid or fibrates, are the recommended treatments for patients exhibiting the lipid triad.[3]

Cholesteryl ester transfer protein and HDL-C. Novel drug develop-ment aimed at raising HDL-C include strategies for inhibiting the CETP. CETP facilitates the exchange of cholesteryl ester with triglycer-ides during HDL reverse cholesterol transport, but it is unclear whether its actions are pro- or antiatherogenic. Trials with the CETP inhibitor torcetrapib were halted because of excess mortality and morbidity, possibly caused by molecule-specific increases in BP; a decrease in serum potassium; and increases in serum sodium, bicarbonate, and aldosterone.[34] Two other CETP inhibitors are currently in clinical trials: dalcetrapib, which raises HDL-C but has little effect on LDL-C concentrations, and anacetrapib, which raises HDL-C and lowers LDL-C.[35,36] Other experimental approaches to exploiting the protective properties of HDL center on mimetic and naturally occurring variants of apo A-I, the primary protein in HDL, and stimulation of apo A-I synthesis.[37]

Blood triglycerides. Although triglyceride levels are commonly high in patients with coronary artery disease, the specific role of hypertriglyceridemia in atherogenesis remains controversial because it often occurs in conjunction with the lipid triad of obesity, hypertension, and diabetes mellitus. Epidemiologically, an elevated triglyceride level can be an independent risk factor, even with adjustment for HDL-C.[38] Values of more than 150 mg/dL are considered elevated (1.69 mmol/L; versus the prior cutoff of 200 mg/dL)[3], and values below that level are associated with reduced cardiovascular risk even after major reduction of the LDL-C.[38] Levels of more than 1000 mg/dL (11.3 mmol/L) confer increased risk for pancreatitis and require treatment with prescription-strength ω-3 fatty acids, nicotinic acid, or a fibrate. A recent statement from the AHA suggests that fasting triglycerides less than 100 mg/dL are optimal and recommends treatment with intensive dietary and lifestyle therapy, which can lower triglyceride levels by 50% or more.[39] An elevated triglyceride level (>200 mg/dL; 2.3 mmol/L) may be viewed with special concern when combined with high blood LDL-C or low blood HDL-C values. Elevated triglyceride and low HDL-C levels are believed to directly increase cardiovascular risk and should be treated initially with lifestyle modification, followed by niacin, a fibrate, or intensification of LDL-C lowering therapy if necessary.[31]

Metabolic syndrome. The ATP III guidelines recognize as a secondary target of treatment the cluster of risk factors known as the *metabolic syndrome*. According to ATP III, metabolic syndrome can be diagnosed when three or more of the five basic ingredients are present (see Table 11-1), and it greatly enhances the risk for coronary morbidity and mortality at any level of LDL-C. The underlying pathologic findings of the metabolic syndrome appears to be linked to obesity and insulin resistance. After appropriate control of LDL-C, if elevated, first-line therapy is weight control and increased physical activity. Achieving a significant increase in HDL-C, although very desirable, may require fibrates or nicotinic acid or the development of future therapies.

Non-HDL cholesterol. Non-HDL cholesterol is a secondary target of treatment in patients with triglyceride levels greater than 200 mg/dL (2.26 mmol/L) and may aid in cardiovascular risk stratification.[3,40] Measuring non-HDL cholesterol is believed to capture the risk associated with triglyceride-rich particles such as very-low-density lipoprotein (VLDL) and to include all of the apo B–containing particles. The non-HDL cholesterol value is calculated by subtracting the HDL-C value from the total cholesterol value. Treatments that target non-HDL cholesterol include intensified lifestyle measures and possibly drug therapy in high-risk persons. The treatment goals for non-HDL cholesterol are determined by adding 30 mg/dL (0.76 mmol/L) to the LDL-C goals specified in Table 10-2.

Apolipoprotein B and other risk markers. Apo B, a key atherogenic lipoprotein, is a more sensitive measure of lipid-based risk than LDL-C.[40] The apo B level reflects the total number of atherogenic apo B–containing lipoproteins and provides information on LDL particle size, which is difficult to measure directly. The ratio of apo B to apo A-I has been shown to be directly related to the risk for myocardial infarction (MI) in a very large 52-country study,[41] and it has outperformed total cholesterol: HDL-C ratios in cardiovascular risk stratification.[42] The apo B: apo A-I ratios are particularly valuable in patients with the metabolic syndrome or type 2 diabetes, which can be characterized by normal LDL-C levels but small LDL particles. High levels of lipoprotein(a) and homocysteine are two other emerging risk factors. Overall, in practice, LDL-C remains the major aim of lipid-lowering therapy, although these alternative measures can help determine the intensity of treatment for patients who appear to be at borderline risk based on traditional risk factors alone.

Cholesterol in Special Population Groups

Secondary hyperlipidemias. Diabetes mellitus, hypothyroidism, nephrotic syndrome, and alcoholism should be excluded and remedied if possible. Among drugs causing adverse lipid changes are diuretics, β-blockers, progestogens, and oral retinoids.

Diabetic patients. Patients with diabetes constitute a high-risk group and warrant aggressive risk reduction. Increasingly, type 2 diabetes is regarded as a risk category in its own right and, hence, as a CHD equivalent (see Table 10-1). In recent years, there has been growing awareness of the overlapping pathophysiologic characteristics of CHD and type 2 diabetes, with increased coordination between cardiologists and diabetologists in addressing the joint risk.[43] In patients with type 2 diabetes, there may be a preponderance of smaller, denser, atherogenic LDL particles, even though the LDL-C level may be relatively normal. Metaanalysis of 14 randomized trials with a follow-up of at least 2 years indicates that lipid-lowering drug treatment significantly reduces cardiovascular risk in both diabetic and nondiabetic patients.[44] In terms of absolute risk, it is likely that diabetic patients benefit more than nondiabetic patients in both primary and secondary prevention.

The Diabetes Association Intervention Study (DAIS) reported increased LDL particle size and increased angiographic coronary lumen size in diabetic patients who responded to fenofibrate.[45] The Collaborative Atorvastatin Diabetes Study (CARDS) was a multicenter, randomized, placebo-controlled primary-prevention trial in patients with type 2 diabetes with at least one other risk factor who were treated with atorvastatin, 10 mg/day, compared with placebo. The trial was stopped early because of a favorable clinical benefit of the statin.[46] Taken together with a large subgroup analysis from the Heart Protection Study (HPS),[47] there are strong arguments for considering statin therapy, in addition to lifestyle modification and BP control, in all patients with type 2 diabetes. In the ACCORD Lipid study in patients with type 2 diabetes, combination therapy with simvastatin and fenofibrate did not show increased benefit in cardiovascular event reduction compared with simvastatin alone; however, a subgroup analysis suggests that combination therapy may be beneficial in diabetic patients with both high triglycerides and low HDL-C.[48]

Older adult patients. Although the relation between cholesterol and coronary disease weakens with age, physicians should continue to consider lipids as a modifiable risk factor in older adults. The absolute risk for clinical coronary disease in older adults is much higher because age is a powerful risk factor and because BP, another risk factor, often increases with age. Furthermore, consider the cumulative effect of lifetime exposure to a coronary risk factor on an older adult patient. The PROSPER study found coronary but no overall mortality benefit with statin treatment in older adults (see section on pravastatin), although this trial may have been too short (3 years) to show major decreases in cerebrovascular disease.[28] The SAGE study confirmed the safety and benefit of intensive treatment with atorvastatin, 80 mg/day, in older adult patients with stable coronary syndromes, but failed to demonstrate the superiority of intensive versus moderate treatment in reaching the primary end point of total ischemia duration from baseline to 1 year.[49] While awaiting further research, judicious application of statin therapy to higher-risk older adults is appropriate.

Women. Women have a lower baseline risk for CHD than men at all ages except perhaps beyond 80 years.[3] Risk lags by about 10 to 15 years, perhaps because of a slower rate of increase in LDL-C, higher levels of HDL-C, or ill-understood, protective genetic factors in the heart itself. It is not simply a question of being pre- or postmenopausal. In large statin trials such as the HPS, women experience relative risk reduction comparable to that seen in men.[47] In the MEGA trial, low-dose pravastatin was given to low-risk Japanese patients; 69% were women, who had marginally less CHD risk reduction than men, possibly because of their lower initial risk.[14] The JUPITER trial, which enrolled 6801 women (38% of study population), showed that women experienced similar risk reduction as men, primarily because of reductions in risk for revascularization and unstable angina.[50] A metaanalysis conducted by the JUPITER investigators found that statins reduced cardiovascular events in women in primary prevention trials by one-third.[50]

Pregnant women. As a group, lipid-lowering drugs are either totally or relatively contraindicated during pregnancy because of the essential role of cholesterol in fetal development. Bile acid sequestrants may be safest, whereas statins must not be used (see Table 12-10; also see "Contraindications and Pregnancy Warning" in the later section on statins).

Dietary and Other Nondrug Therapy

Lifestyle and risk factors. Nondrug dietary therapy is basic to the management of all primary hyperlipidemias and frequently suffices as basic therapy when coupled with weight reduction, exercise, ideal (low) alcohol intake, and treatment of other risk factors such as smoking, hypertension, or diabetes. Regular exercise may also increase insulin sensitivity and lessen the risk of type 2 diabetes. If lifestyle recommendations, including diet, were rigorously followed, CHD would be largely eliminated in those younger than age 70.[51] However, high-intensity lifestyle modification is required to prevent progression or even to achieve regression of CHD.

Diet. Changes in diet are an absolute cornerstone of lipid-modifying treatment. As a general aim, saturated fats should be less than 7% of the calories, and total fat less than approximately 30% (Table 10-4). Monounsaturates, such as *olive oil*, are relatively beneficial within the framework of total lipid reduction, and patients, especially hypertensive older adults, should limit sodium intake (see Chapter 7). The dietary fatty acid recommendations can be simplified to reducing *trans*-fatty acids and saturated fatty acids, which are largely of animal origin, and increasing other fatty acids from plants or fish oils. Exceptions are coconut oil and crustacean flesh, such as lobsters and prawns, which are high in saturated fatty acids.

A *Mediterranean-type diet* confers increased postinfarct protection,[52] as discussed under post-MI management in Chapter 12. Patients are told to eat more bread, more fiber (10 to 25 g/day), more fresh vegetables, more fish, and less meat, with "no day without fruit" and canola margarine to replace butter and cream. Olive oil is often used. The better the adherence to this diet, the better the survival rate[53] (see "ω-3 Fatty Fish Oils" later). Higher-risk individuals may require a stricter diet with reduced intake of cholesterol-raising nutrients, saturated fats less than 7% of total calories, and dietary cholesterol less than 200 mg/day. Vegetable oils containing polyunsaturated linoleic acid are not as ideal as once thought, and total lipid intake must be restricted. *In brief, the ideal diet is low in total fat and cholesterol, high in fiber, and high in fresh vegetables and fruit, with modest sodium restriction.* Much the same

Table 10-4

Suggested Nutrient Composition for Diet	
Nutrient	**Recommended Intake**
Saturated fat	<7% of total calories
Polyunsaturated fat	Up to 10% of total calories
Monounsaturated fat	Up to 20% of total calories
Total fat*	25%-35% of total calories
Carbohydrate	50%-60% of total calories
Fiber	20-30 g/day
Protein	≈15% of total calories
Cholesterol	<200 mg/day
Total calories (energy)	Balance energy intake and expenditure to maintain desirable body weight and prevent weight gain

*US guidelines suggest a range of total fat consumption, provided saturated fats and trans-fatty acids are kept low. A higher intake of unsaturated fats can help reduce triglycerides and raise high-density-lipoprotein cholesterol in patients with the metabolic syndrome.
From Expert Panel on Detection, Evaluation, and Treatment of High Blood Cholesterol in Adults.[3]

diet benefits hypertensives (see Chapter 7) and is recommended by the AHA, the American Diabetes Association, and the American Cancer Society.[54]

Drug-Related Lipidemias

Cardiac Drugs and Blood Lipid Profiles

β-Blockers and diuretics may harmfully influence blood lipid profiles (Table 10-5), especially triglyceride values. Diuretics, in addition, tend to increase total cholesterol unless used in low doses. Nonetheless, cardiac drugs known to be protective, such as β-blockers, should not be withheld on the basis of their lipid effects alone, especially in postinfarct patients when there is clear indication for the expected overall benefit. Statins appear to counter some of the effects of β-blockers on blood lipids.

β-Blockers. β-Blockers tend specifically to reduce HDL-C and to increase triglycerides. β-Blockers with high intrinsic sympathomimetic activity or high cardioselectivity may have less or no effect (as in the case of carvedilol with added α-blockade). The fact that β-blockers also impair glucose metabolism is an added cause for concern when giving these agents to young patients (see Chapter 7, p. 250). Nonetheless, note the strong evidence for protective effects of β-blockers in postinfarct and heart failure patients (see Chapter 1, pp. 10-13). In stable effort angina, calcium channel blockers may have a more favorable effect on triglycerides and HDL-C than β-blockers. In hypertensives, angiotensin-converting enzyme (ACE) inhibitors, angiotensin receptor blockers, and calcium channel blockers are all lipid neutral.

Diuretics. Doses should be kept low (see Chapter 7, p. 239). In ALLHAT, chlorthalidone, 12.5 to 25 mg daily over 5 years increased total cholesterol by 2 to 3 mg/dL.[55] In the ALPINE study, hydrochlorothiazide, 25 mg, combined with atenolol in most patients, increased blood triglycerides and apo B, while decreasing HDL-C.[56]

Lipid-neutral cardiac drugs. Cardiac drugs that have no harmful effects on blood lipids include the ACE inhibitors; the angiotensin receptor blockers; the calcium channel blockers; vasodilators such as the nitrates and hydralazine; and the centrally acting agents, such as reserpine, methyldopa, and clonidine. The α-blockers, including prazosin and doxazosin, favorably influence the lipid profiles.

Table 10-5

Effects of Antihypertensive Agents on Blood Lipid Pr (Percentage Increase or Decrease)			
Agent	**TC**	**LDL-C**	**HDL-C**
Diuretics			
Thiazides[126]	14	10	2
Low-dose TZ[127]*	0	0	0
Indapamide[128]	0 (+9)	0	0
Spironolactone[129]	5	?	?
β-Blockers			
Grouped (>1 year)[130]	0	0	−8
Propranolol[126]	0	−3	−11
Atenolol[126]	0	−2	−7
Metoprolol[126]	0	−1	−9
Acebutolol[127]*	−3	−4[†]	−3
Pindolol[126]	−1	−3	−2
α-Blockers			
Grouped	−4	−13	5
Doxazosin[127]*	−4[†]	−5[†]	2
αβ-Blocker			
Labetalol[126]	2	2	1
Carvedilol[131]	−4	?	7
CCBs			
Grouped[126]	0	0	0
Amlodipine[127]*	−1	−1	1
ACE Inhibitors			
Grouped	0	0	0
Enalapril[127]	−1	−1	3
Angiotensin Receptor Blockers			
Losartan[128]	(0)[†]	(0)	(0)
Central Agents			
MD + TZ	0	0	0

ACE, Angiotensin-converting enzyme; CCBs, calcium channel blockers; HDL-C, high-density-lipoprotein cholesterol; LDL-C, low-density-lipoprotein cholesterol; MD, methyldopa; TC, total cholesterol; TG, triglyceride; TZ, thiazide.
  *Chlorthalidone 15 mg/day; acebutolol 400 mg/day; doxazosin 2 mg/day; amlodipine 5 mg/day; enalapril 5 mg/day; data placebo-corrected.
  [†]<0.01 versus placebo over 4 years.
  [‡](0) = no long-term data.

Oral contraceptives. When oral contraceptives are given to patients with ischemic heart disease or with risk factors such as smoking, possible atherogenic effects of high-estrogen doses merit attention. In postmenopausal women, the cardiovascular benefits of hormone replacement therapy (HRT) have not been supported by clinical trials (see "Estrogens" later).

The Statins: 3-Hydroxy-3-Methylglutaryl Coenzyme A Reductase Inhibitors

The currently available lipid-lowering drugs can be divided into the statins, the bile acid sequestrants, nicotinic acid, the fibrates, and cholesterol absorption inhibitors. These all reduce LDL-C. Of these drugs, statins are now usually the first drugs of choice because of their relatively

...cts and predictable benefits for treating LDL-C. All of the few side ...ease hepatic cholesterol synthesis by inhibiting 3-hydroxy-statins ...lutaryl coenzyme A (HMG-CoA) reductase (Fig. 10-3). They 3-...ly effective in reducing total cholesterol and LDL-C, they usually ...se HDL-C, and long-term safety and efficacy are now established. ...y are now available in generic form. The landmark Scandinavian ...nvastatin Survival Study (4S) showed that simvastatin used in second-...ry prevention achieved a reduction in total mortality and in coronary events.[57] This was soon followed by a successful primary prevention study with pravastatin in high-risk men.[58] Successful primary prevention of common events has been found in patients with LDL-C values near the U.S. national average.[59] An interesting recent concept is that lipid-lowering drugs may act in ways beyond regression of the atheromatous plaque, for example, by improving endothelial function, stabilizing platelets, reducing fibrinogen (strongly correlated with triglyceride levels), or inhibiting the inflammatory response associated with atherogenesis.[60] These *non-lipid or pleiotropic* benefits have primarily been extrapolated to humans based on experimental studies showing substantial nonlipid cardiovascular protection with statins. One proposed mechanism for the antiinflammatory effects of statins following ACS is reduction of phospholipase A2 biomarkers.[61] Statins have also been investigated for potential beneficial effects on disease states unrelated to atherosclerosis, such as arrhythmias, cancer, and Alzheimer's and other neurodegenerative disorders. A possible example is the reduction of stroke by statins. In 61 studies with 55,000 vascular deaths, statins reduced the incidence of stroke, sometimes strikingly, despite a lack of association with blood cholesterol levels.[62] Currently, the dominant view is that apparent pleiotropic effects can largely be explained by lipid reduction, especially of LDL-C (Fig. 10-4).

WHERE LIPID-LOWERING DRUGS ACT
Opie 2012

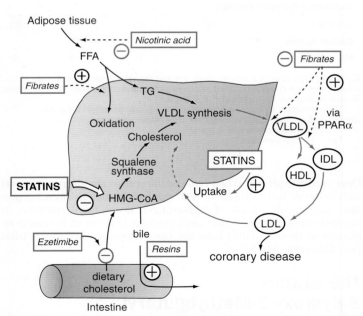

Figure 10-3 Hepatic import and export of lipids is crucial to the sites of action of lipid-lowering drugs. Proposed mechanism of action of statins, fibrates, and nicotinic acid. *FFA*, Free fatty acids; *HDL*, high-density lipoproteins; *HMG-CoA*, 3-hydroxy-3-methylglutaryl coenzyme A; *IDL*, intermediate-density lipoproteins; *LDL*, low-density lipoproteins; *PPAR-α*, peroxisome proliferator–activated receptor-α; *TG*, triglycerides; *VLDL*, very-low-density lipoproteins. (Figure © L.H. Opie, 2012.)

EFFECTS OF LDL-LOWERING

The LDL - hypothesis: the lower, the better

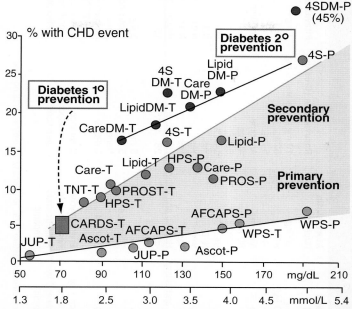

Figure 10-4 The lower the low-density-lipoprotein cholesterol (LDL-C), the fewer the events and the greater the benefit. Relation between LDL-C lowering and coronary heart disease (CHD) events in major trials for primary and secondary prevention. Note greater effects with secondary than with primary prevention and especially marked effects in diabetics. Trials include those in Table 10-7. *P*, Placebo arm of the trial indicated; *T*, treatment arm of the trial indicated. (Figure © L.H. Opie, 2012; modified from Fisher M. Diabetes and atherogenesis. *Heart* 2004;90:336–40 by addition of new trials.)

Class Indications for Statins

Cardiovascular prevention. In general, depending on the drug chosen (Table 10-6), the large statin trials show beyond doubt that cardiovascular end points are reduced, that total mortality is reduced in primary and secondary prevention, and that the number needed to treat (NNT) to prevent any given major end point makes their use cost effective, especially in secondary prevention (Table 10-7). In patients with clinical *CHD,* statins may be used to slow the progression of coronary atherosclerosis, again as part of an overall treatment strategy. In patients with primary *hypercholesterolemia and mixed dyslipidemias,* statins reduce levels of total cholesterol, LDL-C, apo B, and triglycerides. Some are licensed to increase HDL-C. In *homozygous familial hypercholesterolemia,* statins are indicated to reduce total cholesterol and LDL-C levels. If at the time of hospital discharge from an *acute coronary event* the LDL-C level equals or exceeds 130 mg/dL (3.4 mmol/L), then statin therapy may be considered. Of note, and as indicated in the package insert for fluvastatin, in hypertriglyceridemic patients the LDL-C may be low or normal despite elevated total cholesterol; statins are not indicated for this situation. In addition, the results of a metaanalysis suggest that *perioperative cardiovascular prevention* in vascular surgery is not another potential indication for statins.[63]

How intensive should statin therapy be? A metaanalysis of trials comparing intensive versus moderate statin therapy in patients with

Table 10-6

Pharmacologic Properties of Commonly Used Statins

Characteristic	Pravastatin (Pravachol)	Simvastatin (Zocor)	Fluvastatin (Lescol)	Atorvastatin (Lipitor)	Rosuvastatin (Crestor)	Pitavastatin (Livalo)
Usual starting dose (mg/day)	40 mg	20-40 mg	20-40 mg	10 mg	10 mg (in Asians: 5 mg)	2 mg
Expected LDL fall, this dose	34%	38%	25% (40 mg)	39%	52%	38%
Older adult starting dose	40 mg start	20 mg or less	→	→	5 mg	→
Timing of dose	Any time	Evening	Bedtime	Any time	Any time	Any time
Maximum daily dose	80 mg	40 mg	80 mg	80 mg	40 mg	4 mg
LDL reduction, max dose	37%	41%	36%	60%	63%	45%
HDL-C increase, max dose	13%	8%	5.6%	5%	14.7%	8%
Mortality reduction in trials	Yes	Yes	N/D	N/D	Yes	N/D
CV end point ↓	Yes	Yes	Probable	Yes	Yes	N/D
Stroke reduction	Yes	Yes	N/D	Yes	Yes	N/D
Elimination route, chief	Hepatic and biliary	Hepatic and biliary	Hepatic and biliary	Hepatic and biliary	Hepatic and biliary	Hepatic and biliary
Renal excretion of absorbed dose (%)*	20	13	<6	<2	28	15
Dose in severe renal failure	10 mg	5 mg	→	→	5 mg	1 mg
Dose with cyclosporine	10 mg	Contraindicated	→	? Reduce†	5 mg	Contraindicated
Digoxin effect	None	Small ↑	Small ↑	↑ 20%	None	None
Mechanism of hepatic metabolism*	Not by CYP by sulfation	CYP3A4	CYP2C9	CYP3A4	CYP2C9	Glucuronidation; CYP2C9 marginal
Hepatic interactions	No	Conazoles, some antibiotics, antiretrovirals, nefazodone, gemfibrozil, danazol, cyclosporine, verapamil, diltiazem, amlodipine, ranolazine	Clearance ↓ by cimetidine, ranitidine; ↑ by rifampin	Erythromycin Ketoconazole Antiretrovirals Verapamil	Clearance ↓ by cyclosporine, gemfibrozil	Clearance ↓ by erythromycin, rifampin

→, Dose unchanged; ↓, decrease; ↑, increase; CV, cardiovascular; CYP, cytochrome P-450; HDL-C, high-density-lipoprotein cholesterol; LDL, low-density lipoprotein; N/D, no data.

*Source: Package inserts.

†No clear information in package insert, but warning against myopathy during co-therapy.

Table 10-7

Key Statin Trials with Major Significant Outcomes

Trial, Statin, 1° or 2° Prevention	Initial Blood Cholesterol (Mean)	Duration and Numbers	Comparator Events per Trial (%)	Statin Events per Trial (%)	Absolute Risk Reduction per Trial	Number Needed to Treat per Trial
4S[57] Simvastatin 40 mg 2° prevention	260 mg/dL (6.75 mmol/L)	5.4 yr, median (Placebo: 2223; statin: 2221)	Total deaths 1° end point: 256 (11.5%) 2° end point: 502 (22.6%)	182 (8.2%) 353 (15.9%)	74 (3.3%) 149 (30%)	30 (162/yr) 15 (80/yr)
WOSCOPS[58] Pravastatin 1° prevention	272 mg/dL (7.03 mmol/L)	4.9 yr (mean) (Placebo: 3293; statin: 3302)	Deaths: 135 (4.1) 1° end point: 248 (7.5%)	106 (3.2) 174 (5.3%)	29 (0.9%) 74 (2.2%)	114 (558/yr) 45 (217/yr)
AFCAPS/TexCAPS[59] Lovastatin 1° prevention	221 mg/dL (5.71 mmol/L)	5.2 yr (mean) (Placebo: 3301; statin: 3304)	CAD deaths: 15 (0.5%) AMI* 81 (2.5%) 1° end point: 183 (5.5%)	11 (0.3%) 45 (1.4) 116 (3.5%)	4 (0.12%) 39 (1.3%) 67 (2.0%)	826 (4295/yr) 85 (441/yr) 49 (256/yr)
HPS[47] Simvastatin 40 mg 65% with CHD	228 mg/dL (5.9 mmol/L)	5 yr (mean) (Placebo: 10,267; statin: 10,269)	Mortality: 1507 (14.7%) Vascular deaths: 937 (9.1%) Total MI: 1212 (11.8%)	1328 (12.9%) 781 (7.6%) 898 (8.7%)	179 (1.8%) 156 (1.5%) 314 (3.1%)	56 (280/yr) 66 (330/yr) 32 (160/yr)
PROSPER[80] Pravastatin High-risk older adults	221 mg/dL (5.7 mmol/L)	3.2 yr (mean) (Placebo: 2913; statin: 2891)	Primary end point CHD death, nonfatal MI, + stroke: 473 (16.2%)	408 (14.1%)	65 (2.1%)	48 (152/yr)
ASCOT-LLA[86] Atorvastatin 10 mg 1° prevention; hypertensive	212 mg/dL (5.48 mmol/L)	3.3 yr (median) (Placebo: 5137; statin: 5168)	Primary end point nonfatal MI + CHD death: 154 (3.0%)	100 (1.9%)	54 (1.1%)	90 (297/yr)

Continued

Table 10-7

Key Statin Trials with Major Significant Outcomes (Continued)

Trial, Statin, 1° or 2° Prevention	Initial Blood Cholesterol (Mean)	Duration and Numbers	Comparator Events per Trial (%)	Statin Events per Trial (%)	Absolute Risk Reduction per Trial	Number Needed to Treat per Trial
PROVE-IT[22][†] Atorvastatin 80 mg; pravastatin 40 mg Recent ACS, 2° prevention	180 mg/dL (4.65 mmol/L)	2 yr (median) (Pravastatin: 2063; atorvastatin 2099)	Primary composite endpoint (death plus cardiovascular events): pravastatin, 543 (26.3%)	Atorvastatin, 470 (22.4%)	73 (3.7%)	29 (58/yr)
JUPITER[5] Rosuvastatin 20 mg 1° prevention	186 mg/dL (4.81 mmol/L)	1.9 yr (median) (Placebo: 8901; rosuvastatin: 8901)	Primary composite endpoint (MI, stroke, revascularization, hospitalization for angina, CV death): 251 (2.8%)	142 (1.6%)	109 (1.2%)	29 (5/yr)[‡]

ACS, Acute coronary syndrome; *AMI*, (nonfatal) acute myocardial infarction; *CAD*, coronary artery disease; *CHD*, coronary heart disease; *CV*, cardiovascular; *MI*, myocardial infarction.

[*]Estimated.

[†]PROVE-IT compares atorvastatin versus pravastatin, not versus placebo.

[‡]Endpoint of myocardial infarction, stroke, or death.[132]

chronic stable angina and ACS suggests that intensive lipid lowering provides benefit over standard-dose therapy, with a significant reduction in coronary death or MI.[22] A more recent metaanalysis found significant benefit with intensive over standard-dose therapy in risk reduction for nonfatal MI but not for mortality, except for in a subgroup analysis of ACS trials that did show significant reductions in all-cause and cardiovascular mortality with intensive therapy.[64] It remains unclear whether *routine* intensive statin therapy or *goal-directed* target LDL reduction should be used to guide treatment decisions. A third option, based on a metaanalysis of more than 90,000 subjects on standard statin therapy, is to regard all patients with *clinical vascular disease* (including all diabetics) as strong candidates for statins, irrespective of their initial lipid profile.[65] The authors estimated that, for every 1-mmol/L decrease in LDL-C (approximately 40 mg/dL), the 5-year relative risk for major coronary events is reduced by about one-fifth, with the absolute risk reduction dependent on the initial level of risk, and they projected that sustained statin therapy over a period of 5 years might reduce the incidence of major vascular events by approximately one-third. An updated metaanalysis from this same group that included 170,000 subjects found that intensive statin treatment further reduced the risk of major vascular events, so that the relation between absolute LDL-C reduction and proportional risk reduction remained consistent in the trials of intensive statin therapy.[21] Based on these findings, their proposed strategy is to achieve the largest LDL-C reduction possible in high-risk patients without increasing risk for myopathy.

Benefit versus possible harm with very-high-dose statins. The first metaanalysis comparing intensive versus moderate therapy discussed previously found a 16% odds reduction in coronary death and MI in trials lasting between 2 and 5 years, which corresponds to approximately a 3% reduction per year for patients with stable coronary artery disease and approximately an 8% reduction per year for patients with prior ACS.[22] In contrast, a retrospective analysis of possible adverse effects with very-high-dose statin therapy suggested a small increased risk of cancer, equivalent to only 1.5% per 5 years.[66] However, in an analysis of more than 6000 patients with LDL-C levels less than 60 mg/dL, those with very low levels ($<$40 mg/dL) had improved survival without any risk of increased cancer or rhabdomyolysis.[67] Myopathy remains a definite risk, especially in the case of high-dose simvastatin, whereas new diabetes is more common in high- than in medium-dose statin therapy (see "Class Warnings").

Stroke prevention and transient ischemic attack. Patients with a history of stroke or who have a new coronary artery disease equivalent should be considered for statin therapy. In CARDS, stroke in diabetics was reduced by 48% with only a 10-mg daily dose of atorvastatin.[46] In the SPARCL study, high-dose atorvastatin (80 mg/day) reduced fatal and nonfatal strokes (2.2% absolute risk reduction; hazard ratio [HR], 0.84) and major cardiovascular events (3.5% absolute risk reduction; HR, 0.80) in patients with a history of stroke or transient ischemic attack (TIA), but no clinical ischemic heart disease.[68] These benefits outweighed the slight increase in nonfatal hemorrhagic stroke (22 in 2365 patients; absolute increase, 0.9%).[68] A metaanalysis on more than 120,000 persons found a powerful statin-related reduction of ischemic stroke and associated mortality that could not simply be linked to the degree of LDL-C reduction.[69]

Class Warnings

Liver damage, myopathy, new diabetes, and cognitive side effects. The package inserts for statins were revised by the Food and Drug Administration (FDA) in early 2012.[70,71] Pretreatment *liver function tests* are recommended, but routine periodic monitoring of liver enzymes is not, as it was in the past, because serious liver injury with statins rarely occurs. Warnings regarding myopathy and rhabdomyolysis remain in place. Skeletal muscle effects range from muscle pains to objective myopathy to severe myocyte breakdown that in turn can cause potentially fatal renal failure by way of myoglobinuria. *Myopathy* is diagnosed when the creatine kinase (CK) blood levels exceed 10 times normal. The patient is in advance warned that muscle pain, tenderness, or weakness must immediately be reported to the physician and the statin stopped. Abnormal enzyme values usually resolve with cessation of treatment. Thereafter follows a monitored rechallenge at a lower dose or a change to low-dose fluvastatin or alternate-day low-dose rosuvastatin (possibly these cause less myopathy) or nonstatin therapy.[72] A trial of added coenzyme Q10 may help. However, in a very large trial with more than 10,000 patients in each group, enzyme-diagnosed myopathy over 5 years only occurred in 0.11% versus 0.06% in controls, and rhabdomyolysis in only 0.05% versus 0.03% in controls.[47] The absolute rates of myopathy, much less rhabdomyolysis, are low in reported clinical surveys,[73] although in clinical practice they seem fairly common.[66,72] Fatal cases are extremely rare, occurring in only 0.2 or fewer instances per million prescriptions.[74] Predisposing to myopathy is high-dose simvastatin (see section on simvastatin) and co-therapy with fibrates, niacin, cyclosporine, erythromycin, or azole antifungal agents. Although not contraindicated, the combination of a statin and a fibrate increases the risk for myopathy to an incidence of approximately 0.12%,[75] and physicians are cautioned to be mindful of this risk.

Interactions with protease inhibitors are potentially myopathic. The FDA warns as follows (statins in alphabetical order):[71]

- **Atorvastatin:** add telaprevir to list to avoid ritonavir, use lowest dose with lopinavir + ritonavir, care with others
- **Lovastatin:** contraindicated: human immunodeficiency virus (HIV) protease inhibitors, boceprevir, telaprevir
- **Pitavastatin:** no dose limitations
- **Pravastatin:** no dose limitations
- **Rosuvastatin:** limit dose to 10 mg/day with atazanavir + ritonavir, lopinavir + ritonavir
- **Simvastatin:** contraindicated: HIV protease inhibitors, boceprevir, telaprevir

Thus of the commonly used agents in the United States, pravastatin is the safest and simvastatin the least safe to use with HIV and hepatitis C protease inhibitors.

New diabetes is a recently discovered side effect, first reported with rosuvastatin and now recognized as a generalized problem of high-dose statins. There have been at least two metaanalyses. In the larger analysis of 91,140 persons in 13 trials, statin therapy was associated with a slightly increased risk of new diabetes (9%, odds ratio 1.09; confidence interval [CI], 1.02-1.17).[76] Taking together all the data, statin therapy for 255 patients for 4 years gave one extra case of diabetes, whereas 5.4 coronary events were prevented (coronary deaths, nonfatal MI). The other metaanalysis compared intensive- with moderate-dose statin therapy in five studies on 32,752 persons without diabetes at baseline.[77] The NNT annually to harm was 498 for new-onset diabetes versus a NNT of 155 for reduced cardiovascular events. Thus the approximate ratio of benefit to harm for high versus medium doses was approximately 3:1. Another analysis found a greater degree of increased risk for diabetes in an observational study of 161,808 postmenopausal women (48%, multivariate-adjusted HR, 1.48; 95% CI, 1.38-1.59).[78] As a result of this cumulative evidence, the FDA has added information concerning an effect of statins on incident diabetes and increases in hemoglobin A1c and fasting plasma glucose to all statin labels.[70] On the other hand, *nuclear cataracts,* the most common age-related form of cataracts, may be lessened by statin therapy, possibly by an antioxidant mechanism.[79]

Additional information about potential nonserious and reversible *cognitive side effects* (memory loss, confusion, etc.) has also been added to statin labels, based on postmarketing reports.[70] Onset of cognitive problems can range from 1 day to years, and symptoms generally resolve within a median of 3 weeks following cessation of statin therapy. Despite the label changes regarding these adverse effects, the FDA stated that it believes that the increased risks for new diabetes and cognitive problems are small and outweighed by the cardiovascular benefits of statin therapy.

Contraindications and pregnancy warning. Statins are contraindicated in patients with active liver disease or unexplained persistent elevations of serum transaminases. Statins must not be prescribed to women who are pregnant or who are planning to become pregnant (see Table 12-10) because cholesterol is essential to fetal development. Statins are excreted in the mother's milk, so women taking it should not breast feed. Women desiring to become pregnant should stop statins for approximately 6 months before conception. If a patient becomes pregnant when taking such drugs, therapy should be discontinued and the patient apprised of the potential hazard to the fetus (pravastatin package insert).

Lovastatin (Mevacor) and Fluvastatin (Lescol, Lescol XL)

Lovastatin (Altocor) was the first statin to be approved and marketed in the United States and was the first generically available. In the landmark AFCAPS/TexCAPS primary prevention study, it reduced clinical cardiac events, including heart attacks, by 37% in individuals with baseline LDL-C values considered "normal" within the general American population (221 mg/dL; 5.71 mmol/L), but with low HDL-C levels (36 mg/dL; 1.03 mmol/L).[59] The Lescol Intervention Prevention Study showed benefit with early initiation of fluvastatin in patients with average cholesterol levels following percutaneous coronary intervention.[80]

Dose, effects, and side effects. The usual starting dose for lovastatin is 20 mg once daily with the evening meal, going up to 80 mg in one or two doses. The dosing range of fluvastatin is 20 to 80 mg/day, taken in the evening or at bedtime, and the recommended starting dosage may be determined by the degree of LDL-C reduction needed. In 2012 the FDA revised the labeling of lovastatin with new contraindications and dose limitations for concomitant medications, because of an increased risk for myopathy with strong inhibitors of the hepatic cytochrome P-450 3A4 (CYP3A4) substrate.[70] Lovastatin is contraindicated with itraconazole, ketoconazole, posaconazole, erythromycin, clarithromycin, telithromycin, HIV protease inhibitors, boceprevir, telaprevir, and nefazodone. Regarding *drug interactions,* concomitant therapy with cyclosporine and gemfibrozil should be avoided; a 20-mg dose of lovastatin should not be exceeded when the patient is taking danazol, diltiazem, or verapamil; and the 40-mg dose should not be exceeded with amiodarone. Large quantities of grapefruit juice should also be avoided. There are no significant interactions between lovastatin and the common antihypertensive drugs, nor with digoxin. Fluvastatin is metabolized mainly by the CYP2C9 isoenzyme, making it less likely to interact with drugs commonly co-administered with those statins that compete for the CYP3A4 pathway, such as the fibrates (see Table 10-6). However, phenytoin and warfarin share metabolism by CYP2C9, raising the risk for interactions. The same cautions concerning hepatoxicity, myopathy, and rhabdomyolysis that affect other statins also apply to lovastatin and fluvastatin.

Pravastatin (Pravachol, Lipostat)

In the primary prevention WOSCOPS trial, pravastatin reduced the risk for coronary morbidity and mortality in high-risk men.[58] In the secondary prevention LIPID trial, pravastatin therapy reduced the risk for death from any cause by 22% ($P < 0.001$) and also decreased the risks for nonfatal MI or CHD death, stroke, and coronary revascularization.[81] In another secondary prevention trial, PROVE-IT, pravastatin at 40 mg daily was inferior to 80 mg of atorvastatin daily in the reduction of LDL-C and clinical events.[22] The PROSPER trial, which enrolled older adult patients with a mean cholesterol of 5.7 mmol/L (212 mg/dL) and high coronary risk, found that pravastatin, 40 mg/day, reduced the relative risk for CHD death by 24% ($P = 0.043$), chiefly when given for secondary prevention; results for primary prevention were nonsignficant.[82] There was, however, an increased incidence of cancer. Longer-term pravastatin therapy over 10 years was not associated with cancer in the WOSCOPS study.[4] (For MEGA trial, see p. 407.)

Indications. Besides its class indications (see previously), pravastatin is licensed for primary prevention in patients with hypercholesterolemia to reduce the risk for MI, revascularization, and cardiovascular mortality. In patients with previous MI, it is indicated to reduce total mortality by reducing coronary deaths and to reduce recurrent MI, revascularization, and stroke or TIA.

Dose and effects. The recommended starting dose is 40 mg at any time of the day, increasing to 80 mg if needed. As with the other statins, liver damage and myopathy are rare but serious *side effects. Cautions and contraindications* are also similar to other statins. There is no drug interaction with digoxin. Pravastatin is not metabolized by the CYP3A4 pathway, so there may be a lower risk for interactions with agents such as erythromycin and ketoconazole (see Table 10-6). Importantly, there is no interaction with antiretrovirals.

Simvastatin (Zocor)

Major trials. The landmark Scandinavian 4S study paved the way to widespread acceptance of statins as the cornerstone of lipid-lowering drug therapy. In this study of 4444 patients with increased cholesterol levels, mostly men with past MI, simvastatin reduced LDL-C by 35% over 4 years, total mortality by 30%, cardiac death rate by 42%, and revascularization by 37%.[57] There was no evidence of increased suicide or violent death, previously thought to be a potential hazard of cholesterol reduction. Differences between simvastatin and placebo arms started to emerge after 1 to 2 years of treatment, and most curves were still diverging at 4 years. Longer-term follow-up after the trial suggested that benefits were maintained.

The landmark HPS evaluated the role of simvastatin versus placebo in 20,536 high-risk patients for whom guidelines at the time would not have recommended drug intervention.[47] Included patients were 40 to 80 years of age and had total serum cholesterol concentrations of at least 135 mg/dL (3.49 mmol/L). Only 65% of the patients had a history of CHD at baseline, and HPS included many high-risk "primary prevention" individuals who had never had a coronary event (n = 7150), although a significant number had a CHD-equivalent risk profile: diabetes, peripheral vascular disease, or cerebrovascular disease. Simvastatin reduced the risk for any major vascular event by 24% ($P < 0.0001$) and all-cause mortality by 13% ($P = 0.0003$), with a 17% reduction in deaths attributed to any vascular cause. There were no safety issues with treatment and an incidence of myopathy of only 0.01%. Because there was a similar good response in patients with an initial LDL-C level of less than 3 mmol/L (116 mg/dL) or total cholesterol below 193 mg/dL (5.0 mmol/L) compared with those with higher values, *the intriguing interpretation emerges that selection for statin therapy should be by the degree of clinical risk, so that those at high risk should receive a statin irrespective of the initial lipid levels.* In the SEARCH study, 12,064 participants were randomized to either 80 mg or 20 mg simvastatin daily.[83] The 6% reduction in major vascular events with a further 0.35 mmol/L reduction in LDL-C was consistent with previous trials. However, myopathy was increased with 80 mg simvastatin daily, which led to new FDA recommendations (see later).

Indications. Simvastatin has additional, specific indications in patients with CHD and hypercholesterolemia, for (1) reduction of coronary and total mortality, (2) reduction of nonfatal MI, (3) reduction of myocardial revascularization procedures, and (4) reduction of stroke or TIA. Simvastatin also has a license to increase HDL-C in patients with hypercholesterolemia or combined lipidemias, without claiming an effect independent of LDL-C lowering. Based on the results of the HPS, the FDA approved a revised labeling for simvastatin in 2003 that emphasized high-risk status rather than LDL-C alone as the primary determinant of treatment. Essentially, the labeling states that simvastatin may be started simultaneously with dietary therapy in patients with coronary disease or at high risk for coronary disease.

Dose, side effects, and safety. The usual starting dosage is 20 mg once daily in the evening. In the 4S study, the initial dose was 20 mg once daily just before the evening meal, increased to 40 mg if cholesterol lowering was inadequate after 6 weeks.[57] A daily dose of 20 mg has almost exactly the same effect on blood lipids as atorvastatin, 10 mg (manufacturers' information). For patients at high risk, the starting dosage is 40 mg/day as in the HPS. The previous top dosage of 80 mg daily is now linked to a substantial risk of myopathy, so the FDA recommends that patients should not be started on or switched to this dose, and patients already on this dose should be carefully monitored for myopathy. *FDA recommendations to reduce myopathy with simvastatin,* which is broken down by the hepatic enzyme CYP3A4 system, are that simvastatin should not be used with the conazole group of drugs (itraconazole, ketoconazole, posaconazole), some antibiotics (erythromycin, clarithromycin, telithromycin), nefazodone, gemfibrozil, cyclosporine, and danazol.[70,71] Specifically contraindicated by the FDA are the HIV protease inhibitors, boceprevir, and telaprevir.[71] The 10-mg dose should not be exceeded in patients taking amiodarone, verapamil, and diltiazem. The 20-mg dose should not be exceeded with amlodipine and ranolazine (Ranexa). The 80-mg dose should not be started.[70,84]

The 11-year follow up study of the HPS found that simvastatin reduced the risk of cardiovascular disease by almost one-quarter without any increase in cancer or other nonvascular causes.[85] The original concerns about the long-term safety of statins have thus been dispelled.[86]

Atorvastatin (Lipitor)

Secondary prevention. Atorvastatin is one of the best tested and most prescribed of the statins. The Myocardial Ischemia Reduction and Aggressive Cholesterol Lowering trial[87] and the PROVE-IT[22] trial examined the premise that early treatment with high-dose (80 mg daily) atorvastatin therapy following ACS would give clinical benefits. Versus placebo, atorvastatin produced modestly significant relative risk reductions for symptomatic ischemia.[87] Versus pravastatin, in a large study of more than 4000 patients, atorvastatin reduced LDL-C to only 62 mg/dL (1.60 mmol/L) and decreased the composite primary endpoint. In those with stable coronary disease, a similar vigorous reduction of LDL-C versus pravastatin decreased the atheroma volume.[23] In the Treating to New Targets trial, top doses of atorvastatin (80 mg daily) reduced mean LDL-C from approximately 2.6 to 2 mmol/L, and major cardiovascular events fell by 22% versus a low dose (10 mg daily).[19] In the Incremental Decrease in Endpoints through Aggressive Lipid lowering study on 8888 patients with a prior MI, atorvastatin 80 mg daily reduced the secondary endpoint of any coronary event, when compared with simvastatin, taken at mostly 20 mg daily. However, the primary endpoint was not different nor was mortality reduced. The final lower LDL-C level of 2.1 mmol/L in the atorvastatin group versus 2.6 mmol/L in the simvastatin group modestly supports the "lower is better" hypothesis, at the cost of approximately double the drug-discontinuing adverse events (9.6% for atorvastatin versus 4.2% for simvastatin).[20]

Primary prevention. The lipid-lowering arm of the Anglo-Scandinavian Cardiac Outcomes Trial (ASCOT) assessed the clinical effect of atorvastatin, 10 mg/day, versus placebo in 10,305 hypertensive patients with mean total cholesterol of 212 mg/dL (5.5 mmol/L), mean LDL-C of 130 mg/dL (3.4 mmol/L), and a high-risk profile.[88] Originally planned with a follow-up of 5 years, ASCOT ended early because of clear benefit. Atorvastatin reduced the relative risk for cardiovascular events by 36% ($P = 0.0005$) and for stroke by 27% ($P = 0.024$). There was no effect on the low total mortality rate, and the adverse event rates did not differ between the treatment groups. The CARDS of high-risk diabetics was similarly stopped because of improved clinical endpoints in those treated with atorvastatin, 10 mg daily, versus placebo.[46] Recent evidence suggests that atorvastatin may improve glomerular filtration rate in patients with kidney disease.[89]

Indications. Besides class indications (see previously), atorvastatin is licensed by the FDA for primary prevention in patients with multiple risk factors to reduce the risk for MI, stroke, revascularization, or angina. For primary prevention in those with type 2 diabetes and multiple risk factors, atorvastatin is indicated for reduction of MI and stroke. For patients with CHD, atorvastatin is indicated for reduction of nonfatal MI, stroke, revascularization, hospitalization for congestive heart failure, and angina.

Dosage, effects, and side effects. Atorvastatin is available as 10-, 20-, 40-, and 80-mg tablets, which can be given once daily at any time of the day, with or without food. The ASCOT and CARDS trials suggested that a dosage of only 10 mg daily may help prevent clinical events.[46,88] The PROVE-IT study showed that high-dose atorvastatin, 80 mg/day, reduces LDL-C to very low levels and reduces clinical events in patients with recent ACS.[22] A 10-mg starting dose of atorvastatin gives good reductions in total cholesterol, LDL-C, apo B, and triglyceride, and a modest increase in HDL-C. Blood lipid levels should be checked 2 to 4 weeks after starting therapy and the dosage adjusted accordingly. As with the other statins, liver damage and myopathy are rare but serious *side effects*.

Drug interactions. Patients on potent inhibitors of hepatic CYP3A4, such as ketoconazole, erythromycin, or HIV protease inhibitors, should in principle not be given any statin that is metabolized through this enzyme (atorvastatin, fluvastatin, lovastatin; see Table 10-6). Specifically, the FDA warns as follows: avoid atorvastatin with tipranavir and ritonavir, use lowest dose with lopinavir and ritonavir, and use care with other antiteroviral.[71] *Erythromycin* inhibits hepatic CYP3A4 to increase blood atorvastatin levels by approximately 40%. The interaction with clopidogrel has not been clinically evident.[90] Atorvastatin increases blood levels of some *oral contraceptives*. There is no interaction with warfarin. Other drug interactions are similar to the other statins, including co-therapy with fibrates and niacin.

Rosuvastatin (Crestor)

Rosuvastatin is claimed to be exceptionally potent in reducing cholesterol and LDL-C levels. It is a hydrophilic compound with a high uptake into and selectivity for its site of action in the liver. Rosuvastatin's half-life is approximately 19 hours, and it can be taken at any time of the day. It is not metabolized by the CYP3A4 system, thus lessening the risk for certain key drug interactions (see Table 10-6). However, there are interactions with antiretrovirals.

Major trials. The ASTEROID study, an experimental study of 349 patients with coronary atherosclerosis, found that high-intensity rosuvastatin, 40 mg/day, achieved a mean LDL-C of 60.8 mg/dL (1.57 mmol/L) and increased HDL-C by 14.7%, with regression of coronary atherosclerosis as measured by intravascular ultrasound.[91] In METEOR, in low-risk men with modest carotid intimal-medial thickening and mean LDL-C values of 154 mg/dL, 40-mg/day rosuvastatin for 2 years substantially reduced the rate of progression of the carotid changes.[92] Results from the JUPITER study have established the efficacy of rosuvastatin in primary prevention, particularly for individuals at increased risk because of elevated levels of CRP but with low levels of LDL-C.[5] The trial, which enrolled 17,802 middle-aged adults free of heart disease and diabetes with LDL-C less than 130 mg/dL and CRP or at least 2 mg/L, compared rosuvastatin 20 mg versus placebo and was stopped after 1.9 years because of efficacy. Rosuvastatin reduced LDL-C levels by 50% to a median of 55 mg/dL and decreased high-sensitivity CRP levels by 37%, which translated to a 44% relative reduction in major cardiovascular events and a 20% reduction in all-cause mortality compared with placebo. Based on the results of JUPITER, the FDA approved a new indication for rosuvastatin, discussed in the following section.

Indications. In addition to its class indications, rosuvastatin has a favorable effect on triglycerides in patients with elevated serum triglyceride levels and is licensed to slow the progression of atherosclerosis. Its newest indication for primary prevention, approved on the basis of JUPITER, is to reduce the risk for stroke, MI, and revascularization in patients at increased risk because of age, CRP of at least 2 mg/L, and one additional cardiovascular risk factor. Rosuvastatin can be safely used in systolic heart failure without any specific antifailure benefit.[93]

Dose, effects, and side effects. Rosuvastatin is supplied in 5-, 10-, 20-, and 40-mg tablets. The usual starting dosage is 10 mg/day (5 mg for Asian patients) taken any time with or without food. At this dosage, there is an expected 52% reduction in LDL-C in patients with primary hypercholesterolemia. In these same patients, rosuvastatin produces approximately a 10% increase in HDL-C and a 24% decrease in triglycerides. For patients of advanced age or with renal insufficiency, the recommended starting dose is 5 mg/day. Renal patients may be titrated up to 10 mg/day; at this dose, rosuvastatin did not increase adverse events and reduced lipid parameters in patients with end-stage renal disease, although it had no effect on cardiovascular outcomes.[94] Patients receiving concomitant cyclosporine should be limited to rosuvastatin, 5 mg/day. In combination with gemfibrozil, rosuvastatin should be limited to 10 mg/day. Its *side effects* and warnings are similar to those of other statins. The maximum 40-mg dose of rosuvastatin is reserved for patients who have an inadequate response to 20 mg/day. Findings of increased risk for new diabetes were first observed with rosuvastatin in the JUPITER trial and subsequently extended to the other statins.[5] Whereas the results of a large metaanalysis found a 9% increased risk for incident diabetes over a 4-year period, the risk with rosuvastatin was 18%, based on the results of JUPITER and two other clinical trials.[76] Uncommon instances of proteinuria with microscopic hematuria have been reported, and the frequency may be greater at the 40-mg dose (distribution of which is limited in the United States), compared with lower doses. In clinical studies of 10,275 patients, 3.7% were discontinued because of adverse experiences attributable to rosuvastatin. The most frequent adverse events ($\geq$2%) included hypertension, myalgia, constipation, asthenia, and abdominal pain.

Drug interactions. Like fluvastatin, it is metabolized by way of the CYP2C9 isoenzyme and therefore may be less likely to interact with common drugs that use the CYP3A4 pathway, such as ketoconazole or erythromycin (see Table 10-6). The FDA warns regarding antiretrovirals that the dose should be limited to 10 mg daily with atazanavir with or without ritonavir, or lopinavir with ritonavir.[71] Warfarin interaction is a risk. Nonetheless, the standard statin warnings against co-therapy with fibrates or niacin remain, although fenofibrate appears safe. Co-administration of cyclosporine or gemfibrozil with rosuvastatin results in reduced clearance of this drug from the circulation, so that the rosuvastatin dose is reduced. An antacid (aluminium and magnesium hydroxide combination) decreases plasma concentrations of rosuvastatin and should be taken 2 hours after and not before rosuvastatin.

Pitavastatin (Livalo)

Pitavastatin is the newest statin to be approved by the FDA. A low-dose statin, it is also available in several Asian countries and is currently under regulatory review in Europe. Noninferiority studies indicate that pitavastatin is comparable to atorvastatin and simvastatin in terms of LDL-C reduction and that it achieves greater LDL-C reductions than pravastatin at equivalent doses.[95] It also favorably affects HDL-C and triglycerides. Clinical outcome studies, primarily in Asia, are ongoing and will help to determine pitavastatin's effects on morbidity and mortality.

Indications, dose, effects, and side effects. Pitavastatin is indicated as an adjunct to diet to reduce elevated total cholesterol, LDL-C, apo B, and triglyceride levels and to increase HDL-C in patients with primary hyperlipidemia or mixed dyslipidemia. It is supplied in 1-, 2-, and 4-mg tablets, with a usual starting dose of 2 mg/day taken at any time of day and a maximum dose of 4 mg/day. For patients with renal disease, the recommended starting dose is 1 mg/day up to a maximum of 2 mg/day. Depending on the dose, pitavastatin can be expected to reduce LDL-C by 31%-45%, reduce triglycerides by 13%-22%, and increase HDL-C by 1%-8%. The *side effects* and warnings for pitavastatin are similar to those of other statins.

Drug interactions. Pitavastatin is not a substrate for CYP3A4, so it may be less likely to interact with drugs that inhibit the CYP3A4 system. It is minimally metabolized by CYP2C9, which appears to have little clinical effect on drug clearance. Importantly, there is no interaction with antiretrovirals. It is primarily metabolized via glucuronidation, so concomitant treatment with gemfibrozil and other fibrates should only be used with caution, as gemfibrozil has the potential to inhibit the glucuronidation and clearance of statins.[96] Co-administration of cyclosporine is contraindicated because of reduced clearance of pitavastatin, and dosages of pitavastatin should be reduced with co-administration of erythromycin and rifampin for the same reason. Pitavastatin has not been studied with the protease inhibitor combination lopinavir-ritonavir, so should not be used with this combination. As with other statins, combination treatment with niacin and fibrates increases risk for myopathy.

Bile Acid Sequestrants: The Resins

Bile acid sequestrants—*cholestyramine (Questran), colesevelam (Welchol),* and *colestipol (Colestid)*—bind to bile acids to promote their secretion into the intestine. There is increased loss of hepatic cholesterol into bile acids and hepatic cellular cholesterol depletion, the latter leading to a compensatory increase in the hepatic LDL receptor population so that the blood LDL is more rapidly removed and total cholesterol falls (see Fig. 10-4). There may be a transitory compensatory rise in plasma triglycerides that is usually ignored, but may require co-therapy. Colesevelam received an additional FDA indication in 2008 for improved glycemic control in the treatment of type 2 diabetes, as combination therapy with metformin, sulfonylureas, or insulin. The major trial conducted with resins was the Lipid Research Clinics Coronary Primary Prevention Trial, in which cholestyramine modestly reduced CHD in hypercholesterolemic patients and improved blood lipid profiles, yet without effect on overall mortality.[97] Regarding *drug interactions,* watch for interference with the absorption of digoxin, warfarin, thyroxine, and thiazides, which need to be taken 1 hour before or 4 hours after the sequestrant. Impaired absorption of vitamin K may lead to bleeding and sensitization to warfarin. Poor palatability is the major problem. *Combination therapy* is often undertaken, and coadministration with a statin may exploit the complementary mechanisms of action of these two drug classes. Resins may increase triglycerides, so a second agent such as nicotinic acid or a fibrate may be required to adequately lower triglycerides. Resins should be used with caution in patients with hypertriglyceridemia. Long-term therapy with resins may result in a compensatory increase in HMG-CoA reductase activity that tends to increase cholesterol levels.

Inhibition of Lipolysis by Nicotinic Acid (Niacin)

Nicotinic acid was the first hypolipidemic drug to reduce overall mortality.[98] It is the cheapest compound and can be bought over the counter. The basic effect of nicotinic acid may be decreased mobilization of free fatty acids from adipose tissue, so that there is less substrate for hepatic synthesis of lipoprotein lipid (see Fig. 10-3). Consequently there is less secretion of lipoproteins so that LDL particles, including triglyceride-rich VLDL, are reduced. Nicotinic acid is the drug that best increases HDL-C, and is recommended for the *lipid triad* (small dense LDL, high triglycerides, low HDL-C).[3] The lipid-lowering effects of nicotinic acid are not shared by nicotinamide and have nothing to do with the role of that substance as a vitamin.

The AIM-HIGH study, an outcomes study examining the effect of adding extended-release niacin to simvastatin in patients with cardiovascular disease, was stopped early because of lack of efficacy.[99] Niacin demonstrated no incremental benefit in cardiovascular event reduction for patients already optimally treated with lipid-lowering therapy to a mean LDL-C of 71 mg/dL at baseline; in addition, there was an unexplained increase in ischemic stroke in the niacin arm. After 36 months, there was only a 4 mg/dL difference in HDL-C between treatment groups, and it may be that the study was underpowered to show benefit with niacin on top of statin therapy. Interestingly, niacin was found to induce carotid plaque regression in a small study using intravascular ultrasound and was superior to ezetimibe, which did not.[100] Prescribing patterns with niacin should not be altered; the ongoing HPS2-THRIVE study with similar design and endpoints will provide further information on the effects of increasing HDL-C levels and reducing triglycerides with niacin.

Dose, side effects, and contraindications. The dosage required for lipid lowering is up to 4 g daily, achieved gradually with a low starting dose (100 mg twice daily with meals to avoid gastrointestinal discomfort) that is increased until the lipid target is reached or side effects occur. A lower target dosage (1.5 to 2 g daily) still has a marked effect on blood lipids with better tolerability and only two daily doses. If taken with meals, flushing is lessened. *Niaspan* is an extended-release formulation with an initiation starter pack that titrates up the dose to reduce side effects. The recommended maintenance dose is 1 to 2 g once daily at bedtime.

On the debit side, this drug has numerous subjective *side effects*, although these can be lessened by carefully building up the dose. Through ill-understood mechanisms, nicotinic acid causes prostaglandin-mediated symptoms such as flushing, dizziness, and palpitations. Flushing, which is very common, lessens with time and with use of the extended-release formulation. *Caution* should be used in patients with peptic ulcer, diabetes, liver disease, or a history of gout. Impaired glucose tolerance and increased blood urate are reminiscent of thiazide side effects, also with an unknown basis. Hepatotoxicity may be linked to some *long-acting preparations* (extended-release capsules or tablets), whereas flushing and pruritus are reduced. Myopathy is rare. Use in pregnant women is questionable. Nicotinic acid and statin co-therapy gives a better effect on the lipid levels at the cost of an increased (albeit low) risk of hepatotoxicity and of myopathy.

The Fibrates

As a rule, none of the fibrates reduces blood cholesterol as much as do the statins or nicotinic acid. Their prime action is to decrease triglyceride, thereby increasing HDL-C, and to increase the particle size of small, dense LDL. Like nicotinic acid, they are therefore suitable for use in atherogenic dyslipidemia.[3] They are first-line therapy to reduce the risk for pancreatitis in patients with very high levels of plasma triglycerides and may be useful with more modest triglyceride elevations or when the prime problem is a low HDL-C.[101] At a molecular level, fibrates are agonists for the nuclear transcription factor peroxisome proliferator–activated receptor-α (PPAR-α) that stimulates the synthesis of the enzymes of fatty acid oxidation, thereby reducing VLDL triglycerides.[3] Although all belong to the same group, structural differences between the compounds seem important because of the very different results of large-scale trials on clofibrate (unfavorable) and gemfibrozil (favorable).

Class warnings. There are five warnings or reservations for this class of drugs, as found in the fenofibrate package insert. First, the early experience with clofibrate suggested that fibrates may increase mortality. This fear has not been borne out by trials of other fibrates, and gemfibrozil has significant coronary benefits. Second, hepatotoxicity may occur, with a pooled analysis of 10 placebo-controlled trials showing elevated transaminases in 5.3% of patients given fenofibrate compared to 1.1% on placebo. Third, cholelithiasis is a risk, because fibrates act in part by increasing biliary secretion of cholesterol; however, again this was not found in the Veterans Affairs Cooperative Studies Program High-density lipoprotein cholesterol Intervention Trial (VA-HIT) study. Fourth, there is an important drug interaction with concomitant oral anticoagulants, so that the warfarin dose needs to be reduced. Fifth, combined therapy with statins should be avoided unless the potential beneficial effects on lipids outweigh the increased risk for myopathy (see later section on "Combination Therapy").

Gemfibrozil (Lopid)

Major trials. This agent was used in the large Helsinki Heart Study in a primary prevention trial on 2000 apparently healthy men with modest hypercholesterolemia observed for 5 years.[102] With a dose of 600 mg twice daily, there was a major increase in HDL-C (12%), a decrease in total cholesterol and LDL-C (8% to 10%), and a substantial reduction in triglycerides with an overall reduction in coronary events. Although the total death rate was unchanged, the study was not powered to assess mortality. An open-label follow-up found mortality reduction after 13 years.[103] Despite the theoretical risk of gallstone formation, none was found.

Benefit in men with low HDL-C. The VA-HIT was a secondary intervention trial in men with CHD whose primary abnormality was a low HDL-C: less than 40 mg/dL (1 mmol/L), with a mean of 32 mg/dL.[101] The LDL-C was 140 mg/dL (3.6 mmol/L) or less, with a mean of 112 mg/dL. Over 5 years, the mean HDL-C was 6% higher, the mean triglyceride 31% lower, and the total cholesterol 4% lower, whereas the mean LDL-C level did not change. There was a 24% reduction in the outcome of death from CHD, nonfatal MI, and stroke. The 5-year NNT to prevent one major outcome event was 23, which compared well with the major statin trials. This trial showed that major reduction of total cholesterol or LDL-C was not essential to achieve outcome benefit.

Dose, side effects, contraindications. This agent is currently licensed in the United States for treatment of the lipid triad. The dose is 1200 mg given in two divided doses 30 minutes before the morning and evening meals. *Contraindications* are hepatic or severe renal dysfunction, preexisting gallbladder disease (possible risk of increased gallstones, not found in the HIT study), and simvastatin. There are *drug interactions* to consider. Because it is highly protein bound, gemfibrozil potentiates warfarin. When combined with statins, there is an increased risk for myopathy with myoglobinuria and a further rare risk for acute renal failure (for perspective, see "Combination Therapy" section).

Bezafibrate

This agent (*Bezalip* in the United Kingdom; not available in the United States) resembles gemfibrozil in its overall effects, side effects, and alterations in blood lipid profile. Uniquely among fibrates, it is also a PPAR-γ agonist, thereby theoretically stimulating the enzymes that regulate glucose metabolism. Hence plasma glucose tends to fall with bezafibrate, which may be useful in diabetics or those with abnormal glucose metabolic patterns. In patients with coronary artery disease, bezafibrate slows the development of insulin resistance.[104] As with other fibrates, warfarin potentiation is possible, and co-therapy with statins should ideally be avoided. In addition, myositis, renal failure, alopecia, and loss of libido have occurred. The dose is 200 mg two to three times daily; however, once daily is nearly as good, and there is now a slow-release formulation available (*Bezalip-Mono*, 400 mg once daily). Some increase in plasma creatinine is very common and of unknown consequence. The major problem with this agent is that, unlike gemfibrozil and the statins, there are as yet no major long-term outcome trials with clear results. In the Bezafibrate Infarction Prevention (BIP) study, patients with a low HDL-C and modest elevations of LDL-C experienced trends in favor of bezafibrate, but no clear advantage was observed except post hoc in a subgroup of patients with initial triglyceride levels greater than 250 mg/dL.[105]

Fenofibrate (Tricor, Trilipix, Lipofen, Antara, Lofibra)

Fenofibrate is a prodrug converted to fenofibric acid in the tissues. The licensed indications are as adjunctive therapy to diet to reduce LDL-C and total cholesterol, triglycerides, and apo B and to increase HDL-C. Fenofibrate is also indicated for treatment of hypertriglyceridemia, although the effect on the risk for pancreatitis in patients with very high triglyceride levels, typically exceeding 2000 mg/dL, has not been well studied. The Trilipix formulation, which contains fenofibric acid rather than the ester, has an indication for mixed dyslipidemia in combination with statin therapy. Tablets are 48 or 145 mg for Tricor, but other formulations have slightly altered dosing. The dose for Tricor is 48 to 145 mg once daily (half-life of 20 hours), taken with food to optimize bioavailability. Predisposing diseases such as diabetes and hypothyroidism need to be excluded and treated. The DAIS suggests that treatment with fenofibrate in patients with type 2 diabetes reduces progression of atherosclerosis, with a nonsignificant trend to cardiovascular event reduction.[45] The FIELD study similarly attempted to assess the effect of fenofibrate on cardiovascular disease events in patients with type 2 diabetes, but failed to reach the primary endpoint of reduction in coronary events, possibly because the study design allowed for initiation of statin therapy in both the placebo and fenofibrate treatment arms.[106] Despite these null findings, FIELD did show a decrease in total cardiovascular events, primarily caused by significant reductions in nonfatal MI and revascularizations. However, the ACCORD Lipid study, which examined the effects of fenofibrate in patients with type 2 diabetes treated with simvastatin, found no cardiovascular benefit with the drug, except in a subgroup of individuals with low baseline HDL-C and high triglycerides.[48] Post hoc analyses of three other fibrate trials, including the Helsinki Heart Study, BIP, and FIELD, similarly suggested benefit with a fibrate in a subgroup of patients with atherogenic dyslipidemia.[48] Thus the cumulative body of evidence indicates that the prime lipid-lowering therapy for prevention of macrovascular complications in most diabetic patients remains a statin.

Weight reduction, increased exercise, and elimination of excess alcohol are recognized in the package insert as essential steps in the overall control of triglyceride levels. In addition, there is a warning that cyclosporine co-therapy may cause renal damage with decreased excretion of fenofibrate and increased blood levels. Note risk of bleeding in patients given warfarin (bold warning in package insert). Animal data suggest a deleterious effect in pregnancy. Avoid in nursing mothers (carcinogenic potential in animals). Use with caution in older adults or patients with renal dysfunction (renal excretion).

Cholesterol Absorption Inhibitors: Ezetimibe

Cholesterol absorption inhibitors selectively interrupt intestinal absorption of cholesterol and other phytosterols. The first of this drug class to reach the market, ezetimibe (*Zetia*), acts at the brush border of the small intestine and inhibits the absorption of cholesterol, leading to decreased delivery of intestinal cholesterol to the liver,[107] which reduces hepatic cholesterol and increases cholesterol clearance from the blood. This mechanism is complementary to that of the statins. This drug has a half-life of 22 hours and is not metabolized by the CYP system.

Ezetimibe monotherapy is an option for patients with statin intolerance, and combination therapy with statins is effective in those requiring large LDL-C reductions. Its clinical benefit in primary and secondary prevention has yet to be established.

Indications. As monotherapy in primary hypercholesterolemia, ezetimibe is indicated as adjunctive therapy to diet for the reduction of elevated total cholesterol, LDL-C, and apo B. Combination therapy with simvastatin is approved in the United States for lipid indications similar to ezetimibe alone, but is also licensed to increase HDL-C (which it modestly elevates). In homozygous familial hypercholesterolemia, ezetimibe may be combined with atorvastatin or simvastatin, used as an adjunct to other lipid-lowering treatments (e.g., LDL apheresis), or used if such treatments are unavailable. Ezetimibe is indicated as adjunctive therapy to diet for the reduction of elevated sitosterol and campesterol levels in patients with homozygous familial sitosterolemia.

Dosage and effect. The recommended dosage of ezetimibe is 10 mg once daily, administered with or without food. The daily dose of ezetimibe may be taken at the same time as the HMG-CoA reductase inhibitor, according to the dosing recommendations for the statin. As fixed-dose monotherapy, ezetimibe produces an approximate 12% reduction in total cholesterol, an 18% reduction in LDL-C, and modest beneficial effects on triglycerides and HDL-C, with no apparent safety concerns. No dosage adjustment is necessary in patients with mild hepatic insufficiency, but the effects of ezetimibe have not been examined in patients with moderate or severe hepatic insufficiency. No dosage adjustment is necessary in patients with renal insufficiency or in geriatric patients. As *co-therapy*, the lipid effects of ezetimibe and a statin appear to be additive. For example, with pravastatin, 10 to 40 mg, LDL-C fell by 34% to 41% and triglycerides by 21% to 23%, and HDL-C rose by 7.8% to 8.4%, with a safety profile similar to pravastatin alone.[108] Coadministration of a resin may dramatically decrease the bioavailability of ezetimibe; therefore its dosing should occur either 2 or more hours before or 4 or more hours after administration of the resin.

Combination Therapy

Combined statin plus fibrate. Statins alone are not the answer to all lipid problems.[3] In secondary prevention, the currently ideal lipid levels may be difficult to achieve with only a statin, and the increase in HDL-C is especially limited. In primary prevention, for patients with severe hypercholesterolemia or familial combined hyperlipidemia with marked triglyceride elevations, combination of a statin with a fibrate is increasingly seen as an option. The statin is very effective in the reduction of LDL-C, whereas the fibrate reduces triglycerides, increases LDL particle size, and increases HDL-C. Two reservations are, first, the lack of any unambiguously favorable large-scale outcome studies with such combinations and, second, the fear of myopathy. The latter is now increasingly seen as a rather rare event during combination therapy.[74,109,110] When statins are metabolized through CYP3A4 (see Table 10-6), the risk of adverse interaction with fibrates is greater during co-therapy with erythromycin, azole antifungals, and antiretrovirals.[109] A logical combination would be a statin and a fibrate that are metabolized by noncompeting pathways, for example, fluvastatin or rosuvastatin with fenofibrate. Hepatotoxicity seems to be a consistent but rare side effect of statins, also during statin-fibrate therapy.[111]

Combined statin plus resin or nicotinic acid. Another choice is between a statin plus a resin, or a statin plus nicotinic acid. In the FATS angiographic trial, men with coronary disease at high risk for cardiovascular events received either lovastatin or nicotinic acid, combined with colestipol. Both regimens were equally effective on blood lipids, and angiographically measured coronary stenosis was lessened, although side effects were worse on the nicotinic acid regimen.[112] A combination preparation has reached the market that pairs extended-release nicotinic acid at doses of 500, 750, and 1000 mg with lovastatin, 20 mg (*Advicor*). This agent is indicated for treating primary hypercholesterolemia and mixed dyslipidemias where the lipid triad is present.

Ezetimibe plus statin. Two studies on carotid arterial lesions found that ezetimibe plus a statin (Vytorin) does less well than expected[111] or has adverse effects.[98] When ezetimibe was added to a statin in patients with a well-controlled lipid profile to decrease LDL-C, which it did, the carotid-media thickness paradoxically increased; when niacin was added to the statin, HDL-C was increased, triglycerides decreased, and there were fewer major cardiovascular events than with ezetimibe.[98] On the benefit side, the combination of simvastatin plus ezetimibe reduced the risk of major atherosclerotic events in a wide range of patients with chronic kidney disease in the SHARP trial.[113,114] Note that this study could equally well argue for lipid-lowering with a statin in dialysis patients.[115] The FDA updated the prescribing information for Vytorin to include data from SHARP[116] Although it approved the ezetimibe-simvastatin combination for use in chronic kidney disease as a new indication, ezetimibe without simvastatin was not approved because the relative contributions of simvastatin and ezetimibe were not assessed in the trial. Also for this reason, the prescribing information for ezetimibe alone (Zetia) does not contain data from SHARP. *FDA recommendations to reduce myopathy with simvastin are also applicable to Vytorin.* In brief, Vytorin should not be used with the conazole group of drugs, some antibiotics, HIV protease inhibitors, cyclosporine, and gemfibrozil. The 10-mg dose should not be exceeded in patients taking amiodarone, verapamil, and diltiazem. The 20-mg dose should not be exceeded with amlodipine and ranolazine (Ranexa). The 80-mg dose should not be started.[84]

Niacin plus laropiprant. Niacin plus laropiprant (Tredaptive) is approved in the European Union as a modified-release tablet in a dose of 1 g nicotinic acid and 20 mg laropiprant for dyslipidemia and primary hypercholesterolemia. Laropiprant minimizes the flushing side effect of using niacin alone.[117] Tredaptive is approved for use in combination with statins, but may be used as monotherapy if statins are inappropriate or not tolerated. However, it is not approved by the FDA and is being tested for clinical event reduction in the large HPS2-THRIVE trial.

Other combinations. Because of the enormous popularity of the statins, it is likely that various other combinations will be considered in the future, such as a statin with low-dose aspirin and other cardioprotective drugs. Some experts have put forth the concept of a "polypill" that combines several heart-beneficial agents as a potential approach.

Natural Antiatherosclerotic Agents

Estrogens. Despite observational studies that noted an association between HRT and reduced coronary risk in women, prospective, randomized clinical trials, including the secondary prevention Heart Estrogen/Progestin Replacement Study and the primary prevention Women's Health Initiative, have reported no clinical cardiovascular benefits with HRT compared with placebo.[118,119] An increased risk for thrombotic complications in the early years of HRT makes such therapy even less attractive for cardiovascular risk management. Caveats are the following: (1) in younger women closer to menopause there was no increase in cardiovascular disease and short-term use for relief of vasomotor symptoms can be justified;[120] and (2) the lipid pattern matters, in that a high LDL-C/HDL-C of 2.5 or more is associated with an increased CVD risk (odds ratio 1.83) whereas those with a low ratio less than 2.5 had no increase when given conjugated equine estrogen with or without medroxyprogesterone.[121]

Dietary antioxidants. In the light of the negative mega-studies showing no cardiovascular protection by vitamin E, either as primary or secondary prevention (see Chapter 12, p. 464), enthusiasm for antioxidant supplements has cooled. A Mediterranean diet, which in the United States is associated with decreased all-cause mortality, is likely to contain adequate amounts of antioxidants mixed in the right proportions.

ω-3 fatty fish oils. Prescription-strength fish oil (*Lovaza*) is FDA approved to decrease triglycerides 500 mg/dL or more at a dose of 4 g/day. Nonprescription fish oil may also be protective, at least in the postinfarct period and when the benefit is largely independent of any change of blood lipid levels and may relate to sodium channel blockade.

Several good epidemiologic studies relate intake of ω-3 fish oils to decreased sudden death or increased life span.

Plant sterol and stanol margarines. Plant sterols can be converted to the corresponding stanol esters that interfere with the intestinal uptake of cholesterol, to cause "cholesterol malabsorption." Daily intake of 2 to 3 g reduces LDL-C by approximately 6% to 15%.[3] In the United States, *Benecol* margarine is available (dose, 2 to 2.5 g/day).

Folic acid. The role of homocysteine as a risk factor remains controversial.[3] Nonetheless, convincing studies show that reducing homocysteine with folic acid fails to lower the coronary risk[122,123] so that there is little point in searching for homocysteinemia (unless genetic excess is suspected).

Alcohol. There is a U-shaped relation between alcohol intake and coronary artery disease, with modest intake rates having a protective effect and higher rates an adverse effect, the latter probably by elevation of triglycerides and BP. Modest quantities of alcohol may promote protection by giving a more favorable blood lipid profile and, in particular, increasing HDL-C. In addition, red wine contains flavonoids that give experimental coronary vascular protection, perhaps by an antioxidant effect. However, the potential for abuse makes it difficult to give a whole-hearted endorsement to alcohol consumption as a preventive measure. Dealcoholized red wine has favorable vascular compliance effects when given to humans.[124] For teetotallers, a liberal intake of red grape juice or cranberry juice could be equally protective.

Juices, tea, and nuts. In a variety of studies, red fruit juices such as cranberry juice, purple or red grape juice, black tea, and nuts have shown varying degrees of benefit on lipid profiles or vascular function. Almonds are well-studied, with a dose-response benefit.[125] Full-dose unblanched almonds (approximately 75 g/day) reduced LDL-C of hyperlipidemic subjects by 9%, reduced conjugated dienes (evidence of oxidized LDL) by 14%, and raised HDL-C by 4%. Herbal remedies are unsupported by data.

SUMMARY

1. *Primary prevention.* In primary prevention of cardiovascular disease, global risk factor assessment and correction is the current favored approach. The atherogenic components of blood lipids and especially LDL are an important part of an overall risk factor profile that includes factors that cannot be changed, such as age, sex, and family history of premature disease, and those that can, such as BP, diet, smoking, exercise, and weight. Elevated CRP can help identify individuals at increased risk despite having low to normal LDL-C. The ideal blood cholesterol and LDL-C levels appear to be falling lower and lower, and a Mediterranean diet is a currently recommended dietary approach.

2. *Secondary prevention.* In secondary prevention, strict LDL-C lowering (recent ultralow aim for very high risk: LDL-C <70 mg/dL or 1.8 mmol/L) is an essential part of a comprehensive program of risk-factor modification. Strict dietary modification is required. Among the cardiac drugs tending to cause hyperlipidemias are β-blockers (especially propranolol) and thiazide diuretics; however, when these drugs are indicated, their protective effect overrides the relatively small changes in blood lipids, especially with statin co-therapy.

3. Increasing use of statins. The decisive 4S and several other studies have shown substantial total and cardiac mortality reduction when statins (HMG-CoA reductase inhibitors) are given to postinfarct patients with modest to severe hypercholesterolemia. The HPS extends the benefits of statins to all high-risk patients defined by any clinical vascular disease or by diabetes, regardless of baseline total cholesterol or LDL-C. Statins have few serious side effects or contraindications.

4. Statins in primary prevention. Although lifestyle and dietary measures remain the basis of primary prevention, the impressive results of one large statin trial (JUPITER), in individuals with blood cholesterol levels that are within the normal range, without known coronary disease, but with elevated levels of CRP, raise important issues for the future prevention of coronary disease.

5. Fibrates. Fibrates act differently from statins at a molecular level to modify tissue fatty acid metabolism by stimulation of PPAR-α, and clinically to decrease triglyceride, increase HDL-C, and decrease LDL particle size, with only a modest fall in LDL-C. Fibrates appear to have the most benefit in patients with low HDL-C and high triglyceride levels, which is part of the adverse risk profile (lipid triad) of the metabolic syndrome.

6. Combination therapy. Combination therapy is now increasingly used to achieve goal lipid levels. The principle is to combine two different classes of agents with different mechanisms of action, such as a statin and a fibrate or nicotinic acid. Most sources warn against these combinations because of the fear of muscle or renal damage or hepatotoxicity. Nonetheless, there is a growing consensus that judicious use of combination therapy, when required, is likely to confer more benefits than harm. Caution is still required, with regular clinical observation, patient education about side effects, and monitoring of CK and blood liver enzymes. An additional combination, approved for use in chronic kidney disease, is that of simvastatin with a cholesterol absorption inhibitor, ezetimibe.

7. Interactions with antiretrovirals. Recent FDA warnings relate to all statins except pravastatin and pitavastatin. Specifically, there are dose limitations for atorvastatin and rosuvastatin, with major contraindications for use with simvastatin and lovastatin.

8. Side effects. Hyperglycemia and new diabetes, first noted with rosuvastatin, are now recognized. Although this metabolic harm is more than outweighed by the overall cardiovascular benefits of statin therapy, periodic checks for glycemia are strongly advised.

9. HRT. HRT in postmenopausal women can no longer be linked to major cardiovascular benefit. *Dietary antioxidants* may be obtained in adequate amounts by following the Mediterranean-type diet, whereas vitamin E supplements, in particular, have not given protection either in secondary prevention or as primary prevention in high-risk individuals.

Acknowledgment

We are greatly indebted to Dr. Jennifer Moon, whose superb and professional editorial work was invaluable.

References

1. White PD. *Heart disease.* 3rd ed. New York: Macmillan, 1944.
2. Domanski MJ. Primary prevention of coronary artery disease. *N Engl J Med* 2007;357: 1543–1545.
3. Expert Panel on Detection, Evaluation, and Treatment of High Blood Cholesterol in Adults. Executive Summary of the Third Report of the National Cholesterol Education Program (NCEP) (Adult Treatment Panel III). *JAMA* 2001;285:2486–2497.
4. Ford I, et al. Long-term follow-up of the West of Scotland Coronary Prevention Study. *N Engl J Med* 2007;357:1477–1486.
5. Ridker PM, et al. Rosuvastatin to prevent vascular events in men and women with elevated C-reactive protein. *N Engl J Med* 2008;359:2195–2207.
6. Hsia J, et al. Cardiovascular event reduction and adverse events among subjects attaining low-density lipoprotein cholesterol <50 mg/dL with rosuvastatin. *J Am Coll Cardiol* 2011;57:1666–1675.
7. Gustafsson M, et al. Mechanism of lipoprotein retention by the extracellular matrix. *Curr Opin Lipidol* 2004;15:505–514.
8. Sherer Y, et al. Mechanisms of disease: atherosclerosis in autoimmune diseases. *Nature Clin Pract Rheumatol* 2006;2:99–106.
9. Libby P, et al. Inflammation in atherosclerosis: from pathophysiology to practice. *J Am Coll Cardiol* 2009;54(23):2129–2138.
10. Libby P, et al. Progress and challenges in translating the biology of atherosclerosis. *Nature* 2011;473(7347):317–325.
11. Pearson TA, et al. Markers of inflammation and cardiovascular disease: application to clinical and public health practice. A statement for healthcare professionals from the Centers for Disease Control and Prevention and the American Heart Association. *Circulation* 2003;107:499–511.
12. Devaraj S, et al. The evolving role of C-reactive protein in atherothrombosis. *Clin Chem* 2009;55(2):229–238.
13. Elliott P, et al. Genetic loci associated with C-reactive protein levels and risk of coronary heart disease. *JAMA* 2009;302(1):37–48.
14. Nakamura H, et al. MEGA Study Group. Primary prevention of cardiovascular disease with pravastatin in Japan (MEGA Study): a prospective randomised controlled trial. *Lancet* 2006;368:1155–1163.
15. Taylor F, et al. Statins for the primary prevention of cardiovascular disease. *Cochrane Database Syst Rev* 2011;Jan 19(1):CD004816.
16. Grundy SM, et al. Implications of recent clinical trials for the National Cholesterol Education Program Adult Treatment Panel III Guidelines. *J Am Coll Cardiol* 2004;44:720–732.
17. Graham I, et al. European guidelines on cardiovascular disease prevention in clinical practice: executive summary. Fourth Joint Task Force of the European Society of Cardiology and Other Societies on Cardiovascular Disease Prevention in Clinical Practice (constituted by representatives of nine societies and by invited experts). *Eur Heart J* 2007;28:2375–2414.
18. Smith Jr SC, et al. AHA/ACCF secondary prevention and risk reduction therapy for patients with coronary and other atherosclerotic vascular disease: 2011 update. *Circulation* 2011;124:2458–2473.
19. LaRosa JC, et al. Intensive lipid lowering with atorvastatin in patients with stable coronary disease. *N Engl J Med* 2005;352:1425–1435.
20. Pedersen TR, et al. High-dose atorvastatin vs usual-dose simvastatin for secondary prevention after myocardial infarction. The IDEAL study: a randomized controlled trial. *JAMA* 2005;294:2437–2445.
21. Cholesterol Treatment Trialists' Collaboration. Efficacy and safety of more intensive lowering of LDL cholesterol: a meta-analysis of data from 170,000 participants in 26 randomised trials. *Lancet* 2010;376(9753):1670–1681.
22. Cannon CP, et al. Intensive versus moderate lipid lowering with statins after acute coronary syndromes. *N Engl J Med* 2004;350:1495–1504.
23. Nissen SE, et al. Effect of intensive compared with moderate lipid-lowering therapy on progression of coronary atherosclerosis: a randomized controlled trial. *JAMA* 2004;291:1071–1080.
24. von Birgelen C, et al. Relation between progression and regression of atherosclerotic left main coronary artery disease and serum cholesterol levels as assessed with serial long-term (>12 months) follow-up intravascular ultrasound. *Circulation* 2003;108:2757–2762.
25. O'Keefe JH, et al. Optimal low-density lipoprotein is 50 to 70 mg/dl. *J Am Coll Cardiol* 2004;43(11):2142–2146.
26. Rohrer L, et al. High density lipoproteins in the intersection of diabetes mellitus, inflammation and cardiovascular disease. *Curr Opin Lipidol* 2004;15:269–278.
27. Pfeffer MA, et al. Influence of baseline lipids on effectiveness of pravastatin in the CARE trial. *J Am Coll Cardiol* 1999;33:125–130.
28. Collins R, et al. High-risk elderly patients PROSPER from cholesterol-lowering therapy. *Lancet* 2002;360:1618–1619.
29. Barter P, et al. HDL cholesterol, very low levels of LDL cholesterol, and cardiovascular events. *N Engl J Med* 2007;357:1301–1310.
30. Ridker PM, et al. HDL cholesterol and residual risk of first cardiovascular events after treatment with potent statin therapy: an analysis from the JUPITER trial. *Lancet* 2010;376:333–339.
31. Chapman MJ, et al. Triglyceride-rich lipoproteins and high-density lipoprotein cholesterol in patients at high risk of cardiovascular disease: evidence and guidance for management. *Eur Heart J* 2011;32:1345–1361.

32. The AIM-HIGH Investigators. Niacin in patients with low HDL cholesterol levels receiving intensive statin therapy. *N Engl J Med* 2011;365(24):2255–2267.

33. Arca M, et al. Usefulness of atherogenic dyslipidemia for predicting cardiovascular risk in patients with angiographically defined coronary artery disease. *Am J Cardiol* 2007; 100:1511–1516.

34. Barter PJ, et al. Effects of torcetrapib in patients at high risk for coronary events. *N Engl J Med* 2007;357:2109–2122.

35. Cannon CP, et al. Safety of Anacetrapib in patients with or at high risk for coronary heart disease. *N Engl J Med* 2010;363(25):2406–2415.

36. Fayad ZA, et al. Safety and efficacy of dalcetrapib on atherosclerotic disease using novel non-invasive multimodality imaging (dal-PLAQUE): a randomized clinical trial. *Lancet* 2011;378(9802):1547–1559.

37. Hovingh GK, et al. Apolipoprotein A-I mimetic peptides. *Curr Opin Lipidol* 2010;21(6): 481–486.

38. Miller M, for the PROVE IT-TIMI 22 Investigators, et al. Impact of triglyceride levels beyond low-density lipoprotein cholesterol after acute coronary syndrome in the PROVE IT-TIMI 22 Trial. *J Am Coll Cardiol* 2008;51:724–730.

39. Miller M, et al. Triglycerides and cardiovascular disease. *Circulation* 2011;123(20): 2292–2333.

40. Ramjee V, et al. Non-high-density lipoprotein cholesterol versus apolipoprotein B in cardiovascular risk stratification: do the math. *J Am Coll Cardiol* 2011;58(5):457–463.

41. Yusuf S, et al. Effect of potentially modifiable risk factors associated with myocardial infarction in 52 countries (the INTERHEART study): case-control study. *Lancet* 2004; 364:937–952.

42. Mudd JO, et al. Beyond low-density lipoprotein: defining the role of low-density lipoprotein heterogeneity in coronary artery disease. *J Am Coll Cardiol* 2007;50:1735–1741.

43. Ryden L, et al. Guidelines on diabetes, pre-diabetes, and cardiovascular diseases: executive summary. The Task Force on Diabetes and Cardiovascular Diseases of the European Society of Cardiology (ESC) and of the European Association for the Study of Diabetes (EASD). *Eur Heart J* 2007;28:88–136.

44. Cholesterol Treatment Trialists' (CTT) Collaborators. Efficacy of cholesterol-lowering therapy in 18,686 people with diabetes in 14 randomised trials of statins: a meta-analysis. *Lancet* 2008;371:117–125.

45. Vakkilainen J, et al. Relationships between low-density lipoprotein particle size, plasma lipoproteins, and progression of coronary artery disease: the Diabetes Atherosclerosis Intervention Study (DAIS). *Circulation* 2003;107:1733–1737.

46. Colhoun HM, et al. Primary prevention of cardiovascular disease with atorvastatin in type 2 diabetes in the Collaborative Atorvastatin Diabetes Study (CARDS): multicentre randomised placebo-controlled trial. *Lancet* 2004;364:685–696.

47. Heart Protection Study Collaborative Group. MRC/BHF heart protection study of cholesterol lowering with simvastatin in 20,536 high-risk individuals: a randomised placebo-controlled trial. *Lancet* 2002;360:7–22.

48. ACCORD Study Group, et al. Effects of combination lipid therapy in type 2 diabetes mellitus. *N Engl J Med* 2010;362(17):1563–1574.

49. Deedwania P, et al. Effects of intensive versus moderate lipid-lowering therapy on myocardial ischemia in older patients with coronary heart disease: results of the Study Assessing Goals in the Elderly (SAGE). *Circulation* 2007;115:700–707.

50. Mora S, et al. Statins for the primary prevention of cardiovascular events in women with elevated high-sensitivity C-reactive protein or dyslipidemia. *Circulation* 2010;121: 1069–1077.

51. Kromhout D, et al. Prevention of coronary heart disease by diet and lifestyle: evidence from prospective cross-cultural, cohort, and intervention studies. *Circulation* 2002;105:893–898.

52. de Lorgeril M, et al. Mediterranean diet: traditional risk factors, and the rate of cardiovascular complications after myocardial infarction. Final report of the Lyon Diet Heart Study. *Circulation* 1999;99:779–785.

53. Trichopoulou A, et al. Adherence to a Mediterranean diet and survival in a Greek population. *N Engl J Med* 2003;348:2599–2608.

54. Lichtenstein AH, et al. Diet and lifestyle recommendations revision 2006: a scientific statement from the American Heart Association Nutrition Committee. *Circulation* 2006; 114:82–96.

55. ALLHAT Collaborative Research Group. Major outcomes in high-risk hypertensive patients randomized to angiotensin-converting enzyme inhibitor or calcium channel blocker vs diuretic. The Antihypertensive and Lipid-Lowering Treatment to Prevent Heart Attack Trial (ALLHAT). *JAMA* 2002;288:2981–2997.

56. Lindholm LH, et al. Metabolic outcome during 1 year in newly detected hypertensives: results of the Antihypertensive Treatment and Lipid Profile in a North of Sweden Efficacy Evaluation (ALPINE study). *J Hypertens* 2003;21:1563–1574.

57. Scandinavian Simvastatin Survival Study Group. Randomised trial of cholesterol lowering in 4444 patients with coronary heart disease: the Scandinavian Simvastatin Survival Study (4S). *Lancet* 1994;344:1383–1389.

58. Shepherd J, for the West of Scotland Coronary Prevention Study Group, et al. Prevention of coronary heart disease with pravastatin in men with hypercholesterolemia. *N Engl J Med* 1995;333:1301–1307.

59. Downs JR, et al. Primary prevention of acute coronary events with lovastatin in men and women with average cholesterol levels: results of AFCAPS/TexCAPS. Air Force/Texas Coronary Atherosclerosis Prevention Study. *JAMA* 1998;279:1615–1622.

60. Sadowitz B, et al. Basic science review: statin therapy—part I: the pleiotropic effects of statins in cardiovascular disease. *Vasc Endovascular Surg* 2010;44(4):241–251.

61. Ryu SK, et al. Phospholipase A2 enzymes, high-dose atorvastatin, and prediction of ischemic events after acute coronary syndromes. *Circulation* 2012;125(6):757–766.
62. Lewington S, et al. Prospective Studies Collaboration. Blood cholesterol and vascular mortality by age, sex, and blood pressure: a meta-analysis of individual data from 61 prospective studies with 55,000 vascular deaths. *Lancet* 2007;370:1829–1839.
63. Kapoor AS, et al. Strength of evidence for perioperative use of statins to reduce cardiovascular risk: systematic review of controlled studies. *Brit Med J* 2006;333:1149.
64. Mills EJ, et al. Intensive statin therapy compared with moderate dosing for prevention of cardiovascular events: a meta-analysis of >40,000 patients. *Eur Heart J* 2011;32: 1409–1415.
65. Baigent C, et al. Cholesterol Treatment Trialists' (CTT) Collaborators. Efficacy and safety of cholesterol-lowering treatment: prospective meta-analysis of data from 90,056 participants in 14 randomised trials of statins. *Lancet* 2005;366:1267–1278.
66. Silva M, et al. Meta-analysis of drug-induced adverse events associated with intensive-dose statin therapy. *Clin Ther* 2007;29:253–260.
67. Leeper NJ, et al. Statin use in patients with extremely low low-density lipoprotein levels is associated with improved survival. *Circulation* 2007;116:613–618.
68. Amarenco P, et al. High-dose atorvastatin after stroke or transient ischemic attack. *N Engl J Med* 2006;355:549–559.
69. O'Regan C, et al. Statin therapy in stroke prevention: a meta-analysis involving 121,000 patients. *Am J Med* 2008;121:24–33.
70. US Food and Drug Administration. *FDA Drug Safety Communication: important safety label changes to cholesterol-lowering statin drugs.* <http://www.fda.gov/Drugs/DrugSafety/ucm293101.htm>; 2012 [accessed 29.02.12].
71. US Food and Drug Administration. *FDA Drug Safety Communication: interactions between certain HIV or hepatitis C drugs and cholesterol-lowering statin drugs can increase the risk of muscle injury.* <http://www.fda.gov/Drugs/DrugSafety/ucm293877.htm>; 2012 [accessed 09.03.12].
72. Jacobson TA: Toward "pain-free" statin prescribing: clinical algorithm for diagnosis and management of myalgia. *Mayo Clin Proc* 2008;83:687–700.
73. Gaist D, et al. Lipid-lowering drugs and risk of myopathy: a population-based follow-up study. *Epidemiology* 2001;1:565–569.
74. Staffa JA, et al. Cerivastatin and reports of fatal rhabdomyolysis. *N Engl J Med* 2002; 539–540.
75. Shek A, et al. Statin-fibrate combination therapy. *Ann Pharmacother* 2001;35:908–917.
76. Sattar N, et al. Statins and risk of incident diabetes: a collaborative meta-analysis of randomised statin trials. *Lancet* 2010;375:735–742.
77. Preiss D, et al. Risk of incident diabetes with intensive-dose compared with moderate-dose statin therapy. *JAMA* 2011;305:2556–2564.
78. Culver AL, et al. Statin use and risk of diabetes mellitus in postmenopausal women in the Women's Health Initiative. *Arch Intern Med* 2012;172(2):144–152.
79. Klein BE, et al. Statin use and incident nuclear cataract. *JAMA* 2006;295:2752–2758.
80. Serruys PW, et al. Fluvastatin for prevention of cardiac events following successful percutaneous coronary intervention: a randomized controlled trial. *JAMA* 2002;287: 3215–3222.
81. LIPID Study Group. Prevention of cardiovascular events and death with pravastatin in patients with coronary heart disease and a broad range of initial cholesterol levels. *N Engl J Med* 1998;339:1349–1357.
82. Shepherd J, et al. Pravastatin in elderly individuals at risk of vascular disease (PROSPER): a randomised controlled trial. *Lancet* 2002;360:1623.
83. Armitage J, et al. Intensive lowering of LDL cholesterol with 80 mg versus 20 mg simvastatin daily in 12,064 survivors of myocardial infarction: a double-blind randomised trial. *Lancet* 2010;376:1658–1669.
84. Egan A, et al. Weighing the benefits of high-dose simvastatin against the risk of myopathy. *N Engl J Med* 2011;365:285–287.
85. Heart Protection Study Collaborative Group. Effects on 11-year mortality and morbidity of lowering LDL cholesterol with simvastatin for about 5 years in 20,536 high-risk individuals: a randomized controlled trial. *Lancet* 2011;378(9808):2013–2020.
86. Kohli P, et al. Statins and safety: can we finally be reassured? *Lancet* 2011;378(9808): 1980–1981.
87. Schwartz GG, et al. Effects of atorvastatin on early recurrent ischemic events in acute coronary syndromes, The MIRACL study: a randomized controlled trial. *JAMA* 2001;285: 1711–1718.
88. Sever PS, et al. Prevention of coronary and stroke events with atorvastatin in hypertensive patients who have average or lower-than-average cholesterol concentrations, in the Anglo-Scandinavian Cardiac Outcomes Trial–Lipid Lowering Arm (ASCOT-LLA): a multicentre randomised controlled trial. *Lancet* 2003;361:1149–1158.
89. Shepherd J, et al. Effect of intensive lipid lowering with atorvastatin on renal function in patients with coronary heart disease: the Treating to New Targets (TNT) study. *Clin J Am Soc Nephrol* 2007;2(6):1131–1139.
90. Bates ER, et al. Clopidogrel-drug interactions. *J Am Coll Cardiol* 2011;57:1251–1263.
91. Nissen SE, et al. Effect of very high-intensity statin therapy on regression of coronary atherosclerosis: the ASTEROID trial. *JAMA* 2006;295:1556–1565.
92. Crouse 3rd JR, et al. Effect of rosuvastatin on progression of carotid intima-media thickness in low-risk individuals with subclinical atherosclerosis: the METEOR Trial. *JAMA* 2007;297:1344–1353.
93. Kjekshus J, et al. Rosuvastatin in older patients with systolic heart failure. *N Engl J Med* 2007;357:2248–2261.

94. Fellström BC, et al. Rosuvastatin and cardiovascular events in patients undergoing hemodialysis. *N Engl J Med* 2009;360:1395–1407.

95. Gotto AM, et al. Pitavastatin for the treatment of primary hyperlipidemia and mixed dyslipidemia. *Exp Rev Cardiovasc Ther* 2010;8(8):1079–1090.

96. Prueksaritanont T, et al. Mechanistic studies on metabolic interactions between gemfibrozil and statins. *J Pharm Exp Ther* 2002;301(3):1042–1051.

97. The Lipid Research Clinics Coronary Primary Prevention Trial Results 1. Reduction in incidence of coronary heart disease. *JAMA* 1984;251:351–364.

98. Canner PL, et al. Fifteen year mortality in Coronary Drug Project patients: long-term benefit with niacin. *J Am Coll Cardiol* 1986;8:1245–1255.

99. The AIM-HIGH Investigators. Niacin in Patients with Low HDL Cholesterol Levels Receiving Intensive Statin Therapy. *N Engl J Med* 2011;365(24):2255–2267.

100. Villines TC, et al. The ARBITER 6-HALTS Trial (Arterial Biology for the Investigation of the Treatment Effects of Reducing Cholesterol 6-HDL and LDL Treatment Strategies in Atherosclerosis): final results and the impact of medication adherence, dose, and treatment duration. *J Am Coll Cardiol* 2010;55(24):2721–2726.

101. Rubins HB, for the Veterans Affairs Cooperative Studies Program High-Density Lipoprotein Cholesterol Intervention Trial Study Group, et al. Gemfibrozil for the secondary prevention of coronary heart disease in men with low levels of high-density lipoprotein cholesterol. *N Engl J Med* 1999;341:410–418.

102. Frick MH, et al. Helsinki Heart Study: primary prevention trial with gemfibrozil in middle-aged men with dyslipidemia. *N Engl J Med* 1987;317:1237–1245.

103. Tenkanen L, et al. Gemfibrozil in the treatment of dyslipidemia: an 18-year mortality follow-up of the Helsinki Heart Study. *Arch Intern Med* 2006;166:743–748.

104. Tenenbaum A, et al. Attenuation of progression of insulin resistance in patients with coronary artery disease by bezafibrate. *Arch Intern Med* 2006;166:737–741.

105. Haim M, et al. Decrease in triglyceride level by bezafibrate is related to reduction of recurrent coronary events: a Bezafibrate Infarction Prevention substudy. *Coron Artery Dis* 2006;17:455–461.

106. Keech A, et al. Effects of long-term fenofibrate therapy on cardiovascular events in 9795 people with type 2 diabetes mellitus (the FIELD study): randomised controlled trial. *Lancet* 2005;366:1849–1861.

107. Shepherd J. Combined lipid lowering drug therapy for the effective treatment of hypercholesterolaemia. *Eur Heart J* 2003;24:685–689.

108. Melani L, et al. Efficacy and safety of ezetimibe coadministered with pravastatin in patients with primary hypercholesterolemia: a prospective, randomized, double-blind trial. *Eur Heart J* 2003;24:717–728.

109. Law M, et al. Statin safety: a systematic review. *Am J Cardiol* 2006;97:52C–60C.

110. Shepherd J, et al. Safety of rosuvastatin: update on 16,876 rosuvastatin-treated patients in a multinational clinical trial program. *Cardiology* 2007;107:433–443.

111. Athyros VG, et al. Safety and efficacy of long-term statin-fibrate combinations in patients with refractory familial combined hyperlipidemia. *Am J Cardiol* 1997;80:608–613.

112. Brown G, et al. Regression of coronary artery disease as a result of intensive lipid-lowering therapy in men with high levels of apolipoprotein B. *N Engl J Med* 1990; 323:1289–1298.

113. Kastelein JJ, et al. Simvastatin with or without ezetimibe in familial hypercholesterolemia. *N Engl J Med* 2008;358:1431–1443.

114. Baigent C, et al. The effects of lowering LDL cholesterol with simvastatin plus ezetimibe in patients with chronic kidney disease (Study of Heart and Renal Protection): a randomized placebo-controlled trial. *Lancet* 2011;377(9784): 2181–2192.

115. Stevens KK, et al. SHARP: a stab in the right direction in chronic kidney disease. *Lancet* 2011;377:2153–2154

116. New FDA approved labeling for VYTORIN® (Ezetimibe/Simvastatin) includes results from the Study of Heart and Renal Protection (SHARP) in patients with moderate to severe chronic kidney disease [press release]. Whitehouse Station, NJ: Merck; January 25, 2012.

117. Paolini JF, et al. Effects of laropiprant on nicotinic acid-induced flushing in patients with dyslipidemia. *Am J Cardiol* 2008;101:625–630.

118. Grady D, et al. Cardiovascular disease outcomes during 6.8 years of hormone therapy: Heart and Estrogen/progestin Replacement Study follow-up (HERS II). *JAMA* 2002; 288:49–57.

119. Writing Group for the Women's Health Initiative Investigators. Risks and benefits of estrogen plus progesterone in healthy postmenopausal women: principal results from the Women's Health Initiative randomized controlled trial. *JAMA* 2000;288: 321–333.

120. Rossouw JE, et al. Postmenopausal hormone therapy and risk of cardiovascular disease by age and years since menopause. *JAMA* 2007;297:1465–1477.

121. Bray PF, et al. Usefulness of baseline lipids and C-reactive protein in women receiving menopausal hormone therapy as predictors of treatment-related coronary events. *Am J Cardiol* 2008;101:1599–1605.

122. Albert CM, et al. Effect of folic acid and B vitamins on risk of cardiovascular events and total mortality among women at high risk for cardiovascular disease: a randomized trial. *JAMA* 2008;299:2027–2036.

123. Baigent C, et al. B vitamins for the prevention of vascular disease: insufficient evidence to justify treatment. *JAMA* 2007;298:1212–1214.

124. Opie LH, et al. The red wine hypothesis: from concepts to protective signaling molecules. *Eur Heart J* 2007;28:1683–1693.

125. Jenkins DJ, et al. Dose response of almonds on coronary heart disease risk factors: blood lipids, oxidized low-density lipoproteins, lipoprotein(a), homocysteine, and pulmonary nitric oxide. A randomized, controlled, crossover trial. *Circulation* 2002;106: 1327–1332.

126. Frishman WH, editor. *Medical management of lipid disorders: focus on prevention of coronary artery disease.* New York: Futura; 1992.

127. Neaton JD, et al. Treatment of Mild Hypertension study (TOMH): final results. *JAMA* 1993;270:713–724.

128. Lerch M, et al. Effects of angiotensin II-receptor blockade with losartan on insulin sensitivity, lipid profile, and endothelin in normotensive offspring of hypertensive parents. *J Cardiovasc Pharmacol* 1998;31:576–580.

129. Plouin P-F, et al. Are angiotensin enzyme inhibition and aldosterone antagonism equivalent in hypertensive patients over fifty? *Am J Hypertens* 1991;4:356–362.

130. Kasiske FL, et al. Effects of antihypertensive therapy on serum lipids. *Ann Intern Med* 1995;122:133–141.

131. Giugliano D, et al. Metabolic and cardiovascular effects of carvedilol and atenolol in non-insulin-dependent diabetes mellitus and hypertension: a randomized, controlled trial. *Ann Intern Med* 1997;126:955–959.

132. Ridker PM, et al. Number needed to treat with rosuvastatin to prevent first cardiovascular events and death among men and women with low low-density lipoprotein cholesterol and elevated high-sensitivity C-reactive protein: Justification for the Use of Statins in Prevention: an Intervention Trial Evaluating Rosuvastatin (JUPITER). *Circ Cardiovasc Qual Outcomes* 2009;2:616–623.

11

Metabolic Syndrome, Hyperglycemia, and Type 2 Diabetes

LIONEL H. OPIE · JURIS MEIER

"The goal of many clinicians who manage diabetes is to achieve optimum glucose control alongside weight loss and a minimum number of hypoglycemic episodes."

Bergenstal, *Lancet,* 2010[1]

This chapter starts with prevention at the level of obesity and the metabolic syndrome, precursors of overt type 2 diabetes. We then cover overall management of diabetes and the standard glycemia-controlling drugs, before emphasizing the incretins which are specifically covered in greater detail. Then follow new sections on new drugs such as bromocriptine and inhibitors of renal sodium-glucose cotransport. The chapter closes with the need for multifactorial intervention.

Obesity has become a common problem in Western society, and it is a strong predictor of type 2 diabetes.[2] In the United States it is estimated that almost one third of the population has a lifetime risk of diabetes. Diabetes, in turn, predisposes to cardiovascular abnormalities, such that persons with diabetes without known coronary heart disease (CHD) have the same prognosis as a patient without diabetes who has CHD.[3] An increased waistline is one of the five criteria of the metabolic syndrome (MetSyn) in addition to fasting hyperglycemia and blood pressure (BP) elevation, increased circulating triglycerides, and decreased circulating high-density lipoprotein (HDL) cholesterol.[4] Three of these are required for the diagnosis of the MetSyn (Fig. 11-1; Table 11-1).[5,6] The three main factors relating to the metabolic risk of cardiovascular disease are the body mass index (BMI), abdominal girth, and insulin resistance (IR) and response.[7] However, waist circumference rather than obesity reflected by the BMI is the better predictor of the risk of myocardial infarction (MI).[8]

Abdominal adipose tissue is now recognized as a metabolically active organ and regarded as the basic abnormality in the MetSyn by the International Diabetes Federation.[6] There are strong links between excessive abdominal fat leading to excessive circulating free fatty acids (FFAs) and cytokines, which hypothetically lead to the other four features of the MetSyn and could explain IR.[9] Nonetheless, the links between visceral abdominal fat and IR are challenged, the alternate culprit being subcutaneous fat, especially in the upper body.[10] The MetSyn is of clinical importance in that it increases the risk of cardiovascular disease and especially type 2 diabetes.[11] Currently an increasing number of patients with the MetSyn obesity or type 2 diabetes are being treated by cardiologists, often in close collaboration with diabetologists.

METABOLIC SYNDROME

Opie 2012

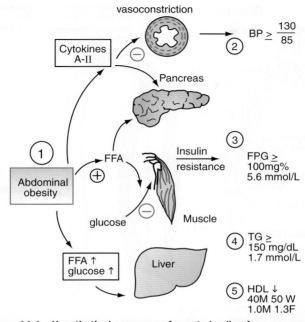

Figure 11-1 Hypothetical sequence of events leading from excess abdominal adiposity to the five features of the metabolic syndrome, of which three are required for diagnosis. The adipose tissue releases increased free fatty acids (FFAs) into the circulation, thereby inhibiting the uptake of glucose by muscle. Plasma glucose rises and elicits an insulin response. However, the pancreas is damaged by the high FFA levels and increased cytokines. The net effect is increased fasting plasma glucose (FPG) despite the increased circulating insulin (insulin resistance). Increased plasma FFA and glucose predispose to increased hepatic synthesis of triglycerides (TGs) and increased blood levels of TG, which in turn decrease levels of high-density lipoprotein (HDL) cholesterol. Increased release of angiotensin II (A-II) from the abdominal fat causes vasoconstriction and increases the blood pressure (BP). For details see Opie LH. Metabolic syndrome, *Circulation* 2007;115:e32. (Figure © L.H. Opie, 2012.)

Table 11-1

Clinical Diagnosis of the Metabolic Syndrome		
Risk Factor	**Defining Level**	**Level, Metric Units**
Abdominal obesity; waist		
Men	>40 inches	>102 cm
Women	>35 inches	>88 cm
Triglycerides	≥150 mg/dL	≥1.7 mmol/L
HDL cholesterol		
Men	< 40 mg/dL	<1.03 mmol/L
Women	< 50 mg/dL	<1.3 mmol/L
Fasting glucose	≥100 mg/dL	≥5.6 mmol/L
Blood pressure	≥130/85 mm Hg	≥130/85 mm Hg

HDL, High-density lipoprotein.
For those on prior therapy see Table 2 of AHA/NHLBI statement.[5] Note important ethnic variations and lower waistline standards of International Diabetes Federation.[6]

NORMAL RENAL GLUCOSE FILTRATION

Opie 2012

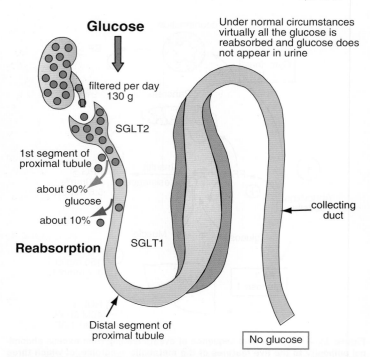

Figure 11-2   Normal renal glucose filtration. Under normal conditions virtually all the glucose that is filtered through the glomeruli is reabsorbed, mostly in the first segment of the proximal tubule by the sodium-glucose transporter (SGLT2) (Figure © L.H. Opie, 2012.)

Risks of metabolic syndrome. MetSyn comprises a group of cardiovascular risk factors, each of which individually may be of only borderline significance, but when taken together indicate enhanced risk of development of overt diabetes or cardiovascular disease. Influential authorities have questioned the predictive value of the MetSyn for the future development of diabetes and stress the role of one of the five components alone (glucose; Fig. 11-2).[12] Others emphasize the predictive value of two components of the MetSyn, modest elevations of glucose and BP, which were mostly responsible for increasing the cardiovascular risk by 71% in one study.[13] For cardiologists, becoming alert to risk-factor clustering, including abdominal obesity, high triglycerides, low HDL cholesterol, prehypertension, and hyperglycemia, is an important widening of vision.[5] The risk of developing future cardiovascular problems is proportional to the number of MetSyn features.[14] With four or five features, the risk of diabetes was 25-fold greater than with no features and still much more than with only one feature.[15] In an analysis of 172,573 persons in 37 studies, MetSyn had a relative risk of 1.78 for future cardiovascular events, and the association remained after adjusting for traditional cardiovascular risk factors (relative risk [RR], 1.54; confidence interval [CI], 1.32-1.79).[16] The International Day for Evaluation of Abdominal Obesity study measured waistlines in 168,000 primary care patients spread worldwide to confirm an association between waist and cardiovascular disease (RR 1.36) and more so with diabetes (RR 1.59 in men and 1.83 in women).[11]

Insulin resistance. IR leads to the MetSyn[7] and increased circulating FFA and glycemia (see Fig. 11-1), plus elevated glucose production in the liver, which are the precursors of type 2 diabetes mellitus (T2DM).[17] There is a dose-response effect of elevated plasma FFA on insulin signaling.[9] The dietary routes to IR were studied in more than 7000 young Finns.[18] There were specific circulating metabolic clues, namely increased branched-chain and aromatic amino acids, intermediates of gluconeogenesis, ketone bodies, and fatty acids abnormal in composition and saturation. Taken together, these 20 metabolite measures were strongly associated with the homeostasis model of IR (P < 0.0005). Thus early life dietary patterns already predispose to IR.

Where does obesity enter the picture? Obese persons have high blood FFA levels, which even at modest elevations inhibit insulin signaling[9] and stimulate nuclear factor kappa B (NFκB) to promote IR (Fig. 1 in Kim, 2012).[19] NFκB in turn stimulates macrophages to provoke the chronic low-grade inflammatory response (Fig. 2 in Kim, 2012)[19] with increased plasma levels of C-reactive protein, and inflammatory cytokines such as tumor necrosis factor–alpha (TNFα), interleukin (IL) 6, monocyte chemotactic protein (MCP) 1, and IL-8, and the multifunctional proteins leptin and osteopontin.[17] Macrophages in human adipose tissue are the main, but not the only, source of these inflammatory mediators that stimulate IR in multiple organs.[19] Hypothalamic microglia are macrophage-like cells that are also activated by proinflammatory signals causing local production of specific interleukins and cytokines. The "Western" high-fat diet experimentally enhances such cytokine production, whereas exercise diminishes it.[20] The overall sequence is:

$$\text{Obesity} \rightarrow \text{high FFA} \rightarrow \text{NF}\kappa\text{B} \rightarrow \text{macrophages} \rightarrow$$
$$\text{inflammatory cytokines} \rightarrow \text{insulin resistance}$$

A simple therapeutic attack on the inflammatory response is by high-dose aspirin in impractical doses (approximately 7 g/day).[21]

From Metabolic Syndrome to Overt Diabetes and Cardiovascular Disease

Lifestyle changes to slow the onset of diabetes. The transition from MetSyn to full-blown diabetes can be significantly lessened by lifestyle intervention. Thus walking only approximately 19 km per week can be beneficial in treating MetSyn.[22] However, more intense intervention is needed for real change. Tuomilehto et al.[23] studied a group of overweight subjects with impaired glucose tolerance who, on average, also had the features of the MetSyn. Dietary advice and exercise programs were individually tailored. The five aims were weight reduction, decreased fat intake, decreased saturated fat intake, increased fiber intake, and increased endurance exercise (at least 30 min daily). Of these, increased exercise was achieved in 86% of participants, and the other components less frequently. After a mean duration of 3.2 years, the relative risk for new diabetes in the lifestyle intervention group was 0.4 (p < 0.001). In the Diabetes Prevention Group[24] similar subjects were given lifestyle modification or metformin for a mean of 2.8 years. Lifestyle intervention was very intense with a 16-lesson curriculum covering diet, exercise, and behavior modification taught by case managers on a one-to-one basis during the first 24 weeks after enrollment. Lifestyle intervention was more effective than metformin in delaying the onset of diabetes, and both were more effective than placebo in preventing new diabetes. The physical exercise in these two preventative studies was intense, and cannot readily be achieved in the average clinic. Please see Update for premature termination of Look-AHEAD study (no change in major cardiovascular outcomes).

Sustainability of lifestyle changes. Is the protection from diabetes found in the Diabetes Prevention Group study sustained? The 10-year follow-up says no, with an equal incidence of new diabetes in placebo, former lifestyle, and metformin groups. Yet the cumulative incidence of diabetes remained lowest in the lifestyle group. Thus prevention or delay of diabetes with lifestyle intervention or metformin can persist for at least 10 years.

Long-term diet-induced weight loss. Wadden et al. write, "Physical activity appears to be critical for long-term weight management."[25] However, weight loss is no easy task. Even in a motivated group receiving in-person support over 2 years, only 41% lost 5% or more of their weight from an initial mean of 103.8 kg.[26] From an excellent review of 21 lifestyle modification studies,[25] only 4 are above average: a 2-year meal replacement program (−10.4 kg); a low-carbohydrate ketogenic diet with nutritional supplements (−12.0 kg) but only over 6 months, when weight loss often peaks; a center-based Jenney Craig diet (−10.1 kg at 12 months); and a Weight Watchers diet plus individual counseling (−9.4 kg at 12 months). However, the standard pattern was weight regain after 12 months, equal to the low-fat and low-carbohydrate diets, and less weight regain in those who are exercising vigorously (300 min or more weekly). Increasingly, "personalized" programs are conducted electronically.

Physical disability in adults with type 2 diabetes. Could weight loss reduce mobility-related problems in adults with type 2 diabetes who have a high prevalence of disability? The ongoing Action for Health in Diabetes (Look AHEAD) study enrolled more than 5000 overweight or obese persons with type 2 diabetes and mean initial weight was 100.9 kg.[27] At year 4, the lifestyle-intervention group had a relative reduction of 48% in the risk of loss of mobility (odds ratio [OR], 0.52; CL: 0.44-0.63; P < 0.001). Both weight loss and improved fitness (assessed on treadmill testing) were significant mediators of this effect (P < 0.001 for both variables). Those with the greatest initial disability had correspondingly less benefit. Provisional results of Look-AHEAD, were disappointing. The study had to be stopped because there was no emerging difference in the hard cardiovascular endpoints. See On-line update for details.

Drugs for weight loss. Few are approved and without danger. Current interest lies in the *naltrexone slow-release (SR)/bupropion SR combination* (Contrave). Bupropion has effects (μ-opioid receptor antagonist and catecholamine inhibitor) that lead to reduced energy intake and increased energy expenditure, whereas naltrexone may potentiate these effects. On June 2, 2011, the Food and Drug Administration (FDA) requested a large safety study of naltrexone before its approval, and the FDA plans an advisory committee for 2012 to discuss the need for cardiovascular safety of all obesity drugs.[28]

The following drugs have been turned down by the FDA:[28] In the *combined phentermine and topiramate* (PHEN/TPM), phentermine induces central norepinephrine release and promotes weight loss by reducing food intake. Topiramate has complex central effects and is approved for treatment of seizures and for migraine prophylaxis. Among the reasons for refusal were depression and cognitive-related complaints. *Lorcaserin* (Lorqess), is a novel serotonergic agent approved by the FDA in 2012, expected to have a reduced cardiac valve risk profile compared with earlier serotonergic agents, such as fenfluramin. However, neuropsychiatric and cognitive-related side effects occurred with approximately double the frequency in patients treated with lorcaserin. *Sibutramine* (Meridia) has sympathomimetic properties, acting centrally to block the neuronal uptake of norepinephrine and serotonin, as well as stimulating peripheral β3-adrenergic receptors to induce satiety, yet with notable increases in systolic and diastolic BP and heart rate. On October 8, 2010, the FDA asked for the voluntary withdrawal of sibutramine from the US market, a request with which Abbott, the maker of sibutramine, complied.

Orlistat is available over the counter in the USA, European Union, and Australia. The review committee of the European Medicines Agency (February 13-16 2012) evaluated the risk of liver injury with orlistat drugs, such as Xenical and Alli with the conclusion that the weight-loss drug's benefits outweigh the risks in patients with a BMI of more than 28 kg/m^2.[29]

DRUG-RELATED NEW DIABETES
Lam and Andrew, 2007

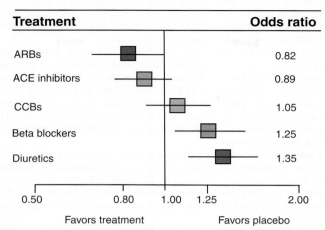

Figure 11-3   Drug-related new diabetes. Note protective effect of angiotensin receptor blockers (ARBs) and angiotensin-converting enzyme (ACE) inhibitors, and deleterious effects of β-blockers and diuretics. Network metaanalysis of 22 trials with 143,153 patients, using placebo as referent agent, and including earlier higher-dose diuretic trials. *CCB,* Calcium channel blocker. From Lam SKH, et al. Incident diabetes in clinical trials of antihypertensive drugs. *Lancet* 2007;369:1513.

Gastric surgery for weight loss. Although lacking long-term outcome studies, the impressive and often sustained weight loss after gastric bypass surgery seems to be one way to counter recalcitrant obesity for those who have failed in weight loss programs.[30] Further data are awaited.

Blood pressure and lifestyle. Modest BP elevation, a component of the MetSyn, is often associated with overweight and obesity. Loss of weight and exercise in the setting of intensive behavioral intervention in the MetSyn can reduce systolic BP in the range of 8 mm Hg with small additional reductions if the Dietary Approaches to Stop Hypertension diet is added.[31] However, in a parallel study, similar reductions in BP were not observed at 18 months.[32] When added drugs are required, β-blockers and diuretics should be considered second-line agents and avoided except when there are compelling indications. There is now growing but controversial evidence that new diabetes may develop during the therapy of hypertension, more so with β-blockers and diuretics than with angiotensin-converting enzyme (ACE) inhibitors and angiotensin receptor blockers (ARBs) (Fig. 11-3).[33-36] There is a "weight of evidence against β-blockers" as first choice for obese patients with hypertension.[37] A network metaanalysis linked diuretic and β-blocker therapy separately to new diabetes in hypertension (Fig. 11-3).[38] Thus current European Hypertension Guidelines counsel against initial use of a β-blocker in MetSyn.[39] Nebivolol may be an exception,[40] but lacks outcome studies. In view of the potential increased risk of new diabetes with β-blockers and diuretics in the therapy of hypertension, and as new diabetes is the major risk of the MetSyn, it seems prudent to give preference to antihypertensive therapy initially based on ACE inhibitors or ARBs, with low-dose diuretics (hydrochlorothiazide 12.5 to 25 mg) as needed (unless there are compelling indications for β-blocker–diuretic therapy).

Which drugs halt the slide to diabetes? *Metformin* 850 mg twice daily when given in the Diabetes Prevention Study[24] reduced future diabetes, albeit less than vigorous lifestyle changes. *Glitazones* increase hepatic and peripheral insulin sensitivity by activation of peroxisome proliferator–activated receptor–γ (PPAR-γ) receptors. Rosiglitazone helps limit the evolution of prediabetic state into overt diabetes.[41] However, rosiglitazone has the risk of precipitating heart failure or MI (see later). In the ACT NOW trial, pioglitazone, as compared with placebo, reduced the risk of conversion of impaired glucose tolerance to T2DM by 72%, but was associated with significant weight gain and edema.[42]

Acarbose inhibits the gastric absorption of glucose. Although often poorly tolerated because of gastrointestinal symptoms, it has well-documented reduction in MI and it reduces the incidence of new hypertension (RR reduction 34%).[43] *Rimonabant* is a selective central cannabinoid-1 receptor blocker, initially highly promising because it reduced body weight, triglyceride levels, glycemia, and increased HDL cholesterol.[44] However, psychiatric side effects have led to rejection by the FDA and other bodies.

Comparative choices. Because there have been no comparative studies between metformin, acarbose, and glitazones, it is difficult to say with certainty which would be most effective in preventing progression to new diabetes should lifestyle modifications prove inadequate. However, metformin and pioglitazone have convincing data.

What can be achieved? For lifestyle by itself to be effective in preventing transition to diabetes as well as reducing BP, major changes have to be effected, requiring intense input from professional personnel such as nutritionists and exercise physiologists. Although this intensive counseling may not be a cost-effective approach when applied to the general population, it is undeniable that the ideal strategy for the whole population is a broad behavior modification that avoids obesity. Drug therapy to prevent the transition to type 2 diabetes is both feasible and effective in selected patients, yet not widely applied.

Cardiovascular Control in Established Type 2 Diabetes

In general, control of BP and of blood lipids improves macrovascular disease and clinical outcome, whereas the control of glycemia limits microvascular disease (retina, kidneys, nerves). Both are important endpoints of effective therapy. Macrovascular disease predominates in type 2 diabetes.[45] However, with the increasing life expectancy of patients with type 2 diabetes, microvascular complications may well become increasingly prevalent. Of note, agents with equivalent glucose-lowering properties may be very different in their ability to improve cardiovascular outcomes.

Weight Loss

Intense lifestyle intervention aimed at a less calorie intake and more exercise over 1 year gave improved diabetic control and decreased cardiovascular risk factors such as BP and lipid profiles; mean hemoglobin A1c (HbA1c) dropped from 7.3% to 6.6%.[46]

Blood Pressure Control

In the prospective observational UKPDS 36 Study over a mean of 8.4 years, reduction of systolic pressure toward or even less than 120 mmHg, was associated with a decreased incidence of both macrovascular and microvascular events.[47] However, prospective data are required to validate outcomes at such low levels. In the ADVANCE study[48] the mean BP in high-risk diabetic patients in the placebo group (on existing treatment) was 140/77 mm Hg, and was further reduced to a mean of 137/75 mm Hg by the addition of an ACE inhibitor, perindopril, together with a diuretic, indapamide. Over the study period, the mean reduction of systolic pressure was 5.6 mm Hg systolic, whereas the diastolic fell by 2.2 mm Hg. Risk of death from cardiovascular disease fell by 18% (p = 0.03) and all-cause mortality by 14% (RR 0.86; CI 0.75-0.98, p = 0.03), in addition to strong trends toward reductions in macrovascular- and microvascular disease. Future trials will hopefully prospectively test the hypothesis that additional reduction of BP toward a target systolic BP of 120 mm Hg will yield greater reduction of microvascular and macrovascular events. In the meantime ADVANCE teaches us that greater reduction of BP can give mortality benefits.

Control of intraglomerular pressure. Third-generation dihydropyridine calcium channel blockers such as manidipine inhibit T-type calcium channels on vascular muscular cells such as those localized on postglomerular arterioles.[49] In the DEMAND study on 380 subjects for a mean of 3.8 years, combined manidipine and ACE-inhibitor therapy reduced both macrovascular events and albuminuria in hypertensive patients with T2DM, whereas the ACE inhibitor did not. Worsening of IR was almost fully prevented in those on combination therapy.

Statin Therapy: Impressive Overall Benefits

The benefits of adding atorvastatin 10 mg to diabetic therapy were shown in the CARDS study (see Chapter 10, p. 406). Entry criteria were type 2 diabetes and at least one other cardiovascular risk factor such as hypertension, smoking, or diabetic complications. Atorvastatin 10 mg daily taken by patients with type 2 diabetes reduced the low-density lipoprotein (LDL) cholesterol from a mean of approximately 118 mg/dL to approximately 72 mg/dL, as well as decreasing major cardiovascular events including, surprisingly, a reduction in stroke of 48%.[50] Although LDL levels remain the major indication for statins, there can be normal LDL cholesterol levels but small LDL particles. However, in practice the standard indices for statin therapy remain valid.[51]

Statin-induced diabetes. Goldfine states, "Statins may simply be unmasking disease in people who were likely to develop diabetes anyway"—those in older age, with high baseline fasting glucose levels, and other features of the MetSyn.[52] Although a large metaanalysis found a 9% increased risk for incident diabetes over a 4-year period, the risk with rosuvastatin was 18%, based on the results of JUPITER and two other clinical trials. Logically, the more powerful the statin, the greater the risk of diabetes.[53] The other metaanalysis compared intensive- with moderate-dose statin therapy in five studies on 32,752 persons without diabetes at baseline. The number needed to treat (NNT) annually to harm was 498 for new-onset diabetes versus a NNT of 155 for reduced cardiovascular events. Thus the approximate ratio of benefit to harm for high versus medium doses was approximately 3:1.[54]

Glycemic control: how tight? Selection of drugs from a large number of oral agents to obtain glycemic control or when to use insulin are decisions optimally made by close collaboration between diabetologists and cardiologists. As the blood glucose increases, so does cardiovascular risk and total mortality, as shown in the large DECODE Study in 29,714 persons over 11 years,[55] so that reduction of glycemia should be equally beneficial. In general, guidelines recommend an HbA1c level of less than 7,[56] largely on the basis of the UK series of studies.[57] German guidelines advise less than 6.5%. However, "the cardiovascular safety and efficacy of available glucose-lowering strategies remain to a large degree uncertain."[58] Thus there is an increasing need for trials with cardiovascular outcomes and mortality, reaching beyond glycemic control. One large study, ADVANCE, which aimed at intense glucose lowering by a regimen based on gliclazide, succeeded in reducing both cardiovascular events and glycated hemoglobin (HbA1c) from 7.5 to 6.53.[59] In patients with diabetes at high cardiovascular risk, perhaps similar to those that a cardiologist might see, the National Institutes of Health–supported Action to Control Cardiovascular Risk in Diabetes (ACCORD) study compared intense versus standard glycemic control. Mean HbA1c levels were 6.4% in the intense and 7.5% in the standard arms. Unexpectedly, mortality increased after 3.7 years yet without reducing major cardiovascular events as compared with standard therapy.[60] After termination of the intensive therapy, the target HbA1c level was eased to 7 to 7.9. Although reduced 5-year nonfatal MIs decreased, 5-year mortality increased. The ACCORD study researchers write, "Such a strategy cannot be recommended for high-risk patients with advanced type 2 diabetes."[61] Also, another prospective-randomized trial in patients with advanced type 2 diabetes (VADT) failed to demonstrate a significant benefit in terms of overall or cardiovascular mortality from lowering HbA1c to 6.9% in the intensive-therapy group versus 8.4% in the standard-therapy group.[62]

A high-quality metaanalysis assessed the effects of intensive glycemic versus conventional glycemic control on all-cause and cardiovascular mortality, microvascular complications, and severe hypoglycemia in patients with type 2 diabetes.[63] All-cause mortality was unchanged, nonfatal MI was reduced (RR 0.85; P = 0.004; 28,111 participants, eight trials), as was the composite microvascular outcome (RR 0.88, P = 0.01; 25,600 participants, three trials) and retinopathy (RR 0.80, P = 0.009; 10,793 participants, seven trials). However, strict statistical testing by trial sequential analyses showed insufficient evidence for any beneficial conclusions except that hypoglycemia increased by 30%.

The updated 2012 recommendation of the American Diabetes Association (ADA) and European Association for the Study of Diabetes (EASD) is to individualize treatment targets.[64] In older adults, often with comorbidities and vascular complications, less stringent control is advocated (e.g., 7.5%-8% HbA1c [59-64 mmol/mol]); nonetheless, the ideal goal remains less than 7 (<53 mmol/mol) to reduce microvascular disease.

The *bottom line* is that an HbA1c of 7% to 7.9% is often appropriate for cardiovascular patients, but consider less than 7% for younger, newly diagnosed patients.

Insulin. After failed oral therapy, insulin clearly is the remaining requirement, as in the current guidelines.[64] The major problem with insulin is that control hyperglycemia may be bought at the cost of hypoglycemia. The long-acting flat profile of new *degludec insulin* forms a deposit of soluble subcutaneous multihexamers from which insulin is slowly and continuously absorbed into the circulation, thus being "not a revolution but an evolution" of insulin therapy for type 1 and type 2 diabetes.[65] The often presumed increased risk of heart failure caused by fluid retention with insulin treatment has not been translated into a consistent increase in the rate of mortality or hospitalization for heart failure.[66] Overall, the paucity of well-controlled studies in this area do not allow any final conclusion about the potential effects of insulin therapy on patients with diabetes and heart failure.

Metformin. Singly or in combination, metformin is standard to promote glycemic control. Metformin reduces glucose production by the liver and increases glucose uptake by muscle by increasing glucose transporter–4 mediated glucose uptake (Fig. 11-4). Importantly, it also suppresses appetite and appears to be devoid of cardiovascular harm and may benefit when given to patients with diabetes and heart failure.[66] In the prolonged UKPDS study, metformin was the only drug to reduce diabetes-related and all-cause mortality.[45] Since then, it has been the first-line treatment in overweight patients with type 2 diabetes.

Metformin versus secretogogues. In a large UK general practice research database on 91,521 people with a mean follow up of 7.1 years, metformin had a favorable risk of mortality as compared with sulphonylureas.[67] In a German primary care study, sulfonylureas doubled the risk of hypoglycemia.[68]

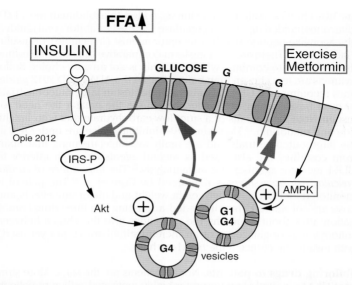

Figure 11-4 Site of action of metformin. Molecular steps leading from increased free fatty acid (FFA) to insulin resistance. Excess FFA entering the muscle cell is activated to long-chain acyl coenzyme A, which inhibits the insulin signaling pathway so that there is less translocation of glucose transporter vesicles (GLUT-4 and GLUT-1glucose) to the cell surface. Glucose uptake is decreased and hyperglycemia promoted. The increased uptake of FFA promotes lipid metabolites accumulation in various organs, including the heart and pancreas. Metformin and exercise, by stimulating adenosine monophosphate protein kinase (AMPK), promote the translocation of transport vesicles to the cell surface to promote glucose entry and to oppose insulin resistance. Protein kinase B, also called *Akt,* plays a key role. G, Glucose; *IRS-P,* insulin receptor substrate–phosphatidyl. (Modified from Opie LH. *Heart Physiology, from Cell to Circulation.* 4th ed. Philadelphia: Lippincott, Williams & Wilkins; 2004. p. 313.)

First stop, metformin? Of 11 quality guidelines, 7 favor metformin as the first-line agent.[69] Yet the guidelines, normally taking months or years to finalize, could not have taken into account the 2012 metaanalysis on 13 controlled trials that showed no evidence that metformin has any clear beneficial or harmful effect on all-cause mortality, nor on cardiovascular mortality or morbidity among patients with type 2 diabetes.[70] In yet another metaanalysis, when combined with insulin, metformin reduced HbA1c by 0.5% and weight gain by 1 kg, whereas the insulin dose fell by 5 U/day.[71] Of note, metformin remains the first agent recommended by the influential 2012 ADA-EASD guidelines[64] and remains the usual first choice in clinical practice.

Metformin and kidney disease. Metformin is renally excreted. Bearing in mind that moderate to severe renal disease with estimated glomerular filtration rate (eGFR) less than 60 mL/min occurs in 20%-30% of patients with T2DM, the dose of metformin must be reduced. Suggested cut-off eGFR values are the following: if more than 60, no problems; if 45-60, use but monitor renal function; if 30-45, don't start, and if already giving metformin, use with care, decrease dose, and repeat eGFR every 3 months; and if less than 30 don't use.[72] In the UK, the policy is less tight, allowing use of metformin with monitoring down to 30 mL/min (see reference 14 in Inzuchi et al., 2012[64]).

The *bottom line* is that ideal evidence-based first-line therapy is not yet established. In practice, metformin stays the standard for comparators.

Two or three drug combinations: 2012 guidelines. Starting with metformin, what comes next? *To achieve glycemic control,* 2012 guidelines recommend that after initiation of therapy with metformin, there are five choices: added sulfonylureas, added thiazolidinedione (TZD; glitazones), added dipeptidyl peptidase (DPP)–4 inhibitor (oral), added glucagon-like peptide (GLP)–1 receptor agonist (injectable), or insulin (Table 11-2).[73] There are few long-term comparative trials available; thus the best agent to combine with metformin is not an easy choice. Sulfonylureas are less chosen than before. Rather, the ADA-EASD 2012 guidelines recommend a GLP-1 agonist as under test in large outcome trials, or even basal insulin; the higher the HbA1c, the greater the need for insulin. Note the benefits of a strict low-carbohydrate diet with liraglutide and metformin.[74] However, DPP-4 inhibitors also are under test in the large outcome trials and are orally available, meaning that, apart from cost, they are also used as second agents although inferior to GLP-1 receptor agonists in a metaanalysis.[75] The *importance of cardiovascular risk assessment* is reinforced by Gore et al.[76] The patient is monitored for HbA1c, hypoglycemia, weight, and major side effects, and costs are considered. Then, if needed, advancing to a three-drug combination after about 3 months, the guidelines give the choice between sulfonylureas or glitazones or an incretin stimulator (if not yet used), with insulin the choice if the HbA1c is high.

Tailoring drugs to patients. Not all patients are the same. More stringent HbA1c control is proposed for highly motivated, adherent patients who are capable of self-care, often newly diagnosed, with long life expectancy and without established vascular complications (Fig. 1 in Inzucchi et al., 2012[64]). Self-management of type 2 diabetes, including avoidance of hypoglycemia, is complex, but the effect of cognition on safe self-management is not well understood. Poor *cognitive function* increases the risk of severe hypoglycemia in patients with type 2 diabetes.[77] Prospective cohort analysis of data from the ACCORD trial included 2956 adults aged 55 years and older with type 2 diabetes and additional cardiovascular risk factors.[78] After a median 3.25-year follow-up, a 5-point-poorer baseline score on the cognitive tests was predictive of a first episode of hypoglycemia requiring medical assistance. Cognitive decline over 20 months increased the risk of subsequent hypoglycemia to a greater extent in those with lower baseline cognitive function (P for interaction: 0.037).

Sulfonylureas. These are insulin secretagogues that stimulate insulin secretion act by inhibiting adenosine triphosphate (ATP)–sensitive potassium channels of β-cells. Because the sulphonylurea receptor SUR2a is also expressed on cardiomyocytes, it has long been held that these drugs might also interfere with cardiac function. Indeed, several smaller-scale clinical trials and experimental studies have suggested an impairment of ischemic preconditioning with sulphonylurea drugs.[79]

Besides these potential direct effects of sulphonylureas on cardiac and vascular functions, hypoglycemia, as commonly seen during sulphonylurea therapy, is associated with cardiac arrhythmias, thereby providing an additional potential mechanism linking these drugs to increased cardiovascular events.[80]

There are few prospective studies on the long-term major clinical effect of these agents on outcomes in type 2 diabetes. The UGDP study from the 1960s has initially suggested a high incidence of cardiovascular mortality in patients treated with the sulfonylurea agent tolbutamide.[81]

In contrast, the UKPD study revealed no significant effect of glibenclamide on either mortality or the incidence of cardiovascular events.[57]

There are few prospective studies on the long-term major clinical effect of these agents on outcomes in type 2 diabetes. Monotherapy with the most used agents, including glimepiride, glibenclamide, glipizide, and tolbutamide, was associated with increased mortality and cardiovascular risk compared with metformin in a large prospective registry trial.[82] Gliclazide and repaglinide were not statistically different from metformin in patients both without and with previous MI. A gliclazide modified release (MR)–based regimen together with BP lowering by perindopril-indapamide in 11,140 persons with type 2

Table 11-2

Choices in the Further Management of Hyperglycemia in Type 2 Obese Diabetic Already on Metformin

	Pioglitazone	Exenatide/Liraglutide	DPP-4 Agonists	Insulin
Mechanism	PPAR-γ ↑ Glucose metabolism ↑ Liver fat ↓	Incretin: insulin release ↑; glucagon ↓ Gastric emptying ↓	Prevent the rapid breakdown of endogenous GLP-1	Glucose metabolism ↑
Daily dose	15-45 mg	Weekly or daily injections	Oral	One or more daily injections
Advantages	**Versus Insulin:** Oral; Hypoglycemia ↓ Weight gain same HDL-C ↑	**Versus Insulin:** Weight loss; Glucose better; Less hypoglycemia CV protection under study in large trials	**Oral** Controls glycemia CV protection under study in large trials	**Versus Glitazones:** Lower cost **Versus Exenatide:** More injections No GI side effects **Injections** Hypoglycemia Weight gain
Disadvantages	Cost ↑ versus insulin Bone density ↓ Weight gain versus exenatide	Expensive Injections Side effects: Nausea; ?pancreatitis	**Oral Expensive** No weight loss	

CV, Cardiovascular; DPP, dipeptidyl peptidase; GI, gastrointestinal; GLP, glucagon-like peptide; HDL-C, high-density-lipoprotein cholesterol; PPAR-γ, peroxisome proliferator–activated receptor-γ.
Modified from Goldberg et al.[73]

HDL & TG IN METABOLIC SYNDROME & DIABETES
Opie 2012

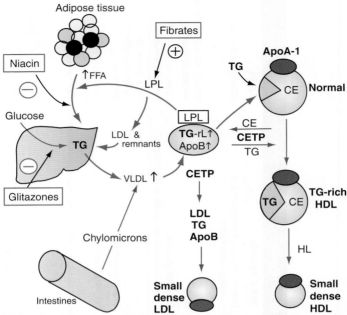

Figure 11-5 Proposed patterns of dyslipidemia in metabolic syndrome and type 2 diabetes. Consistent features (see *right side* of the figure) are the increased circulating levels of triglycerides (TGs) and decreased high-density lipoprotein (HDL) cholesterol. The basic problem lies in increased levels of the atherogenic particles: very-low density lipoproteins (VLDLs), triglyceride-rich lipoprotein (TG-rL) and apolipoprotein (Apo) B. (Apos have detergent-like properties that solubilize the hydrophobic lipoproteins.) Levels of TG-rL and Apo B are increased by (1) excess hepatic synthesis of VLDL, (2) high postprandial TG concentrations after a fatty meal, and (3) low levels of lipoprotein lipase activity. Adipose tissue releases excess free fatty acids (FFAs), which with hyperglycemia leads to increased hepatic production of VLDL. Cholesterol-ester transfer protein (CETP) increases the transfer of TG to HDL particles to form TG-rich HDL, with a simultaneous transfer of cholesteryl esters (CE) from the HDL particles to TG-rL. TG-rich HDL is broken down by hepatic lipase (HL) to form small, dense HDL particles. A similar process leads to increased formation of small dense low-density lipoprotein (LDL) particles. For further details see Syvanne and Taskinen, 1997. *LPL,* lipoprotein lipase. (Figure © L.H. Opie, 2012.)

diabetes reduced the risk of new or worsening nephropathy by 33%, new onset of macroalbuminuria by 54%, and of microalbuminuria by 26%, together with an 18% reduction in the risk of all-cause death.[83]

Thiazolidinediones. TZDs, also called the *glitazones,* are drugs that activate the PPAR-γ (gamma) transcriptional system, thereby promoting the metabolism of glucose. The main drugs are rosiglitazone, the first, but now suspended in Europe, and the safer pioglitazone.[84] The FDA restricted access to rosiglitazone in September 2010. Glitazones favorably increase HDL by 19%, potentially offsetting an LDL increase of 8%, while reducing triglycerides and glycemia (Fig. 11-5).[85] More specifically, pioglitazone reduced LDL-particle concentration, whereas rosiglitazone increased it.[86] Both drugs increased LDL-particle size with pioglitazone having the greater effect. Pioglitazone increased HDL particle size, decreased by rosiglitazone. Total LDL cholesterol rose more with rosiglitazone, whereas pioglitazone increased HDL levels much more than rosiglitazone.[87] Pioglitazone decreased fasting triglyceride, which was increased by rosiglitazone.[87] These changes help to explain

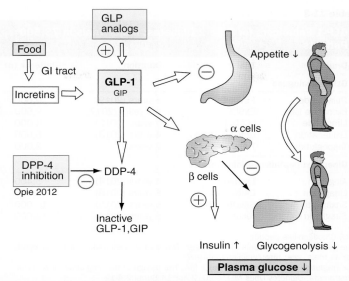

Figure 11-6 Site of action of incretins. *DPP,* Dipeptidyl peptidase; *GI,* gastro-intestinal; *GIP,* glucose-dependent insulinotropic polypeptide; *GLP,* glucagon-like peptide. (Figure © L.H. Opie, 2012.)

why rosiglitazone but not pioglitazone monotherapy was associated with increased MI[88,89] and mortality.[84] Pioglitazone has also improved clinical outcomes in type 2 diabetes in the PROactive study.[90] In the ACT NOW trial, pioglitazone, reduced the risk of conversion of impaired glucose tolerance to T2DM by 72%, but, and thereby lies the snag, was associated with significant weight gain and edema.[42] Overall, based on a General Practice Research Database (206,940 patients), higher risks for death (overall and caused by cardiovascular disease) and heart failure were found for rosiglitazone compared with pioglitazone. These excess risks were twofold for ages 65-74, threefold for 75-84, and sevenfold for older ages. The European regulatory decision to suspend rosiglitazone is supported by this study.[84]

The incretin system. This is the focus of major current attention. Major trials on 73,500 patients are underway. Incretins are gastrointestinal peptide hormones released during absorption of nutrients to augment insulin secretion. GLP-1 is a hormone secreted into the circulation by the intestinal L-cells in response to ingested food (Fig. 11-6). Besides acting on blood glucose, "targeting the incretin axis might address the elusive goal of an antidiabetic agent that improves cardiovascular disease."[91] The incretin response system is disturbed in T2DM. The incretin axis also includes the enzyme DPP-4, a serine protease that rapidly degrades GLP-1 and other proteins. Ultimately, this "arc of discovery" has led to new approved antidiabetic therapies: GLP-1 analogs (exenatide, liraglutide, and others) and DPP-4 inhibitors (saxagliptin, sitagliptin, and others).[91] More than 73,000 patients are in various trials (Table 11-3).

GLP-1–based therapies could potentially target both diabetes and cardiovascular disease.[92] They regulate glucose metabolism through multiple mechanisms and have beneficial cardiovascular effects, possibly independent of the glucose-lowering activity, which include changes in BP, endothelial function, body weight, cardiac metabolism, lipid metabolism, left ventricular function, atherosclerosis, and the response to ischemia-reperfusion injury.

Incretin mimetics. Incretin mimetics are GLP-1 receptor agonists. GLP-1 regulates glucose levels by stimulating glucose-dependent insulin secretion and biosynthesis, and by suppressing glucagon secretion, delayed gastric emptying and promoting satiety. In view of the somewhat

Table 11-3

GLP-1 Enhancers for Type 2 Diabetes: Major Trials in 73,500 Patients

Drug	Trial	Duration	Patients (n)
GLP-1 analogues			
Dulaglutide	REWIND	8 years (2019)	9,600
Exenatide LAR	EXSCEL	5.5 years (2017)	9,500
Liraglutide	LEADER	5 years (2016)	9,000
Lixisenatide	GetGoal-Mono	4 years (2013)	6,000
Taspoglutide	T emerge 8	2 years	2,000
Dipeptidyl peptidase-4 inhibitors			
Alogliptin	Examine	4 years (2014)	5,400
Linagliptin	CAROLINA	8 years (2018)	6,000
Saxagliptin	SAVOR-TIMI 53	5 years (2015)	12,000
Sitagliptin	Tecos	5 years (2014)	14,000

GLP, Glucagon-like peptide.
The generous help of Troels Munk Jensen, NovNordisk, Denmark, is acknowledged.
For all trials, see: http://clinicaltrials.gov/.
For liraglutide clinical trials, see Nauck MA. The design of the liraglutide clinical trial programme. *Diabetes Obes Metab* 2012 Apr;14 Suppl 2:4-12.
For lixisenatide in monotherapy, see Fonseca VA, et al. on behalf of the EFC6018 GetGoal-Mono Study Investigators. Efficacy and safety of the once-daily GLP-1 receptor agonist lixisenatide in monotherapy: a randomized, double-blind, placebo-controlled trial in patients with type 2 diabetes. *Diabetes Care* 2012 Mar 19.
For alogliptin versus pioglitazone, see Defronzo RA, et al. Efficacy and tolerability of the DPP-4 inhibitor alogliptin combined with pioglitazone, in metformin-treated patients with Type 2 Diabetes. *J Clin Endocrinol Metab* 2012 Mar 14.
For linagliptin, see Toth PP. Linagliptin: a new DPP-4 inhibitor for the treatment of type 2 diabetes mellitus. *Postgrad Med* 2011;123:46–53.
For saxagliptin, see Scirica BM, et al. The design and rationale of the saxagliptin assessment of vascular outcomes recorded in patients with diabetes mellitus-thrombolysis in myocardial infarction (SAVOR-TIMI) 53 study. *Am Heart J* 2011;162:818–25.

disappointing results of adding sulfonylureas (exception: gliclazide) to metformin and the risk for heart failure with the glitazones, attention is now shifting to combining metformin with incretin-based therapy.[93] This combination efficiently improves glycemia patients with type 2 diabetes, and within 16-30 weeks there is a more pronounced reduction in HbA1c with long-acting GLP-1 receptor agonists (liraglutide and exenatide long-acting release) than with DPP-4 inhibitors, both with a very low risk of adverse events, including hypoglycemia.

The Cochrane analysis reported that GLP-1 agonists in use or in the licensing process include exenatide and liraglutide as the most extensively studied, the others being albiglutide, dulaglutide, lixisenatide, and taspoglutide.[94] In comparison with placebo, all GLP-1 agonists reduced glycosylated HbA1c levels by approximately 1%. Both exenatide and liraglutide led to greater weight loss than most active comparators. Vagal-induced nausea, which can be regarded as an exaggerated form of appetite suppression, is a relatively common side effect of the GLP-1 agonists. These adverse events were strongest at the beginning and then subsided. β-cell function was improved with GLP-1 agonists, but the effect did not persist after treatment stopped. Exenatide 2 mg once weekly and liraglutide 1.8 mg reduced HbA1c by 0.20% and 0.24% respectively more than insulin glargine. Major outcome trials are still in the offing (see Table 11-3).

Assessment of incretin-based drugs. Incretin-based drugs seem to offer several benefits in terms of improving cardiovascular risk factors. Thus in addition to reducing hyperglycaemia, the GLP-1 receptor agonists and DPP-4 inhibitors are associated with moderate reductions in BP and some reduction in triglyceride levels.[95]

Furthermore, body weight is typically lowered during GLP-1 receptor agonist treatment. On the other hand, a consistent trend toward a higher pulse rate (approximatley 4-6 beats per minute) has been seen with liraglutide[96] and exenatide-LAR.[97] Increased heart rate might require readjustment of antianginal drugs, but there are no clinical studies on this issue.

This increase in heart rate is less obvious with the DPP-4 inhibitors. Several smaller-scale studies have also suggested improvements in endothelial function in patients with type 2 diabetes and coronary disease,[98] and in those with class III/IV heart failure.[99]

Exenatide. Exenatide *(Bydureon)* is a degradation-resistant GLP-1 pep- tide analog (incretin mimetic) that reduces HbA1c as well as produc- ing moderate weight loss and is given by injection. The FDA has ap- proved a once-weekly extended-release formulation as an adjunct to diet and exercise to improve glycemic control in adults with type 2 diabetes. There is a boxed warning on the possible risk of medullary thyroid carcinoma (MTC) as found in animal studies, and the FDA required a 15-year registry on this and other risks such as acute pancre- atitis. The boxed warning also states that the drug is contraindicated in patients with a personal or family history of MTC and in patients with multiple endocrine neoplasia syndrome type 2.

Exenatide 2 mg once weekly reduced HbA1c more than exenatide 10 mcg twice daily, sitagliptin, and pioglitazone.[94] In the DURATION-2 trial, 514 patients receiving metformin were randomized to receive 2 mg exenatide injected once weekly; 100 mg oral sitagliptin once daily; or 45 mg oral pioglitazone once daily.[100] After 26 weeks, addition of exenatide once weekly to metformin achieved the goal of optimum glucose control plus weight loss and with minimal hypoglycemic epi- sodes more often than did addition of maximum daily doses of either sitagliptin or pioglitazone. Hypoglycemia is uncommon except when combined with sulfonylureas (but not with metformin). Exanitide is also cardioprotective by decreasing reperfusion-induced cell death.[101] It decreased final infarct size by 30% only in patients within a short delay of 132 minutes or less from symptom onset to reperfusion. How- ever, this finding must be confirmed in larger studies.

Liraglutide. Liraglutide *(Victoza)* is another incretin mimetic given once a day that also reduces HbA1c with weight loss. Liraglutide is an effective GLP-1 agent to add to metformin, superior to sitagliptin for reduction of HbA1c, and well tolerated with minimum risk of hypogly- cemia.[96] It is approved by the FDA in combination with metformin for adults with type 2 diabetes who require more than one medication to lower blood glucose. There are similar FDA warnings and postmar- keting cancer registry requirements to those on exenatide regarding the possible risk of MTC and its implications. Pancreatitis also occurred more often, although still rarely in patients given liraglutide than with other antidiabetic medications, so that it should be stopped if there is severe abdominal pain. The most common side effects observed with liraglutide have been headache, nausea, and diarrhea.

A small but important proof-of-concept study tested the effect of dietary carbohydrate restriction in conjunction with liraglutide and metformin on metabolic control in patients with type 2 diabetes.[74] Insulin or oral antidiabetic drugs (excluding metformin) were stopped. After 6 months of liraglutide and metformin, body weight fell by 10% and HbA1c fell from 9% to 6.7%. Longer-term and larger outcome studies would cement this approach.

Dipeptidyl peptidase–4 inhibitors. DPP-4 inhibitors are chemically –derived, selective, competitive inhibitors of DPP-4 and can be adminis- tered orally. Of note, not only GLP-1, but also other potentially important peptides, such as glucose-dependent insulinotropic polypeptide (GIP), B-type natriuretic peptide, neuropeptide Y, peptide YY, and so on, are subject to DPP-4 cleavage, thereby suggesting that the metabolic and cardiovascular effects of the DPP-4 inhibitors might not be exclusively mediated via GLP-1. As a second-line treatment, DPP-4 inhibitors were inferior to GLP-1 agonists and similar to pioglitazone in reducing HbA1c, and had no advantage over sulfonylureas in a metaanalysis.[75] As a group, they are well tolerated as found in a review of 45 clinical trials, and rates of weight gain, gastrointestinal adverse effects, and hypoglycemia were minimal.[102] They counteract the degradation of plasma GLP-1 and GIP after eating. Like GLP-I agonists, these agents have antidiabetic activity by stimulating the release of insulin from the pancreas and by inhibiting that of glucagon. However, they differ from the GLP-I agonists in that there are few gastrointestinal side effects such as nausea and no marked inhibition of gastric emptying. Also in contrast to GLP-1 agonists they are weight neutral rather than promoting weight loss.[75,103,104] Furthermore, insulin secretion decreases if the plasma concentration falls to less than 70 mg/dL, thus lessening the risk of hypoglycemia.

Trial data. Typically, in randomized clinical trials, DPP-4 inhibitors achieved HbA1c reduction from 0.6% to 0.9% and, so far, have shown an optimal safety profile, not being associated with serious adverse effects. Importantly, the incidence of hypoglycemia in DPP-4 inhibitor–treated patients in clinical trials was similar to placebo and thus significantly lower than with other insulin-secretagogues, such as sulphonylureas and meglitinides. For these reasons, and for ease of oral administration, DPP-4 inhibitors are increasingly used in the treatment of type 2 diabetes.[105] Nasopharyngitis was more prevalent with the DPP-4 inhibitors than with placebo, but rates of pancreatitis were lower than with other oral antihyperglycemic agents.[102] Besides the control of glycemia, in experimental models of ischemia and reperfusion injury, GLP-1 is cardioprotective and reduces myocyte death.[106]

Currently, most DPP-4 inhibitors have been approved for the combination with insulin as well as for monotherapy in Europe.

Alogliptin given to type 2 diabetic patients inadequately controlled by metformin, in doses of 12.5 and 25 mg daily combined with pioglitazone, gave additive reduction in HbA1c and improved measures of β-cell function.[107] Thus far it is not FDA approved.

Linagliptin has a unique xanthine-based structure that experientially promotes wound healing and thus should benefit diabetic ulceration.[108] It was FDA approved in May 2011. A new treatment option, also FDA approved, combines linagliptin and metformin in a single tablet taken twice daily in adults with type 2 diabetes who require more than one medication to lower blood glucose. Phase 3 clinical trials on more than 4000 patients have demonstrated the efficacy of linagliptin as monotherapy or in combination with other antidiabetic agents.[109]

Saxagliptin is approved by the FDA and by the European Union for use as monotherapy or in combination regimens for the treatment of T2DM. It is the drug chosen (5 mg daily, 2.5 mg in moderate or severe renal impairment) by the TIMI Harvard-based group for the SAVOR-TIMI 53 outcome study that aims to examine cardiovascular complications.[106] The trial will continue until approximately 1040 primary endpoints accrue, providing 85% power to identify a 17% relative reduction of the primary cardiovascular endpoints.

Sitagliptin is licensed in the United States for use with diet and exercise to control glycemia alone or with metformin, glitazones, or sulfonylureas. It also exerts direct, DPP-4–independent effects on intestinal L-cells, activating cyclic adenosine monophosphate (AMP) and extracellular signal-regulating kinase 1 and 2 (ERK1/2) signaling and stimulating total GLP-1 secretion.[110]

Vildagliptin is available in combination with metformin. It is registered for use in the European Union but not in the United States. Vildagliptin add-on (50 mg twice daily) had similar efficacy to glimepiride (up to 6 mg/day) in reducing HbA1c levels after 2 years' treatment, with markedly reduced hypoglycemia risk and no weight gain.[111]

Meglitinide analogs. Meglitinide analogs such as *repaglinide* and *nateglinide* act on the pancreatic β-cells where, similarly to the sulfonylureas, they regulate ATP-dependent potassium channels to induce insulin secretion.[112] These agents affect chiefly early insulin release, reducing postprandial hyperglycemia, whereas the sulfonylureas improve late insulin release to act more on the fasting glucose level. Repaglinide has an FDA license rather similar to that of sitagliptin. The ability of these short-acting insulin secretagogues to reduce the risk of diabetes or cardiovascular events in people with impaired glucose tolerance remains unknown. There are few outcome studies. Nateglinide up to 60 mg thrice daily for 5 years did not reduce the incidence of diabetes or the co-primary composite cardiovascular outcomes in those with impaired glucose tolerance.[113]

Bromocriptine. Bromocriptine acts on the hypothalamus of the brain as a dopamine D2 receptor agonist. It is the first of its class of agents approved by the FDA that acts at the level of the brain. Bromocriptine-QR provides a short-duration dopamine pulse to brain centers that regulate peripheral fuel metabolism. It is administered in the morning, within 2 hours of waking, to increase central dopaminergic tone at that time of day when that tone normally peaks in healthy but not in diabetic persons, thereby improving glycemic control and lessening postprandial hyperglycemia that is thought to be an independent risk factor for macrovascular and microvascular complications.[114]

Sodium-glucose cotransporter-2 inhibition (Fig. 11-7). In patients with type 2 diabetes inadequately controlled with metformin monotherapy, dapagliflozin was compared with glipizide.[115] Despite similar 52-week glycemic efficacy, dapagliflozin reduced weight and produced less hypoglycemia. In patients with type 2 diabetes inadequately controlled on pioglitazone, the addition of dapagliflozin further reduced

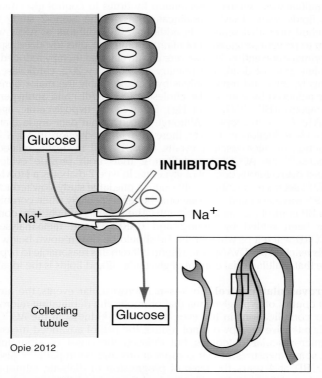

Figure 11-7   Site of action of inhibitors of glucose reuptake. These agents, not yet widely available for clinical use, inhibit the reuptake of glucose by sodium-glucose exchange in the collecting tubule. (Figure © L.H. Opie, 2012.)

HbA1c levels and mitigated the pioglitazone-related weight gain without increasing the risk of hypoglycemia.[116] A side effect in both studies was that genital infection increased.

Ideal Control of Glycemia, Blood Pressure, and Lipids: Multifactorial Intervention

The ACCORD studies. The ACCORD trials examined whether ultraintense cardiovascular risk-factor reduction could improve clinical outcomes. To improve on the impressive baseline control of risk factors in the patients assigned to standard therapy in ACCORD was a formidable task, illustrating the synergistic effects of the multifactorial risk-reduction regimen. The respective intense arms achieved a more than 1% absolute difference in HbA1c, a 14.2-mm Hg lower systolic pressure, and plasma triglycerides of approximately 145 mg/dL. For each of the three separate questions, further reduction of BP or glycemia or triglycerides, despite the more intense therapies, the primary clinical composite was not significantly reduced, as assessed in a *Circulation* editorial.[117]

Hypoglycemia. Avoiding hypoglycemia and its possible cerebral effects is a major aim in vigorous glycemic control. Less often appreciated is that preexisting cognitive impairment can predispose to hypoglycemia, because poor cognitive function increases the risk of severe hypoglycemia in patients with type 2 diabetes. Clinicians should consider the cognitive function of their patients in assessing whether safe diabetes self-management is realistically possible.[118,119]

As control of BP and of blood lipids independently reduce major events and mortality in those with type 2 diabetes, a logical aim would be multifactorial intense intervention by drugs to control glycemia, BP, and lipids, with lifestyle modification, as in the Steno-2 study that stretched over 13.3 years.[120] In addition, ACE inhibitors or ARBs were given to prevent progression of microalbuminuria, plus low-dose aspirin for primary prevention. Intense versus conventional therapy reduced the absolute risks of death, the primary endpoint, by 20%, cardiovascular events by 29%, and renal dialysis by 6.3%. Probably the major benefits were achieved by statins (LDL cholesterol 83 mg/dL) and antihypertensive agents (BP 131/73 mm Hg), followed by hypoglycemic agents (HbA1c 7.9%) and aspirin. Although observational data argue that for each 1% reduction in HbA1c, there is a 14% reduction in MI, a 37% reduction in microvascular events, and 21% fall in deaths related to diabetes,[121] the ACCORD and Steno-2 trials both provide evidence against overvigorous control of glycemia. In type 2 diabetes, a HbA1c of 7%-7.9% seems reasonable,[122] although in one large study slow reduction to 6.9% was associated with outcome benefit especially when combined with BP control (see next paragraph). The benefits of tight LDL control have been settled by Steno-2 and CARDS[123] and metaanalyses.[124] ACCORD will tell us whether the BP should be driven down below the levels reached in ADVANCE and Steno-2. It remains reasonable to hypothesize that multifactorial control of glycemia, BP, and lipids is the ideal.

Microvascular control. To lessen microvascular events, the aim is tight control of hyperglycemia that promotes the debilitating microvascular complications in the eyes, nerves, and kidneys. In the ACCORD study, intensive therapy did not reduce the risk of advanced measures of microvascular outcomes, but delayed the onset of albuminuria and some measures of eye complications and neuropathy.[125] Also in ACCORD, at 4 years, the rates of progression of diabetic retinopathy was slowed from 10.4% with standard therapy to 7.3% with intensive glycemia treatment (OR, 0.67; P = 0.003) with a similar decrease with fenofibrate for intensive dyslipidemia therapy.[126]

Macro- and microvascular control. Both macro- and microevents were the targets in BP lowering and intensive glucose control in patients with long-standing type 2 diabetes.[127] Therapy was perindopril-indapamide and a gliclazide MR–based regimen (with target HbA1c < or = 6.5%) in 11,140 participants with type 2 diabetes. Combination treatment by routine BP lowering and intensive glucose control on macrovascular and microvascular outcomes in patients with type 2 diabetes reduced the risk of new or worsening nephropathy by 33% (CI 12-50%, P = 0.005), new onset of macroalbuminuria by 54% (35%-68%, P < 0.0001), and new onset of microalbuminuria by 26% (17%-34%). Combination treatment was associated with an 18% reduction in the risk of all-cause death (P = 0.04). Of note, this degree of control was achieved over 4.3 years of follow up, whereas the disastrous sudden drop of HbA1c in ACCORD was over weeks and months.

Diabetes and Coronary Disease Requiring Intervention

Regarding prevention, as already discussed, the emphasis must be on tight control of BP and blood lipids. Although generally recommended, one study suggests that low-dose aspirin may be less effective than expected.[128] Regarding percutaneous coronary interventions (PCI), observational and cohort studies suggest that diabetes is a risk factor for stent thrombosis, especially among patients with multivessel disease and complex lesions.[129] In patients with diabetes and multivessel coronary disease, PCI with drug-eluting stents was less effective than coronary artery bypass graft (CABG),[130] and among randomized patients, balloon angioplasty was inferior to CABG when an arterial conduit was used.[131]

Acute MI poses special problems for the diabetic patient. Tight glycemic control has been recommended either by insulin low-dose glucose[132] or by oral agents.[133] The IMMEDIATE trial, which started glucose-insulin-potassium (GIK) in the ambulance with positive outcome data, suggests that the GIK regimen gives specific protection to patients without diabetes by decreasing infarct size.[134]

Diabetes and Heart Failure

Revival of the fatty heart concept. Atherogenic lifestyle may eventually evoke a fatty heart as follows.[135] Excessive adipose tissue, associated with less exercise and excess calories, leads to increased blood levels of FFAs, which waste myocardial oxygen[136] and may also be deposited in the heart of overweight subjects as triglyceride.[137] Cardiomyocyte fat, now measured by magnetic resonance spectroscopy, correlates well with BMI and is increased even in uncomplicated obesity. It is associated with impaired diastolic filling in apparently asymptomatic obese subjects and is more severe in the presence of glucose intolerance or diabetes.[135] Supporting the lipid-heart link, a marked increase in plasma FFA and in myocardial triglyceride after only 3 days of a very-low-calorie diet was associated with decreased diastolic function.[138]

Myocardial steatosis. Metabolically, in humans with heart failure there is increased myocardial triglyceride.[139] Thus overall data support the existence of a diabetic cardiomyopathy with diastolic heart failure in type 2 diabetes. The origin is multifactorial, with contributions from hypertension and coronary disease. Whenever heart failure is established, then the adrenergic–fatty acid load is likely to worsen the situation, therefore arguing for therapy by β-blockade added to BP control.[140] In contrast, in type 1 diabetes the influence of hypertension and coronary disease is very much less, so that there is a "pure" metabolic cardiomyopathy resulting from the increased blood fatty acids in poorly controlled diabetes,[141] leading to increased myocardial uptake of toxic FFAs, mitochondrial oxygen wastage, and increasing risk of systolic heart failure. Here tight diabetes control should be protective.[139]

Prevention of heart failure? Can tight glycemic control prevent later heart failure in type 2 diabetes? No, says a 37,229 patient analysis.[142] Furthermore, intensive glycemic control with TZDs increased the risk of heart failure. More surprisingly, and inexplicably, in a small cohort with very advanced heart failure and diabetes, a higher HbA1c seemed to be associated with better outcomes protective.[143]

Glitazones and heart failure. A series of metaanalyses,[66,89,144-147] have confirmed a higher incidence of congestive heart failure (CHF), a previously known major side effect of glitazones.[90] In ADOPT rosiglitazone was associated with more cardiovascular events, specifically heart failure, and bone fractures than glyburide, the sulfonylurea,[148] and with more heart failure than pioglitazone.[84] A proposed mechanism of the CHF is that PPAR-γ acts on the distal nephron to promote sodium and fluid retention,[149] which in the presence of lipid-induced incipient diastolic heart failure,[137] precipitates CHF.[144] This issue has caused widespread concern, which led the FDA to insert a black box warning about heart failure for the glitazones.

Glitazones and myocardial infarction. The Nissen and Singh metaanalyses,[89,147] focusing on rosiglitazone, also found significantly increased MI. By contrast, pioglitazone (Actos) although found to increase CHF, was associated with decreased mortality, MI, and stroke.[85,145] A large Canadian case-control retrospective cohort study on an entire population of older adults with diabetes, confirmed that rosiglitazone but not pioglitazone monotherapy increased heart failure and MI.[88] Similarly, in a large UK general practice research database on 91,521 people with a mean follow up of 7.1 years, pioglitazone was associated with reduced all-cause mortality compared with metformin and with rosiglitazone.[67] The increased MI with rosiglitazone in these studies may be related to the changes in the lipid profile previously reviewed.[73,86] Of 11 quality guidelines, 10 agreed that TZDs as a group are associated with higher rates of edema and CHF compared with other oral medications to treat type 2 diabetes.[69] In a trial on 224 type 2 diabetic patients with class I or II heart failure, rosiglitazone improved glycemic control without adversely affecting left ventricular function despite more fluid-related events (dyspnea, edema).[150]

SUMMARY

1. *MetSyn*. The MetSyn is rapidly increasing in incidence worldwide. It conveys increased risk for type 2 diabetes and for cardiovascular disease. To prevent the transition to these two entities, the ideal therapy is intensive lifestyle modification. Failing that, metformin and, when indicated, other medications to control hypertension and dyslipidemia should be considered. In view of the known increased risk of new diabetes with β-blockers and diuretics in the therapy of hypertension, and because new diabetes is the major risk of the MetSyn, it seems prudent to give preference to antihypertensive therapy initially based on ACE inhibitors or ARBs, either with low-dose diuretics as needed (unless there are compelling indications for β-blocker–diuretic therapy).

2. *Cardiovascular disease*. In established type 2 diabetes there is increased risk of vascular disease with coronary and cerebral complications. The key to prevention lies in tight BP and lipid control. The role of very tight glycemic control is not as well established and argued against by the cessation of this arm of ACCORD.

Furthermore, the cardiovascular advantages of weight loss and the antidiabetic drugs that promote weight loss must be emphasized.

3. *Multivessel coronary artery disease.* Multivessel coronary artery disease in type 2 diabetics often needs assessment for intervention. Among patients with multivessel disease and complex lesions, PCI is less successful than in nondiabetics and there is a stronger case for CABG using an arterial conduit.

4. *Glycemic control.* To achieve glycemic control, 2012 guidelines suggest starting off with metformin, followed by one of five add-on choices: sulfonylureas, TZDs (glitazones), DPP-4 inhibitors, GLP-1 receptor agonists, or insulin. Sulfonylureas are less favored than previously. However, there are few long-term comparative trials; thus the best agent to combine with metformin is not an easy choice. Of the add-ons, the 2012 guidelines recommend a GLP-1 agonist or insulin; the higher the HbA1c, the greater the need for insulin. Advancing to the third agent, any one of the five not yet used could follow, but insulin is often preferred.

5. *TZDs (glitazones).* TZDs improve insulin sensitivity at the cost of side effects: weight gain, edema, bone fractures, and heart failure. Nonetheless, they are among the five guideline choices to follow metformin. Whereas pioglitazone is associated with improved lipid profiles, rosiglitazone has the reverse effects so that its use is now being restricted. The proposed mechanism for heart failure is fluid retention added to diabetic diastolic heart failure caused by lipid overload. The current proposal that excess adiposity tissue can lead to clinical heart failure requires further study, including validation of effective treatment strategies.

6. *Agents acting on the incretin system.* This is an extremely active area of investigation, with approximately 73,500 patients currently in nine mega trials. *GLP-1* is a natural incretin postprandial hormone that is secreted by the gut in response to a meal. It stimulates insulin release from the pancreas. These therapeutic effects can be magnified by inhibiting its breakdown by DPP-4 inhibitors or by agonists acting on the pancreatic receptor (exenatide, liraglutide, and others). In patients with difficult to control type 2 diabetes who are already on metformin or other oral hypoglycemics, these agents when added have advantages over insulin. In view of better weight and lipid control than with sulfonylureas, and less risk of heart failure than with the glitazones, a current trend is to use exenatide or liraglutide after lifestyle and metformin. A once-weekly formulation of exenatide has FDA approval.

7. *How tight to control?* Observational studies have suggested reductions of diabetic complications, both microvascular and macrovascular, by tight control of glycemia and of BP, with outcome studies arguing for tight LDL cholesterol lowering. ACCORD argues against very tight HbA1c control, at least in established patients with diabetes at high cardiovascular risk. Decreased BP less than 140/90 mm Hg is argued for by two outcome trials (ADVANCE, Steno-2) but ultratight BP control gave no outcome benefit in ACCORD. Guidelines strongly suggest tight control for younger patients at the onset of their disease, to prevent microvascular complications. Overall, multifactorial intervention remains the ideal.

Acknowledgments

We gratefully acknowledge the help and expertise of John M. Miles, MD, Mayo Clinic.

References

1. Bergenstal RM, et al. for the DURATION-2 Study Group. Efficacy and safety of exenatide once weekly versus sitagliptin or pioglitazone as an adjunct to metformin for treatment of type 2 diabetes (DURATION-2): a randomised trial. *Lancet* 2010;376:431–439.
2. Flegal KM, et al. Cause-specific excess deaths associated with underweight, overweight, and obesity. *JAMA* 2007;298:2028–2037.
3. Haffner SM, et al. Mortality from coronary heart disease in subjects with type 2 diabetes and in nondiabetic subjects with and without prior myocardial infarction. *N Engl J Med* 1998;339:229–234.
4. Grundy SM, et al. Definition of metabolic syndrome: report of the National Heart, Lung, and Blood Institute/American Heart Association conference on scientific issues related to definition. *Circulation* 2004;109:433–438.
5. Grundy SM, et al. Diagnosis and management of the metabolic syndrome: an American Heart Association/National Heart, Lung, and Blood Institute Scientific Statement. *Circulation* 2005;112:2735–2752.
6. Alberti KG, et al. The metabolic syndrome—a new worldwide definition. *Lancet* 2005;366:1059–1062.
7. Ferrannini E, et al., RISC Investigators. Insulin resistance, insulin response, and obesity as indicators of metabolic risk. *J Clin Endocrinol Metab* 2007;92:2885–2892.
8. Yusuf S, et al., on behalf of the INTERHEART Study Investigators. Obesity and the risk of myocardial infarction in 27,000 participants from 52 countries: a case-control study. *Lancet* 2005;366:1640–1649.
9. Belfort R, et al. Dose-response effect of elevated plasma free fatty acid on insulin signaling. *Diabetes* 2005;54:1640–1648.
10. Miles JM, et al. Counterpoint: visceral adiposity is not causally related to insulin resistance. *Diabetes Care* 2005;28:2326–2328.
11. Balkau B, et al. International Day for the Evaluation of Abdominal Obesity (IDEA): a study of waist circumference, cardiovascular disease, and diabetes mellitus in 168,000 primary care patients in 63 countries. *Circulation* 2007;116:1942–1951.
12. Kahn R, et al. The metabolic syndrome: time for a critical appraisal. Joint statement from the American Diabetes Association and the European Association for the Study of Diabetes. *Diabetologia* 2005;48:1684–1699.
13. Mancia G, et al. Metabolic syndrome in the Pressioni Arteriose Monitorate E Loro Associazioni (PAMELA) study: daily life blood pressure, cardiac damage, and prognosis. *Hypertension* 2007;49:40–47.
14. Malik S, et al. Impact of the metabolic syndrome on mortality from coronary heart disease, cardiovascular disease, and all causes in United States adults. *Circulation* 2004;110:1245–1250.
15. Sattar N, et al. Metabolic syndrome with and without C-reactive protein as a predictor of coronary heart disease and diabetes in the West of Scotland Coronary Prevention Study. *Circulation* 2003;108:414–419.
16. Gami AS, et al. Metabolic syndrome and risk of incident cardiovascular events and death: a systematic review and meta-analysis of longitudinal studies. *J Am Coll Cardiol* 2007;49:403–414.
17. Zeyda M, et al. Obesity, inflammation, and insulin resistance—a mini-review. *Gerontology* 2009;55:379–386.
18. Würtz P, et al. Metabolic signatures of insulin resistance in 7,098 young adults. *Diabetes* 2012;61:1372–1380.
19. Kim JK. Endothelial nuclear factor κB in obesity and aging: is endothelial nuclear factor κB a master regulator of inflammation and insulin resistance? *Circulation* 2012;125:1081–1083.
20. Yi CX, et al. Exercise protects against high-fat diet-induced hypothalamic inflammation. *Physiol Behav* 2012;106:485–490.
21. Hundal RS, et al. Mechanism by which high-dose aspirin improves glucose metabolism in type 2 diabetes. *J Clin Invest* 2002;109:1321–1326.
22. Johnson JL, et al. Exercise training amount and intensity effects on metabolic syndrome (from Studies of a Targeted Risk Reduction Intervention through Defined Exercise). *Am J Cardiol* 2007;100:1759–1766.
23. Tuomilehto J, et al. Prevention of type-2 diabetes mellitus by changes in lifestyle among subjects with impaired glucose tolerance. *N Engl J Med* 2001;344:1343–1350.
24. Diabetes Prevention Program Research Group. Reduction in the incidence of type 2 diabetes with lifestyle intervention and metformin. *N Engl J Med* 2002;346–393.
25. Wadden TA, et al. Lifestyle modification for obesity: new developments in diet, physical activity, and behavior therapy. *Circulation* 2012;125:1157–1170.
26. Appel LJ, et al. Comparative effectiveness of weight-loss interventions in clinical practice. *N Engl J Med* 2011;365:1959–1968.
27. Rejeski WJ, et al., Look AHEAD Research Group. Lifestyle change and mobility in obese adults with type 2 diabetes. *N Engl J Med* 2012;366:1209–1217.
28. Hiatt WR, et al. What cost weight loss? *Circulation* 2012;125:1171–1177.
29. *www.ema.europa.eu/ema/index.jsp?curl=pages/.../**Orlistat**/...jsp*
30. Zimmet P, et al. Surgery or medical therapy for obese patients with type 2 diabetes? *N Engl J Med* 2012;366:1635–1636.
31. Lien LF, et al. Effects of PREMIER lifestyle modifications on participants with and without the metabolic syndrome. *Hypertension* 2007;50:609–616.
32. Elmer PJ, et al. Effects of comprehensive lifestyle modification on diet, weight, physical fitness, and blood pressure control: 18-month results of a randomized trial. *Ann Intern Med* 2006;144:485–495.

33. Dahlöf B, et al. Prevention of cardiovascular events with an antihypertensive regimen of amlodipine adding perindopril as required versus atenolol adding bendroflumethiazide as required, in the Anglo-Scandinavian Cardiac Outcomes Trial-Blood Pressure Lowering Arm (ASCOT-BPLA): a multicentre randomised controlled trial. *Lancet* 2005;366:895–906.

34. Mason JM, et al. The diabetogenic potential of thiazide-type diuretic and beta-blocker combinations in patients with hypertension. *J Hypertens* 2005;23:1777–1781.

35. Opie LH, et al. Old antihypertensives and new diabetes. *J Hypertens* 2004;22:1453–1458.

36. Zanchetti A, et al. Prevalence and incidence of the metabolic syndrome in the European Lacidipine Study on Atherosclerosis (ELSA) and its relation with carotid intima-media thickness. *J Hypertens* 2007;25:2463–2470.

37. Williams B. The obese hypertensive: the weight of evidence against beta-blockers. *Circulation* 2007;115:1973–1974.

38. Lam SK, et al. Incident diabetes in clinical trials of antihypertensive drugs. *Lancet* 2007;369:1513–1514; author reply 1514–1515.

39. Mancia G, et al. 2007 guidelines for the management of arterial hypertension: The Task Force for the Management of Arterial Hypertension of the European Society of Hypertension (ESH) and of the European Society of Cardiology (ESC). *J Hypertens* 2007;25:1105–1187.

40. Kaiser T, et al. Influence of nebivolol and enalapril on metabolic parameters and arterial stiffness in hypertensive type 2 diabetic patients. *J Hypertens* 2006;24:1397–1403.

41. DREAM Trial Investigators, Gerstein HC, et al. (Diabetes REduction Assessment with ramipril and rosiglitazone Medication). Effect of rosiglitazone on the frequency of diabetes in patients with impaired glucose tolerance or impaired fasting glucose: a randomised controlled trial. *Lancet* 2006;368:1096–1105.

42. DeFronzo RA, et al. ACT NOW Study. Pioglitazone for diabetes prevention in impaired glucose tolerance. *N Engl J Med* 2011;364:1104–1115.

43. Chiasson JL, et al. Acarbose treatment and the risk of cardiovascular disease and hypertension in patients with impaired glucose tolerance: the STOP-NIDDM trial. *JAMA* 2003;290:486–494.

44. Despres JP, et al. Effects of rimonabant on metabolic risk factors in overweight patients with dyslipidemia. *N Engl J Med* 2005;353:2121–2134.

45. UKPDS 34. UK Prospective Diabetes Study Group. Effect of intensive blood-glucose control with metformin on complications in overweight patients with type 2 diabetes. *Lancet* 1998;352:854–865.

46. Pi-Sunyer X, et al. Reduction in weight and cardiovascular disease risk factors in individuals with type 2 diabetes: one-year results of the look AHEAD trial. *Diabetes Care* 2007;30:1374–1383.

47. Adler AI, et al. On behalf of the UK Prospective Diabetes Study Group. Association of systolic blood pressure with macrovascular and microvascular complications of type 2 diabetes (UKPDS 36): prospective observational study. *Brit Med J* 2000;321:412–419.

48. Patel A, et al. Effects of a fixed combination of perindopril and indapamide on macrovascular and microvascular outcomes in patients with type 2 diabetes mellitus (the ADVANCE trial): a randomised controlled trial. *Lancet* 2007;370:829–840.

49. Ruggenenti P, et al. For the DEMAND Study Investigators. Effects of manidipine and delapril in hypertensive patients with type 2diabetes mellitus: The Delapril and Manidipine for Nephroprotection in Diabetes (DEMAND) randomized clinical trial. *Hypertension* 2011;58:776–783.

50. Colhoun HM, et al. Problems of reporting genetic associations with complex outcomes. *Lancet* 2003;361:865–872.

51. Mora S, et al. On-treatment non-high-density lipoprotein cholesterol, apolipoprotein B, triglycerides, and lipid ratios in relation to residual vascular risk after treatment with potent statin therapy: JUPITER (Justification for the Use of Statins in Prevention: An Intervention Trial Evaluating Rosuvastatin). *J Am Coll Cardiol* 2012;59:1521–1528.

52. Goldfine AB. Statins: is it really time to reassess benefits and risks? *N Engl J Med* 2012;366:1752–1755.

53. Sattar N, et al. Statins and risk of incident diabetes: a collaborative meta-analysis of randomised statin trials. *Lancet* 2010;375:735–742.

54. Preiss D, et al. Risk of incident diabetes with intensive-dose compared with moderate-dose statin therapy. *JAMA* 2011;305:2556–2564.

55. DECODE Study Group. Is the current definition for diabetes relevant to mortality risk from all causes and cardiovascular and noncardiovascular disease? *Diabetes Care* 2003;26:688–696.

56. Qaseem A, et al. Glycemic control and type 2 diabetes mellitus: the optimal hemoglobin A1c targets. A guidance statement from the American College of Physicians. *Ann Intern Med* 2007;147:417–422.

57. UKPDS 33. UK Prospective Diabetes Study (UKPDS) Group. Intensive blood-glucose control with sulphonylureas or insulin compared with conventional treatment and risk of complications in patients with type 2 diabetes. *Lancet* 1998;352:837–853.

58. Inzucchi SE, et al. New drugs for the treatment of diabetes: part II: incretin-based therapy and beyond. *Circulation* 2008;117:574–584.

59. ADVANCE Collaborative Group, Patel A, et al. Intensive blood glucose control and vascular outcomes in patients with type 2 diabetes. *N Engl J Med* 2008;358:2560–2572.

60. Action to Control Cardiovascular Risk in Diabetes (ACCORD) Study Group, Gerstein HC, et al. Effects of intensive glucose lowering in type 2 diabetes. *N Engl J Med* 2008;358:2545–2559.

61. ACCORD Study Group, Gerstein HC, et al. Long-term effects of intensive glucose lowering on cardiovascular outcomes. *N Engl J Med* 2011;364:818–828.

62. Duckworth W, et al., VADT Investigators. Glucose control and vascular complications in veterans with type 2 diabetes. *N Engl J Med* 2009;360:129–139.
63. Hemmingsen B, et al. Intensive glycaemic control for patients with type 2 diabetes: systematic review with meta-analysis and trial sequential analysis of randomised clinical trials. *Brit Med J* 2011 Nov 24;343:d6898.
64. Inzucchi SE, et al. Management of hyperglycemia in type 2 diabetes: a patient-centered approach. Position statement of the American Diabetes Association (ADA) and the European Association for the Study of Diabetes (EASD). *Diabetes Care* 2012;DOI:10.2337/dc12- 0413. *Diabetologia* 2012; DOI 10.1007/s00125-012-2534-0.
65. Tahrani AA, et al. Insulin degludec: a new ultra long-acting insulin. *Lancet* 2012;379: 1465–1467.
66. Eurich DT, et al. Benefits and harms of antidiabetic agents in patients with diabetes and heart failure: systematic review. *Brit Med J* 2007;335:497.
67. Tzoulaki I, et al. Risk of cardiovascular disease and all cause mortality among patients with type 2 diabetes prescribed oral antidiabetes drugs: retrospective cohort study using UK general practice research database. *Brit Med J* 2009;339:b4731.
68. Tschöpe D, et al. Antidiabetic pharmacotherapy and anamnestic hypoglycemia in a large cohort of type 2 diabetic patients–an analysis of the DiaRegis registry. *Cardiovasc Diabetol* 2011;10:66.
69. Bennett WL, et al. Evaluation of guideline recommendations on oral medications for type 2 diabetes mellitus: a systematic review. *Ann Intern Med* 2012;156(1 Pt 1):27–36.
70. Boussageon R, et al. Reappraisal of metformin efficacy in the treatment of type 2 diabetes: a meta-analysis of randomised controlled trials. *PLoS Med* 2012;9:e1001204.
71. Hemmingsen B, et al. Comparison of metformin and insulin versus insulin alone for type 2 diabetes: systematic review of randomised clinical trials with meta-analyses and trial sequential analyses. *Brit Med J* 2012;344:e1771.
72. Lipska KJ, et al. Use of metformin in the setting of mild-to-moderate renal insufficiency. *Diabetes Care* 2011;34:1431–1437.
73. Goldberg RB, et al. Clinical decisions. Management of type 2 diabetes. *N Engl J Med* 2008;358:293–297.
74. Müller JE, et al. Carbohydrate restricted diet in conjunction with metformin and liraglutide is an effective treatment in patients with deteriorated type 2 diabetes mellitus: proof-of-concept study. *Nutr Metab* (Lond) 2011;8:92.
75. Karagiannis T, et al. Dipeptidyl peptidase-4 inhibitors for treatment of type 2 diabetes mellitus in the clinical setting: systematic review and meta-analysis. *Brit Med J* 2012 Mar 12;344:e1369.
76. Gore MO, et al. Resolving drug effects from class effects among drugs for type 2 diabetes mellitus: more support for cardiovascular outcome assessments. *Eur Heart J* 2011; 32:1832–1834.
77. Punthakee Z, et al. Poor cognitive function and risk of severe hypoglycemia in type 2 diabetes: post hoc epidemiologic analysis of the ACCORD trial. ACCORD-MIND Investigators. *Diabetes Care* 2012;35:787–793.
78. Launer LJ, et al. ACCORD MIND investigators. Effects of intensive glucose lowering on brain structure and function in people with type 2 diabetes (ACCORD MIND): a randomised open-label substudy. *Lancet Neurol* 2011;10:969–977.
79. Meier JJ, et al. Is impairment of ischaemic preconditioning by sulfonylurea drugs clinically important? *Heart* 2004;90:9–12.
80. Desouza CV, et al. Hypoglycemia, diabetes, and cardiovascular events. *Diabetes Care* 2010;33:1389–1394.
81. Meinert CL, et al. A study of the effects of hypoglycemic agents on vascular complications in patients with adult-onset diabetes. II. Mortality results. *Diabetes* 1970;19(Suppl): 789–830.
82. Schramm TK, et al. Mortality and cardiovascular risk associated with different insulin secretagogues compared with metformin in type 2 diabetes, with or without a previous myocardial infarction: a nationwide study. *Eur Heart J* 2011;32:1900–1908.
83. Zoungas S, et al. Combined effects of routine blood pressure lowering and intensive glucose control on macrovascular and microvascular outcomes in patients with type 2 diabetes: new results from the ADVANCE trial. *Diabetes Care* 2009;32:2068–2074.
84. Gallagher AM, et al. Risk of death and cardiovascular outcomes with thiazolidinediones: a study with the general practice research database and secondary care data. *PLoS One* 2011;6:e28157.
85. Erdmann E, et al. The effect of pioglitazone on recurrent myocardial infarction in 2,445 patients with type 2 diabetes and previous myocardial infarction: results from the PROactive (PROactive 05) Study. *J Am Coll Cardiol* 2007;49:1772–1780.
86. Deeg MA, et al. Pioglitazone and rosiglitazone have different effects on serum lipoprotein particle concentrations and sizes in patients with type 2 diabetes and dyslipidemia. *Diabetes Care* 2007;30:2458–2464.
87. Ratner R, et al. Impact of intensive lifestyle and metformin therapy on cardiovascular disease risk factors in the diabetes prevention program. *Diabetes Care* 2005;28: 888–894.
88. Lipscombe LL, et al. Thiazolidinediones and cardiovascular outcomes in older patients with diabetes. *JAMA* 2007;298:2634–2643.
89. Nissen SE, et al. Effect of rosiglitazone on the risk of myocardial infarction and death from cardiovascular causes. *N Engl J Med* 2007;356:2457–2471.
90. Dormandy JA, et al. Secondary prevention of macrovascular events in patients with type 2 diabetes in the PROactive Study (PROspective pioglitAzone Clinical Trial In macroVascular Events): a randomised controlled trial. *Lancet* 2005;366:1279–1289.
91. Plutzky J. The incretin axis in cardiovascular disease. *Circulation* 2011;124:2285–2289.

92. Sivertsen J, et al. The effect of glucagon-like peptide 1 on cardiovascular risk. *Nat Rev Cardiol* 2012;9:209–222.
93. Deacon CF, et al. Glycaemic efficacy of glucagon-like peptide-1 receptor agonists and dipeptidyl peptidase-4 inhibitors as add-on therapy to metformin in subjects with type 2 diabetes—a review and meta analysis. *Diabetes Obes Metab* 2012;14:762–767.
94. Shyangdan DS, et al. A glucagon-like peptide analogues for type 2 diabetes mellitus. *Cochrane Database Syst Rev* 2011;10:Art CD006423.
95. Ussher JR, et al. Cardiovascular biology of the incretin system. *Endocr Rev* 2012;33: 187–215.
96. Pratley RE, et al. Liraglutide versus sitagliptin for patients with type 2 diabetes who did not have adequate glycaemic control with metformin: a 26-week, randomised, parallel-group, open-label trial. *Lancet* 2010;375:1447–1456.
97. Diamant M, et al. Once weekly exenatide compared with insulin glargine titrated to target in patients with type 2 diabetes (DURATION-3): an open-label randomised trial. *Lancet* 2010;375:2234–2243.
98. Nyström T, et al. Effects of glucagon-like peptide-1 on endothelial function in type 2 diabetes patients with stable coronary artery disease. *Am J Physiol Endocrinol Metab* 2004;287:E1209–1215.
99. Sokos GG, et al. Glucagon-like peptide-1 infusion improves left ventricular ejection fraction and functional status in patients with chronic heart failure. *J Card Fail* 2006;12: 694–699.
100. Bergenstal RM, et al., DURATION-2 Study Group. Efficacy and safety of exenatide once weekly versus sitagliptin or pioglitazone as an adjunct to metformin for treatment of type 2 diabetes (DURATION-2): a randomised trial. *Lancet* 2010;376:431–439.
101. Lønborg J, et al. Exenatide reduces final infarct size in patients with ST-segment-elevation myocardial infarction and short-duration of ischemia. *Circ Cardiovasc Interv* 2012;5: 288–295.
102. Richard KR, et al. Tolerability of dipeptidyl peptidase-4 inhibitors: a review. *Clin Ther* 2011;33:1609–1629.
103. Drucker DJ, et al. The incretin system: glucagon-like peptide-1 receptor agonists and dipeptidyl peptidase-4 inhibitors in type 2 diabetes. *Lancet* 2006;368:1696–1705.
104. Duffy NA, et al. Effects of antidiabetic drugs on dipeptidyl peptidase IV activity: nateglinide is an inhibitor of DPP IV and augments the antidiabetic activity of glucagon-like peptide-1. *Eur J Pharmacol* 2007;568:278–286.
105. Fadini GP, et al. Cardiovascular effects of DPP-4 inhibition: beyond GLP-1. *Vascul Pharmacol* 2011;55:10–16.
106. Scirica BM, et al. The design and rationale of the saxagliptin assessment of vascular outcomes recorded in patients with diabetes mellitus-thrombolysis in myocardial infarction (SAVOR-TIMI) 53 study. *Am Heart J* 2011;162:818–825.
107. Defronzo RA, et al. Efficacy and tolerability of the DPP-4 inhibitor alogliptin combined with pioglitazone, in metformin-treated patients with type 2 diabetes. *J Clin Endocrinol Metab* 2012;97:1615–1622.
108. Schurmann C, et al. The dipeptidyl peptidase-4 inhibitor linagliptin attenuates inflammation and accelerates epithelialization in wounds of diabetic ob/ob mice. *J Pharmacol Exp Ther* 2012;342:71–80.
109. Toth PP. Linagliptin: a new DPP-4 inhibitor for the treatment of type 2 diabetes mellitus. *Postgrad Med* 2011;123:46–53.
110. Sangle GV, et al. Novel biological action of the dipeptidylpeptidase-IV inhibitor, sitagliptin, as a glucagon-like peptide-1 secretagogue. *Endocrinology* 2012;153:564–573.
111. Matthews DR, et al. Vildagliptin add-on to metformin produces similar efficacy and reduced hypoglycaemic risk compared with glimepiride, with no weight gain: results from a 2-year study. *Diabetes Obes Metab* 2010;12:780–789.
112. Black C. Cochrane data base of systematic reviews 2007; Issue 2.
113. NAVIGATOR Study Group, Holman RR, et al. Effect of nateglinide on the incidence of diabetes and cardiovascular events. *N Engl J Med* 2010;362:1463–1476. Erratum in *N Engl J Med* 2010;362:1748.
114. Gaziano JM, et al. Randomized clinical trial of quick-release bromocriptine among patients with type 2 diabetes on overall safety and cardiovascular outcomes. *Diabetes Care* 2010;33:1503–1508.
115. Nauck MA, et al. Dapagliflozin versus glipizide as add-on therapy in patients with type 2 diabetes who have inadequate glycemic control with metformin: a randomized, 52-week, double-blind, active-controlled noninferiority trial. *Diabetes Care* 2011;34:2015–2022.
116. Rosenstock J, et al. Effects of dapagliflozin, a sodium-glucose cotransporter-2 inhibitor, on hemoglobin A1c, body weight, and hypoglycemia risk in patients with type 2 diabetes inadequately controlled on pioglitazone monotherapy. *Diabetes Care* 2012;35:1473–1478.
117. Pfeffer MA. ACCORD(ing) to a trialist. *Circulation* 2010;122:841–843.
118. Funnell MM, et al. National standards for diabetes self-management education. *Diabetes Care* 2011;34(Suppl 1):S89–S96.
119. Punthakee Z, et al. Poor cognitive function and risk of severe hypoglycemia in type 2 diabetes: post hoc epidemiologic analysis of the ACCORD trial. ACCORD-MIND Investigators. *Diabetes Care* 2012;35:787–793.
120. Goede P, et al. Effect of a multifactorial intervention on mortality in type 2 diabetes. *N Engl J Med* 2008;358:580–591.
121. Stratton IM, et al. On behalf of the UK Prospective Study Diabetes Group. Association of glycaemia with macrovascular and microvascular complications of type 2 diabetes (UKPDS 35): prospective observational study. *Brit Med J* 2000;321:405–412.
122. Opie LH, et al. Controversies in the cardiovascular management of type 2 diabetes. *Heart* 2011;97:6–14.

123. Colhoun HM, et al. Primary prevention of cardiovascular disease with atorvastatin in type 2 diabetes in the Collaborative Atorvastatin Diabetes Study (CARDS): multicentre randomised placebo-controlled trial. *Lancet* 2004;364:685–696.

124. Baigent C, et al. Efficacy and safety of cholesterol-lowering treatment: prospective meta-analysis of data from 90,056 participants in 14 randomised trials of statins. *Lancet* 2005;366:1267–1278.

125. Ismail-Beigi F, et al. ACCORD trial group. Effect of intensive treatment of hyperglycaemia on microvascular outcomes in type 2 diabetes: an analysis of the ACCORD randomised trial. *Lancet* 2010;376:419–430.

126. ACCORD Study Group, ACCORD Eye Study Group, Chew EY, et al. Effects of medical therapies on retinopathy progression in type 2 diabetes. *N Engl J Med* 2010;363:233–244.

127. Zoungas S, et al. ADVANCE. Combined effects of routine blood pressure lowering and intensive glucose control on macrovascular and microvascular outcomes in patients with type 2 diabetes: new results from the ADVANCE trial. *Diabetes Care* 2009; 32:2068–2074.

128. Evangelista V, et al. Prevention of cardiovascular disease in type-2 diabetes: how to improve the clinical efficacy of aspirin. *Thromb Haemost* 2005;93:8–16.

129. Machecourt J, et al. Risk factors for stent thrombosis after implantation of sirolimus-eluting stents in diabetic and nondiabetic patients: the EVASTENT Matched-Cohort Registry. *J Am Coll Cardiol* 2007;50:501–508.

130. Javaid A, et al. Outcomes of coronary artery bypass grafting versus percutaneous coronary intervention with drug-eluting stents for patients with multivessel coronary artery disease. *Circulation* 2007;116:1200–1206.

131. BARI Trial Participants. Comparison of coronary bypass surgery with angioplasty in patients with multivessel disease. *N Engl J Med* 1996;335:217–225.

132. DIGAMI Study, Malmberg K, et al. Randomized trial of insulin-glucose infusion followed by subcutaneous insulin treatment in diabetic patients with acute myocardial infarction (DIGAMI Study): effects on mortality at 1 year. *JACC* 1995;26:57–65.

133. Malmberg K, et al. Intense metabolic control by means of insulin in patients with diabetes mellitus and acute myocardial infarction (DIGAMI 2): effects on mortality and morbidity. *Eur Heart J* 2005;26:650–661.

134. Selker HP, et al. Out-of-hospital administration of intravenous glucose-insulin-potassium in patients with suspected acute coronary syndromes: the IMMEDIATE randomized controlled trial. *JAMA* 2012;307:1925–1933.

135. Szczepaniak LS, et al. Forgotten but not gone: the rediscovery of fatty heart, the most common unrecognized disease in America. *Circ Res* 2007;101:759–767.

136. How OJ, et al. Increased myocardial oxygen consumption reduces cardiac efficiency in diabetic mice. *Diabetes* 2006;55:466–473.

137. McGavock JM, et al. Cardiac steatosis in diabetes mellitus: a 1H-magnetic resonance spectroscopy study. *Circulation* 2007;116:1170–1175.

138. van der Meer RW, et al. Short-term caloric restriction induces accumulation of myocardial triglycerides and decreases left ventricular diastolic function in healthy subjects. *Diabetes* 2007;56:2849–2853.

139. Opie LH. Glycaemia and heart failure in diabetes types 1 and 2. *Lancet* 2011;378:103–104.

140. Opie LH, et al. The adrenergic-fatty acid load in heart failure. *J Am Coll Cardiol* 2009;54:1637–1646.

141. Belfort R, et al. Dose-response effect of elevated plasma free fatty acid on insulin signaling. *Diabetes* 2005;54:1640–1648.

142. Castagno D, et al. Intensive glycemic control has no impact on the risk of heart failure in type 2 diabetic patients: evidence from a 37,229 patient meta-analysis. *Am Heart J* 2011;162:938–948.

143. Tomova GS, et al. Relation between hemoglobin A(1c) and outcomes in heart failure patients with and without diabetes mellitus. *Am J Cardiol* 2012;109:1767–1773.

144. Lago RM, et al. Congestive heart failure and cardiovascular death in patients with pre-diabetes and type 2 diabetes given thiazolidinediones: a meta-analysis of randomised clinical trials. *Lancet* 2007;370:1129–1136.

145. Lincoff AM, et al. Pioglitazone and risk of cardiovascular events in patients with type 2 diabetes mellitus: a meta-analysis of randomized trials. *JAMA* 2007;298:1180–1188.

146. Richter B, et al. Rosiglitazone for type 2 diabetes mellitus. *Cochrane Database Syst Rev* 2007;(3):CD006063.

147. Singh S, et al. Long-term risk of cardiovascular events with rosiglitazone: a meta-analysis. *JAMA* 2007;298:1189–1195.

148. Martin TL, et al. Diet-induced obesity alters AMP kinase activity in hypothalamus and skeletal muscle. *J Biol Chem* 2006;281:18933–18941.

149. Zhang H, et al. Collecting duct-specific deletion of peroxisome proliferator-activated receptor gamma blocks thiazolidinedione-induced fluid retention. *Proc Natl Acad Sci U S A* 2005;102:9406–9411.

150. Dargie HJ, et al. A randomized, placebo-controlled trial assessing the effects of rosiglitazone on echocardiographic function and cardiac status in type 2 diabetic patients with New York Heart Association Functional Class I or II Heart Failure. *J Am Coll Cardiol* 2007;49:1696–1704.

12

Which Therapy for Which Condition?

BERNARD J. GERSH · LIONEL. H. OPIE

"Stop it at the start, 'tis late for medicine to be prepared when disease has grown strong through long delays."

Ovid, Remedia Amoris

Angina Pectoris

The general approach to angina or any other manifestation of coronary disease has become both more interventional (with increasing use of stents) and more preventional, in that lifestyle modification and aggressive risk factor reduction are now regarded as crucial. Every patient with coronary artery disease requires an assessment of predisposing factors such as diet, smoking, obesity, and lack of exercise, with a search for the metabolic syndrome and diabetes. In exertional angina pectoris, the long-term objectives of treatment are first to improve survival primarily by the prevention of myocardial infarction (MI) and death, and second to improve the quality of life by relief of symptoms.[1] Initial examination requires attention to any precipitating factors (hypertension, anemia, congestive heart failure [CHF], and valve disease). A cornerstone of the management of patients with established coronary artery disease who comprise a population at high risk of subsequent cardiovascular events is aggressive risk-factor reduction.[2-4] The key risk factors are hypertension, hyperlipidemia, smoking, obesity, lack of exercise, and diabetes; more recently, chronic kidney disease has been considered as a coronary heart disease risk equivalent.[5]

Although depression is not established as a major risk factor for the *development* of coronary heart disease, it frequently coexists in patients with symptomatic disease and its recognition and treatment may improve the quality of life.

Role of Education in Risk-Factor Modification

Risk-factor modification is a critical component of the integrative management of chronic stable angina as emphasized by the following mnemonic modified from the American College of Cardiology (ACC)–American Heart Association (AHA) guidelines:

A = Aspirin and angiotensin-converting enzyme (ACE) inhibitor

B = β-blocker and blood pressure (BP)

C = Cigarette smoking and cholesterol

D = Diet and diabetes

E = Education and exercise

Therapeutic Targets

Lipids. Regarding a low *high-density lipoprotein (HDL) cholesterol*, our previous advice was to add niacin, but in patients with stable coronary disease and a well-controlled low-density lipoprotein (LDL) cholesterol, the current AIM/HIGH trial found no change in cardiovascular and mortality outcomes even though niacin both increased HDL and decreased triglyceride levels.[6] Furthermore, a large genetic study on more than 100,000 persons found that those with genetically high HDL levels were at the same risk of MI as those with lower HDL values.[7] On the other hand, hereditary factors had no influence on the very strong (p $< 10^{-9}$) relationship between LDL levels and MI.[7] Thus strong evidence suggests concentrating on lowering the LDL cholesterol.

LDL cholesterol. In regard to the goal LDL cholesterol, the 2007 ACC-AHA guidelines concluded that a goal of less than 70 mg/dL (1.8 mmol/L) was reasonable in patients with non–ST-elevation acute coronary syndromes (ACS), but there is no reason that this should not apply to all patients with established coronary disease.[8] In patients with an LDL cholesterol of less than 40 mg/dL (1.03 mmol/L) the role of exercise, smoking cessation, and weight loss in obese subjects makes sense and requires further study

Goal blood pressures. Goal BPs are more controversial, but the recent ACCORD trial demonstrated no compelling reason to support a goal of less than 130/80 mm Hg in patients with established cardiovascular disease and in any event irrespective of the goal, BP reduction should be gradual.[9] ACE inhibitors or angiotensin receptor blockers (ARBs) are indicated in patients with cardiovascular disease who need antihypertensive therapy.[10] In all patients with chronic stable angina, β-blockers are an established therapy. In diabetics, strict glycemic control is recommended, but "how low one should go" is also controversial, as discussed elsewhere in Chapter 11, p. 454).

Diet and Supplements

We do not recommend supplemental vitamin E or other antioxidants. The trial data in regard to vitamin E are largely neutral or even negative in two large studies in high-risk or postinfarct patients.[2] Long-term follow-up in the HOPE trial showed an increased risk of heart failure with vitamin E. Rather, we recommend the Mediterranean diet, rich in ω-3 fatty acids.[11] Testosterone improved angina in only one trial.[12] Side effects and lack of data limit its use.

Aspirin is strongly indicated in patients without contraindications, and its efficacy in reducing cardiovascular events in stable angina has been confirmed by a metaanalysis of 287 randomized trials.[13] Clopidogrel is the recommended alternative in patients intolerant to aspirin, although never tested in patients with chronic stable angina. Moreover, for chronic angina its combination with aspirin is unlikely to be more effective than aspirin alone.[14] Low-intensity anticoagulation with warfarin may give benefit similar to that obtained with aspirin,[15] but this approach is rarely employed. Despite the established links between inflammatory markers and coronary artery disease, there is as yet no role for antibiotic therapy.[16] Of note, both statins and aspirin have antiinflammatory properties.

Antianginal Drugs

Sublingual nitroglycerin. Of the various agents that give pain relief (see Fig. 2-2), nitrates are among the most effective, although there is no evidence that nitrates reduce mortality in patients with chronic coronary artery disease. Nonetheless, their efficacy in relieving symptoms and improving exercise tolerance justifies their use as standard therapy in conjunction with a β-blocker or calcium channel blocker (CCB). The prophylactic use of sublingual nitroglycerin prior to activity may be very effective and is probably underused. Thereafter, the addition of long-acting nitrates is indicated. Nitrate tolerance remains a major problem, although the precise mechanisms remain unclear. Eccentric dosage schedules with 8- to 12-hour nitrate-free intervals are the most practical method of avoiding tolerance. Alternatively, a long-acting mononitrate may be given once a day in the morning; its duration of action is supposedly long enough to see the patient through the day, yet short enough to provide a nitrate-free interval at night. All long-acting nitrates appear to be equally effective provided that an adequate nitrate-free interval is provided.

β-Blockers versus calcium channel blockers. Deciding whether to choose a β-blocker or CCB for first-line treatment of angina pectoris is not always easy. Each is combined with nitrates. The metaanalysis of 90 randomized or crossover studies comparing β-blockers, CCBs, and long-acting nitrates demonstrated no significant difference in the rates of cardiac death and MI between β-blockers and CCBs.[17] Nevertheless, there are groups of patients for whom, on the whole, one of these agents might be preferable. First, in the presence of left ventricular (LV) dysfunction, β-blockers are much preferred because of their capacity to confer postinfarction protection and their favorable effects on outcomes in trials of patients with heart failure.[18] Specifically, there are strong data favoring carvedilol, metoprolol *(Toprol XL)*, and bisoprolol in heart failure. All β-blockers appear to be effective in chronic stable angina irrespective of their pharmacologic properties, and the best advice is to become familiar with one or two drugs (e.g., atenolol, metoprolol, propanolol, and carvedilol, and although rarely used pindolol and acebutolol) that have sympathomimetic activity that may be helpful in patients with a resting sinus bradycardia. Of the β-blockers, only atenolol, metoprolol, nadolol, and propranolol are approved by the US Food and Drug Administration (FDA) for chronic stable angina, leaving metoprolol as the common denominator. Second, in those at risk of acute myocardial infarction (AMI), β-blockers protect in the acute and chronic phases. Third, in patients with angina associated with a relatively high heart rate (anxiety), β-blockade is more logical, or if CCBs are used they should be of the nondihydropyridine variety (heart rate–lowering agents). β-Blocker downsides include quality-of-life problems such as impaired exercise capacity, erectile dysfunction, and weight gain, besides risk of glucose intolerance (see Fig. 11-3), the latter being less likely with carvedilol, nebivolol, and especially the CCBs.

Absolute contraindications to β-blockers. Absolute contraindications are severe bradycardia, preexisting high-grade or second-degree atrioventricular (AV) block, sick sinus syndrome, asthma that is at least moderate in severity, or class IV heart failure. In patients with chronic obstructive pulmonary disease without frank bronchospasm, cardioselective β-blockers should be used.[19] Most diabetics will tolerate β-blockers, but particular care is needed in patients with insulin-dependent diabetes mellitus with symptomatic hypoglycemia. CCBs may be more effective in hypertensives; in the large ASCOT study, amlodipine combined with an ACE inhibitor reduced the development of unstable angina, MI, and heart failure.[20] When coronary spasm is the established cause of the angina, as in Prinzmetal's variant angina, β-blockers are ineffective and probably contraindicated, whereas CCBs work well.

Which drug and when? Despite such guidelines, the choice between these two types of agents often cannot readily be resolved. β-Blockers are logical initial therapy in the absence of contraindications in those with prior MI or LV dysfunction. Then, if needed, CCBs should be combined with β-blockers and long-acting nitrates. In the ACTION study, combination of long-acting nifedipine with prior β-blockade reduced major endpoints, particularly in patients with persisting modest hypertension.[21] If side effects from β-blockers are substantial, CCBs in combination with nitrates are the substitute, and long-acting nondihydropyridine CCBs should be used preferentially. "Triple therapy" with nitrates, CCBs, and β-blockers should not be automatically equated with maximal therapy because of new metabolic modulators such as ranolazine (see next section). Furthermore, patients' reactions vary. In particular, excess hypotension should be avoided.

Other antianginal agents. *Nicorandil,* a combined nitrate and adenosine triphosphate–dependent potassium channel activator, reduced major coronary events in patients with stable angina in the IONA trial, but there has been no application for its use in the United States.[22] *Ranolazine,* a metabolic agent that is thought to inhibit fatty acid oxidation and the slow sodium channel, improves exercise tolerance and is currently approved for chronic effort angina in the United States (see Fig. 2-8).[23] The drug is effective in reducing symptoms and improving exercise capacity and its role as an antiarrhythmic and glycometabolic agent is currently under investigation.[24] *Trimetazidine* is another metabolic agent, also free of hemodynamic effects, widely used as an antianginal in Europe. *Ivabradine,* approved for use in Europe, acts specifically on the pacemaking hyperpolarization-activated current (I_f) in the sinoatrial node to cause bradycardia. It gives a dose-dependent improvement in exercise tolerance with a lower side effect profile than atenolol.[25,26] The efficacy of ivabradine in regard to the composite endpoint of cardiovascular death, MI, and hospitalization for heart failure was evaluated in the BEAUTIFUL trial of 10,000 patients with stable coronary artery disease and an ejection fraction of less than 40%, and there was no difference between ivabradine and placebo except in a specific subgroup of patients with heart failure and a rate of 70 beats per minute.[27] However, in the subsequent trial of patients with symptomatic heart failure who are in sinus rhythm with heart rates of 70 beats or higher, ivabradine was associated with a reduction in the composite of cardiovascular death or hospital admission for worsening heart failure.[28] *Allopurinol* decreases myocardial oxygen demand per unit of cardiac output in patients with heart failure, and in a small study of patients with documented coronary disease high-dose allopurinol showed promise as antianginal agent but needs to be tested further.[29] In patients with stable coronary disease treated with conventional antiischemic and vasculoprotective agents, high-dose allopurinol creates vascular oxidative stress and improved endothelial-dependent vasodilatation.[30] *Perhexiline* was shown to be effective in older trials but is little used to hepatotoxicity and peripheral neuropathy. It has however been used in Australia and Europe in patients with refractory angina.[31]

Revascularization or Optimal Medical Therapy for Chronic Stable Angina?

In stable effort angina, even with multivessel disease, two important trials have not demonstrated any benefit with regard to death or MI of percutaneous coronary intervention (PCI) over medical therapy in patients with preserved LV function in the main, and symptoms of mild to moderate severity.[32,33] In addition, the BARI IID trial in patients with type 2 diabetes and stable coronary disease demonstrated no benefit for a strategy of revascularization over medical therapy, although in patients with severe coronary artery disease there was a benefit from coronary bypass surgery (but not PCI) on major cardiac events, driven mainly by a reduction in nonfatal MI.[34] In summary, based on the COURAGE and BARI IID trials, in *angiographically selected patients with chronic stable angina and preserved LV function, there is no benefit from coronary revascularization on death and MI.* Unresolved questions are how to extrapolate this to the population at large and the role of stress testing. Another key question is the role of revascularization in patients with moderate to severe ischemia and mild to moderate angina, and this is the objective of the recently initiated National Institutes of Health Heart, Lung, and Blood Institute (NHLBI) ISCHEMIA trial (David Maron, personal communication, 2011). These results are consistent with almost 3 decades of trials and emphasize that current mortality rates in patients with chronic stable angina on intensive medical therapy receiving aggressive secondary prevention are low and unlikely to be improved by revascularization. Thus decisions about the indications for, timing, and type of intervention must be tailored to the individual and need to take into account all these complex cardiac factors and, in addition, the patient's lifestyle, occupation, other medical conditions, and tolerance of optimal medical therapy. In general the concept of "the greater the risk, the greater the benefit from revascularization over medical therapy" applies to patients with left main coronary artery disease, multivessel disease, and in particular in conjunction with LV dysfunction, severe angina, and proximal left anterior descending coronary disease in conjunction with multivessel disease.[35]

Percutaneous coronary intervention. Major advances have occurred in the use of drug-eluting stents, new antiplatelet agents, new anticoagulants including low-molecular-weight heparin (LMWH) and bivalirudin, and the concept of physiologically directed PCI using measurements of fractional flow reserve as demonstrated by the FAME trial.[36] The introduction of drug-eluting stents (Fig. 12-1) has further decreased the

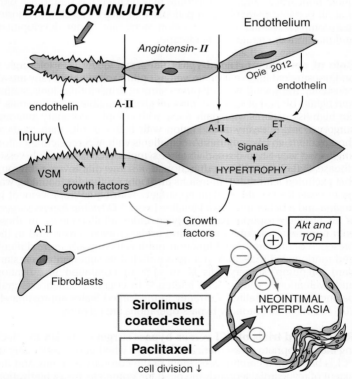

Figure 12-1   Molecular events in restenosis and prevention by drug-eluting stents. The balloon-induced injury damages both endothelium and vascular smooth muscle (VSM) with release of endothelin (ET) and penetration of angiotensin II (A-II). These act to promote growth of both VSM cells and fibroblasts. Growth signals include protein kinase B (Akt) and target of rapamycin (TOR). The result is neointimal hyperplasia that predisposes to restenosis. Drug-eluting stents diminish restenosis. Sirolimus (rapamycin) inhibits growth pathways at the site of TOR, whereas paclitaxel inhibits neointimal hyperplasia. (Figure © L.H. Opie, 2012.)

rate of in-stent restenosis and the need for target lesion revascularization by 30%-70% compared with bare-metal stents (BMS), but a metaanalysis of 14 randomized clinical trials failed to demonstrate any differences in rates of death or MI.[37] Several studies have demonstrated the slight increase in very late (greater than 1 year) stent thrombosis, but this has not been associated with any increase in mortality.[38] Despite registry reports demonstrating both increased and decreased late mortality with drug-eluting stents,[39] a randomized trial demonstrated no difference in mortality at all in patients with AMI, suggesting that baseline differences may have played a role in the impact of the registry studies.[40,41] There were four articles in the *Journal of the American College of Cardiology* in 2007, and five in *Circulation*. The *Lancet* focused on cost-effectiveness of BMS versus drug-eluting stents (if results are the same for some categories of patients, chose the cheaper option). *Reasonable conclusions* to be drawn at present are that the major risk of drug-eluting stents is late thrombosis and that of BMS is restenosis needing revascularization.[40] *Thus drug-eluting stents reduce the need for repeat PCI and improve the quality of life, at the cost of late stent thrombosis that, although infrequent, is unpredictable and has catastrophic consequences.* For on-label indications, there is no increase in death or MI with drug-eluting stents, and for off-label indications where drug-eluting stents are generally used for more complex lesions, several but not all registry studies show no increase in mortality.[42] Crucial to the decision to implant a drug-eluting stent is an assessment of the patient's compliance and ability to tolerate prolonged dual antiplatelet therapy. In the event that a subsequent noncardiac surgical procedure may be likely, it is best to use BMS if at all possible, particularly in patients with larger vessels and shorter, less complex lesions. Third-generation stents are under development and may further change the landscape.

Role of coronary artery bypass surgery. Techniques for surgical and nonsurgical intervention as well as optimal medical therapy are all constantly improving, with off-pump surgery, drug-eluting stents, statins, and tighter BP and glycemic control all giving tangible improvements.[43] For high-risk patients, especially those with complex coronary anatomy, surgery remains a very good option with better results than medical therapy.[44,45] High risk includes some patients with ACS, recalcitrant effort angina, left mainstem disease whether symptomatic or not, triple-vessel disease, diabetes, and LV dysfunction. In a somewhat lower risk group that excluded left mainstem lesions and poor LV function, stenting was more cost-effective than off-pump surgery with equal improvement in angina and a better quality of life after 1 year.[46] *Off-pump bypass surgery* is an attractive option, particularly in older adult patients, in those with peripheral vascular disease and aortic atherosclerosis, and in the presence of impaired renal function, but it is technically more difficult and randomized trials have not demonstrated its superiority over standard "on-pump" surgery. This is an area of continued investigation and evaluation,[47] with special reference to cognitive function,[48] graft patency,[49] and mortality.[50] Currently in the United States approximately 20% to 25% of all coronary bypass operations are off-pump.

Randomized trials of PCI versus bypass surgery. The key to selecting the appropriate revascularization strategy, whether bypass surgery or PCI, is based on a careful assessment of the coronary anatomy and the extent of myocardial jeopardy, the need for "complete" revascularization, LV function, the technical suitability of the lesions for a transcatheter technique, and realistic expectations from the patient of what can be achieved by each procedure. Worldwide, the trend is toward PCI for revascularization.[51] In an older patient population, it is particularly important to screen for comorbid conditions, which can have a crucial effect on procedural success and complications, but also on the long-term outcome. Furthermore, stent insertion has become more adventurous; for example, multiple stent insertion is common and selected stenting

FACTORS FAVORING CABG OVER PCI IN PATIENTS WITH MULTIVESSEL DISEASE
Gersh 2012

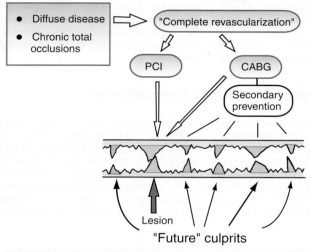

Figure 12-2 **Advantages of coronary artery bypass grafting (CABG) over percutaneous coronary intervention (PCI) in severe multivessel coronary artery disease.** CABG gives added protection by bypassing future "culprit lesions." Whereas PCI is directed to the culprit lesion or lesions that are considered responsible for the patient's symptoms, CABG and secondary prevention are directed toward the entire epicardial vessel, including potential "future culprits," defined by nonobstructive lesions that may be the sites of future plaque rupture. (Figure © B.J. Gersh, 2012.)

for unprotected left mainstem disease is under study.[52] *The ability of coronary artery bypass grafting to bypass the entire vessel as opposed to a single culprit lesion treated by stenting is probably an important predictor of prognosis in the intermediate term* (Fig. 12-2).[53] In clinical practice, it appears that physician judgment and patient preference result in the appropriate bias toward referral of the more complex forms of multivessel disease to surgery as opposed to PCI. Ongoing trials such as FREEDOM in diabetics and the long-term follow-up data from the SYNTAX trial will provide important information regarding the efficacy of drug-eluting stents versus coronary bypass surgery in patients with complex three-vessel and left main coronary disease but against a backdrop of aggressive risk factor reduction. Data from the SYNTAX trial using an angiographic grading tool, namely the SYNTAX score, emphasized the superiority of bypass surgery in patients with more complex and diffuse disease, but approximately one third of patients with three-vessel and left main disease may be appropriately treated with PCI with outcomes that are at least equivalent to coronary artery bypass grafting (CABG). Additional trials in patients with left main coronary disease are needed.[54] It is important in interpreting the results of registry and randomized trials to understand the strengths and limitations of each as the data may be complimentary if used in the correct context.

Mechanical therapies for refractory angina. Revascularization is the key when the effort angina is more than mild, especially if symptoms are escalating. The patient population with refractory angina not amenable to revascularization is growing and constitutes a difficult clinical problem. Alternative therapies such as chelation and acupuncture, ineffective in controlled trials, should be avoided. Of the promising mechanical therapies, the best studied is enhanced external counterpulsation.[55] The multicenter study MUST-EECP trial[56] and several registries have demonstrated both efficacy and tolerability, although the mechanisms of benefit are unclear.[55,57-59] Spinal cord stimulation in which an electrode is inserted into the epidural space at C7-T1 level is thought to function via the "gate theory" and has been shown to be effective in reducing symptoms and improving the quality of life.[60] Other techniques include transcutaneous electrical nerve stimulation and the intramyocardial implementation of stem cells.[61,62] All of these modalities require the rigorous scrutiny of large placebo-controlled trials[55]; translaser myocardial revascularization failed this test.[63]

Acute Coronary Syndromes

MI as redefined by cardiac troponin elevation has become much more common in patients with chest pain.[64,65] Further classification of ACS is based on the presence or absence of electrocardiographic ST-segment elevation at presentation, giving two clear divisions. ST-elevation ACS requires urgent revascularization by early fibrinolysis or PCI. The sooner revascularization takes place, the better. In non–ST-elevation myocardial infarction (NSTEMI) and unstable angina, management is determined by the degree of risk (Fig. 12-3), with the emphasis in the low-risk groups

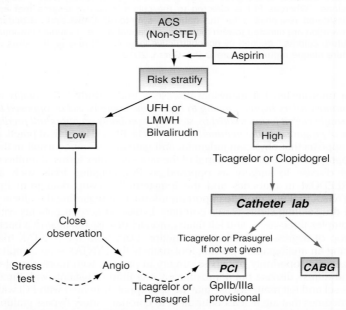

ACUTE CORONARY SYNDROMES: TRIAGE

Gersh 2012

Figure 12-3   Principles of triage for acute coronary syndromes (ACS) with non–ST elevation (non-STE). All receive aspirin. Patients are stratified according to the risk are given unfractionated heparin (UFH) or low-molecular-weight heparin (LMWH) and bivalirudin (no glycoprotein [Gp] IIb/IIIa, as below). Those at high risk are given ticagrelor or clopidogrel, and taken to the catheter laboratory. Then they either undergo coronary artery bypass grafting (CABG) or percutaneous coronary intervention (PCI). Those undergoing PCI are given ticagrelor (or prasugrel), if not yet given, and some are selected to be given GpIIb/IIIa inhibitors (see text, Chapter 9, p. 352). Those at low risk are closely observed and if requiring an angiogram (angio) given ticagrelor or prasugrel to be followed by PCI. Those at lower risk and stable are subject to an effort stress test. (Figure © B.J. Gersh, 2012.)

on prevention of complete thrombosis by antiplatelet and antithrombotic agents, with symptomatic management followed in medium and higher-risk groups by rapid revascularization by PCI.[66] In the current era of new and more powerful antithrombotic agents in conjunction with older and sicker patients, the risk of bleeding is of increasing importance.[67,68] *General measures* include bed rest and immediate relief of ischemia by nitroglycerin (sublingual, spray, or intravenously) with added β-blockers to reduce the myocardial oxygen demand (Table 12-1). Morphine sulfate is given intravenously if the pain persists or if the patient is agitated or pulmonary congestion is present. Supplemental oxygen is required for hypoxemia or respiratory distress (class IB in the ACC-AHA guidelines),[8] and although in practice it is given routinely to all patients, only three randomized controlled clinical trials have been performed in just 387 patients and no benefit in terms of mortality or pain relief has been demonstrated. In fact, a recent systematic review suggested a trend toward harm from the administration of oxygen, but this could be due to chance.[69]

Non–ST-Segment Elevation ACS

Aspirin and clopidogrel. Evidence for the efficacy of combined aspirin and heparin is strong.[70] Aspirin should be started immediately and continued indefinitely. The key to effective therapy is to institute

Table 12-1

ACCF-AHA Guidelines for Management of Unstable Angina and Non–ST-Elevation Myocardial Infarction[589]

Early Antiischemic and Analgesic Therapy

1. Oxygen if low arterial saturation (<90%) or respiratory distress (class 1B).*
2. IV nitroglycerin if persistent ischemia, heart failure, or hypertension (class 1B). (Oral nitroglycerin 0.4 mg every 5 min.)
3. Oral β-blockade if no C/I (class 1B).
4. If β-blockade C/I, nondihydropyridine CCB (class 1B).
5. Oral ACE inhibitor within 24 h if LV failure if BP > 100 mm Hg or not >30 mm Hg less than baseline (class 1A); oral ARB if ACE intolerant (class 1A).

Antiplatelet Therapy

1. Aspirin on arrival or before, continue indefinitely (class 1A), nonenteric 162-325 mg; long-term 75-162 mg daily, higher disease after stenting.
2. If aspirin intolerant, clopidogrel loading dose 300 mg, then 75 mg daily (class 1A).
3. Proton pump inhibition if gastric intolerance to aspirin or clopidogrel (class 1B).
4. Initial invasive strategy: upstream clopidogrel or GpIIb/IIIa blocker (class 1A). Abciximab only if rapid PCI likely, otherwise eptifibatide or tirofiban (class 1B).
5. Initial conservative strategy: upstream before urgent diagnostic angiography, clopidogrel loading dose or GpIIb/IIIa (eptifibatide or tirofiban) (class 1A).

Anticoagulant Therapy

1. Initial invasive strategy: enoxaparin or UFH (class 1A) as soon as possible; fondaparinux or bivalirudin (class 1B).
2. Initial conservative strategy: enoxaparin or UFH (class 1A); fondaparinux (class 1B) especially if increased risk of bleeding (1B).

ACCF, American College of Cardiology Foundation; *ACE,* angiotensin-converting enzyme; *AHA,* American Heart Association; *ARB,* angiotensin receptor blocker; *BP,* blood pressure; *CCB,* calcium channel blocker; *C/I,* contraindication; *Gp,* glycoprotein; *IV,* intravenous; *LV,* left ventricular; *PCI,* percutaneous coronary intervention; *UFH,* unfractionated heparin.

*Classes of Recommendations (1-3) and levels of evidence (A-C).

all other components in the emergency room as rapidly as possible. In patients who are unable to take aspirin, the case for clopidogrel is self-evident. In addition, there is now compelling evidence for combining clopidogrel and aspirin on admission, irrespective of whether catheterization and PCI is planned. Clopidogrel 75 mg daily should be added (class IA in guidelines)[71] for at least 7 days.[72] In centers in which bypass surgery is performed soon after angiography, it is reasonable to withhold clopidogrel until the coronary anatomy and the revascularization strategy have been determined. Before PCI, a loading dose of clopidogrel (class IA) 300 or 600 mg should be given at least 6 hours before the procedure and continued thereafter for at least 1 month, and ideally up to 12 months for drug-eluting stents depending on the type of stent used (see Table 12-3 later), while checking for the bleeding risk, which is increased by combining with aspirin. The ACC-AHA guidelines recommend that troponin-positive high-risk ACS patients needing PCI should be covered both by upstream clopidogrel and by glycoprotein (Gp) IIb/IIIa inhibition besides aspirin and an anticoagulant.[4] Although there appears to be an interaction between clopidogrel and proton pump inhibitors (PPIs), the clinical significance of this is uncertain.[73] Furthermore, in regard to clopidogrel there is considerable controversy over the effect of CYP2C19 loss-of-function carrier status. In regard to clinical responses and outcomes, in one recent study of patients with ACS and also atrial fibrillation (AF), the effect of clopidogrel over placebo was consistent, irrespective of CYP2C19 status.[74]

Moreover, the recent GRAVITAS trial demonstrated no benefit from double-dose clopidogrel in patients with higher on-treatment platelet reactivity after PCI, suggesting that clinical, procedural, and genetic predictors of the early resolution of high-on-treatment platelet reactivity after PCI requires further investigation. Current evidence suggests that clopidogrel responsiveness is a clinically relevant factor, but we are not sure how to deal with this therapeutically.[75]

Limitations of clopidogrel include its delayed onset of action; marked patient variability; the drug responsiveness, which may be genetically mediated; and the irreversibility of its inhibitory effect. This has led to the development of growth that has higher efficacy but more bleeding.[76] Ticagrelor binds reversibility with $P2Y_{12}$ platelet receptor and has a more rapid onset of action than clopidogrel. Its antiplatelet inhibiting effects appear greater than with clopidogrel, but it is not yet approved for clinical use.[77] In the PLATO trials, ticagrelor was superior overall to clopidogrel in patients treated both invasively and noninvasively.[78] The new European Society of Cardiology (ESC) guidelines recommend *ticagrelor* 180 mg loading dose and 90 mg twice daily in all patients at moderate to high risk of ischemic events (e.g., elevated troponins) regardless of initial treatment strategy. Clopidogrel should be discontinued at the time of *ticagrelor* initiation. In patients in whom the coronary anatomy is known and who are proceeding directly to PCI, *prasugrel* is recommended depending on the risk of bleeding. If fondaparinux is used and the patient proceeds to PCI, a single bolus of unfractionated heparin (UFH) should be added at the time of PCI (and the dose depends on the concomitant use of IIB/IIIA inhibitor.[79]

Cangrelor. Cangrelor is an intravenous nonthiepyridine $P2Y_{12}$ receptor blocker. It has a rapid onset of action and a short half-life, but has not been shown to be superior to clopidogrel in the CHAMPION trials and is still under evaluation.[80] *Atopaxar* (E555) is a reversible protease-activated receptor-1 thrombin receptor antagonist that interferes with platelet signaling and was shown in a recent trial of patients treated with clopidogrel to reduce early ischemia on Holter monitoring without any increase in bleeding. The drug is not available for clinical use.[81] Clearly, the therapeutic armamentarium in regard to platelet inhibitor therapy is expanding, but it remains to be seen how this plays out depending on the trade-off between efficacy and bleeding.

Heparin versus low-molecular-weight heparin. The optimum dose of UFH is not established, but a weight-adjusted regimen with frequent monitoring to maintain the activated partial thromboplastin time (aPTT) between 1.5 and 2 times controlled is probably the most reasonable.[82] Although the optimal duration of anticoagulant therapy remains undefined, in the majority of trials, UFH was continued for 2 to 5 days. There is a lower incidence of heparin-associated thrombocytopenia with LMWH. The introduction of LMWH has been an advance given the ease of subcutaneous administration and the absence of a need for aPTT monitoring. This allows for a longer period of treatment and consequently offers some protection against the "rebound" phenomenon seen soon after heparin withdrawal. Theoretically, LMWH offers other potential benefits by acting on both thrombin generation and thrombin activity (see Chapter 9, p. 369).

Which LMWH should be used? Because there are no direct head-to-head comparative trials, definitive conclusions cannot be drawn. Two trials with enoxaparin, ESSENCE and TIMI IIB, have demonstrated a moderate benefit over UFH,[83,84] one trial with dalteparin[85] was neutral, and the FRAXIS trial with nadroparin showed an unfavorable trend.[86] Hence enoxaparin is preferred in guidelines.

LMWH and PCI. Because the level of anticoagulant activity cannot easily be measured in patients receiving LMWH, concern has been expressed regarding its use in patients undergoing coronary angiography. Three studies have shown, however, that PCI can be performed safely in this setting,[87-89] as now confirmed in the large SYNERGY study, although at the cost of a modest increase in bleeding.[90] A subsequent comprehensive review of seven relevant trials found no difference between the two treatments in regard to mortality, recurrent angina, and bleeding, although LMWH significantly reduced the risk of MI, revascularization, and thrombocytopenia.[91] Thus LMWH is safe and effective with PCI and GpIIb/IIIa inhibitors, but in many institutions, particularly in the United States, is used less frequently than UFH, with which clinical experience is greater.

Direct thrombin and factor Xa inhibitors. *Bivalirudin,* a direct thrombin inhibitor, is approved in the United States for clinical use in patients with unstable angina undergoing PCI, as summarized in Chapter 9 (see Fig. 9-11). In patients with moderate- to high-risk ACS and planned early catheterization, bivalirudin infusion with upstream aspirin is superior to UFH or enoxaparin plus GpIIb/IIIa antagonists, with less bleeding and similar clinical outcomes.[92]

Fondaparinux (see Chapter 9, p. 374) is a synthetic pentasaccharide that is an antithrombin-dependent indirect inhibitor of activated factor X (Xa) without inhibition of the thrombin molecule itself (see Fig. 9-10). The specific anti-Xa activity is approximately sevenfold higher that that of LMWHs. It has a longer half-life (approximately 17 hours) than UFH or LMWH, and needs no monitoring. Fondaparinux is superior to placebo but not to UFH in ST-elevation myocardial infarction (STEMI) (treated with thrombolytic agent or without reperfusion) and is superior to LMWH in non–ST-elevation ACS (lower bleeding and fewer deaths). The ESC guidelines favor fondaparinux in non–ST-elevation ACS unless the patient is planned for early intervention.[93] ACC-AHA guidelines, however, support fondaparinux for both invasive and conservative strategies as class IB, below class IA for UFH or enoxaparin.[8] Before PCI, adjunctive UFH is added to lessen the risk of catheter thrombosis.

Platelet GpIIb/IIIa receptor antagonists. Smith et al. state, "A challenge for current guidelines is the integration of GpIIb/IIIa studies from the 1990s with more recent studies using preangiography clopidogrel loading and newer anticoagulants."[4] As shown in Fig. 12-3, GpIIb/IIIa blockers combined with aspirin and clopidogrel and heparin (UFH/ LMWH) benefit patients who have ACS without ST-segment elevation but are also at high risk (high risk score or elevated troponin levels), in whom intervention by PCI is likely or indicated. The ACC-AHA guidelines recommend that troponin-positive high-risk ACS patients needing PCI should be covered both by upstream clopidogrel and by GpIIb/IIIa inhibition besides aspirin and an anticoagulant (class I).[4] For such use "upstream" of PCI, the "small-molecule" agents eptifibatide or tirofiban are FDA approved in the United States, whereas abciximab is not. In low-risk patients, the guidelines suggest that either a GpIIb/IIIa blocker *or* clopidogrel should be added to aspirin and anticoagulation before angiography.[4] However, the more recent results of the ACUITY study show that bivalirudin monotherapy can replace heparin plus GpIIb/IIIa inhibitors with less bleeding[94] and similar outcomes at 1 year.[94,95]

The window of opportunity for new anticoagulants in the acute syndromes is narrow, particularly because many patients are on dual antiplatelet therapy and the risk of bleeding with a third drug is higher. In the ACS2-TIMI 51 trial rivaroxaban increased the risk of major bleeding and intracranial hemorrhage but not the risk of fatal bleeding. It did, however, reduce the risk of the composite endpoint of death from cardiovascular causes, MI, or stroke.[96] A previous trial on the ACS with apixaban was stopped prematurely because of a lack of benefit and an increased risk of bleeding.[97]

In a nonrandomized subgroup analysis of the PLATO trial, the use of PPI was independently associated with a higher rate of cardiovascular events in ACS patients receiving clopidogrel and also during ticagrelor treatments. The conclusion is that the association between PPI use and adverse events may be confounding with PPI use more of marker for than a cause of a higher rate of cardiovascular events.[98]

Thrombolytic therapy to be avoided. Despite its beneficial role in patients with AMI presenting with ST-segment elevation, thrombolytic therapy is absolutely contraindicated in patients with unstable angina or NSTEMI. Not only is the complication rate increased, but in some studies, overall mortality was higher.

Antiischemic Drugs for ACS

Intravenous nitroglycerin. Intravenous nitroglycerin (Fig. 12-4) is part of the standard therapy, although sometimes it is held in reserve for patients with recurrent pain despite oral nitrates.

β-Blockers. β-Blockers, even though lacking good prospective trial data, are standard therapy, and should be started early in the absence of contraindications. Arguments for β-blockade largely rest on first principles (reduced myocardial demand). For higher-risk patients or those with ongoing rest pain, intravenous β-blockers are followed by oral administration, whereas oral β-blockers will suffice for patients at lower risk. In hemodynamically unstable patients, ultra-short-acting esmolol may be used.[99]

Calcium channel blockers and other drugs. Nondihydropyridine CCBs (diltiazem or verapamil) are used when β-blockers are contraindicated or are inadequate; contraindications include clinically significant LV dysfunction. Diltiazem compared well with nitrates during the acute phase of unstable angina, with better event-free survival at 1 year.[100] An *ACE inhibitor* should be administered orally within 24 hours in patients with pulmonary congestion or an LV ejection fraction of 40% in the absence of hypotension or other contraindications.[8] Although not available in the United States, *nicorandil,* a K_{ATP} channel opener, could be useful (see Chapter 2). *Ranolazine* (see Fig. 2-9; p. 55) was tested in the large MERLIN-TIMI 36 randomized trial in 6560 patients with non–ST-elevation ACS.[101] The primary endpoint (composite of cardiovascular death, MI, or recurrent ischemia) was

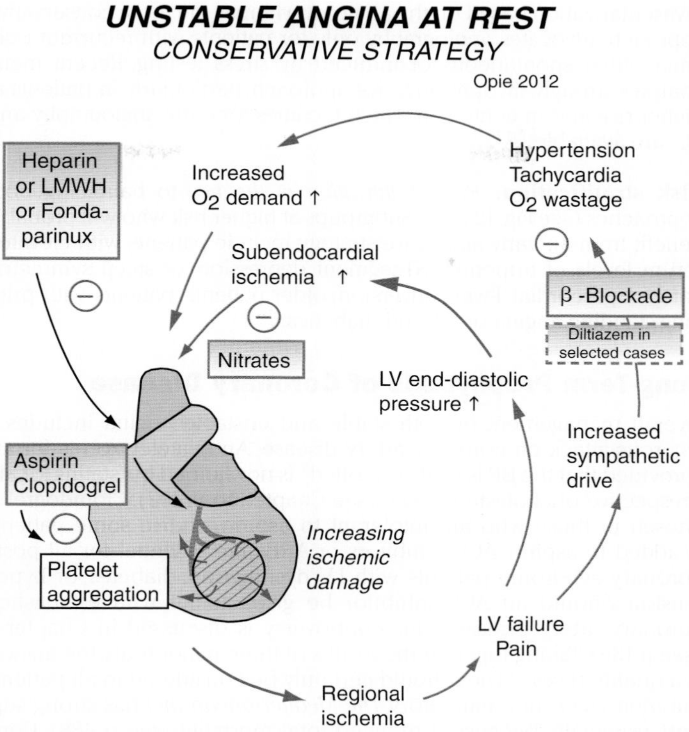

UNSTABLE ANGINA AT REST
CONSERVATIVE STRATEGY
Opie 2012

Figure 12-4 Hypothetical mechanisms in acute coronary syndrome presenting as unstable angina at rest, and for proposed conservative therapy. Note major role of anticoagulants, including fondaparinux and antiplatelet agents (aspirin plus clopidogrel). Nitrates and β-blockade are standard. β-Blockade should be particularly effective against sympathetic activation with increased heart rate and blood pressure. Calcium channel blockers such as diltiazem (heart-rate lowering) may be used intravenously or orally if β-blockade is contraindicated or fails or with care added to β-blockade. Dihydropyridines such as amlodipine and nifedipine should generally not be used unless vasospastic angina is strongly suspected. *LMWH,* Low-molecular-weight heparin; *LV,* left ventricular; O_2, oxygen. (Figure © L.H. Opie, 2012.)

not achieved, yet recurrent ischemia was reduced. In patients with refractory angina on maximal medical therapy, the potential antiarrhythmic effects of ranolazine are currently under investigation.[102] Ranolazine has also been shown to significantly improve hemoglobin A1c (HbA1c) and recurrent ischemia in patients with diabetes and reduce the incidence of increased HbA1c in those without evidence of previous hyperglycemia in the MERLIN-TIMI 36 randomized controlled trial of patients with ACS. The mechanisms of these glycometabolic effects are under investigation.[103] Intraaortic balloon counterpulsation may be helpful in hemodynamically unstable patients pending angiography and PCI.

Invasive versus Conservative Strategy in ACS

Although there is general agreement that the first step is to stabilize the patient, there has been considerable debate as to whether the subsequent strategy should be invasive or conservative (see Fig. 12-3). The former involves coronary angiography with a view toward coronary revascularization based on the anatomy, whereas the more conservative approach advocates angiography only for patients with recurrent ischemia, either spontaneous or induced by stress testing. Recent meta-analyses strongly favor an invasive approach, particularly in patients at higher risk and in centers in which facilities for early angiography and PCI are available.[104-108]

Risk stratification. *Risk stratification is the key* to balancing both approaches (see Fig. 12-3).[109] Subgroups at higher risk who will probably benefit from an early aggressive strategy include patients with elevated serum levels of troponins, ST-segment depression, or steep symmetric anterior precordial T-wave inversion; older patients; patients with prior long-standing angina or MI; and diabetics.[110-112]

Long-Term Prophylaxis of Coronary Disease

Overall management of both stable and unstable angina includes a vigorous attack on coronary artery disease. "Antiplatelet agents for all" (provided that the BP is well controlled) is now joined by "statins for all," irrespective of cholesterol level (see Chapter 10, p. 402). Clopidogrel is chosen in those who are intolerant to aspirin, and in some patients is added to aspirin. ACE inhibitors or ARBs are essential for all post–coronary syndrome patients with LV dysfunction, diabetes, or hypertension. Should an ACE inhibitor be given to all with established coronary artery disease? This controversy is discussed in Chapter 5 (see p. 136). Taking together the results of three major trials, the answer is a qualified yes.[10] They should certainly be considered in all patients but their use is not mandatory. *The Mediterranean diet* has strong support, especially because it reduced total mortality (see p. 488). Combined laboratory, epidemiologic, and clinical trial data strongly suggest that increased dietary ω-3–rich fish oils help to protect from sudden cardiac death (SCD).[113] Tight BP and glycemia control is logical although not evidence based. Other risk factors also need optimizing, including weight loss, increased exercise, and smoking cessation. Long-term β-blockade is generally recommended, although without firm supporting contemporary trial data, and with potential side effects of fatigue, erectile dysfunction, and weight gain that mitigate against an optimal lifestyle.

Prinzmetal's Vasospastic Angina

Prinzmetal's vasospastic angina is a relatively rare condition, which is much more common in Japan, that often manifests as acute ischemic pain with ST-segment elevation but without MI, although MI and malignant arrhythmias may occur.[114] It requires relief of coronary spasm rather than thrombolytic therapy. *β-Blockers are inferior to CCBs* and may theoretically aggravate the spasm. However, in one study of active cocaine users, β-blockers were associated with a reduced risk of MI.[115] Coronary spasm is usually responsive to nitroglycerin, long-acting nitrates, and CCBs, all of which are considered first-line therapies. Short-acting nifedipine, diltiazem, and verapamil all completely abolish the recurrence of angina in approximately 70% of patients, with a substantial improvement in another 20%. Starting doses of CCBs are high (e.g., 240 to 480 mg/day of verapamil, 120 to 360 mg/day of diltiazem, and 60 to 120 mg/day of nifedipine). The relatively vasoselective long-acting dihydropyridine amlodipine is also effective. The next step is to add a CCB from another class or a long-acting nitrate.[116] Smoking cessation is imperative. β-Blockers may be tried, particularly in patients not responding to CCBs and nitrates. In refractory cases of Prinzmetal's angina associated with coronary artery disease, bypass grafting may be combined with cardiac sympathetic denervation (plexectomy).

REPERFUSION TIME, MYOCARDIAL SALVAGE AND MORTALITY

Gersh 2012

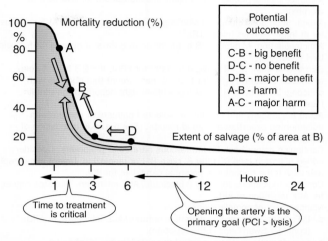

Figure 12-5 **Relationship between mortality reduction and extent of salvage.** Schematic illustrating the relationship between duration of ischemia prior to reperfusion, reduction in mortality *(thick black line)*, and myocardial salvage *(area under the curve)*. During the first 2 to 3 hours *(shaded in pale red)*, potential benefits are large and time to treatment is critical. *The shorter the time, the greater the benefit.* Later, on the "flat" part of the curve, time is less of a factor and the priority is to open the infarct-related artery; in this setting a mechanical approach is preferable. *A-D* illustrates potential outcomes from strategies that alter times to achieve reperfusion. A key issue relates to delays incurred on the steep part of the curve in which transfer to receive a more effective strategy (primary percutaneous coronary intervention [PCI]) might be offset by achieving earlier reperfusion with fibrinolytic agents *(D-C)*. These relationships might be modified by other factors such as myocardial oxygen uptake, collaterals, and preconditioning.

Early Phase Acute Myocardial Infarction

Management of AMI encompasses two different strategies. *The early phase* of evolving MI is dominated by the need for prompt reperfusion therapy because the time for possible salvage is so limited, possibly only up to 3 hours at the most (Fig. 12-5), whereas the *chronic phase* is a multipronged attack on the extent and progression of coronary artery disease, ventricular remodeling, and arrhythmias.

General care. General care is nonetheless also crucial (Table 12-2). Aspirin needs to be given as early as possible, and pain relieved. *Morphine* (4-8 mg IV by slow intravenous push followed by 2-8 mg at 5- to 15-min intervals) combines a potent analgesic effect with hemodynamic actions that are particularly beneficial in reducing myocardial oxygen demand (mixed venous oxygen [MVO_2]), namely a marked venodilator action reducing ventricular preload, a decrease in heart rate, a mild arterial vasodilator action that may reduce afterload, and a decrease in sympathetic outflow. A "hidden" benefit of morphine may be its capacity, shown experimentally, to precondition the heart, thereby protecting against further ischemia. In the presence of hypovolemia, morphine may cause profound hypotension. The administration of *oxygen* by nasal prongs is almost universal practice in AMI, although whether it does any good is not established. Oxygen should

Table 12-2

Early Phase Acute Myocardial Infarction: Principles of Management[589]

1. Minimize pain-to-needle time, urgent hospitalization. Relieve pain by morphine.
2. Aspirin upon suspicion. Add clopidogrel 75 mg daily (class 1A),* continue for at least 14 days (class 1B).[71]
3. Anticoagulation: Minimum 48 h, prefer up to 8 days; if beyond 48 h, avoid UFH (class 1A).[71]
4. Duration of pain: If >3 h, rapid transfer for PPCI. If <2-3 h, or if delay to balloon inflation is greater than 90 min, urgent thrombolysis with anticoagulation by UFH or low-molecular-weight heparin or bivalirudin (see Fig. 12-3).
5. Acute angioplasty and stenting in selected patients at centers with documented expertise and good results. (See previous discussion of delay times.)
6. Continuing pain: Check BP. Intravenous nitrates or β-blockers. Consider added diltiazem (see Chapter 3, page 81) or ranolazine. Urgent angiography and IABP if the patient is a potential candidate for PCI.
7. Consider indications for early β-blockade, ACE inhibition. Diabetes argues for ACE inhibition or ARB.
8. Management of complications:
   a. LVF: Treat aggressively; diuretics, nitrates, ACE inhibitors, or ARBs (consider Swan-Ganz catheterization).
   b. Symptomatic ventricular arrhythmias: Lidocaine; if refractory, amiodarone.
   c. Supraventricular arrhythmias: Adenosine; consider esmolol; avoid verapamil or diltiazem if LVF.
   d. Cardiogenic shock: Acute angioplasty, IABP, bypass surgery.
   e. RV infarction: Fluids, inotropic support. Avoid nitrates.
   f. Rupture of free wall, mitral valve, ventricular septum: Cardiac surgery.
   g. Hyperglycemia: Use insulin whether or not patient is diabetic.
   h. Strongly consider ACE inhibition or ARB for all diabetics.

ACE, Angiotensin-converting enzyme; *ARB*, angiotensin receptor blocker; *BP*, blood pressure; *CCB*, calcium channel blocker; *IABP*, intraaortic balloon pump; *LVF*, left ventricular failure; *PCI*, percutaneous coronary intervention; *PPCI*, primary percutaneous coronary intervention; *RV*, right ventricular; *UFH*, unfractionated heparin.
*Classes of Recommendations (1-3) and levels of evidence (A-C)

be administered to those patients with overt pulmonary congestion or arterial oxygen desaturation ($SaO_2 < 90\%$).[8]

Bradyarrhythmias. *Atropine* (0.3-0.5 mg IV aliquots to a maximum of 2 mg) has a vagolytic effect that is useful for the management of bradyarrhythmias with AV block (particularly with inferior infarction), sinus or nodal bradycardia with hypotension, or bradycardia-related ventricular ectopy. Small doses and careful monitoring are essential because the elimination of vagal inhibition may unmask latent sympathetic overactivity, thereby producing sinus tachycardia and rarely even ventricular tachycardia (VT) or ventricular fibrillation (VF). The role of prophylactic atropine for uncomplicated bradycardia remains questionable.

Sinus tachycardia. Sinus tachycardia is a common manifestation of early phase sympathetic overactivity, which increases MVO_2 and predisposes to tachyarrhythmias. The first step is to treat the underlying cause—pain, anxiety, hypovolemia, or pump failure—and then to use a β-blocker, which is safe and effective provided that there are no contraindications and the patient is carefully observed. If the hemodynamic status is borderline, the very-short-acting esmolol (see next section) may be selected.

Acute hypertension. Acute hypertension must be tightly controlled in all patients in whom thrombolytic therapy is under consideration because elevated BPs increase the risk of bleeding and, in particular, cerebral hemorrhage.[72] Target BPs are in the range of less than 130/80 mm Hg, but without hard data to support these goals. The BP should be lowered gradually, particularly in older patients. In STEMI, the principles of hypertension management are similar to those for the non–ST-elevation ACS.[117] Short-acting β-blockers, usually intravenous, in conjunction with intravenous nitrates, are given to hemodynamically stable patients. ACE inhibitors are indicated in stable patients with persistent hypertension, particularly in the presence of large infarcts, anterior MIs, and LV dysfunction. In patients intolerant to ACE inhibitors, ARBs are a proven alternative. CCBs are untested in the setting of AMI.

Acute Reperfusion Therapy for AMI

How urgent? Reperfusion therapy has revolutionized the management and prognosis of STEMI.[118] The benefit is that more cardiomyocytes are saved from ischemic death than are killed by reperfusion injury.[119] There is a steep relationship during the first 3 hours between the duration of ischemia, mortality reduction, and myocardial salvage (see Fig. 12-5). Thus the window of opportunity is narrow and time to treatment is critical. This relationship between time and salvage may be modified by factors such as myocardial oxygen demands, ischemic preconditioning, the extent of collaterals, age, and infarct location.[120] Thereafter, on the "flat" part of the curve, time dependence of therapy is less urgent in comparison to the primary objective of achieving patency of the infarct-related artery. It is likely that the efficacy of lysis decreases as clots become increasingly resistant with time, whereas the ability of PCI to open arteries probably remains unimpaired, supporting a mechanical approach at this stage in the time course of MI.[121,122] In approximately 60% of hospitals in the United States with facilities for primary percutaneous coronary intervention (PPCI), the mechanical approach is unequivocally the preferred form of therapy, providing this can be carried out 24 hours a day, 7 days a week.

Community management. The approach to the patient presenting in a community hospital without a catheterization laboratory but within 2 to 3 hours of symptoms (Fig. 12-6) is controversial. The crucial question now is whether such patients should receive routine fibrinolytic therapy as opposed to the delay incurred in transferring to a hospital with PPCI facilities. The degree of delay that is acceptable remains controversial. After 2-3 hours, when time to treatment is less of an issue, transfer for PPCI is logical and widely used.[123-125]

Mechanical revascularization in AMI. Despite the undisputed success of early fibrinolysis, especially in the first 2 to 3 hours, there are considerable limitations to the ability of currently available thrombolytics in achieving "optimal" reperfusion. This provides a strong rationale for the mechanical approaches using PPCI with angioplasty and stents. Several metaanalyses comparing PPCI with thrombolytic therapy have demonstrated 30-day and 1-year benefits for PPCI in terms of death and particularly reinfarction and stroke. This was noted in each period after symptom onset, but these analyses do not address the effect of incremental delay prior to transport for PPCI.[126] Thus there is now consensus that PPCI is the preferred form of reperfusion therapy providing the time delay between balloon inflation versus administration of lytic drug is less than 90 minutes. Stents lessen the high rates of restenosis and reocclusion after balloon angioplasty but without any overall difference in mortality.[127] For any program using PPCI, constant auditing of individual and institutional outcomes is mandatory. It is not good enough to rely on the results of randomized trials in large registries, composed of individuals with expertise and enthusiasm for this particular approach.[128] In the HORIZONS trial, patients receiving a paclitaxel-eluting stent had a slightly but statistically significantly lower

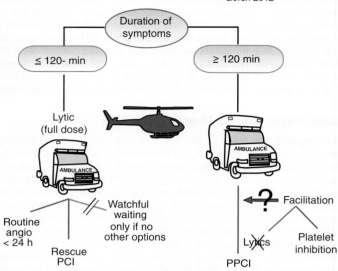

REPERFUSION FOR STEMI IN COMMUNITY HOSPITALS
Gersh 2012

Figure 12-6 Reperfusion therapy for ST-elevation myocardial infarction in community hospitals, according to duration of symptoms. If less than 120 to 180 minutes have passed, lytic therapy is started and the patient transferred to a percutaneous coronary intervention (PCI) center by ambulance or helicopter, followed by routine angiography (angio) and, if needed, rescue PCI. If more than 120 to 180 minutes have passed, the patient is transported to a PCI center for primary percutaneous coronary intervention (PPCI). Facilitation by thrombolytic therapy en route gives no benefit. In the long term, one solution is the development of PCI facilities at peripheral hospitals even without on-site surgery. (Figure © B.J. Gersh, 2012.)

rate of ischemia-driven revascularization at 3 years with no differences in rates of death, MI, and stroke.[129] Given the drive to shorten door-to-balloon times, many patients will present for PPCI without crucial information on comorbidities, the ability to continue platelet inhibitors for at least 1 year, and the need for noncardiac surgical procedures in the future, and in this situation, BMS may be a better option depending on lesion length, complexity, and vessel diameter.[128,130-132] Intracoronary thrombectomy and distal protection devices, although logical and at times clinically useful, have not had any beneficial effects on outcomes, and their routine use is not recommended.[133] Intracoronary β-blockade may be a simple procedure to protect the distal myocardium during PCI.[134]

How to do it faster. The quicker the better, whether the reperfusion is by fibrinolysis or by PCI: a delay of only 30 minutes increases 1-year mortality by 7.5%.[94] Three major time delays are (1) onset of patient's pain to first medical contact; (2) home-to-hospital time; and (3) door-to-needle or door-to-balloon time in the hospital. The greatest delay is from symptom onset to emergency room, and this has changed little over the last decade, being in the range of 85 minutes.[135] The next delay is the door-to-balloon time, with the benchmark being less than 90 minutes.[136] There have been marked improvements in door-to-balloon times in the United States and elsewhere, but the Achilles heel of reperfusion therapy remains the delay between symptom onset and first medical contact and prolonged delays incurred in transferring patients to PCI-capable facilities.[137-141] The major advances in the delivery of reperfusion therapy will arise from steps taken outside the PCI-capable hospitals, which already have streamlined systems in place.[142-144] In large cities, the optimal approach is achieved by having paramedics available to triage and transport patients directly to designated PPCI centers.

Regional systems of care. To rapidly reperfuse patients who present to hospitals without PCI capability, rapid transfer to sites with PPCI can be streamlined.[128] To reduce the overall "ischemic time" (symptom onset to reperfusion), effective and integrated prehospital systems (including paramedic ambulance with telemetry of the electrocardiogram and rapid coordination with the PCI center) can substantially reduce prehospital delays.[128,141,144] Another approach to early reperfusion, which has been effective in some countries, particularly in Europe, is prehospital thrombolytic therapy, which requires intense community organization to get the paramedic team trained and on site in time.[145,146] The key to the establishment of successful STEMI networks is to understand that "one size does not fit all" and that factors such as weather, distance (rural or urban), resources, and the organization of ambulance services play a determining role.[128,147] As recently pointed out in a French registry, the key is to keep it simple and avoid the involvement of too many people.[148,149]

Facilitated PCI or pharmacoinvasive approach. Facilitated PCI is defined by the initial use of fibrinolytic drugs followed by routine immediate PCI after transfer to a PCI-capable institution.[124,130,150]

The "pharmacoinvasive approach" is characterized by full-dose fibrinolytic therapy followed by transfer either for rescue PCI or, if the patient is stable with evidence of successful reperfusion, there is a general consensus that angiography with a view to PCI should be performed within 3 to 24 hours of admission (the so called "drip and ship" approach).[128,151,152] Facilitated PCI is now not recommended following the results of the FINESSE[153] and ASSENT–4 studies.[154,155] Although the pharmacoinvasive strategy is currently the objective of an ongoing trial, this approach is widely practiced and recommended by the ESC guidelines for systems in which transfer times result in door-to-balloon times of greater than 90 minutes.[72]

Which thrombolytic agent? Worldwide, most patients with AMI are given fibrinolytic therapy. The first GUSTO trial[156] demonstrated the superiority of the accelerated regimen of tissue plasminogen activator (tPA; *Alteplase*) over streptokinase. Nonetheless, this came at two prices: increased cost (see Table 9-8) and a slightly but significantly greater risk of intracranial hemorrhage (see Table 9-9), especially in women older than 75 years.[157] Single-bolus *tenecteplase* (TNK) is now the most widely used thrombolytic agent in North America and Europe because of its efficacy and ease of administration. TNK and alteplase are equivalent in regard to 30-day mortality, but noncerebral bleeding and blood transfusions were less with TNK.[158] The dose of TNK is weight adjusted and administered as a single bolus over 5 seconds (versus 90 minutes of variable-rate infusion with tPA). *Reteplase* (rPA) is a more fibrin-specific agent administered as two 10-unit boluses given 30 minutes apart. Alteplase and rPA are equivalent in both mortality and hemorrhage.[159] Overall, we appear to have reached a plateau in that the new fibrinolytics do not result in increased reperfusion rates or reduced mortality. The major strength of the bolus agents (TNK, rPA) lies in their ease of administration, resulting in fewer dosing errors.

Limited benefit of GpIIb/IIIA inhibitors plus reperfusion therapy. The initial promise of GpIIb/IIIa inhibitors for acute STEMI has not been translated into a major long-term clinical benefit. In the early trials totaling more than 22,000 patients, there was a modest benefit on rates of reinfarction, no mortality benefit, and a significant increase in bleeding that is especially marked in the case of abciximab.[160] In the setting of PPCI, a metaanalysis of six randomized trials suggested that the early administration of the GpIIb/IIIa inhibitors abciximab or tirofiban in patients receiving UFH was associated with a nonsignificant 28% reduction in mortality and significant improvements compared with placebo in TIMI flow grades.[161] However, no bivalirudin was used and two of the four studies refer only to abstracts. The largest study,[162] not included in this metaanalysis, did not show any benefit from abciximab and stenting. In HORIZON's AMI trial, bivalirudin with provisional GpIIb/IIIA use was equivalent in efficacy to heparin plus Gp IIab/IIIa use prior to PPCI, but major non–CABG-related bleeding was less.[163] Despite the lack of decisive data, in current practice GpIIb/IIIa inhibitors are usually administered on arrival in the catheterization laboratory or during transfer unless bivalirudin is used.

Reperfusion injury and microvascular dysfunction. Considerable experimental evidence points to a spectrum of reperfusion events, including ventricular arrhythmias, mechanical stunning, and microvascular injury. Reperfusion-induced apoptosis has now been added to this list.[119] Reperfusion injury occurs on reperfusion, not later. Microvascular dysfunction, however, may precede or follow arterial reperfusion. There is now increasing realization that, despite restoration of flow to the epicardial infarct-related artery, there remains a persistent impairment of myocardial reperfusion and microvascular dysfunction[164,165] that has stimulated multiple trials of widely diverse agents aimed at modifying these pathophysiologic consequences of coronary occlusion and reperfusion. Initially optimistic expectations that myocardial cooling, the use of aqueous oxygen, erythropoietin, delta protein kinase C inhibition, antiinflammatory agents, and compliment inhibitors, among many others, would be effective adjuncts to reperfusion therapy by enhancing myocardial salvage have not been met.[166-170] Although distal mechanical protection devices have been shown to be ineffective, the use of adjunctive manual thrombectomy devices is associated with better epicardial and myocardial perfusion, less distal embolization, and a lower mortality.[171] More recently, a number of novel strategies such as ischemic preconditioning,[172-174] human atrial natriuretic peptide,[175] cyclosporine A,[176] and remote ischemic preconditioning[177] have been shown to reduce infarct size in smaller trials that illustrate proof of the concept that reperfusion injury can be modified. A recent addition to the list of promising agents is exenatide, which is a drug initially used for glycemic control.[178,179] Whether this drug that appears to enhance myocardial salvage can also improve clinical outcomes remains to be determined. This has been an area of considerable frustration and the failure to translate the animal models into the clinical setting could be due to multiple factors including inappropriate animal models, species differences, the different natural history between experimental occlusion and reperfusion versus the dynamic nature of an evolving MI, and poorly designed clinical studies. The problem is that, even if these approaches were effective, they are often given too late to make a difference. Conversely, if used very early in the course of MI, the preexisting low mortality rates and high rates of salvage would make it difficult to "demonstrate" a difference—a real "Catch-22" situation.

Aspirin and clopidogrel. All patients with AMI need both aspirin and clopidogrel. For the initial aspirin dose, 160 mg was used in the first large AMI trial in 1988[180] and also favored by a recent retrospective analysis,[181] although some guidelines recommend 160-325 mg for the initial dose.[182] The first tablet should be chewed or crushed and as indefinite maintenance therapy, the dose should be 75-162 mg per day. Clopidogrel is given whether AMI is treated by fibrinolysis or PPCI, provided that the added risk of bleeding is acceptable (see Tables 12-1 and 12-2; see also Chapter 9, p. 348). In patients receiving fibrinolytic drugs, the 2007 focus update of the 2004 ACC-AHA guidelines advocate

300 mg of clopidogrel followed by 75 mg per day for 14 days and no loading dose in patients older than the age of 75.[183] Although there are no trials specifically addressing the efficacy of clopidogrel plus aspirin versus aspirin alone in STEMI patients treated with PPCI, subset analyses from other trials strongly favor the use of clopidogrel and most would advocate a loading dose of 600 mg.[184] The first perspective randomized trial to compare a 600-mg loading dose of clopidogrel with a 300-mg dose in patients with STEMI undergoing PPCI demonstrated a reduction in infarct size and in clinical events at 30 days[185] and support the recommendations of the latest European guidelines in the context of primary PCI for STEMI.[186]

Prasugrel and ticagrelor. Depending on the risk bleeding, prasugrel 60 mg given as early as possible after presentation may be superior to clopidogrel, particularly in patients with diabetes as shown in the Triton-TIMI 38 trial.[187,188] The role of ticagrelor in STEMI remains to be determined.

Heparin prophylaxis. Reocclusion, which occurs both early and late (weeks or months) after thrombolysis, remains the "Achilles heel" of reperfusion therapy. In a metaanalysis of more than 20,000 patients, the frequency of symptomatic recurrent MI during the index hospitalization was 4.2%, together with a two- to threefold increase in 30-day mortality.[189] Irrespective of the timing, reocclusion has markedly deleterious effects on LV function and long-term outcomes. There are many contributory factors, including the severity of the underlying residual stenosis, the persistence of the initial thrombogenic substrate (plaque fissure), and activation of platelets and of the clotting cascade. *Intravenous UFH* has an established place in fibrinolysis alongside tPA, TNK, or rPA, and should be used in the initial 24 to 48 hours to prevent further thrombin generation and reduce the risk of reocclusion. The dose should be adjusted to keep the aPTT between 60 and 80 seconds, taking care to avoid wide swings in the aPTT values. The aPTT should be evaluated 4 to 6 hours following a heparin bolus and then checked every 6 to 8 hours thereafter.

Duration of heparin therapy. Appropriate duration of heparin therapy is uncertain, but up to 48 hours has a class I recommendation, the limit existing because of increasing risk of heparin-induced thrombocytopenia (see Chapter 9 p. 368); thereafter other anticoagulant regimens are recommended.[72] In patients presenting with AMI and already on chronic warfarin therapy, the use of intravenous heparin should be similar to that in those not on warfarin. In patients receiving streptokinase, added intravenous heparin is controversial. (For our positive recommendations, see section on streptokinase, Chapter 9, p. 394).

Low-molecular-weight heparins. Enoxaparin is increasingly used because of the heparin deficiencies as an antithrombotic agent. In fibrinolytic therapy of AMI, dose-adjusted enoxaparin continued up to 8 days has class IA evidence.[72] Reduce doses for those aged 75 years or older or for renal impairment (see Table 9-5). For PCI, a single dose of enoxaparin gave less bleeding than heparin (see Chapter 9).

In the randomized ATOLL trial intravenous enoxaparin compared with UFH significantly reduced clinical ischemic outcomes without differences in bleeding and procedural success in 910 patients undergoing primary PCI.[190]

Direct thrombin and factor Xa inhibitors. Fondaparinux and bivalirudin (see Fig. 9-10 for sites of action) both cause less bleeding than heparin, with fondaparinux best tested for fibrinolytic therapy and bivalirudin for early invasive PCI (see Table 9-5). Bivalirudin has excellent data for use in an invasive strategy (PCI), especially when bleeding should be avoided (see Chapter 9, p. 371). For thrombolytic or no reperfusion therapy for STEMI, fondaparinux was superior to placebo and to UFH in the OASIS-6 trial.[191] However, when primary PCI was chosen, there was an increase in guiding catheter thrombosis with no overall benefit. Thus we do not recommend fondaparinux for STEMI treated by primary PCI.

Protecting the Ischemic Myocardium

Prophylactic early β-blockade. Pooled data on trials of β-blockers given early to approximately 29,000 patients with AMI showed a 13% reduction in acute-phase mortality.[192] Yet almost all of these studies were gathered in the prethrombolytic era. With thrombolysis, there is no hard evidence on the benefits of β-blockers on early mortality in patients receiving reperfusion therapy. Moreover, the COMMIT trial on almost 46,000 patients, half of whom had received thrombolytics, raised serious questions about the routine use of intravenous β-blockers; mortality increased in patients with hemodynamic instability with a balancing trend in the other direction in stable patients.[193] Furthermore, in the only study comparing early intravenous β-blockade with delayed oral β-blockade (6 days later), early reinfarction decreased with early therapy but mortality was unchanged at 1 year.[194] Overall, *early intravenous β-blockade should be used only selectively* for sinus tachycardia, tachyarrhythmias such as AF, hypertension, and recurrent ischemia. Despite the lack of definitive clinical trial evidence, several studies from a variety of databases suggested the mortality benefit of β-blockers persists during the reperfusion era[195-197] and that the benefit is similar or greater in older patients.[198] For patients undergoing primary PCI, observational analyses (but no prospective studies) suggest that early intravenous β-blocker therapy may be beneficial and may reduce 6-month mortality.[199-201] Although there have been no randomized trials of β-blockers specifically in patients with NSTEMI, nonetheless, based on pathophysiologic considerations and evidence of efficacy in unselected patients with ACS and chronic coronary disease, the 2011 ACC-AHA focus update on the management of patients with unstable angina and non–ST-elevation ACS do recommend use of β-blockers in all patients with ACS who do not have contraindications.[202] β-blockers are particularly indicated in patients with ongoing chest pain, hypertension, or tachycardia.[117] Ideally β-blockade can more easily be introduced later, when there is hemodynamic stabilization (late intervention, 25 studies, 24,000 patients) to bring about a 23% reduction in late-phase mortality.[192] The drugs with US licenses are metoprolol and atenolol, whereas the short-acting esmolol is preferred when the hemodynamic situation is potentially unstable.

Early use of ACE inhibitors or ARBs in AMI. Early oral ACE inhibitors in patients at high risk (hypertension, diabetes, chronic renal disease, clinical LV failure or LV ejection fraction less than 40%) followed by treatment continued indefinitely is strongly advised (class IA).[72] A logical policy would be to start the ACE inhibitor as soon as the patient is hemodynamically stable and to watch for hypotension or new renal impairment. An ARB is the therapy of choice if there is ACE inhibitor intolerance. Intravenous ACE inhibitors are not recommended because of the risk of hypotension.

Limitation of infarct size. Because MI is ultimately the consequence of a serious imbalance between myocardial oxygen supply and demand, it is logical and prudent to employ measures aimed at redressing this imbalance. These measures include the treatment of arrhythmias, hypoxia, heart failure, hypertension, and tachycardia. Hypokalemia should be sought and treated. Despite much laboratory evidence that numerous pharmacologic agents such as β-blockers, nitrates, metabolic agents, and free radical scavengers will reduce infarct size, clinical evidence of benefit has been difficult to prove, perhaps because such therapy has inevitably been started after the first 2 to 3 hours, whereafter the infarct size is relatively fixed (see Fig. 12-5).

Early intervention before PCI. Logically timing is important and the earlier the better as shown experimentally[203] and in patients by the benefits of early metabolic intervention by exenatide or glucose-insulin-potassium (GIK). Exenatide, a glucagon-like peptide–1 agonist (see Fig. 11-6), reduced infarct size by 30%.[204] In the IMMEDIATE trial, 871 patients with suspected ACS were given GIK in the ambulance, which reduced rates of the composite outcome of cardiac arrest or in-hospital mortality, although the primary endpoint was not achieved.[205] That timing is crucial was shown as follows. Exenatide reduced reperfusion infarct size by 30% when given within 132 minutes or less of the time delay from first medical contact to first balloon.[204] In another early study in the ambulance, intervention by remote conditioning (pumping up and down a BP cuff), increased the myocardial reperfusion salvage index by approximately one-third from 0.55 to 0.75 (p = 0.33).[206] Thus in the future there will be more emphasis on ideal management in the ambulance whether by metabolic therapy or by conditioning.

Timing of metabolic therapy is critical. A recent metaanalysis of nine randomized trials that involved more than 28,000 patients did not reveal any mortality benefit for GIK given for ST-segment elevation AMI.[207] However, all the studies were on AMI 3 or more hours after the onset of symptoms except for GIPS-1, which accounted for only 3% of the total and had a relative risk (RR) of 0.83, whereas more than 20,000 of the patients were in one large trial, CREATE-ECLA, which accounted for 70% of the patients and in which the mean delay time was 4.7 hrs.[207]

Intravenous magnesium. Intravenous magnesium, otherwise discredited, remains indicated for patients with a torsades de pointes type of VT and in patients who have low serum magnesium or potassium levels frequently associated with chronic diuretic therapy.

Intravenous erythropoietin. Experimental data suggesting a variety of potentially cardioprotective mechanisms from the use of erythropoietin led to the REVEAL trial of 222 patients in which there was no difference in infarct size at 10-14 weeks, but there was a significantly increased risk of death, recurrent MI, stroke, or stent thrombosis in erythropoietin-treated patients.[208]

Arrhythmias in AMI

Therapy of ventricular arrhythmias in AMI. Primary VF and VT are associated with a sixfold increased mortality.[209] Although infrequent, recurrent ventricular arrhythmias pose a difficult management problem. *Lidocaine* (lignocaine) should not be given prophylactically but only against documented serious ventricular arrhythmias. A metaanalysis of 14 trials showed that prophylactic lidocaine reduces VF by approximately one-third, but may increase mortality by approximately the same percentage.[210] *Amiodarone* is now the preferred intravenous antiarrhythmic agent for life-threatening VTs when lidocaine fails. *Interventional techniques* such as atrial or ventricular pacing, stellate ganglion blockade, or radiofrequency catheter ablation may occasionally be life saving. Treatment of LV failure is an essential adjunct to antiarrhythmic therapy. The possibility of drug-induced VT or of hypokalemia should always be borne in mind.

Supraventricular tachyarrhythmias in AMI. AF, atrial flutter, or paroxysmal supraventricular tachycardia (PSVT) is usually transient, yet may be recurrent and troublesome.[211] Such arrhythmias may increase myocardial oxygen demands with an adverse prognosis. Precipitating factors requiring treatment include heart failure with atrial distention, hypoxia, acidosis, and pericarditis. Recurrent AF is best treated with intravenous amiodarone, particularly in the face of hemodynamic compromise, but in some patients the careful use of β-blockers may achieve adequate rate slowing. In the presence of hemodynamic instability, the ultra-short-acting β-blocker esmolol may be chosen. Intravenous digoxin may have a role especially in patients with heart failure. Class IC antiarrhythmic drugs should be avoided in place of supraventricular tachycardia. Initial therapy should be carotid sinus massage or other vagal maneuvers, and intravenous adenosine. If this fails, try intravenous metoprolol, amiodarone, or cardioversion depending on hemodynamic instability. In the case of supraventricular tachycardia, initial therapy should be carotid sinus massage or other vagal maneuvers. In the absence of LV failure, intravenous diltiazem or verapamil is effective in controlling the ventricular rate. Although intravenous diltiazem is licensed in the United States for acute conversion of supraventricular tachycardia, experience in AMI is limited and concurrent use of intravenous β-blockade is a contraindication. In the presence of LV failure, intravenous adenosine (*Adenocard*) or the careful use of esmolol may be tried. Adenosine cannot be used for AF or atrial flutter because of its ultrashort action. *Cardioversion* may be required in the face of compromised hemodynamics or severe ischemia, starting with a low threshold. To avoid systemic embolization after cardioversion for AF, heparin should be restarted or continued.

LV Failure and Shock in AMI

The first step is to exclude a reversible cause such as volume depletion, papillary muscle or ventricular septal rupture, or transient LV apical ballooning. Acute emotional stress can precipitate acute LV failure.[211,212] Swan-Ganz catheterization to measure LV filling pressure and cardiac output allows a rational choice between various IV agents that reduce both preload and afterload or chiefly the preload. Although for diverse reasons the use of the Swan-Ganz catheterization has declined, the concepts of pre- and afterload reduction remain important.

Load-reducing agents in AMI. In the intensive care unit setting, intravenous nitroglycerin is the most appropriate preload-reducing agent, particularly in the early hours of acute infarction when ischemia may contribute to LV dysfunction. For pulmonary edema, excess diuresis with excess preload reduction and relative volume depletion must be avoided, because reduced ventricular compliance requires higher filling pressures to maintain cardiac output. Where there are no intensive care facilities, intravenous unloading agents such as nitroprusside and nitrates are best avoided. Sublingual agents that reduce the preload (short-acting nitrates) should be useful. The diuretic furosemide, although standard therapy and acting by rapid vasodilation as well as by diuresis, may sometimes paradoxically induce vasoconstriction.

Nitrates in AMI. Current indications for nitrate therapy in AMI include recurrent or ongoing angina or ischemia, hypertension, and load reduction in patients with CHF and mitral regurgitation. Nitrates should not be administered to patients with a systolic BP of less than 90 mm Hg, patients with right ventricular infarction, or those who received sildenafil (or its equivalent) in the last 24 hours.

Low cardiac output in AMI. Monitoring the hemodynamic response invasively is indispensable. When cardiac output is low in the absence of an elevated wedge pressure or clinical and radiographic evidence of LV failure, it is crucial to exclude hypovolemia (possibly drug induced) or right ventricular infarction. In the absence of these conditions, acute positive inotropes such as norepinephrine, dopamine, or dobutamine (see Fig. 6-3) are used to bring the systolic BP up to 80 mm Hg. However, it is often forgotten that dobutamine, by stimulating peripheral β$_2$-receptors, can drop the diastolic BP. Nitrates are usually contraindicated because their main effect is reduction of the preload. Intraaortic balloon counterpulsation may be extremely helpful in the temporary stabilization of the patient, particularly if angiography and revascularization are being considered.[213] The benefit-to-harm ratio of digoxin in AMI is doubtful, so that its use is restricted to patients with atrial tachyarrhythmias in whom diltiazem or verapamil or esmolol fails or is contraindicated.

Cardiogenic shock. Cardiogenic shock is the leading cause of death in AMI. A crucial aspect of the management of cardiogenic shock is the diagnosis and prompt treatment of potentially *reversible mechanical complications* such as rupture (free wall, septum, or papillary muscle), tamponade, and mitral regurgitation. Underlying hypovolemia or dominant right ventricular infarction also needs to be excluded.[214] Another paradigm postulates that activation of inflammatory cytokines leads to increased activity of inducible nitric oxide (NO) synthase with excess production of NO and toxic peroxynitrite.[215,216] Unfortunately, the large TRIUMPH trial testing the NO synthase inhibitor tilarginine did not reduce mortality despite the presence of an open infarct artery.[217] Probably the best strategy in cardiogenic shock is *intraaortic balloon counterpulsation* followed by prompt revascularization. With either PCI or in some patients CABG, one of the few indications for acute multivessel primary PCI is in the hemodynamically compromised or shocked patient without significant improvement after PCI of the culprit vessel.[218] Inotropes and vasopressors are frequently required, and the choice of agent may be modified by hemodynamic parameters measured by pulmonary artery (PA) catheterization.[72] Occasionally LV and biventricular assist devices and percutaneous cardiopulmonary bypass support are used. Although hemodynamic and metabolic parameters were reversed more effectively by ventricular assist than by standard treatment with intraaortic balloon counterpulsation in a small trial, there was no difference in mortality or bleeding, and limb ischemic events were more frequent after use of a ventricular assist device.[219]

Recurrent chest pain after STEMI. Distinguishing between recurrent ischemic pain and pericarditis depends on the clinical history, the electrocardiogram, and, often, angiography. Pericarditis may be extremely distressing, and initial recommendations are to use aspirin and discontinue anticoagulation if pericardial effusion develops; if aspirin is ineffective, it is reasonable to try colchicine or acetaminophen. Nonsteroidal antiinflammatory drugs (NSAIDs) as a single dose may be extremely effective, but should not be administered if possible because their use may precipitate cardiac rupture and infarct expansion. *Cardiac tamponade* is an infrequent but life-threatening complication of AMI. Subacute rupture amenable to surgery should be suspected in all patients with recurrent pericardial-like pain and a pericardial effusion.[220]

Long-Term Therapy after AMI

General management. As the early acute-phase MI merges into the chronic phase (Table 12-3), so does the therapeutic approach evolve (Fig. 12-7). Long-term prognosis depends chiefly on the postinfarct LV function, the LV volume, the absence of ischemia, coronary anatomy, and electrical stability.[1] A major aim is to minimize adverse remodeling, specifically by load reduction and renin-angiotensin-aldosterone system (RAAS) inhibitors (Fig. 12-8). On this background, control of risk factors, including lipids and BP, remains essential. Careful choice of long-term protective drugs, giving full reasons, also reassures. For example, those patients receiving statins feel (and do) better.[221] There is increasing realization that psychosocial factors such as depression, social isolation, anger, and marital stress commonly present after MI can carry an adverse prognosis.[222,223] Although psychosocial interventions in drug therapy improve depressive symptoms and their use is logical, the cardiovascular benefits are less clear. Sertraline is at least safe,[224]

Table 12-3

Postinfarct Follow-up: Principles of Management[589]

1. Risk factor modification.
   - No smoking, full lipogram, control of hypertension, aerobic exercise, psychological support.
   - Diabetics: Control of weight, blood pressure, glycemia, lipids.
   - For all: Strongly consider statin therapy, aggressive, to LDL ≤70–100 mg/dL (1.8-2.6 mmol/L); if triglycerides ≥200 mg/dL: lifestyle modification, more intense LDL reduction (class 1B),*[71] then consider fibrate or niacin.
2. Assess extent of coronary disease.
   - Residual ischemia (symptoms, exercise test): Revascularize depending on extent and estimated viability of ischemic tissue.
3. Assess LV function and size. Avoid LV dilation.
   - If LV dysfunction (low EF) or anterior MI or diabetes: ACE inhibitor or ARB. Consider aldosterone antagonists (watch serum K⁺).
4. Prevention of reinfarction.
   - Aspirin indefinitely.
   - Clopidogrel added for 14 days (no stent), 1 month or more (BMS), 12 months or longer (DES) (all class 1B).[71]
   - β-Blockade also to prevent SCD, if not contraindicated (e.g., severe respiratory disease). If contraindicated, verapamil or diltiazem if no clinical LV failure.
   - ACE inhibition or ARB (consider for all, especially if high risk).
   - Oral anticoagulation for selected patients.
5. Complications that may need revascularization.
   - *Postinfarct angina:* Cardiac catheterization; nitrates, add CCB to β-blocker, consider revascularization.
   - *Severe LV dysfunction: Identify hibernating myocardium*—assess viability; consider revascularization after dobutamine echocardiography or stress scintigraphy or positron emission tomography.
6. Complex ventricular arrhythmias (VA).
   - Exclude significant coronary disease; assess LV function.
   - LV preserved: Effort stress test, exercise rehabilitation.
   - Complex symptomatic VA: Consider ICD (covered by amiodarone and β-blockade); data for EF <35%.[381]
7. Advanced heart failure.
   - Maximal medical therapy (see Fig. 6-8).
   - Primary prevention of SCD: For NYHA classes II & III—EF <35%, strongly consider ICD, must wait for 40 days post-MI; add CRT if QRS prolongation >120 msec (CRT, defibrillator).

ACE, Angiotensin-converting enzyme; *ARB,* angiotensin receptor blocker; *BMS,* bare metal stent; *CCB,* calcium channel blocker; *CRT,* cardiac resynchronization therapy; *DES,* drug-eluting stent; *EF,* ejection fraction; *ICD,* implantable cardioverter defibrillator; *LDL,* low-density lipoprotein; *LV,* left ventricular; *MI,* myocardial infarction; *NYHA,* New York Heart Association; *SCD,* sudden cardiac death; *VA,* ventricular arrhythmia.
Classes of Recommendations (1-3) and levels of evidence (A-C).

unlike the tricyclic antidepressants, which may cause orthostatic hypotension in addition to potential proarrhythmia.[225] A heightened awareness of the frequency and prognostic implication of psychosocial factors is a key component of cardiac rehabilitation and post MI care.

Lifestyle changes. Lifestyle changes are often much needed. A rehabilitation exercise program combines social support with the specific benefits of exercise. To stop smoking, patients need enough education and encouragement to become determined in their efforts. Then, if needed, the antidepressant drug bupropion (Wellbutrin) helps them to stop.[226] Even better is varenicline tartrate (Chantix in the United States), newly approved by the FDA. Multifactorial cardiac rehabilitation, which addresses the medical and psychosocial complications of MI, exercise training, and risk-factor modification, is a proven value but for a variety of reasons remains underused.[227-229]

Mediterranean diet, wine, and cocoa. Epidemiologically, Mediterranean countries have a low incidence of coronary heart

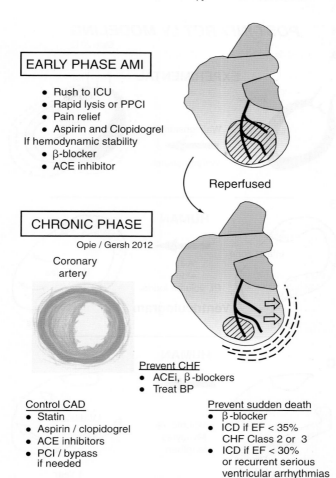

EARLY PHASE AMI

- Rush to ICU
- Rapid lysis or PPCI
- Pain relief
- Aspirin and Clopidogrel

If hemodynamic stability

- β-blocker
- ACE inhibitor

Reperfused

CHRONIC PHASE

Opie / Gersh 2012

Coronary
artery

Prevent CHF
- ACEi, β-blockers
- Treat BP

Control CAD
- Statin
- Aspirin / clopidogrel
- ACE inhibitors
- PCI / bypass
  if needed

Prevent sudden death
- β-blocker
- ICD if EF < 35%
  CHF Class 2 or 3
- ICD if EF < 30%
  or recurrent serious
  ventricular arrhythmias

Figure 12-7 Contrasting management of early and chronic phases of acute myocardial infarction (AMI). In the early phase, the major aim is to achieve reperfusion either by rapid thrombolysis or by primary percutaneous coronary intervention (PPCI), while protecting from pain and starting cardioprotective drugs such as aspirin plus clopidogrel and, when hemodynamically stable, β-blockers and angiotensin-converting enzyme inhibitors (ACEi). In the chronic phase, for secondary prevention, three major aims are to control coronary artery disease, to inhibit adverse remodeling with congestive heart failure (CHF), and to prevent sudden cardiac death. ACEi may be indicated for all or selected for higher-risk patients (controversial). (For implantable cardioverter defibrillator [ICD] management, see Chapter 8 and Fig. 8-16.) *BP,* Blood pressure; *EF,* ejection fraction; *ICU,* intensive care unit; *PCI,* percutaneous coronary intervention. (Figure © L.H. Opie & B.J. Gersh, 2012.)

disease. In the Lyon Diet Heart Study of Infarct Survivors, a Mediterranean-type diet with a high intake of linolenic acid (the precursor of ω-3 long-chain fatty acids found in fish oils), vegetables, fruits, and oils (olive and canola) but with reduced butter and red meat, gave striking protection. Total mortality, cardiac death, and non-fatal MI fell for up to 4 years of follow-up.[230] In a population-based study in Greece, the closer the adherence to the traditional Mediterranean diet, the greater the longevity.[231] In postinfarct survivors, 1 g daily of fish oil gave cardiovascular protection over 3.5 years.[232,233] In line with the *evidence for ω-3 fatty acids,* the Nutrition Committee of the AHA now recommends two fatty fish meals per week or dietary fish oil capsules.[234] A Mediterranean diet supplemented with olive oil or nuts has better effects on

POST-INFARCT LV MODELING
Opie 2012

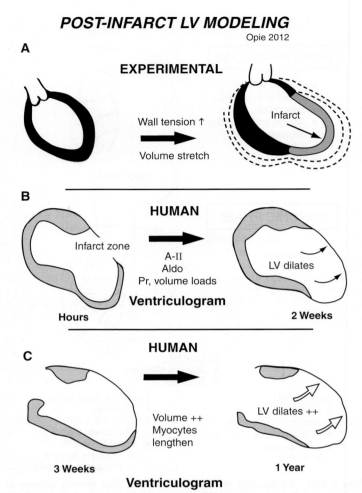

Figure 12-8   Postinfarct remodeling patterns. A, Simplified overall patterns (cartoon style) based on animal models, where *solid black* represents the non-infarcted and *red zones* the infarcted myocardium of the left ventricle (LV). Note potential for considerable remodeling of the infarct zone, thereby increasing the volume of the noninfarcted zone. **B,** Endocardial wall motion outlines of two separate human hearts in the early postinfarct phase with adverse effects of pressure (Pr) or volume loads, angiotensin II (A-II) and aldosterone (aldo). **C,** The late postinfarct phase, derived from contrast ventriculography. Note considerable remodeling in accord with the animal models, with emphasis on progressively increased LV volume. (Modified from Opie LH, et al. Controversies in ventricular remodeling. *Lancet* 2006;367:356–367.)

cardiovascular risk factors than does a low-fat diet.[235] The benefits of red wine have probably been overdramatized, but modest intake of wine with meals, part of the Mediterranean culture, is beneficial.[236] The current dietary rage is cocoa, as found in certain bitter chocolates that contain protective flavonoids; ordinary dark chocolates do not contain these.[237] However, there are no dose-response data, and hard cardiovascular benefits still have to be proven.

No to β-carotene and vitamin E. β-Carotene and vitamin E have not stood the test of time. After 7 years of follow-up in the HOPE study, there was no cardiovascular benefit from vitamin E but rather increased heart failure.[238] Despite indirect evidence associating elevated plasma homocysteine levels to cardiovascular disease, several recent trials have failed to show any benefit from supplementation with folic acid, vitamin B_6, or vitamin B_{12}.[239]

   Hormone replacement therapy: harmful. Large landmark clinical trials have provided firm evidence that combination estrogen and progestin replacement therapy should not be used as either the primary or secondary prevention of cardiovascular disease in women. Postmenopausal women who are already taking hormone replacement therapy at the time of MI should not continue taking the drugs; neither should hormone replacement therapy be given de novo. *Raloxifene*, a selective estrogen receptor modulator, when given to postmenopausal women with coronary artery disease or multiple risk factors for it, did not decrease primary coronary events compared with placebo. There was a reduction in the risk of estrogen receptor–positive invasive breast cancer and vertebral fractures, but an increased risk of fatal stroke and venous thromboembolism. Thus raloxifene, similar to estrogen and progestin replacement therapy, should not be used as either primary or secondary prevention of cardiovascular disease in women.[240]

Postinfarct Cardioprotective Drugs

Postinfarct statins. There no longer is any doubt that statins reduce hard endpoints in patients with coronary disease. Starting statins during the period of acute hospitalization may enhance the continued use of these drugs after discharge. The only remaining issue is how far to reduce LDL cholesterol, with a strong trend favoring aggressive lowering (see Tables 10-2, 10-3, and 12-3; see also Chapter 10). An elegant study with intravascular ultrasound suggests that 75 mg/dL (1.95 mmol/L) is the equilibrium LDL level at which progression and regression of the plaque are, on average, similar.[241]

Postinfarct β-blockade. Solid evidence shows that postinfarct β-blockade provides benefit. In a very large survey on more than 200,000 patients, late mortality fell by approximately 40%.[18,196] The present trend is to continue β-blockers indefinitely, together with aspirin, a statin, and, whenever there is LV dysfunction or diabetes, ACE inhibition, or an ARB. β-Blockers protect from the adverse effects of surges of catecholamines, which may explain their effects on SCD.[242] In a pooled analysis of four intravascular ultrasonography trials, β-blockers slowed the progression of coronary atherosclerosis.[243] In the presence of severe respiratory problems but in the absence of heart failure, verapamil is a viable alternative to β-blockade (see next section). Which subsets of patients are most likely to benefit? Paradoxically, those patients who appear to be at higher risk also benefit most. For example, β-blockade may have its best effects in the presence of heart failure, with all-cause mortality reduced by 23%.[244] The mortality reduction also extends to co-therapy with ACE inhibitors, ARBs, and aspirin.[196] Obvious contraindications to β-blockade remain grade IV heart failure, severe bradycardia, hypotension, overt asthma, and heart block greater than first degree.

ACE inhibitors for all with coronary disease? As already argued in Chapter 5 (see p. 135), prophylactic ACE inhibitors should be considered for all patients with coronary disease even with preserved LV function, and are positively indicated for those with angina pectoris with hypertension, peripheral vascular disease, diabetes, or LV dysfunction.[10]

Aldosterone antagonists. Aldosterone antagonists should be prescribed to all STEMI patients who are receiving an ACE inhibitor, have an ejection fraction of less than 40%, a serum creatinine of less than or equal to 2.5 mg/dL, and a serum potassium of less than 5 mEq/L or have either symptomatic heart failure or diabetes depending on baseline serum potassium levels and renal function (see Chapter 5, p. 161). The risk of hyperkalemia is substantial, and patients need to be monitored carefully.[245] These initial recommendations in the guidelines in 2006 were not changed in the focused updates in 2009.[246]

When to use calcium channel blockers. As a group, CCBs do not give postinfarct protection.[247] No CCB has been shown to reduce mortality in STEMI and they may be harmful in patients with heart failure, significant LV dysfunction, or conduction disease. The major use is for the management of recurrent ischemia despite β-blockers and in patients who are not revascularizable. A case can also be made for the use of verapamil or diltiazem in the absence of LV failure, especially when β-blockade is contraindicated. In the large Danish postinfarct trial (DAVIT-2) in which overt LV failure was prospectively excluded, verapamil 120 mg three times daily decreased reinfarction in cardiac mortality.[247] For BP control, long-acting nifedipine (or amlodipine) added to β-blockade and ACE inhibitors may be helpful.

Aspirin and clopidogrel. Aspirin, the simplest and safest agent, is now established therapy, starting with an oral dose as soon as possible after the onset of symptoms of AMI and continuing indefinitely thereafter (provided that the BP is adequately controlled). It prevents reinfarction, stroke, and vascular mortality as shown in numerous trials. The dose for long-term indefinite aspirin is 75 to 162 mg daily. The updated ACC-AHA recommendations are that, for all post-PCI STEMI stented patients without aspirin resistance, allergy, or increased risk of bleeding, aspirin 162 to 325 mg daily should be given for at least 1 month after BMS, 3 months after sirolimus-eluting stent, and 6 months after paclitaxel-eluting stent implantation, after which the dose is 75 to 325 mg daily (class IB).[72] The lower doses have fewer side effects. Clopidogrel should be used for aspirin intolerance or resistance, and added to aspirin for 14 days (no stent), 1 month or more (BMS), or at least for 12 months (drug-eluting stent) (all class IB).[72] In regard to long-term co-therapy with clopidogrel and aspirin, there are no trials that specifically address this in patients with prior STEMI, other than in patients undergoing PCI and stenting. Many theoretical benefits have to be offset against the risk of bleeding.

Aspirin plus ACE inhibitors. Combined with aspirin, ACE inhibition has an odds ratio for risk reduction of 0.80 versus 0.71 without aspirin.[248]

Nonsteroidal antiinflammatory drugs. Both the cyclooxygenase-2–selective inhibitors and the traditional NSAIDs have been associated with an increase in cardiovascular events. In a metaanalysis and systematic review, low-dose naproxen and ibuprofen appear to be the safest NSAIDS.[249,250] Diclofenac and indomethacin appear to cause the most harm. Celecoxib in doses of 200 mg or more daily is associated with an increase in cardiovascular events. Patients with or at risk of cardiovascular disease are particularly at risk. The combination of aspirin and an NSAID may reduce aspirin's efficacy. Two ex vivo studies have demonstrated a potential interaction of ibuprofen and possibly naproxen, but not diclofenac or rofecoxib, when combined with aspirin.[251,252] The FDA currently recommends that ibuprofen be given 30 minutes after aspirin or at least 8 hours before aspirin to negate this potential interaction.[167] Choice of agent requires a detailed risk evaluation of the potential underlying gastrointestinal and cardiovascular risk profile in the individual patient. The AHA has recommended a stepped-care approach to prescribing these agents.[253]

Warfarin anticoagulation. Warfarin is usually given for 3 to 6 months after an infarct to patients with prior emboli; in those with LV thrombus (echocardiographically proven), or large anterior infarcts (threatened thrombus), or with established AF; and in those with contraindications or hypersensitivity to aspirin. Medium-intensity anticoagulation with an international normalized ratio (INR) of approximately 2.5 seemed effective, albeit in two relatively small studies,[254,255] whereas low-intensity anticoagulation with an INR of 1.8 in the largest study was not.[256] In another large study, mean INR values of approximately 2.2 to 2.8 reduced nonfatal MI and nonfatal embolic stroke.[257] These modest returns need to be balanced against increased bleeding, greater cost, and added inconvenience to the patient. Patients older than 75 years have not been adequately studied. There is some evidence that chronic anticoagulation can reduce the number of adverse cardiovascular events after ACS, but these trials generally antedated the widespread use of clopidogrel and early revascularization for both ST-segment elevation and non–ST-segment elevation AMI.[258] It has been previously widely recommended that either UFH or LMWH should be administered to reduce the risk of deep vein thrombosis until patients become ambulatory. Nonetheless, based on the 2008 American College of Chest Physicians guideline, it is considered that venus thromboembolism prophylaxis is not necessary (unless indicated for some other reason) for complicated STEMI patients who are likely to be on bed rest for less than 24 hours. If longer periods of bed rest are required, than prophylaxis with UFH, LMWH, or fondaparinux is indicated.

Postinfarct antiarrhythmic agents. Complex ventricular ectopy and VT in the late hospital phase of MI are predictors of subsequent sudden death after discharge, independently of their frequent association with LV dysfunction. Nonetheless, the hoped-for benefit of antiarrhythmic therapy on postinfarct mortality is still elusive, with β-blockers the only agents showing clear-cut mortality reduction.[192] The momentum has swung away from amiodarone, given its side effect profile and lack of a consistent mortality benefit in clinical trials, to implantable cardioverter defibrillators (ICDs; see next section).[259] Nonetheless, amiodarone can relieve highly symptomatic premature ventricular extrasystoles or runs of nonsustained VT.

Implantable cardioverter defibrillators. The role of ICDs in the primary prevention of postinfarct SCD in patients with heart failure is well established (see section on Interventions for Severe Stable LV Dysfunction later; see also Fig. 8-16). The use of Holter monitoring and invasive electrophysiologic testing has declined, and the major inclusion criterion is the ejection fraction, albeit an imprecise measurement.

The future. There is an urgent need for new methods of arrhythmia risk stratification. Microvolt T-wave alternans appears the most promising of the new approaches, but its ultimate role requires further clarification.[260,261]

Atrial Fibrillation

The general approach to the therapy of arrhythmias has swung from the widespread use of antiarrhythmic drugs to increasing intervention (Fig. 12-9). As our population ages, the incidence and prevalence of AF is rapidly increasing, giving rise to a "growing epidemic" that has been seriously underestimated.[262] Therapeutic approaches to AF emphasize three main aspects: (1) anticoagulation; (2) cardioversion with maintenance of sinus rhythm by antiarrhythmic agents all having potentially serious side effects or by evolving ablative approaches, primarily catheter based; or (3) accepting chronic AF with the emphasis on rate control and long-term anticoagulation (Table 12-4). Because cardioversion is associated with temporary atrial "stunning," there is definite risk of thrombus formation even if the atrium is not enlarged. Thus whenever possible, anticoagulation is required for either cardioversion or rate control. Newer techniques such as AV nodal ablation followed by

ARRHYTHMIA THERAPY

Opie 2012

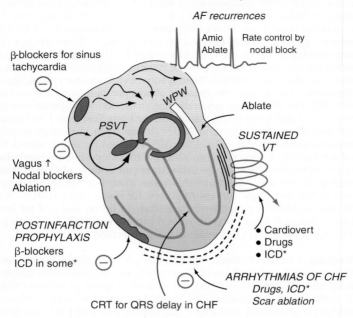

Figure 12-9 Principles of antiarrhythmic therapy, starting from the sinus node (*top left*) and proceeding toward the ventricles. (1) Sinus tachycardia, as in myocardial infarction (MI) or anxiety; treated by β-blockade (after excluding causes such as hypovolemia or fever in MI). (2) Atrial fibrillation (AF) recurrences prevented by amiodarone (Amio), or sotalol and class 1C agents, or ablation, or choosing rate control by nodal blocking agents. (3) Paroxysmal supraventricular tachycardia (PSVT) with nodal reentry paths susceptible to atrioventricular (AV) inhibition by nodal blockers such as vagal maneuvers, calcium channel blockers or β-blockers, or AV ablation. (4) Supraventricular preexcitation tachycardias of the Wolff-Parkinson-White (WPW) syndrome bypass tract are treated either by AV nodal inhibitors or by catheter ablation of the bypass tract. (5) Sustained ventricular tachycardia (VT), especially in the presence of an infarcted or ischemic zone, is based on reentry circuits that require cardioversion if persistent, drug therapy as by amiodarone, and, in selected patients, an implantable cardioverter defibrillator (ICD). (6) Arrhythmias of congestive heart failure (CHF) may require either drugs or, in selected patients, an ICD. (7) For prevention of sudden cardiac death in CHF with QRS prolongation, cardiac resynchronization therapy (CRT) gives excellent results. (8) Postinfarction prophylaxis is best given by β-blockade. (For proposed site of action of amiodarone on pulmonary veins, see Fig. 8-5. *For ICD management, see Fig. 8-16.) (Figure © L.H. Opie, 2012.)

permanent pacemaker implantation, the implantable atrial defibrillator, the maze cardiac surgical procedure, and, in particular, catheter-based techniques of AF ablation, are changing traditional approaches to management. Nonetheless, the management of AF, the most common of all arrhythmias, is often not easy (see Table 12-4).

Acute-Onset Atrial Fibrillation

A thorough history is essential to assess underlying contributory factors, the severity of symptoms, and comorbidities that could interact with AF therapies.

Urgent control of the ventricular rate (see Table 12-4), if needed, is achieved by AV nodal inhibitors, such as (1) verapamil or diltiazem, (2) intravenous β-blockade by esmolol, (3) digoxin, or (4) combinations.

Table 12-4

Acute-Onset AF: Principles of Management[297]

Acute Onset

- Correct precipitating factors (dehydration, alcohol, pyrexia, etc.).
- Use intravenous AV nodal inhibitors to control ventricular rate (diltiazem,* verapamil, or esmolol; sometimes digoxin or drug combinations).
- If duration of AF < 48 h, first observe for 8 h. Spontaneous reversion is common. If not, consider pharmacologic cardioversion by intravenous ibutilide (risk of torsades) or high-dose amiodarone (125 mg/h, up to 3 g/24 h) or if no structural heart disease, flecainide or propafenone.
- Thereafter, electrical cardioversion often required.
- Depending on the local situation, electrical cardioversion may be chosen first.

Urgent Cardioversion

- Required for rapid ventricular response not responding to pharmacologic agents if myocardial ischemia, symptomatic hypotension, or heart failure (class1C).†
- If preexcitation with rapid tachycardia or hemodynamic instability (class 1B).
- Thromboembolism risk if AF > 48 h; start heparin and warfarin.

Elective Cardioversion <7 Days

- Intravenous ibutilide or oral dofetilide (risk of torsades with both). Flecainide or propafenone only when no structural heart disease, with a β-blocker or verapamil to avoid a fast ventricular rate. If AF > 48 h, start heparin and warfarin.

Preparation for Elective Electrical Cardioversion >7 Days

- Prior oral anticoagulation; for 4 consecutive weeks INR must be 2-3; if at any time the INR is subtherapeutic, then start again for another 4 wk. Alternate: TEE-guided approach (see text). Eliminate thyrotoxicosis.
- Pharmacologic facilitation: during fourth week, consider amiodarone at 800-1600 mg/day for 1 wk followed by 200-400 mg/day.
- Other choices: sotalol or ibutilide or (if no structural heart disease) flecainide or propafenone (class 1C).
- Alternate policy: control ventricular rate by AV nodal inhibitors.

Postcardioversion

Search for underlying causes. Congestive heart failure or hypertension, if present, must be vigorously treated. One of three arrhythmia policies:
1. *Rhythm control: Aim to maintain sinus rhythm* by chronic therapy. Follow algorithm in Fig. 8-3. Anticoagulation continued for at least 3-6 mo, but usually indefinitely because many episodes are asymptomatic.
2. *Alternate policy: Leave drug-free,* try "pill-in-the-pocket" and, if recurrence, control ventricular rate (digoxin if CHF, otherwise β-blocker or verapamil or diltiazem). Oral anticoagulation essential.
3. *Third policy: Cardiovert,* observe on anticoagulation, start antiarrhythmics for second episode.
Repetitive recurrent symptomatic AF: Focal pulmonary vein ablation or left atrial isolation; surgical maze procedure.
Under investigation: Dual-site atrial pacing; implantable atrial cardioverter-defibrillator.

AF, Atrial fibrillation; *AV,* atrioventricular; *CHF,* congestive heart failure; *INR,* international normalized ratio; *TEE,* transesophageal echocardiography.
  *Diltiazem preferred because of clearly defined dose guidelines in package insert, including rate for prolonged infusion.
  †Classes of Recommendations (1-3) and levels of evidence (A-C)

Other agents that can also be given intravenously include flecainide, propafenone, sotalol, ibutilide, and high-dose amiodarone.[263] Of these, only ibutilide is registered for use in acute AF and only amiodarone is safe for patients with ischemic heart disease or heart failure.[263] With ibutilide there is the risk of torsades, especially in patients with heart failure.[264] In selected patients without structural heart disease, single loading doses of propafenone[265] or flecainide may also be used, despite their proarrhythmic effects. Vernakalant has been recently approved in Europe but not in the United States.[266-268] If still needed, cardioversion is then undertaken either at the end of the drug infusion, which is logical and effective,[263,264,266-268] or electively once the patient has been anticoagulated. Factors precipitating AF must also be treated (see Table 12-4).

Direct-current cardioversion. Direct-current cardioversion, either guided by transesophageal echocardiography (TEE) or after 3 to 4 weeks of therapeutic anticoagulation, is widely used in newly detected AF. The lowest energy requirements are with biphasic wave forms.[269] Standard practice is not to anticoagulate when the onset of AF can be *precisely* determined and the duration is less than 40 hours. If in doubt, perform TEE (see next section). The use of LMWHs instead of UFH in patients with AF is theoretically attractive from a number of standpoints, but recommendations have been largely based on extrapolation from venous thromboembolic disease states.[270] Following cardioversion, self-administration of LMWHs out of hospital prior to full-dose anticoagulation with warfarin may be cost-effective and requires further study. In the presence of hypokalemia, digitalis toxicity or improper synchronizations, serious ventricular arrhythmias may occur.[79]

Atrial stunning. Following electrical or pharmacologic cardioversion, there may be "temporary stunning" of the atrium, which is probably a function of the duration of AF, but the time cost is variable.[271] There is a risk of thrombus formation, even if the atrium is not enlarged or if echocardiography does not show any atrial appendage thrombus. The risk of systemic thromboembolism is 1%-2%, and this can be reduced by anticoagulation.[79] Consequently, whenever possible, anticoagulation should be started prior to elective cardioversion and continued for at least 3 to 4 weeks thereafter. For urgent cardioversion, logic but no trial data would dictate intravenous heparin to cover the procedure. To reduce the risk of atrial stunning, oral verapamil may be given before and just after the cardioversion.[272]

Role of transesophageal echocardiography. This directly visualizes thrombus in the left atrium or left atrial appendage, which, if found, contraindicates urgent cardioversion without prior prolonged anticoagulation.[273,274] The TEE-guided early approach uses heparin for 24 hours precardioversion and chronic anticoagulation for at least 4 weeks postcardioversion, with the aim of protecting against new left atrial thrombosis during postcardioversion stunning. The advantage of the TEE-guided approach is one of convenience, and, theoretically, it should be safer by reducing the overall time during which a patient is exposed to anticoagulation and the risk of bleeding. Technical expertise and experience are crucial for this approach, because the anatomy of the left atrial appendage is complex and small thrombi can easily be overlooked.

Postoperative atrial fibrillation. In the colchicine for the prevention of post pericardiotomy syndrome (COPPS) trial colchicine was shown to almost halve the incidents of postoperative AF in patients undergoing cardiac surgery.[275]

Chronic Atrial Fibrillation

Rate control versus sinus rhythm. Rather than aiming to maintain sinus rhythm by antiarrhythmic drugs, another major policy is to accept the existence of AF yet control the ventricular response by AV nodal inhibitors (see Chapter 8, pp. 309-314) and to provide oral anticoagulation (see Chapter 8, p. 314). The logic for this line of therapy is that all the drugs that can be used to maintain sinus rhythm (flecainide, propafenone, sotalol, amiodarone, dofetilide, and dronedarone) have potentially serious side effects. The potential advantages of rhythm control are an improvement in the quality of life and exercise tolerance,[276,277] with theoretical effects on endothelial function and platelet activation. However, rhythm control offered no advantage over rate control in the AFFIRM trial that enrolled a total of 4060 patients at high risk for stroke on the basis of either risk factors for stroke or age greater than 65 or both.[278] There was a trend toward more stroke with rhythm control and certainly more hospitalizations. In two other smaller European trials, rate control was again similar in outcome to rhythm control.[279,280] In a recent large multinational registry (RECORD AF), a multivariant analysis suggested that a strategy of rhythm control was associated with superior clinical success and a lower likelihood of AF progression.[281] The choice between rate and rhythm control is not always easy. *A practical policy is to attempt cardioversion for the first episode of AF.*[191] *Then, if this arrhythmia returns and is asymptomatic, rate control is in order.*

Rate control. The drugs inhibiting the AV node are digoxin and β-blockers, especially when there is heart failure, with the CCBs verapamil and diltiazem when heart failure is absent. Other drugs that may be helpful for pharmacologic rate control include dronedarone and amiodarone. In acutely ill patients with CHF, intravenous amiodarone may be helpful, but should not be used long-term for rate control because of side effects. Often several of these drugs must be given in combination. Strict rate control is a resting heart rate less than 80 beats per minute (bpm) and a heart rate less than 110 bpm with minor exercise.[282] In the Rate Control versus Electrical Cardioversion for Persistent AF II trial of strict versus lenient rate control in 614 patients, the latter was achieved by more patients as a result of a higher rate of adverse drug effect in patients assigned to strict rate control. In regard to cardiovascular events, the strategy of lenient rate control was noninferior, suggesting that we should favor a policy of treating the patient and not the rate.[283] Presumably in RACE 2 patients with severe symptoms caused by a high ventricular rate were excluded, and many would be uncomfortable with a resting heart rate of less than 110 bpm as a therapeutic goal in patients being treated with rate-control strategies. More information in this area is needed. When rate control is unsatisfactory, tachycardia-induced ventricular dysfunction is a concern. In this setting, radiofrequency ablation of the AV node causing complete heart block, with implantation of a permanent pacemaker, may markedly improve symptoms and, in some patients, ventricular function.[284,285]

Rhythm control by elective cardioversion. In chronic AF, having achieved control of the ventricular rate by AV nodal inhibitors, the patient is anticoagulated by warfarin while being maintained on drug therapy, which is often amiodarone (see Table 12-4). In persistent AF, once control of the ventricular rate by AV nodal inhibitors has been achieved, the patient is anticoagulated while being loaded and maintained on drug therapy to maintain sinus rhythm, and in this situation the most widely used drug is amidarone (see Table 12-4). Factors favoring drug conversion include a small left atrial size and AF less than 6 months in duration. The risk of embolization at the time of rhythm conversion is approximately 1% to 2%, so that *prophylactic anticoagulation* with an INR greater than 2 for at least 3 consecutive weeks is required. Because the recurrence rate of AF is quite high during the first 3 to 6 months following cardioversion, many cardiologists advocate a much longer period of postcardioversion anticoagulation. Prior to electrical cardioversion, it is reasonable in patients not receiving amiodarone to attempt a pharmacologic cardioversion using intravenous procainamide or ibutilide[286,287] or, less frequently, oral propafenone or flecainide. The latter two drugs should be avoided in the presence of structural heart disease, particularly if significant LV dysfunction is present. For cardioversion failures, repeat after adding prophylactic drugs.

Fish oils. To lessen recurrent AF after cardioversion, prescribe long-chain ω-3 polyunsaturated fatty acids (PUFAs).[288] In patients with persistent AF on amiodarone and a RAAS inhibitor, the daily addition for 1 year of ω-3 PUFAs 2 g of fish oil, 85% or more eicosapentaenoic plus docosahexaenoic acids, improved the probability of the maintenance of sinus rhythm after direct-current cardioversion (hazard ratio [HR] 0.62; confidence interval 0.52-0.72).[289]

Recurrent atrial fibrillation. After one or two attempts at cardioversion or when AF is known to be recurrent, the drug choices are shown in Figure 8-3 and are guided by the presence or absence of structural heart disease. Working down the choices, the final drug is usually amiodarone, failing which catheter ablation follows. Dronedarone is a multichannel blocker that does not have the side effects of amiodarone, although it is also less effective than amiodarone.[290] Somewhat surprisingly in the ATHENA trial, dronedarone reduced cardiovascular mortality and in a post hoc analysis there was a reduction in stroke.[291] The drug should not be used in patients with class III-IV heart failure given the negative results of the ANDRONEDA trial.[292] Dronedarone is currently approved for the treatment of paroxysmal or persistent AF or atrial flutter, but the recent PALLAS trial of patients with permanent AF was prematurely terminated because of a significant increase in rates of death, stroke, and hospitalization for heart failure in patients receiving dronedarone. Both the FDA and the European Medicine Agency are currently conducting reviews.[293] Dronedarone was designed on the basis of the structure of amiodarone, but to reduce toxicity, lipophilicity was reduced and the iodine moieties responsible for thyroid dysfunction in patients on amiodarone were eliminated. Renin-angiotensin blockade helps to reduce recurrences with good theoretical explanations,[294] and benefits comorbidities such as heart failure and hypertension. It is unlikely, however, that these agents will play more than an adjunctive role. A useful drug in patients with paroxysmal or persistent AF include dofetilide (a class III antiarrhythmic drug, I_{Kr} blocker, which is not available in Europe). Dofetilide is well tested in CHF and is well tolerated in the long-term, but there is an increased risk of torsades de pointes necessitating hospital monitoring during admission of the drug. Moreover, there are numerous drug interactions that may prohibit the use of dofetilide.

New pharmacologic options for the maintenance of sinus rhythm. *Vernakalant*, which has been primarily tested for pharmacologic cardioversion[295] may also turn out to be useful for the prevention of recurrent AF based on a single dose-ranging phase 2 study and its pharmacologic properties.[296] The drug is approved in Europe but not in the United States. The antianginal agent *ranolazine* was associated with a reduction in nonsustained VT and AF in the MERLIN TIMI-36 trial.[24] It has atrial-selective, sodium-channel blocking and late I_{Na}-inhibiting properties and an ability to suppress AF in a number of experimental models.[294] Azimilide, which blocks both rapid I_{Kr} and slow I_{Ks} components of potassium channel is still under evaluation, and a wide range of atrial-selective potassium channel blockers are in active development.[296]

Antiplatelet and anticoagulant therapy for stroke prevention. A driving force underlying the recommendations for antiplatelet and anticoagulant therapy is the stratification of patients according to their risk of bleeding and stroke. This has led to the publication of several different risk stratification schemes, the most wisely used being the cardiac failure, hypertension, age, diabetes, stroke (doubled) (CHADS2) and in Europe the CHA2DS-VASC score.[267,297-299]

The Stroke Risk in Atrial Fibrillation Working Group analyzed 12 published schemes for the stratification of risk. The conclusion is that there was substantial differences among the various schemes and none were optimal.[300] The ESC guideline recommendations are based on the CHA2DS-VASC score (for definition see Table 8 in ref 266) and in the United States the CHADS2 score. *The key to therapy is to individualize and balance the risk of stroke versus the risk of bleeding.* High risk for stroke can best be predicted by the CHA2DS2-VASc score.[301] In regard to bleeding, the HAS-BLED score has been developed, and in general those factors that increase the risk of stroke have a similar effect on bleeding (HAS-BLED score: hypertension, abnormal renal/liver function 1 point each, stroke, bleeding history or predisposition, labile INR, elderly drugs/alcohol concomitantly 1 point each]; maximum 9 points.)[302]

In a population-based study of more than 2000 cases of ischemic stroke, 5.2% had an antithrombotic or antiplatelet agent withdrawn within the prior 60 days. The role of bridging therapy is the subject of ongoing trials.[303] Randomized controlled trials have suggested that in patients with AF, aspirin is probably better than placebo, aspirin and clopidogrel are better than aspirin alone,[304] and despite the limitations of warfarin, a metaanalysis of 29 trials involving approximately 28,000 patients demonstrated a 64% reduction in stroke compared with placebo or antiplatelet agents.[305] Moreover, in the ACTIVE-W trial warfarin was superior to aspirin and clopidogrel.[306]

Alternatives to warfarin: a new era. The limitations of vitamin K antagonists are well known, including a narrow therapeutic range, slow "onset" and "offset" of action, numerous food and drug interactions, the inference of genetic variability and clearance, and the effect of concurrent illnesses in pharmacokinetics and pharmcodynamics. This requires constant and frequent monitoring for anticoagulant effect and frequent dose adjustments.[307] The search for an alternatives for warfarin that do not require INR monitoring is an extremely active area of current investigation. The direct thrombin inhibitor *dabigatran etexilate (Pradaxa)* is released in the United States at doses of 150 mg twice a day and 75 mg twice a day in patients with an estimated glomerular filtration rate of less than 30 mL/min, but in Europe and Canada the 110-mg twice-daily dose is also available. In the RE-LY trial, the 150-mg dose was associated with lower rates of systemic embolism and stroke, but similar rates of major bleeding compared with warfarin; the 110-mg dose demonstrated similar risks of stroke but less bleeding; and both doses were associated with lower rates of intracranial hemorrhage.[308] Of concern, however, is a subsequent report demonstrating a higher rate of bleeding in patients older than 75 years receiving the 150-mg twice-daily dose.[309] Advantages of dabigatran include convenience and perhaps efficacy and safety as opposed to the disadvantages of twice-a-day dosing, which may be a problem in the case of patients who are not compliant, in the case of patients with severe chronic renal failure and in patients older than 75 years in whom the dose is uncertain, in the case of gastrointestinal side effects that occur in approximately 10%, because of cost, and because of the lack of an antidote in case of bleeding.

Rivaroxaban, a factor Xa inhibitor, was noninferior to warfarin in the ROCKET AF trial.[308] Noninferiority was demonstrated for the composite primary endpoint of stroke or noncentral nervous system embolism (P < 0.001). Superiority was demonstrated only in analysis that compared "as treated" patients but not in the intention-2-3 analysis. The drug is shortly due to undergo FDA review. *Apixaban,* another factor Xa inhibitor, in the ARISTOTLE trial met the primary efficacy objective of noninferiority to warfarin on the combined outcome of stroke and systemic embolism, but in addition, the drug was associated with a marked reduction in major bleeding, intracranial hemorrhage, and preliminary reports suggest superiority in terms of efficacy.[310] Alternative approaches in patients who cannot take *warfarin* under investigation include left atrial appendage ligation or transvenous closure, amputation, or occlusion at the time of surgery.[311-313] Success of these approaches, however, is predicated on the assumption that the overwhelming proportion of embolic strokes in patients with AF emanates

from thrombi in the left atrial appendage.[314] Counterargument emphasizes that the concept of AF is a more generalized vascular disease,
particularly in the older patients.[315]

**Rhythm control by surgical procedures or percutaneous radio-
frequency ablation.** Surgical procedures and radiofrequency ablation
are invasive approaches to rhythm control that are important advances.
The primary indication for the surgical maze procedure is in patients
undergoing cardiac surgery for other indications.[316] Percutaneous approaches using radiofrequency ablation for focal ablation, pulmonary
vein isolation, or wide atrial circumferential ablation are important advances that continue to evolve. Increasing experience, new imaging
techniques, and advances in electromechanical mapping will likely
result in further improvements to the overall success of the procedure.
Complication rates are declining, but the potential for serious complications such as thromboembolism including stroke, tamponade, pulmonary vein stenosis, phrenic nerve injury, and ateroesophageal fistula
occur in approximately 2%-3% of patients.[267] Of concern is the demonstration of asymptomatic postprocedure intracranial embolic lesions on
magnetic resonance imaging in 4.3% to 37.5% of patients, depending on
the technique for pulmonary vein isolation.[317] This is an area that warrants further investigation and improvement. Operator experience is
probably an important component of overall success and safety.
Multiple small single-center randomized controlled trials ranging from
30 to 245 patients and several multicenter prospective studies in addition to metaanalyses have clearly shown a greater freedom from recurrent AF after radiofrequency ablation compared with antiarrhythmic
drugs,[267,318-320] but many of these studies included patients already refractory to antiarrhythmic drug. Data on comparisons of radiofrequency
ablation versus antiarrhythmic drug therapy as first-line therapy are
scarce, but a large NHLBI-sponsored mortality trial is ongoing.[321] In
regard to the late results of radiofrequency ablation, these are somewhat
disappointing in that there appears to be higher occurrence rate during
the first 5 years in addition to a need for additional procedures.[322,323]

The ideal candidate is the younger patient with paroxysmal AF, no
structural heart disease, and without severe left atrial enlargement, who
is highly symptomatic with drug intolerance or inefficacy. Nonetheless,
the procedure has been extended to higher-risk groups with structural
heart disease and persistent AF but with lower success rates.[320,324-328]
Further trials in specific patient subgroups are needed.

Other Supraventricular Arrhythmias

Atrial flutter. Satisfactory control of the ventricular rate may be
extremely difficult to achieve, but flutter is easily converted by a low-
energy countershock. Although the left atrium still contracts, the potential for embolism does occur and the same rules as those for AF apply
for anticoagulation both in relation to cardioversion and for prevention
of thromboembolism and chronic atrial flutter. Moreover, AF and atrial
flutter may coexist in the same patient. For resistant or recurrent cases,
catheter ablation of the AV node with pacemaker implantation is increasingly used. Patients with "typical atrial flutter" enjoy a very high
success rate with radiofrequency ablation of the flutter circuit. In some
patients with atrial flutter with documented AF at other times, successful
flutter ablation may nonetheless result in recurrences of AF. The combination of AF and atrial flutter either can be treated by drugs or, if refractory, may respond to radiofrequency procedures isolating the pulmonary veins from the left atrium[329] (for details, see Chapter 8, p. 314).

Multifocal atrial tachycardia. Multifocal atrial tachycardia is an uncommon but not rare arrhythmia frequently associated with significant
lung disease, respiratory failure, and pulmonary hypertension. It may

respond to verapamil or β-blockers, but there appear to be no formal drug trials, and the clinical impression is that this is a very difficult arrhythmia to control. Exclude underlying theophylline toxicity. Intravenous magnesium may be effective for rate control and helps in restoration of sinus rhythm in patients with and without serum magnesium levels.[330]

Supraventricular tachycardia. In the standard paroxysmal type (PSVT) with nodal reentry, vagotonic procedures (Valsalva maneuver, facial immersion in cold water, or carotid sinus massage) may terminate the tachycardia (Table 12-5). Always auscultate the carotid arteries before performing carotid sinus massage. If these measures fail, the next step is to use intravenous adenosine followed by intravenous diltiazem, verapamil, or esmolol (see Chapter 8, p. 303). Adenosine with its ultrashort duration of action is safest, especially if there is a diagnostic uncertainty between PSVT with aberrant conduction and wide-complex VT. If these steps fail, vagotonic maneuvers are worth repeating. Thereafter the

Table 12-5

PSVT: Principles of Management[590]

Entry Point

- Narrow QRS complex tachycardia; either AV nodal reentry or WPW (see Fig. 8-14). If *atrial flutter*, proceed straight to DC cardioversion (may consider ibutilide but torsades risk).

Acute Therapy: Hemodynamically Stable

- Vagal maneuvers.
- Intravenous AV nodal blockers (adenosine,* verapamil, diltiazem, esmolol; high success rate).
- Occasionally intravenous propafenone.
- Synchronized DC cardioversion.
- Burst pacing in selected cases (e.g., postbypass surgery).

Acute Therapy: Hemodynamically Unstable

- Intravenous adenosine (not other AV nodal blockers—negative inotropes).
- Must cardiovert if adenosine unsuccessful.

Follow-up: PSVT with AV Nodal Reentry

- Self-therapy by vagal procedures.
- Prevention by long-acting AV nodal blockers (verapamil, diltiazem, standard β-blockers, digoxin).
- If repetitive attacks, perinodal ablation to inhibit reentry through reentry pathways. Small risk of AV nodal damage requiring permanent pacemaker.

Follow-up: Preexcitation (WPW, Delta Wave during Sinus Rhythm)

- RF catheter ablation of bypass tract.
- Rarely, surgery is performed for associated conditions (young children with associated anomalies; multiple paths).
- Occasionally drug therapy: Class IC or class III agents.[†] Digoxin contraindicated, avoid other AV nodal blockers.

Follow-up: Atrial Flutter

- Prevent by sotalol, amiodarone, dofetilide, or RF ablation of flutter circuits.
- Rate control by AV nodal inhibitors (verapamil, diltiazem, β-blocker, digoxin, or combinations).
- Consider RF AV nodal ablation and permanent pacemaker.

Catheter Ablation

- Treatment of choice for recurrent PVST.

AV, Atrioventricular; *DC,* direct-current; *PSVT,* paroxysmal supraventricular tachycardia; *RF,* radiofrequency; *WPW,* Wolff-Parkinson-White syndrome.

　　*Adenosine preferred (ultra-short-acting); esmolol action wears off more slowly but fast enough to allow subsequent safer use of verapamil or diltiazem if needed.

　　†Class refers to class of antiarrhythmic drug (see Fig. 8-1), not to American Heart Association–American College of Cardiology class of recommendation.

choice lies between intravenous digitalization or intravenous amiodarone or direct-current cardioversion, and the decision needs to be tempered by the clinical condition of the patient. (Also, in countries outside
the United States, intravenous flecainide is approved and may be a
choice in the absence of structural heart disease.)

Refractory PSVT. Patients with supraventricular arrhythmias that
are very rapid or refractory to standard drugs, or associated with a wide
QRS complex on the standard electrocardiogram (implying either aberration, antegrade preexcitation, or VT), warrant an invasive electrophysiologic study. In the majority of other patients, drug management is
successful. Nonetheless, the ease of radiofrequency ablation coupled
with its very high success rates and low rates of complications have
increasingly led to its use as first-line therapy, particularly in younger
patients reluctant to commit to lifelong drug therapy, even if the latter is
effective.

Prevention of PSVT. The best measure is often catheter ablation.
Otherwise initiating ectopic beats may be inhibited by β-blockade,
verapamil, diltiazem, or amiodarone. The latter is highly effective for
supraventricular arrhythmias, including paroxysmal AF and arrhythmias involving accessory pathways; potentially severe side effects may
be limited by a low dose (see Chapter 8, p. 319). The class IC drugs
(propafenone and flecainide) are viable alternatives but should not be
used in the presence of structural heart disease.

Wolff-Parkinson-White syndrome. The acute treatment of choice or
Wolff-Parkinson-White syndrome is cardioversion if the patient is hemodynamically compromised. If presenting with narrow-complex PSVT,
the same intravenous therapy as for standard PVST may be followed
(see Table 12-5). For follow-up, because of the risk of antegrade preexcitation via the bypass tract, *digoxin is absolutely contraindicated* (because it shortens the refractory period of the tract). Verapamil, diltiazem,
and β-blockade may also be dangerous by blocking the AV node and
redirecting impulses down the bypass tract. In the prevention of PSVT,
including AF, radiofrequency catheter ablation of the accessory pathway is usually highly successful and is now standard treatment. Otherwise, low-dose amiodarone is probably best, followed by sotalol or
propafenone. Prophylactic ablation in asymptomatic individuals at
high risk may be the best approach—for example, in those age 35 years
or younger, patients with evidence of rapidly conducting pathways with
short refractory periods, or patients with rapid arrhythmias inducible at
the time of an electrophysiologic study, or on the basis of occupational
or other lifestyle circumstances. This is, however, still controversial.[331]

Bradyarrhythmias

Asymptomatic sinus bradycardia does not require therapy and may be
normal, especially in athletes. For *symptomatic sinus bradycardia, sick
sinus syndrome, and sinoatrial disease*, probanthine and chronic atropine are unsatisfactory so that pacing is usually required. First, however,
the adverse effects of drugs such as β-blockers, digitalis, verapamil,
diltiazem, quinidine, procainamide, amiodarone, lidocaine, methyldopa,
clonidine, and lithium carbonate should be excluded. AV block that
was "truly caused by drugs" was found in only 15% of patients during
therapy with β-blockers, verapamil, or diltiazem.[332] In this study 56% of
patients for whom drug discontinuation led to resolution of AV block
had recurrence of AV block in the absence of therapy during follow-
up.[332] In this respect, drugs such as β-blockers and verapamil constituted a "pharmacologic stress test." Second- or third-degree AV block,
which resolved following discontinuation of β-blockers, verapamil, or
diltiazem, 56% had a subsequent recurrence of AV block in the absence
of therapy. In the *tachycardia/bradycardia syndrome,* intrinsic sinus
node dysfunction is difficult to treat and once again may require

permanent pacing. β-Blockers aggravate the bradycardiac component of the syndrome. Patients usually end up with a combination of a permanent pacemaker and antiarrhythmic agents. However, in many patients the combination of radiofrequency ablation of the AV node followed by permanent pacemaker implantation is a highly effective method of controlling refractory tachycardia. For *AV block with syncope* or with excessively slow rates, atropine or isoproterenol or transthoracic pacing is used as an emergency measure, pending pacemaker implantation. In asymptomatic patients with congenital heart block, the role of permanent pacing is debatable, with current trends favoring an aggressive approach at an earlier age.

Ventricular Arrhythmias and Proarrhythmic Problems

The criteria for instituting drug therapy for ventricular arrhythmias are not clear cut, although patients with sustained VT (Table 12-6), survivors of previous arrhythmia-related cardiac arrest, and those with severely symptomatic arrhythmias all require treatment. A full

Table 12-6

Acute Sustained Ventricular Tachycardia[591]

Entry Point: Wide QRS Complex Tachycardia

- Approximately 90% will be wide-complex ventricular tachycardia; the others will include PSVT with aberration or WPW with anterograde conduction.
- DC cardioversion—procedure of choice (ACC/AHA/ESC class 1C*), usually effective.
- If DC cardioversion fails or if patient hemodynamically stable:
  - IV amiodarone often used (class IIA/B).
  - IV procainamide (more effective but less safe) (class IIA/C).
  - IV lidocaine (safe but will revert only a minority) (class IIB/C).
  - If torsades de pointes, IV magnesium sulfate; consider atrial pacing; isoproterenol in an emergency.
  - If VT recurs soon after cardioversion, repeat the latter under cover of lidocaine or other IV drug.
  - (Only if PSVT presents as suspected VT, use IV adenosine for diagnosis but *never* verapamil or diltiazem.)

Follow-up of Acute Attack

- If PSVT, see Table 12-5.
- If VT (majority):
  - Requires thorough cardiologic evaluation.
  - Need accurate diagnosis of rhythm, structural heart disease, and LV function (long QT syndrome); arrhythmogenic RV dysplasia.
- Empirical drug approach (amiodarone) if patient not candidate for ICD.
- Various trials have left unresolved the best way to select antiarrhythmic drugs for patients with ventricular arrhythmias.
- Strong trend toward ICD, away from EPS-guided drug choice.
- Sometimes surgery (LV aneurysm).
- If idiopathic refractory VT, especially RVOT in origin, radiofrequency catheter ablation but verapamil may be effective in RVOT VT and exercise-induced VT in patients without structural heart disease.
- ICD as first-line therapy if high risk of sudden death: in survivors of cardiac arrest, in symptomatic VT, or in asymptomatic VT with a low ejection fraction.
- In patients with recurrent ICD shocks caused by VT, consider amiodarone plus β-blockade—if needed, radiofrequency ablation.

ACC, American College of Cardiology; *AHA,* American Heart Association; *DC,* direct current; *EPS,* electrophysiologic stimulation; *ESC,* European Society of Cardiology; *ICD,* implantable cardioverter defibrillator; *IV,* intravenous; *LV,* left ventricular; *PSVT,* paroxysmal supraventricular tachycardia; *RV,* right ventricular; *RVOT,* right ventricular outflow tract; *VT,* ventricular tachycardia; *WPW,* Wolff-Parkinson-White preexcitation syndrome.
*Classes of Recommendations (1-3) and levels of evidence (A-C).

cardiologic assessment is required. An essential adjunct to antiarrhythmic therapy lies in the management of underlying disease such as LV failure, ischemia, anemia, thyrotoxicosis, or electrolyte imbalance. The potential hazards of antiarrhythmic therapy were emphasized by the CAST study, which warned that the proarrhythmic effects of some class I agents can actually increase mortality in patients with ischemic heart disease. In patients with ICDs, concomitant drug therapy by β-blockade and amiodarone to reduce inappropriate discharges is often administered and the ICD provides "backup" in the event of proarrhythmia. The most effective way to prevent SCD in patients with coronary disease is to eliminate ischemia and to improve LV function, often by coronary revascularization. In the patient who has already survived an episode of cardiac arrest or hemodynamically unstable VT, coronary revascularization alone will usually not suffice, and an ICD is indicated.

Drug choice for ventricular arrhythmias. The choice of drug for chronic use is ideally based on prior demonstration during acute and chronic Holter or electrophysiologic testing that the drug actually works and on its potential for toxicity in the patient under study. Unfortunately, neither the Holter nor the electrophysiologic study is a reliable guide to long-term efficacy of therapy. Class I agents, including quinidine, disopyramide, and mexiletine, are used less and less. Propafenone is possibly the most effective and least harmful of the class IC agents, although not as good as β-blockade or amiodarone in the CASH study,[333] in which the propafenone arm was discontinued. In patients without structural heart disease, the risk of proarrhythmia with both propafenone and flecainide is low. The antiarrhythmic effect of *empirical β-blockade monotherapy* for VT is impressive and reportedly as good as electrophysiologic-guided drug choice. In comparison with other drugs, amiodarone appears to be the most effective antiarrhythmic agent, despite its considerable side effects. Sotalol, a β-blocker with antiarrhythmic class III activity (see Table 1-3), is an alternative, with a reduced dose in renal insufficiency; it should only be given in the hospital under monitoring conditions because QT prolongation and torsades des pointes occur in 1% to 4% of patients.

β-Blockers are among the few antiarrhythmic agents with positive long-term beneficial effects in postinfarct patients.[192] In those not responding to β-blockade, or in whom β-blockade is contraindicated, *low-dose amiodarone* is increasingly used, despite potentially serious side effects. Like β-blockade, amiodarone appears to give postinfarct protection. Deciding between these agents is somewhat of a personal choice and not entirely evidence based. Yet, in comparison with others, amiodarone is the most effective antiarrhythmic agent despite its considerable side effects that are, however, lower at reduced doses.

Implantable cardioverter defibrillators. The treatment of recurrent sustained VT and VF is difficult, and pharmacologic therapy has, in the main, been very disappointing. This failure has stimulated alternative approaches such as surgical or catheter ablation of the VT foci and use of the ICD, which is now mandated for all survivors of SCD, for intractable ventricular arrhythmias, and increasingly for primary prevention of SCD in postinfarct heart failure (for details see section on p. 320). The advent of the ICD has virtually eliminated surgical procedures such as endocardial resection. Prophylactic antiarrhythmic drug therapy is contraindicated except for β-blockade, which can be very helpful, especially in those with coronary-related CHF receiving an ICD, for whom β-blockade is standard therapy, often with amiodarone, to reduce the effect of unpleasant shocks on the patient. Radiofrequency catheter ablation may be very successful in idiopathic or right-ventricular outflow tract VTs. For the vast majority of patients who have VT secondary to coronary artery disease and LV dysfunction, catheter ablation remains an option as newer mapping techniques are improving success rates.

In patients with ICDs, *recurrent discharges* are a major source of morbidity, depression, and anxiety. With the backup of an ICD in place, there is a new role for the use of antiarrhythmic drugs, despite LV dysfunction, whereas these might be contraindicated in patients without devices.[334] Common causes of inappropriate device discharges include supraventricular arrhythmias including AF, electrical noise, inappropriate sensing, and device or lead malfunction. The frequency can be reduced by additional reprogramming, the use of dual-chamber devices, and antitachycardia pacing.[335] Appropriate discharges caused by recurrent VT can be treated with antiarrhythmic drugs to prevent the arrhythmia or slow the rate such that it is more responsive to antitachycardia pacing.[336] Radiofrequency may be effective in reducing the frequency of discharges,[337] and prophylactic ablation of a ventricular arrhythmic substrate was found to reduce the frequency of subsequent ICD discharges in two trials.[338,339]

Congestive Heart Failure

General policy. Despite powerful protective agents (ACE inhibitors, ARBs, β-blockers, spironolactone, eplerenone), the long-term prognosis of CHF remains poor, unless a reversible cause is found. The initial steps in a patient with heart failure include investigation and specific treatment for a cause, including ischemia, hypertension, valvular heart disease, uncontrolled diabetes, thyrotoxicosis, alcohol abuse, cocaine, obstructive sleep apnea, and anemia. It is important to exclude the use of other *drugs that could exacerbate heart failure*, that is, NSAIDs, CCBs, thiazolidinediones, and antiarrhythmic drugs, many of which are negatively inotropic. It is also important to obtain a careful family history as the familial and genetic components of idiopathic dilated cardiomyopathy are increasingly recognized.[340] The effect of lifestyle modification in CHF has not been tested in randomized trials, but makes sense and includes smoking cessation, restriction of salt and alcohol, weight reduction in obese subjects, and regular monitoring to detect fluid build-up.[341-343] Pneumococcal vaccination and an annual influenza vaccination are strongly recommended. The previous policy was to initiate treatment with loop diuretics, salt restriction, and then digoxin before proceeding to conventional vasodilators, but *ACE inhibitors and β-blockers are now the cornerstone of therapy*, increasingly given from the start of symptoms (with diuretics), or even before an asymptomatic LV dysfunction (without diuretics). The key to maximizing the dose of both ACE inhibitors and β-blockers is gradual titration. Although *digoxin* for AF patients with heart failure is less used, meticulous attention must be paid to the new safer blood ranges (see Fig. 6-12); older "therapeutic" ranges were also potentially lethal. As digoxin does not improve mortality, the current trend is to emphasize the agents that do improve mortality (ACE inhibitors, ARBs, β-blockers, aldosterone antagonists) and then to consider digoxin among other options such as nitrate-hydralazine (see Fig. 6-10) for patients remaining symptomatic. Previous combination "triple therapy" with diuretics, ACE inhibition, and digoxin is now replaced by *modern quadruple therapy* (ACE inhibitors or ARBs, β-blockade, diuretics, and spironolactone or eplerenone). How can clinical judgment be aided? Plasma B-type (brain) natriuretic peptide (BNP) is a rapid and sensitive guide that reflects elevated LV filling pressures and is useful in the diagnosis of heart failure in the patient presenting with dyspnea. Studies evaluating the role of BNP measurements in guiding management in both symptomatic and asymptomatic patients are ongoing.

ACE inhibitors versus ARBs. The vast experience gained with ACE inhibitors makes them the "gold standard" for renin-angiotensin inhibition (see Table 5-5). When ACE inhibitors cannot be tolerated (cough), ARBs become a logical replacement, but the combination of these is also being advocated for heart failure.[344] Although the CHARM-Added trial suggested that adding an ARB to an ACE inhibitor may be helpful from a symptomatic standpoint, this was not in patients taking aldosterone antagonists, and the combination of an aldosterone antagonist, ACE inhibitor, and an ARB is not recommended.[345]

β-Blockers. When cautiously added to ACE inhibitors and diuretics in hemodynamically stable patients, β-blockers consistently decrease mortality by approximately 30% or even more. The patient should be closely supervised during this initial titration because there is the risk of transient deterioration. Trial data favor the use of carvedilol, metoprolol, and bisoprolol (see Chapter 1, p. 16). Of these, only carvedilol and long-acting metoprolol XL are licensed for use in the United States (see Chapter 6 for evaluation of these drugs). Only carvedilol is approved for class IV heart failure.[346] Metoprolol XL is only licensed for class II and III heart failure but has an angina license in the United States, which carvedilol does not. β-Blockers are typically initiated after the patient is stabilized on ACE inhibitors, when the watchword is to use low doses and titrate slowly as tolerated. However, the CIBIS-3 trial showed that β-blockade could be instituted *before* ACE inhibition.[347] In practice, many start with a low dose of an ACE inhibitor increasing at 1-2 week intervals followed by the initiation of a β-blocker at very low doses and gradual titration over a period of weeks.

Congestive heart failure. A metaanalysis of double-blind, placebo-controlled trials of β-blockers in heart failure demonstrated a lower magnitude of survival benefit among patients enrolled in the United States versus the rest of the world. Whether this is due to population differences, genetics, cultural or social differences, and disease management or simply chance is uncertain.[348]

Diuretic therapy. Doses and drugs should not be fixed, but loop diuretics are usually the drugs of choice for the treatment of pulmonary or peripheral edema. Diuretics may need to be reduced when the ACE inhibitor is introduced or the dose increased, or diuretic therapy may have to be stepped up in cases of refractory edema. Especially in severe right ventricular failure, the absorption of drugs given orally is impaired and a short course of intravenous furosemide can be very helpful. *Posture* can influence diuretic efficacy. To improve renal perfusion and to increase diuresis, the patient may have to return to bed for 1 to 2 hours of supine rest after taking a diuretic. The principle of *sequential nephron blockade* (see Figs. 4-2 and 4-5) states that different types of diuretics can synergistically be added, such as a thiazide to a loop diuretic.

Aldosterone antagonists. The adverse neurohumoral qualities of diuretic therapy, often forgotten, need to be balanced by an ACE inhibitor or ARB, often with spironolactone. Yet especially in patients with poor renal function, these combinations can precipitate hyperkalemia.

Nonetheless, the RALES study[349] showed that the addition of spironolactone at an average dose of 25 mg daily while watching K can give substantial clinical improvement and save lives in patients with class III or IV heart failure. RALES is complemented by the EPHESUS study that used eplerenone, a selective aldosterone blocker, in post-MI patients with transient heart failure or, in the case of diabetics, an ejection fraction of less than 40%.[245] This too was strongly positive. Subsequently, the EPHESUS-HF trial in sessions with milder symptoms (New York Heart Association [NYHA] class II heart failure) and an ejection fraction of no more than 35% was also resoundingly positive, and aldosterone antagonists are now considered standard therapy.[350]

It remains essential to monitor the serum potassium carefully, particularly when ACE inhibitors or ARBs are also part of the therapeutic attack. In patients treated by both an ACE inhibitor and an ARB, ACC-AHA guidelines warn that aldosterone antagonists should not be used.[351] The remarkable story of aldosterone antagonists for heart failure is backed by experimental evidence suggesting that aldosterone may mediate myocardial fibrosis in remodeling, whereas clinical data suggest that aldosterone antagonism may improve LV function, mass, and volumes (reverse remodeling).[352]

Vasodilators. High-dose nitrates (on-off patches) improve exercise tolerance and LV size and function when added to ACE inhibitors, diuretics, and digoxin.[353] In patients with pulmonary congestion, nitrates given at night can decisively improve sleep. For long-term use, the old combination of nitrates plus hydralazine is logical because the hydralazine appears to counteract nitrate tolerance (see Chapter 2, p. 53), although it is still prudent to maintain a nitrate-free window of 8 to 10 hours depending on whether symptoms occur primarily at night or with exertion during the day. Because black patients appeared to be less responsive to ACE inhibitors in earlier trials, the African-American Heart Failure trial tested the addition of isosorbide dinitrate plus hydralazine to standard therapy, finding increased survival.[354] This trial sparked a controversy about the role of race and ethnicity in clinical trials,[354,355] although settling the issue of how to prevent nitrate tolerance in heart failure. Another byproduct of the African American Heart Failure trial has been a series of investigations aimed at untangling the pharmacogenomic issues underlying the differences between black and white heart failure patients.[356]

Atrial fibrillation in congestive heart failure. AF both contributes to mortality[357] and is a marker for severe disease.[358] Both the AF and the heart failure must be treated as vigorously as possible. In selected patients cardioversion under anticoagulation or new atrial pacing techniques or internal cardioversion may be appropriate, but for most, strict rate control over 24 hours and anticoagulation with warfarin "remain the mainstays of therapy."[358] Failing rate control, the next option is conversion and maintenance of sinus rhythm with amiodarone, which is well tested in CHF although not approved for AF in the United States. Sotalol is an alternative. Dofetilide, approved for highly symptomatic AF, converts to sinus rhythm in CHF but in only approximately 12% of patients.[359] Once sinus rhythm was restored, dofetilide reduced recurrences by 65%. Careful dose adjustment is needed in renal failure. Another major downside is the risk of early torsades de pointes (3.3%). Although dronedarone was associated with reduced heart failure and hospitalization in the ATHENA trial, the results of the ANDROMEDA trial, which compared dronedarone to placebo in patients with symptomatic heart failure and severe LV systolic dysfunction, demonstrated an increased mortality in the dronedarone group. The drug should not be used in patients with NYHA class III-IV heart failure, and great caution should be exercised if the drug is to be given to patients with less severe degrees of heart failure.[291,292]

Rate versus rhythm control. Controversies in patients with LV systolic dysfunction and heart failure will hopefully soon be resolved. The AF-CHF trial found no outcome differences between these policies over 2 years.[360] Although pulmonary vein isolation and wide atrial circumferential ablation can be successful in patients with heart failure, the success rates are reduced, and the option of AV nodal ablation with single or often biventricular pacing is frequently used. One advantage of AV nodal ablation in patients undergoing biventricular pacing is that it ensures 100% paced rhythm and therefore theoretically increases the efficacy of cardiac resynchronization therapy (CRT).[361] In regard to the indications for warfarin therapy in patients with AF and heart failure there are limited data, and the American College of Chest

Physicians' guidelines recommend against the routine use of warfarin or aspirin in patients with heart failure resulting from a nonischemic cause.[362] Nonetheless, many believe that warfarin is indicated in this situation, and it is mandatory in any patients with a history of systemic or pulmonary emboli. In the WATCH trial of 1587 patients in sinus rhythm with symptomatic heart failure there was no benefit from aspirin in regard to the primary endpoint of death, nonfatal MI, or nonfatal stroke.[363] In the WARCEF trial of patients with reduced LVEF who were in sinus rhythm, there was no significant overall difference in the primary outcome between treatment with warfarin and treatment with aspirin. A reduced risk of ischemic stroke with warfarin was offset by an increased risk of major hemorrhage. The choice between warfarin and aspirin should be individualized.[364]

Ventricular arrhythmias in CHF. The incidence of sudden death seems to be falling since the widespread introduction of ACE inhibitors and now β-blockers. For those who still have severe *significantly symptomatic ventricular arrhythmias*, it is first essential to pinpoint precipitating factors such as hypokalemia, hypomagnesemia, or use of sympathomimetics, phosphodiesterase inhibitors, or digoxin. The hemodynamic status of the myocardium must be made optimal because increased LV wall stress is arrhythmogenic. Amiodarone is the most effective drug for preventing AF and complex ventricular ectopy or nonsustained VT, but there was no benefit on SCD or total mortality.[365,366] Patients with class IV symptoms are likely to die of CHF, and an ICD is not indicated unless the patient is a candidate for CRT. *Increasingly, ICDs are considered* for selected high-risk patients with life-threatening arrhythmias, and especially those with an ejection fraction of less than 30% (see Fig. 8-16). Prophylactic class I antiarrhythmic drug therapy is contraindicated. In contrast, prophylactic β-blockade can be very helpful, especially in patients with coronary-related CHF.

Severe intractable CHF. The first steps are to ensure support of oxygenation and ventilation; assess volume status and hemodynamic stability, which may often require the use of a PA catheter; address precipitating factors such as infection, dietary indiscretion, and the administration of nonsteroidal antiinflammatory agents; and to relieve symptoms. In patients with "flash" pulmonary edema, one should be aware of acute hypertension and underlying renal artery stenosis. The next steps are to administer intravenous diuretics (depending on volume status); optimize intravenous vasodilator therapy with nitroprusside, nitroglycerin, or nesiritide; and institute inotropic agents (usually milrinone or dobutamine) for the objective of optimizing hemodynamics. In the DOSE trial, there was no significant difference in efficacy or safety endpoints for bolus versus continuous infusion of furosemide, and high-dose furosemide (2.5 times the previous oral dose) compared with low-dose furosemide produced greater fluid loss, weight loss, and relief from dyspnea, but also more frequent transient worsening of renal function.[367] In this setting, dobutamine has three potential hazards: further β-receptor downgrading, increased arrhythmias,[368] and hypotension. In the current era when most patients are on β-blockers, milrinone may be a better choice. Dopamine remains a useful drug (see Fig. 6-4), although the idea of the renal dose is now discredited.

Nesiritide. Nesiritide is a recombinant human BNP that reduces pulmonary capillary wedge pressure and improves symptoms.[369] In a very large recent trial of more than 7000 patients with acute decompensated heart failure, nesiritide was not associated with an increase or a decrease in the rate of death and rehospitalization and had a small, nonsignificant effect on dyspnea when used in combination with other therapies. Renal function was unchanged, but it was associated with an increase in rates of hypotension, and on the basis of these results nesiritide should not be recommended for routine use in a broad population of patients with acute heart failure.[370] When compared with dobutamine, nesiritide was required for a shorter period and gave a lower 6-month mortality, so that there was an overall saving in health costs.[371] A metaanalysis of five studies in 2005 raised the risk of worsening renal function,[372] which has, however, been discounted by two more recent studies.[373,374]

Other new agents for CHF. The list of promising drugs and therapies for CHF that have failed the rigorous scrutiny of randomized controlled trials makes for lengthy reading and includes *levosimendan* (a calcium sensitizer), *rolofylline* (an adenosine A1 receptor antagonist), *tolvaptan,* endothelin receptor blockers, central sympatholytics, phosphodiasterase-3 inhibitors, immune modulators, erythropoietin, darbepoetin, and vasopeptidase inhibitors. Immune modulators, erythropoietin, and darbepoetin, vasopeptidase inhibitors, and surgical LV reconstruction were studied in the STITCH trial, although better results with this procedure have been reported in nonrandomized studies.[375-377] Ivabradine, which is a selective I_F-channel inhibitor that slows the heart rate (see Fig. 8-4), appears to be of significant benefit based on the randomized SHIFT trial, but the drug is not yet available in the United States.[28] Ongoing studies include trials of direct renin inhibition, combined neutral endopeptidase inhibitor-angiotensin II receptor blocker, the reduction of uric acid with allopurinol, and warfarin versus aspirin in patients with a reduced ejection fraction.[377] Neuregulin-1, which is expressed in the heart and plays a role in the maintenance of adult heart functional integrity, appears to be promising in a recent phase 2 randomized double-blind trial with recombinant neuregulin, but larger trials will be needed.[378]

Omecamtiv mecarbil is a novel investigational myosin-activator given intravenously.[379] Cardiac output is increased not by strengthening contractile force but by prolonging systole, thereby enhancing the efficiency of contraction. The idea of improving cardiac output in a safe way is appealing but further evaluation is needed, and it should be remembered that the field of heart-failure drug development is strewn with casualties.

Interventions for Severe Stable LV Dysfunction

Implantable cardioverter defibrillators. The role of the ICD in the primary prevention of SCD is now well established. In patients with prior MI and nonischemic dilated cardiomyopathy, major trials and current recommendations (reviewed in Chapter 8, p. 320) taken in concert support the use of ICDs in those with class II and III CHF with an ejection fraction of less than 35%, and class I if less than 30%.[259,380,381] Patients with class IV symptoms are likely to die of CHF, and an ICD is not indicated unless the patient is a candidate for CRT. The DINAMIT and IRIS trials confined to high-risk patients 6-40 days postinfarction were completely neutral and supported the recommendation to *delay ICD implantation for primary prevention after MI.*[382,383] Additionally, in our opinion, in patients who have hemodynamically significant sustained ventricular arrhythmias within 24-48 hours of an MI, this is indicative of an arrhythmic substrate and an indication for ICD implantation or an invasive electrophysiologic study, provided that reversible causes such as ischemia have been excluded. Because the ejection fraction may change and improve or deteriorate during the first few weeks post-MI, the current recommendations are to wait at least 40 days before making a definite decision to implant an ICD for primary prevention in post-MI patients. The role of the automatic external defibrillator (AED) during this waiting period has been disappointing.[357] The major cause of the death in the first 18 months postinfarction is probably recurrent MI and ischemic events or heart failure, and during this period, although the device may be effective in terminating arrhythmias, it is unlikely to affect long-term prognosis.[384] The role of Holter monitoring and invasive electrophysiologic testing in identifying candidates for the primary prevention of SCD has declined, and the major inclusion criterion is the ejection fraction, albeit an imprecise measurement. Risk stratification needs to be repeated because interim events such as recurrent ischemia or heart failure are independent risk factors for late SCD.[385]

Cardiac resynchronization therapy. CRT should be considered for patients who have either ischemic or nonischemic cardiomyopathy, an LV ejection fraction EF of 35% or less, class III or IV symptoms, and a QRS duration of greater than 120 msec.[386,387] Recently, the resynchronization R-Defibrillation for Ambulatory Heart Failure Trial (RAFT) has extended the benefits of CRT to patients with minimally symptomatic heart failure, an LV ejection fraction of less than or equal to 30% (mean 22%), and a QRS with equal to or greater than 120 msec (mean 158 msec).[262] The greatest benefit obtained is in patients with a QRS complex of 150 msec or greater (not due to right bundle branch block), and the magnitude of benefit in those with narrower QRS complexes (120-149 msec) is controversial.[388,389] A frustrating aspect of CRT therapy is the relative inability to predict which patients will respond ahead of time and despite a number of echocardiographic and other indices, the magnitude of QRS width still appears to be the best predictors.

Viability testing and revascularization. In moderate to severe ischemic cardiomyopathy, substantial segments of myocardium may be nonfunctioning but hibernating and thus metabolically viable, a state that revascularization could potentially improve.[390,391] Using a variety of modern imaging techniques, including dobutamine magnetic resonance imaging and positron emission tomography, myocardial viability can be recognized and revascularization considered. The recent STITCH trial of coronary bypass surgery versus medical therapy in patients with heart failure and coronary artery disease but without a clear cut indication for CABG is modestly positive, and a viability substudy from this trial is somewhat confusing in that patients with viability appear to do better than those without viability, but the benefit of surgery actually appeared to be greater than those without viability.[392]

Other invasive options. Patients with severe heart failure who are refractory to conventional medical therapy may benefit from extracorporeal ultrafiltration via hemofiltration for the removal of intravascular fluid.[393] An *LV or biventricular assist device* may "bridge" the gap to transplantation, or may even initiate "reverse remodeling" by myocyte unloading.[394] The development of a range of devices for supporting the failing heart has improved outcomes and expanded the use of mechanically assisted circulatory support as both "bridge" and destination therapy.[395,396] A recent randomized trial of treatment with a continuous-flow Heart Mate II device in comparison to the pulsatile flow Heart Mate XVE device demonstrated a significant improvement in the probability of survival free from stroke and device failure at two years, but both devices significantly improved the quality of life and functional capacity.[397] This is a dynamic and evolving field, but despite the improving results the incidence of complications such as infection, bleeding, peripheral emboli, and device failure remain formidable. Most surgical mitral valve repair in patients with heart failure and functional mitral regurgitation does not appear to be beneficial.[398] There is nonetheless understandable interest in the use of percutaneous techniques such as the Mitra Clip system.[399]

General Management of CHF. Sodium restriction and, in severe cases, water limitation are important ancillary measures. It is often forgotten that in severe CHF there is delayed water diuresis. Weight loss and exercise rehabilitation, as well as psychological support, are all positive procedures. Home nursing helps patients with severe limitation of exercise. A short-term high-carbohydrate diet, by allowing muscle glycogen to break down more slowly, can increase endurance exercise, of potential interest to CHF patients who need extra energy for a special occasion.[398] A major advance in the management of CHF is an *extensive, nurse-based outpatient program* that relies on patient education and regular communication between patient and health care provider.[400,401] *Anemia* and its potential as a therapeutic target is increasingly recognized.[402,403] Relatively small-scale studies have shown promising results with the correction of anemia using erythropoietin and darbepoetin, but the final verdict will await the ongoing RED-HF study.[404] As to therapy with intravenous iron, more studies are needed, but the FAIR-HF trial did show an improvement in symptoms and New York Heart Class, quality of life, and exercise capacity.[405]

Summary. In asymptomatic LV dysfunction, initial therapy is by ACE inhibition or ARB. Added β-blockade started in very low doses and titrated upward adds decisive benefit. In patients with symptomatic CHF, a diuretic is required. Spironolactone or eplerenone is being added earlier than before. Of these agents, ACE inhibitors, β-blockers, and spironolactone and eplerenone all improve longevity. Digoxin may be added for AF or to control symptoms, with careful control of the blood levels and without expecting any effect on mortality. The combination of ACE inhibitors or ARBs, β-blockers, diuretics, and spironolactone is now increasingly common, followed by addition of vasodilators such as hydralazine and nitrates. An important advance is the concept of primary prevention of sudden death by prophylactic implantation of an ICD, selected for those with ejection fractions of less than 35% and class II or III heart failure, or below 30% for class I (see Chapter 8, Fig. 8-16). The lot of the individual patient with severe CHF can be improved by searching out underlying causes, by diuretic synergism, by ensuring that there is maximal RAAS inhibition, by checking on serum potassium and magnesium, and by general management including salt restriction, exercise rehabilitation, psychological support ("keep going, you are doing better than you think"), and intensive nurse-based outpatient care of CHF. Team management results in fewer hospital admissions and improved outcomes.[406,407]

Future Directions. A recent NHLBI workshop identified challenges and research opportunities in regard to the emergency department management of cardiac failure, including the development of methods of early detection and hemodynamic and biomarker.[408] The last two decades have been characterized as the era of hemodynamic improvement in neurohormonal modulation. Adjunctive nonpharmacologic approaches included the ICD, cardiac resynchronization, therapy, ventricular assist devices, and the recognition and treatment of sleep apnea. Cardiac transplantation has continued but is limited by donor supply. Future approaches will depend on unraveling the molecular web, underlying altered sarcomeric function, myocardial energetics, signaling, and calcium transport in CHF, and we hope will identify new therapeutic targets. Pharmacogenomic profiling is a field that becomes increasingly complex but is evolving rapidly. Other nonpharmacologic areas under development include biomarker and wireless hemodynamic monitoring, the miniaturization and improvements in the design of ventricular assist devices and the total artificial heart, and in the distant future perhaps a role for xenotransplantation and cardiac cell repair therapy (a field that has captured the imagination of many investigators around the world).

Diastolic Heart Failure

Preserved systolic function and diastolic dysfunction. Differences between proven diastolic heart failure and preserved systolic function (simplistically and variably diagnosed by systolic ejection fractions of less than 40%-50%) are outlined in Chapter 6 (see p. 207), together with definitions.[409] Major causes are increasing age and left ventricular hypertrophy (LVH). Prognosis is serious, similar to that of systolic failure.[410] Therapy trials are scant. Logically, the aim is regression of LVH, which is often the underlying cause. Vigorous therapy of underlying hypertension or aortic stenosis is essential. In clinical heart failure with hypertension, tight 24-hour BP control is mandatory. Other measures are a reduction in central blood volume by diuretics, countering tachycardia, aggressive treatment of AF, and management of concomitant coronary artery disease and ischemic diastolic dysfunction, including revascularization.

Does RAAS blockade give specific benefit? Angiotensin II has powerful profibrotic and proapoptotic properties in the hypertrophic heart.[44] Regarding ARBs, candesartan gave only modest benefit in one arm of the CHARM studies, in which there was heart failure with relatively preserved LV function.[344] The ACE inhibitor perindopril also gave only modest benefits in clinical heart failure in older adults, of whom 79% were hypertensive; therapy decreased the BP and hospitalization.[411] Whether CCBs exert a "lusitropic" effect by enhancing ventricular relaxation is difficult to distinguish from potential benefits from slowing the heart rate. Aldosterone is linked to the development of cardiac hypertrophy and fibrosis, and a large National Institutes of Health–sponsored study (TOPCAT) is currently evaluating the hypothesis that spironolactone could be beneficial in patients with CHF and preserved systolic function (ClinicalTrials.gov/ct2/show/NCT00094302). Other treatments of suggestive but unproven benefit include statins and exercise conditioning.

At present we accept that specific therapies for diastolic heart failure are lacking and that the management is similar to that for CHF with systolic dysfunction. Moreover, in patients with systolic dysfunction, diastolic dysfunction frequently coexists. Specific therapies await a better understanding of the pathophysiologic findings and, in particular, the extent to which this is a cardiac disease versus an imbalance between the heart and the vasculature.[412]

Diastolic dysfunction without clinical heart failure. Here too RAAS inhibition has been studied. In younger hypertensive patients with diastolic dysfunction but without LVH or heart failure, lowering BP by an ARB with an aim of less than 135/80 mm Hg improved diastolic dysfunction, without any specific clinical benefit.[413] In early hypertensive heart disease and diastolic dysfunction but with a mean ejection fraction of 67% and without exercise limitation, aldosterone antagonism improved diastolic function, and modestly decreased LV posterior wall thickness without altering LV mass.[414] Clinically, these studies, albeit imperfect, suggest vigorous BP lowering in hypertensives with diastolic dysfunction even in the absence of clinical heart failure.

Acute Pulmonary Edema

In acute pulmonary edema of cardiac origin, the initial management requires positioning the patient in an upright posture and administering oxygen. The standard triple-drug regimen is morphine, furosemide, and nitrates, to which ACE inhibitors must now be added. If the underlying cause is a tachyarrhythmia, restoration of sinus rhythm takes priority. Morphine sulfate, with both venodilator and central sedative actions, is highly effective in relieving symptoms. Intravenous furosemide, both diuretic and vasodilator, is the other basic therapy. *Acute digoxin* is undesirable in view of the prevailing arrhythmogenic environment, unless there is uncontrolled AF. β-Blockers are contraindicated in the acute phase, but should be initiated before discharge.

Nitrates. Nitrates are excellent for unloading of the left heart and relief of pulmonary congestion. Which is better, repetitive furosemide or repetitive intravenous nitrates? Repeated intravenous boluses of high-dose isosorbide (3 mg every 5 minutes) after a single low dose (40 mg) of furosemide were better than repeated high-dose furosemide with low-dose isosorbide,[415] the former treatment reducing the need for mechanical ventilation and the frequency of MI.

ACE inhibitors. ACE inhibitors such as sublingual captopril or intravenous enalaprilat (1 mg over 2 hours) are logical and achieve load reduction when added to the standard regimen of oxygen, nitrates, morphine, and furosemide.[416,417] In practice, these agents (or ARBs) are rather started orally as soon as the hyperacute phase is over.

Other vasodilators. In patients with pulmonary edema secondary to severe acute or chronic mitral or aortic regurgitation, *intravenous nitroprusside* (see Chapter 6, p. 186) is probably the agent of choice. Whenever vasodilators are contemplated, particular caution is necessary in the patient with a systolic BP of less than 90 mm Hg. In AMI, compounds such as aminophylline and milrinone are best avoided because of their proarrhythmic potential. *Nesiritide* was better than nitroglycerin in small trials, but its effects in renal function were controversial.[418,419] A large recent trial of more than 7000 patients alleviated concerns about nesiritide safety, but its effects on dyspnea were only marginally beneficial, and there was no effect on 30-day mortality or hospitalization.[370] It seems that nesiritide is a second-line agent to fall back on when standard therapies are ineffective in improving symptoms.

Severe hypertension. Use carefully titrated intravenous nicardipine or sodium nitroprusside or nitrates or enalaprilat, together with pressure monitoring. Oral ACE inhibitors are started as soon as feasible, taking care to prevent hypotension. *Bronchospasm* usually responds to diuresis or load reduction. *β-Blockers* should be withheld until hemodynamic stabilization is achieved.

Intravenous positive inotropic agents. The majority of patients will not require positive inotropic agents in the absence of persistent hypotension, cardiogenic shock, severe end-organ dysfunction, or failure to respond to standard therapy.

Refractory cases. In refractory cases, intubate with mechanical ventilation: "When in doubt, intubate." A modest amount of evidence supports the use of continuous positive airway pressure given via a face mask to patients with cardiogenic pulmonary edema.[420] Although noninvasive ventilation resulted in more rapid improvement in respiratory distress and metabolic disturbance, there was no effect on overall mortality.[421] Further studies are needed before general use of increased airway pressures can be recommended.

Hypertrophic Cardiomyopathy

Hypertrophic cardiomyopathy, together with bicuspid aortic valve disease, is one of the commonest forms of inherited cardiac disease and the first ACC-AHA Guidelines for the management of this condition were published in 2011.[422] The principles of management are to screen first-degree relatives for HCM, avoid competitive sport, volume depletion, and isometric exercise, to control symptoms primarily with the use of β-blockers and if necessary the addition of a nondihydropyridine CCB (usually verapamil), and in the event that medical therapy fails septal reduction therapy with surgical myectomy or alcohol septal ablation is indicated. Risk stratification for SCD and prevention with ICD is also the cornerstone of management. Older asymptomatic patients need reassurance, regular surveillance, and exclusion of hypertension.

Principles of pharmacologic therapy. The principles of pharmacologic therapy are (1) to lessen the hypercontractile state by a negative inotrope such as a β-blocker or nondihydropyridine CCB with the combination, and (2) to relieve the outflow tract obstruction with negative inotropes or with septal reduction therapy. The role of ACE inhibitors in aldosterone antagonists is unproven and currently under evaluation. One way to improve diastolic function is to slow the heart rate by prolonging the diastolic filling period. This also serves to reduce myocardial oxygen demands and improve the balance between supply and demand. In patients without outflow tract obstruction, the role of ACE inhibitors, ARB, and aldosterone antagonists is unproven but worth trying in patients with severe symptoms. A new therapeutic approach using metabolic modulation was demonstrated by a small trial of perhexiline maleate, which improved exercise capacity and myocardial energetics in 46 patients with nonobstructive hypertrophic cardiomyopathy.[423]

Is prevention possible? Can the development of hypertrophic cardiomyopathy be prevented? After all, all patients with the genotype have a genetic substrate for the disease, but penetrance is varied and very often the manifestations of hypertrophic cardiomyopathy may be delayed until adolescence or much later in life, or in some patients the phenotype may never become manifested. This does suggest that perhaps the disease could be prevented, and the finding that a statin improves cardiac hypertrophy and fibrosis in an animal model is fascinating and unexpected, but is also far from translation into clinical practice.[424] Likewise are the impressive data with the CCB diltiazem in an animal model,[425] and prospective trials are in the planning phase.

Negative inotropes. Negative inotropes are β-blockers, nondihydropyridine CCBs, and disopyramide. The postulated mechanism of benefit is via a reduction in LV ejection acceleration, which reduces the hydrodynamic force on the protruding mitral leaflet, delaying mitral-septal contact and reducing the outflow tract gradient. Furthermore, the reduction in ventricular afterload and outflow tract gradient may result in a secondary improvement in diastolic function.[426] *High-dose β-blockers,* such as 200-400 mg of propranolol per day or its equivalent, are effective in relieving symptoms such as dyspnea, fatigue, or angina in approximately 50% to 70% of patients. The high doses required may in turn result in dose-limiting side effects. *Calcium channel blockade,* usually verapamil at a dose of 240-320 mg/day, is advocated particularly in patients with asthma and other contraindications to β-blockers or else in combination with β-blockers in patients with continued symptoms. Although CCBs are usually well tolerated, caution needs to be exercised because the peripheral vasodilatory effects can lead to increased hemodynamic obstruction and clinical deterioration. This effect is unpredictable, and the consequences may be rapid and serious. In general, maximum symptomatic benefits are obtained by using β-blockers in combination with verapamil. Nifedipine and other dihydropyridines are contraindicated in patients with resting obstruction. Logically, verapamil and diltiazem may be helpful in relieving the diastolic relaxation problems found in the nonobstructive variety, but clinical evidence is sparse.[427] *Disopyramide,* a class I antiarrhythmic with negative inotropic properties, can be used in patients with significant outflow tract obstruction. Anticholinergic side effects, especially urinary retention, glaucoma, and dry mouth, are frequent.[428]

Relief of outflow tract obstruction. Drug efficacy may decline over the long term, or side effects become a major problem, and in such patients the remaining treatment options are invasive, such as surgical myectomy, *dual-chamber pacing*, or alcohol septal ablation. *Dual-chamber pacing*, programmed with a short AV delay, initially gave encouraging results, but the perceived functional improvement is largely a placebo effect apart from a small subset of patients who might benefit. Nonetheless, a logical application of dual-chamber pacing is with AV nodal ablation for refractory AF. *Alcohol septal ablation* is a very promising technique that needs to stand the test of time. Results may be operator dependent, and there appears to be a steep learning curve. The indications are the same as those for surgery, namely, severe symptoms unresponsive to medical therapy. Alcohol is injected into the first septal perforator branch of the left anterior descending coronary artery, producing a "controlled infarction." Acute and intermediate-term hemodynamic studies show a marked but variable reduction in outflow tract gradients and excellent improvement in symptoms. Short-term results are very similar to surgical myectomy.[428] The most frequent complication is complete heart block requiring a permanent pacemaker. Caution is advocated until the long-term results are available and the potential arrhythmic consequences of creating an MI with an area of transmural necrosis are better understood.[429,430]

Surgery for obstructive cardiomyopathy. When standard therapy fails, surgical myotomy or myectomy is the best choice. Surgery is associated with relief of symptoms and a substantial decrease in gradient and in the degree of mitral regurgitation, but should be reserved for patients with significant obstruction and symptoms. Although there are no trial data to suggest that surgery prolongs life, overall survival is excellent and consistent with that expected in the general population, matched for age and sex. Moreover, rates of SCD and ICD discharge are strikingly reduced. A key, however, to excellent surgical outcomes is a center with documented experience and expertise and a mortality rate approximately less than 1% in patients younger than age 60.[431,432] *Systolic anterior motion of the mitral valve* is an important component of dynamic LV outflow tract obstruction, and mitral regurgitation is common. Thus mitral valve repair and rarely replacement may be combined with surgery. Mitral valve repair is chosen for markedly elongated mitral valve leaflets.[433] A novel repair procedure is grafting a pericardial patch over the center of the anterior leaflet.[434] A subset of patients with markedly hypertrophied and displaced papillary muscles that contribute to the obstruction may require papillary muscle relocation as part of the surgical procedure.

Alcohol septal ablation or surgery? Alcohol ablation avoids the complications of cardiopulmonary bypass and is associated with less expense and a shorter hospital stay. Conversely, surgery appears to provide more immediate and complete relief of outflow tract obstruction, there is a lower incidence of heart block requiring pacemaker insertion, surgery provides the ability to deal with associated abnormalities of the mitral valve apparatus, and it is a procedure of proven durability with a follow-up of up to 20 years. For patients who are not good surgical candidates because of comorbidities or older patients in whom implantation of a pacemaker may be less of an issue, alcohol septal ablation is preferred, but surgery remains the gold standard. This was reaffirmed in the recent ACC-AHA guidelines that recommend surgical septal myectomy as the initial step unless surgery is contraindicated or the risk is considered unacceptable as a result of serious comorbidities.[422] The essence of optimal decision making in hypertrophic cardiomyopathy is a thorough discussion of the risks and benefits with the patient and the performance of either procedure by operators with expertise working within a comprehensive hypertrophic cardiomyopathy clinical program. Randomized trials are needed but for many reasons unlikely to ever be performed.[429]

Management of arrhythmias in hypertrophic cardiomyopathy. Patients at high risk for SCD, usually from VT or VF,[435] include those with documented ventricular arrhythmias, young patients with a history of syncope, a strong family history of SCD,[436] or, highly controversially, certain specific genotypes. The most effective procedure for patients with documented VT or out-of-hospital cardiac arrest is the ICD. Its indications have expanded to asymptomatic patients with a strong family history of SCD.[435] Coexisting coronary artery disease seriously impairs the prognosis.[437] The major complications of ICD implantation are a high rate of inappropriate discharges with their attendant psychological morbidity, particularly in younger patients and patients with AF.[438] AF can be a devastating complication in patients with hypertrophic cardiomyopathy. Treatment options include amiodarone, disopyramide, β-blockers, and CCBs for rate control, and AV nodal ablation plus permanent pacemaker implantation. Anticoagulation with warfarin is essential.

Other Cardiomyopathies

Dilated cardiomyopathy. The basic management of CHF in patients with idiopathic dilated cardiomyopathy in regard to drugs, devices, and transplantation is the same as in patients with ischemic cardiomyopathy (see prior discussion). Patients with idiopathic dilated cardiomyopathy and complete left bundle branch block may respond dramatically to CRT.

Inflammatory and immunologic factors. Specific therapies for inflammatory and immunologic types of myocarditis and dilated cardiomyopathy have not met with clinical success. Ribavirin and interferon have been used in experimental models but clinical data are very limited. A trial of beta-interferon in the clinical setting is ongoing.[439,440] Randomized trials of immunosuppressive therapy for myocarditis have not demonstrated efficacy,[441,442] other than one trial of 84 patients with dilated cardiomyopathy of greater than 6 months' duration and chronic inflammation on biopsy in which 3 months of immunosuppressive therapy had a beneficial effect on ejection fraction and clinical symptoms at 2 years.[443] In a trial of patients with recent-onset dilated cardiomyopathy and an ejection fraction of less than 40%, intravenous immune globulin was no better than placebo.[444] Cytokine inhibitors such as tumor necrosis factor–alpha have also been a disappointment. Unlike the case in dilated cardiomyopathy and lymphocytic myocarditis, *giant cell myocarditis* may respond to immunosuppressive therapy.[445,446] For patients who fail immunosuppressive therapy, cardiac transplantation is a reasonable option,[447] and long-term survival without recurrence has been reported. Another role for immunosuppressive therapy may be for specific disorders such as sarcoid and celiac disease, which may be associated with a dilated cardiomyopathy picture.

Chagas heart disease. The World Health Organization suggests that 15 to 20 million people, primarily in Latin America, are affected by Chagas disease (a *Trypanosoma cruzi* infection). In the acute phase, antitrypanosomal agents (nifurtimox and benznidazole) are helpful in controlling symptoms, in addition to supportive therapy for CHF, arrhythmias, and conduction disturbances. Approximately 20% to 30% of those infected go on to develop the chronic stage of the disease, of which the cardiac form composes 40%.[448] Does acute therapy prevent chronic organ damage? One small trial of benznidazole suggested that specific therapy may have a favorable effect on the chronic phase of Chagas disease. A large, unblinded, nonrandomized trial suggested that benznidazole might reduce the development of progressive disease and deterioration in LV function.[448] Thus the management of Chagas disease remains supportive. Cardiac transplantation may be required in selected cases.[449]

Restrictive cardiomyopathy. Restrictive heart disease is not well understood. It may be idiopathic or associated with other diseases such as amyloidosis or endomyocardial disease with or without hypereosinophilia. First exclude constrictive pericarditis, the treatment of which may be curative, whereas the therapy of the restrictive cardiomyopathy is both difficult and highly unsatisfactory.[450,451] In older adults, restriction may reflect increased myocardial fibrosis, and the latter can perhaps be countered by ACE inhibitors, ARBs, or aldosterone blockers (see Fig. 5-5). Once fibrosis has developed, the most important aspect of treatment is to avoid dehydration and overdiuresis, which impairs the left atrial filling pressure, and to control the heart rate in AF. Pharmacologic therapy of restrictive heart disease is extremely difficult. The fact that amyloid fibrils may bind to both digitalis and nifedipine may lead to increased susceptibility to digitalis toxicity and hemodynamic deterioration after nifedipine, but this can also occur with verapamil. ACE inhibitors may lead to hypotension. Amiodarone is reasonably well tolerated in patients who develop AF. Intracardiac thrombosis and embolism is extremely common in patients with cardiac amyloidosis, but there are also an increased risk of bleeding on anticoagulants.[452] Conduction disease may require a permanent pacemaker. Cardiac transplantation with and without bone marrow transplantation is currently under investigation, as is the role of chemotherapy for some patients with cardiac involvement caused by primary amyloidosis. High-dose melphalan and autologous stem-cell transplantation in patients with amyloid light-chain amyloidosis appears to have a significant benefit on survival in patients without cardiac amyloid.[453] Although long-term follow-up data are not available, cardiac transplantation followed by high-dose chemotherapy and autologous hemopoietic cell transplantation has been associated with symptomatic improvement, although there appears to be a high rate of occurrence.[454,455] Despite the many treatment strategies, none is based on randomized controlled data, nor are randomized trials likely.

Valvular Heart Disease

Rheumatic fever prophylaxis. Treatment should start as soon as a definitive diagnosis of streptococcal infection has been made; the treatment is either a single dose of benzathine penicillin (1,200,000 units for adults and half this dose for children) or a full 10-day course of oral penicillin V (for children, 250 mg two or three times daily[456]; empirically double this for adults). Thereafter, in selected patients in whom recurrences are feared, the penicillin injection is repeated monthly, or penicillin V is given as 125 to 250 mg twice daily continuously. The best route is by injection, which is used for 5 years, followed by oral prophylaxis possibly for life. For *penicillin allergy*, use sulfadiazine,[456] erythromycin, or the cephalosporins.[457]

General approach to valvular heart disease. As surgical techniques for valve repair and the performance of prosthetic valves have improved, so have the surgical indications become less stringent.[458] Now most patients with LV dysfunction are operated on even if asymptomatic. Thus the tendency is to become more aggressive, particularly in the case of mitral regurgitation, where a strong case can be made for surgical repair in asymptomatic patients with severe mitral regurgitation, even in the face of well-preserved LV function. An essential component of this strategy is the local results in regard to mitral valve repair versus mitral valve replacement. Concomitant therapy in patients with valvular heart disease is not based on trial data but may include diuretics, ACE inhibitors, and, especially for certain nonstenotic lesions, vasodilators. Attention to arrhythmias, particularly AF, is essential, and rate control with anticoagulation must be considered.

Aortic Stenosis

In valvular stenosis, the basic problem is obstructive and requires surgical relief. Four advances in understanding are as follows:

1. Increased LV pressure sets in motion a series of signaling pathways that lead not only to myocyte hypertrophy but to fibrosis and progressive myocyte death. The latter promotes deterioration from compensated hypertrophy to failure, arguing for valve replacement while LV function is still relatively preserved.[459]

2. Improved surgical techniques allow valve replacement even in patients with heart failure of such severity that the aortic valve gradient is low.[460] Pseudo–aortic stenosis, in which calculated aortic valve area falsely overestimates the severity of aortic stenosis at low flow rates, must be excluded.[461]

3. Peripheral vasoconstriction can contribute to critically severe heart failure, when careful vasodilator therapy improves the hemodynamic status,[418] so that aortic valve replacement becomes feasible.

4. The potential but unproven role of medical therapy by statins and other drugs is based on the hypothesis that aortic stenosis in older adults has risk factors similar to coronary artery disease[462] and that hypercholesterolemia is associated with disease progression. In the SEAS trial of patients with mild to moderate aortic stenosis, the combination of simvastatin and ezetimibe was no better than placebo in regard to progression to aortic valve replacement.[463]

Afterload reduction remains generally contraindicated, except in highly selected patients,[418] because it increases the pressure gradient across the stenosed valve. Thus CCBs should not be used to treat any accompanying hypertension except in mild degrees of stenosis. In patients with decompensated heart failure caused by systolic dysfunction and severe aortic stenosis, intravenous nitroprusside may play a role as a bridge to valve replacement, but meticulous monitoring is mandatory.[418]

Asymptomatic aortic stenosis. In truly asymptomatic aortic stenosis, which is nonetheless hemodynamically significant, the key to management is careful and regular supervision, with intervention as soon as symptoms appear. Nonetheless, a strong case can be made for surgery for asymptomatic patients with severe aortic stenosis who have LV systolic dysfunction without any evidence of symptomatic cardiac failure and in patients who manifest an abnormal response to exercise (e.g., hypotension). A case, albeit a weaker one, can be made for surgery in asymptomatic patients with documented VT, a valve area of 0.6 cm, or very marked or excessive LVH of 15 mm or greater.[458] Progression of aortic stenosis is unpredictable and may be rapid, so that careful monitoring of a patient on medical therapy is essential. Exercise testing should help to identify asymptomatic patients likely to develop symptoms in the near future.[464]

Aortic valve replacement. Surgical therapy is required for patients with angina, exertional syncope, or symptoms of LV failure (even if early). Surgery can relieve the hypertrophy, improve the coronary perfusion pressure, and often also correct any accompanying coronary artery disease. The combination of aortic stenosis and gastrointestinal bleeding suggests type 2A von Willebrand disease, which improves with aortic valve replacement.[465] Results following aortic valve replacement are excellent in both older and younger patients and in the absence of perioperative CHF, although the latter is not a contraindication to aortic valve replacement.[466] Percutaneous valve replacement, currently generating interest, may be an alternative to conventional open-heart surgery in selected high-risk patients with severe symptomatic aortic stenosis in whom surgical risks are considered excessive.[467]

Transcatheter aortic valve implantation. Transcatheter aortic valve implantation (TAVI) is an exciting and evolving approach that is holding up well in randomized trials.[468] This is the largest consecutively enrolled registry for transcatheter aortic valve procedures and demonstrates excellent 1-year survival in high-risk and inoperable patients. It provides a benchmark against which future TAVI cohorts and devices can be measured.[469] In the PARTNER trial, TAVI with the Edwards-Sapien valve improved survival and functional status in comparison with medical therapy.[470] In 699 high-risk patients, TAVI (either transfemoral or transapical) and surgical aortic valve replacement resulted in similar rates of mortality and major stroke at 30 days and 1 year and 1-year symptomatic improvement was the same.[471] Periprocedural complications including vascular access problems, stroke, subclinical brain injury, and heart block are frequent, but techniques continue to evolve and hopefully will result in improvements.[472-474] The recently published 2-year data from the PARTNER trials are also encouraging.[475,476]

Valvuloplasty for aortic stenosis. The initial enthusiasm for percutaneous aortic balloon valvuloplasty has been tempered by the long-term results, which are disappointing, but it does offer an alternative for patients in whom surgery is contraindicated and in some patients as a bridge to aortic valve replacement, if for one reason or another immediate surgery is inadvisable. Experience with percutaneous balloon valvotomy prior to TAVI is limited. There are also subsets of patients with low gradients and poor ventricular function in whom the symptomatic response to balloon valvuloplasty may provide a guide to the success of surgery in the future.[477] The discouraging results of balloon valvuloplasty in older adults contrast with more positive outcomes in young patients with congenital aortic stenosis.[478]

Bicuspid aortic valve. It has been increasingly recognized that bicuspid aortic valve is a manifestation of an inherited aortopathy and that first-degree relatives should be screened with comprehensive transthoracic echocardiography.[479]

Mitral Stenosis

In mitral stenosis with sinus rhythm, β-blockade improves exercise capacity to lessen possible pulmonary symptoms. This may be particularly helpful in patients with symptomatic mitral stenosis during pregnancy. Prophylactic digitalization is still sometimes used supposedly to avoid a high ventricular rate during intermittent AF; this practice is not supported by the available data. Percutaneous balloon mitral commissurotomy is now well established for relief of symptoms. Excellent long-term results for up to 15 years have been reported, and predictors of event-free survival are the valve echocardiographic score and age.[480] In severely symptomatic patients during pregnancy, balloon valvuloplasty may be extremely effective with minimal or maternal or fetal morbidity. Paroxysmal AF precipitating left-sided failure may require carefully titrated intravenous diltiazem, verapamil, or esmolol, particularly in the presence of LV dysfunction as may be present in patients with associated mitral regurgitation. In established AF, digitalization is usually not enough to prevent an excessive ventricular rate during exercise, so that digoxin, if used, should be augmented by diltiazem, verapamil, or β-blockade. Anticoagulation is essential for patients with AF and merits consideration for those in sinus rhythm thought to be at high risk for AF (marked left atrial enlargement or frequent atrial extrasystoles).

Balloon mitral valvuloplasty gives excellent early and late results in rheumatic mitral stenosis. All patients with symptomatic mitral stenosis should be considered for this procedure. The degree of commissural opening resulting in the larger mitral valve area, the better the patient outcome after balloon valvuloplasty. This can be assessed by use of three-dimensional echocardiography.[481,482] Contraindications include the presence of left atrial thrombus, severe subvalvular fibrosis or valve calcification, and a significant mitral regurgitation, but this can be determined ahead of time by TEE. The surgical alternatives are open mitral commissurotomy or mitral valve replacement. The percutaneous technique is comparable to the more invasive surgical approach.[483]

Aortic Regurgitation

In aortic regurgitation, indications for operation are the development of symptoms or, in the absence of symptoms, evidence of progressive or impending LV dysfunction based on impaired indices of contractility, a LV ejection fraction of less than 55%, or increased LV end-diastolic dimensions.[484] However, "agreement is greatest where data are fewest"[484] because there are no rigorous trials to support any improved survival using such indicators. What is controversial in patients with chronic aortic regurgitation is the degree of severity of LV dysfunction that contraindicates surgery. Substantial long-term improvements in ejection fraction, volumes, and symptoms have been described in patients with both mild (ejection fraction 45% to 50%) degrees of LV dysfunction and in those with ejection fractions of less than 45%.[485] Although aortic valve replacement remains the standard of care, aortic valve repair is increasingly being performed at some centers.[486,487] In patients with systolic hypertension, chronic afterload reduction by long-acting nifedipine is logical[488] and benefits those with asymptomatic aortic regurgitation. Experimental data show that afterload reduction by ACE inhibitors or ARBs, despite increasing the LV ejection fraction, may adversely influence myocardial contractility so that there is no mandate for their use.[484] In asymptomatic patients treated with ACE inhibitors, nifedipine, or placebo, there were no differences in outcomes at 7 years.[489,490] Nonetheless, the guidelines state that there remains a role for vasodilator therapy for symptom relief in patients for whom surgery is not recommended because of additional cardiac or noncardiac factors.[458] β-Blockers are relatively contraindicated in patients in sinus rhythm in that rate slowing could increase regurgitant volume.

Marfan Syndrome

In Marfan syndrome with aortic root dilatation the trend is to be increasingly aggressive with aortic surgery including aortic valve-sparing techniques.[491]

Prosthetic paravalvular regurgitation. Paravalvular leaks, particularly in patients with prosthetic valves, are increasingly being treated by percutaneous transcatheter closure.[492]

Mitral Regurgitation

In mitral regurgitation, the disease is more serious because it affects three primary organs: the left ventricle, the left atrium, and the right ventricle.[484] Hence the criteria for surgery are more stringent, with an LV ejection fraction of less than 60% the best validated predictor of prognosis.[484] Other criteria are persistent AF, a subnormal right ventricular ejection fraction, and an increased LV internal diameter. The current trend is to operate even earlier both to prevent ventricular dilation and to "preserve the atrium," hopefully avoiding AF. Obviously, the development of symptoms is a mandatory indication for surgery, but the best results even in asymptomatic patients are obtained prior to the development of even mild degrees of LV systolic dysfunction.[493] Thus the approach to surgery has become increasingly aggressive, especially if the likelihood of a repair versus valve replacement is high. The ability to perform a mitral valve repair is based on the skill and the experience of the surgeon and on the location and type of mitral valve disease that caused mitral regurgitation. Repair is more likely with degenerative as opposed to rheumatic or ischemic involvement of the mitral valves, and TEE is a critical aspect of pre- and intraoperative strategies. In the United States, for isolated mitral regurgitation the rate of repair is increased steadily, and this has been accompanied by a decline of operative mortality rates.[494] In skilled hands reoperation rates are low but not neglible.[495,496] The EVEREST trial demonstrated that in patients with severe mitral regurgitation percutaneous repair using a clip that grasps and approximates the edges of the mitral leaflets at the origin of the regurgitant jet was less effective at reducing mitral regurgitation than conventional surgery, but safety was said to be superior and clinical outcomes were similar.[497] In the right hands surgical mitral valve repair is a superb operation, and it may be difficult to equal the results percutaneously, but one potential application for the percutaneous device will be in patients with severe heart failure and functional mitral regurgitation, and future trials in this area will be interesting. Currently direct annuloplasty by retrograde catheterization of the left ventricle from the aorta is under test with the aim of reducing the regurgitant orifice.[498]

Cor Pulmonale

The initial step in management is to exclude potentially reversible causes of cor pulmonale and pulmonary hypertension (i.e., obstructive sleep apnea). Many clinical trials attest that ischemic heart disease is a leading but underrecognized cause of death in chronic obstructive pulmonary disease.[499] Retrospective analysis suggests that even low-risk patients receiving ACE inhibitor or ARB plus statin therapy have a major reduction in death or MI and death. Thus prospective studies are now required to test this combination.[500] Therapy of right heart failure is similar to that of left heart failure, except that digoxin appears to be even less effective because of a combination of hypoxemia, electrolyte disturbances, and enhanced adrenergic discharge. Thus when AF develops, cautious verapamil or diltiazem is preferred to reduce the ventricular rate. Multifocal atrial tachycardia is associated with chronic lung disease and is a difficult arrhythmia to treat, although success with verapamil has been reported. In general, all β-blockers should be avoided because of the risk of bronchospasm. Bronchodilators should be β2-selective. For example, albuterol (salbutamol) has relatively little effect on the heart rate while unloading the left heart by peripheral vasodilation. The administration of oxygen has been shown to result in modest reductions in PA pressure and pulmonary vascular resistance in patients with chronic obstructive pulmonary disease complicated by cor pulmonale.[501]

Idiopathic Pulmonary Arterial Hypertension*

Among all subsets of pulmonary arterial hypertension (PAH), idiopathic PAH, familial PAH, and anorectic drug-induced PAH are considered the classical disease manifestations, because patients are commonly young without comorbid conditions and very similar in their clinical disease presentation.

---

*Section cowritten with Irene M Lang, MD

The term *primary pulmonary hypertension* has been replaced by *idiopathic PAH*, both sporadic and familial, and includes pulmonary hypertension secondary to chronic pulmonary disease, congenital heart disease, or left heart disease.[502] Mutations involving the transforming growth factor–β cell signaling family are implicated in the genesis. The three major pathogenetic mechanisms that may influence therapy are an imbalance between vasodilation and vasoconstriction in the pulmonary circulation; vascular smooth muscle and endothelial cell proliferation; and coagulation abnormalities, which may lead to thrombosis in situ.[503] The hallmark of pulmonary hypertension is the histopathologic similarity shared by the different clinical types, and even on lung biopsy the exact pathogenesis may not be apparent. Long-term anticoagulants are frequently used on the assumption that there is thromboembolism or thrombosis in situ. A number of studies, but no randomized trials, suggest a better survival in patients treated with warfarin.[504] Oxygen supplementation should be used as necessary to maintain saturations of 90% at all times, with diuretics for fluid retention and digoxin if the right ventricle begins to fail.

PAH treatment should be initiated exclusively in expert centers. Current treatments are based on the concept of a primarily vasoconstrictive pathophysiologic finding and use three classes of vasodilated drugs: prostacyclins, endothelin receptor antagonists, and phosphodiesterase-5 inhibitors (see Fig. 6-14). Randomized trials with these agents have primarily involved patients with idiopathic PAH but also patients with other forms of PAH and improved quality of life and survival.[505] However, it has become increasingly clear that PAH treatments do not systematically benefit patients with so-called non-PAH pulmonary hypertension (i.e., PAH associated with left heart disease, interstitial lung disease, chronic obstructive pulmonary disease, and chronic thromboembolic pulmonary hypertension [CTEPH]). It is imperative to exclude CTEPH, which is amenable to surgical pulmonary thromboendartectomy, potentially yielding a complete and sustained normalization of pulmonary hemodynamics.[506]

Calcium channel blockers. CCBs are targeted to patients who are hemodynamic responders; in other words, they display a robust drop of at least 10 mm Hg; a drop in mean artery pressure on the acute administration of inhaled NO, intravenous prostacyclin, or adenosine, resulting in a mean PA pressure of less than 40 mm Hg and the presence of a stable cardiac output. Approximately 10%-15% of patients will have a similarly positive response to high-dose CCBs, and only half of these will have a sustained clinical and hemodynamic benefit,[507] but if they do respond, they have an excellent 3-year survival.[508] Systemic hypotension may limit adequate dosing.

Prostacyclin and prostacyclin analogues. A continuous infusion of prostacyclin (epoprostenol sodium) improved hemodynamics, symptoms, and survival in NYHA functional class IV patients.[509] Nonetheless, its use is limited by side effects, the need for continuous intravenous infusion, tachyphylaxis, and rebound pulmonary hypertension on withdrawal. Treprostinol is a prostacyclin analogue that is approved in the United States for both subcutaneous and intravenous use,[510] and its use in Europe is limited to a few centers.[511] Strict evidence for a survival benefit is lacking. Alternatives include oral analogues and inhaled iloprost, neither of which have data for long-term benefit.

Endothelin receptor antagonists. Endothelin-1 levels are elevated in patients with PAH and cause vasoconstriction and myocyte hypertrophy via two receptor subtypes. The orally administered dual endothelin receptor antagonist bosentan improves hemodynamics, clinical status, and echocardiographic variables and is currently approved for patients in NYHA classes III and IV in the United States and for classes II and III in Europe. The major side effect is liver toxicity (i.e., aminotransferase elevations greater than three times the upper limit of normal), which appears in approximately 12% of patients.[512] *Sitaxsentan* is more selective for the ETA receptor, and was recently withdrawn from the market because of liver toxicity.[513] *Ambrisentan*, a nonsulfanimide class endothelin-receptor antagonist has been approved in the United States and Europe after successful phase 3 trials.[503]

Phosphodiesterase-5 inhibitors. Logically, an agent that increases intravascular levels of cyclic guanosine monophosphate (cGMP) should vasodilate in primary pulmonary hypertension. Sildenafil, a selective inhibitor of cGMP-specific phosphodiesterase-5, given as 50 mg every 8 hours, attenuates pulmonary hypertension in animals and improves clinical status over 3 months.[514] Sildenafil is much cheaper than iloprost or bosentan. The largest randomized controlled trial to date demonstrated an improvement in 6-minute walk and lean PA pressure after 12 months of treatment.[515] *Tadalafil*, a longer-acting drug, improved exercise and quality of life[516] and has been approved in the United States and Europe.

Novel emerging therapies. The emerging paradigm shift is addressing the vascular remodeling process with the aim of "reverse remodeling."[517] A host of novel emerging therapies include *imatinib*, a platelet-derived growth factor receptor antagonist, and *fasudil*, a Rho-kinase inhibitor involved in calcium sensitization and vasoconstriction. The data of the large randomized *imatinib* trial are pending. Trials of *simvastatin*, which could enhance endothelial function by actions on the bone morphogenic protein receptive pathway, and endogenous and intestinal vasoactive peptides have been negative.

Among the new vasodilators, *riociguat*, an activator of soluble guanylate cyclase, and the direct prostaglandin receptor antagonist *selexipag* deserve attention. Both drugs are currently undergoing phase 3 clinical randomized evaluations. *Terguride*, a dopamine agonist, and *cicletanine*, an endothelial NO synthase coupling agent, are recruiting.

Bilateral lung transplantation and other surgical interventions. Heart-lung and lung transplantation have been performed for primary pulmonary hypertension for more than 20 years, but this has been hampered by the lack of centers with expertise, shortage of donors, and long waiting times. A more recent trend is clearly toward double- or even single-lung transplantation for PAH. Waiting times remain long and complications such as organ rejection and infections pose formidable obstacles, with survival times with the first transplant of approximately 5 years in approximately 50% of patients. The use of assist devices for the right ventricle (extracorporeal membrane oxygenation [ECMO], Novaloung) is growing. First experience on a wait ECMO and minute-size right-ventricular assist devices has been gained.

Infective Endocarditis*

Infective endocarditis remains potentially fatal if not aggressively treated by antibiotics, with or without surgery.[518] New risk factors have replaced the old. Rheumatic valve disease, long the major predisposing cause, has given way to more modern risk factors such as intravenous drug use; degenerative valve diseases of older adults; prosthetic valves' and healthcare-associated factors, particularly indwelling vascular catheters.[518] In addition, increasing numbers of patients are immunologically compromised by human immunodeficiency virus or acquired immune deficiency syndrome or because they are undergoing therapeutic immune suppression. Drug-resistant endocarditis is increasing,

---

*Section cowritten with Larry M Baddour, MD

whether caused by "old pathogens" outwitting the standard antibiotics or by the more new "exotic organisms" that include fungi. To diagnose infective endocarditis, echocardiography and TEE are very helpful but a negative result does not rule out the diagnosis. Blood cultures remain the key to the diagnosis and treatment of endocarditis. Optimal therapy requires identification of the causative organism, so that appropriate therapy is initiated even though this may delay the start of therapy for a short period. Definitive antibiotic therapy is based on pathogen identification and susceptibility testing and requires the advice of an expert in infectious diseases. In culture-negative endocarditis, therapy is empirical and requires an evaluation of the epidemiologic findings of infection to attempt to define the optimal therapeutic regimen.

Streptococcus viridans* and *Streptococcus bovis. *Streptococcus viridans* and *Streptococcus bovis* are sensitive to penicillin and are still often the causative organisms in community-acquired endocarditis in nonaddicts. Gentamicin may be added to shorten the duration of therapy. If a highly penicillin-resistant streptococcus is suspected, even if not proven, a combination of ampicillin or ceftriaxone with gentamicin is suggested. For highly resistant streptococci[518] or for penicillin allergy, vancomycin is used. In general, the duration of therapy in current responders is 4 weeks for native valve endocarditis and 6 weeks for prosthetic valve endocarditis.

Staphylococcus aureus. *Staphylococcus aureus* is also a common cause of endocarditis, moving up to first place in intravenous drug users, who are also at increased risk of gram-negative bacilli, fungal, and polymicrobial infections, some of which carry a high mortality. *Staphylococcus aureus* is usually penicillin resistant; use naxoline or cefazolin if the infecting strain is methicillin susceptible. Vancomycin is used for methicillin-resistant *S. aureus* infection. If the isolator is vancomycin resistant or the patient is intolerant of vancomycin, then there are few options, including daptomycin or linezolid and co-trimoxazole.[518] Despite optimal diagnostic techniques and appropriate antimicrobial therapy, the mortality in patients infected with the most virulent organisms, such as *S. aureus,* remains high.

Coagulase-negative *staphylococci.* Coagulase-negative *staphylococci* are an important cause of prosthetic valve endocarditis, particularly within the first 2 months of valve placement. Many of these strains are methicillin resistant and require vancomycin, in combination with rifampin, for at least 6 weeks of treatment and 2 weeks of gentamicin. *Enterococcus species, even when fully susceptible to penicillin,* require the addition of a minor glycoside such as gentamicin to achieve an attempted cure. Increasing numbers of enterococci have acquired resistance to vancomycin and penicillin.

The HACEK organisms. Gram-negative bacilli *Haemophilus, Actinobacillus, Cardiobacterium, Eikenella,* and *Kingella* (HACEK organisms) can cause culture-negative endocarditis, which requires empirical therapy for both gram-positive and gram-negative organisms. The AHA recommends treatment with an ampicillin-sulbactam plus gentamicin or with vancomycin plus gentamicin plus ciprofloxacin for 4 to 6 weeks.[519] The ESC recommends combination therapy with vancomycin for 4 to 6 weeks with gentamicin added for the initial 2 weeks of treatment.[520]

Indications for surgery in endocarditis. An increasingly aggressive approach to early cardiac surgery has favorably influenced the outcome of infective endocarditis. In patients with native valve endocarditis, the indications for surgery are CHF resulting from valve dysfunction, new valve regurgitation, systemic embolization to vital organs, refractory infection, and a vegetation on echocardiography.[521] This policy reduces

6-month mortality versus medical therapy alone.[521,522] This policy reduces short-and long-term mortality versus medical therapy alone[521,523] and may improve survival. There is a greater risk of relapses and prosthetic valve dysfunction.[524] EASE, with 134 patients with confirmed endocarditis, is the first prospective trial to demonstrate that early surgery produces better outcomes than conventional therapy in these patients. Surgery outperformed conventional therapy for the primary endpoint of in-hospital death plus embolic events within 6 weeks of randomization (3% versus 23%, P = 0.014).[525] The approach to prosthetic valve endocarditis, particularly within 3 months of the initial operation, is even more aggressive, with surgery for any signs of prosthetic valve dysfunction or any of the indications for surgery in native valves. Infection of a prosthetic valve by *S. aureus*, gram-negative bacilli, or fungi provides an additional indication for early surgery. In the face of hemodynamic decompensation, surgery should not be delayed pending completion of antibiotic therapy. Relative indications for early surgical intervention include apparent failure of medical therapy as evidenced by persistent bacteremia or fever, or an increase in the size of vegetation during treatment. TEE is extremely helpful in the detection of intracardiac vegetations and other complications such as perivalvular extension.

Anticoagulant and antiplatelet therapy. The issues regarding anticoagulant and antiplatelet therapy are complex and characterized by a lack of hard data. The decision to initiate or continue anticoagulant therapy in patients with infective endocarditis is often difficult. In those patients already on anticoagulants (e.g., patients with mechanical prostheses or those in whom there are other indications for anticoagulation, such as thrombophlebitis), anticoagulant therapy should be continued or initiated. In the event of a cerebral thromboembolic complication, the risk of anticoagulant-induced hemorrhage must be balanced against the alternate risk of recurrent embolism. In general, aspirin has not been indicated in the early management of infective endocarditis, being without effect on vegetation resolution and valvular dysfunction.[142] However, one large retrospective study found fewer embolic complications after prior continuous daily antiplatelet therapy (aspirin, dipyridamole, clopidogrel, ticlopidine, or any of combination of these agents).[526]

Antibiotic prophylaxis against infective endocarditis. The AHA recommendations underwent major and controversial revisions in 2007 and were updated in 2008 (Table 12-7) with new underlying pathophysiologic principles very similar to those of the British Society for Antimicrobial Chemotherapy.[527] The changed AHA recommendations reflect the principle that, even if antibiotic prophylaxis were completely effective, of which there is no proof, only a very small number of cases would be prevented. Furthermore, unnecessary antibiotics have possible side effects. Rather, the stress is on sustained prophylactic maintenance of strict oral hygiene. Antibiotic prophylaxis is only indicated for patients with those serious underlying cardiac conditions that are associated with the highest risk of adverse outcomes, such as prosthetic valves, severe congenital heart disease, or cardiac transplantation (Table 12-8). For dental procedures in these individuals, only those procedures that involve manipulation of gingival tissue or perforation of the oral mucosa should be covered by antibiotics. Recommended antibiotics reflect changed organism sensitivities (Tables 12-8 and 12-9).[528] *Updated American recommendations* suggest that, for high-risk patients, only one amoxicillin dose of 2 g be given orally 1 hour before the dental procedure, with specified antibiotic regimens for those unable to take oral medication or allergic to penicillins or amoxicillin (see Table 12-8). *Overall, note that there are no recommendations with Class I and Level of Evidence A.*

Prophylaxis is recommended for procedures on infected respiratory tract or skin, on skin structures, or on musculocutaneous tissue. The new guidelines also simplify antibiotic prophylaxis for patients

Table 12-7

Cardiac Conditions with the Highest Risk of Infectious Endocarditis[592]

Antibiotic prophylaxis during dental procedures recommended by American Heart Association.

1. Prosthetic cardiac valve or prosthetic material used for cardiac valve repair (class 1C).
2. Previous infectious endocarditis (class 1C).
3. Congenital heart disease* (class 1C):
   - Unrepaired cyanotic congenital heart disease, including palliative shunts and conduits.
   - Completely repaired congenital heart defect with prosthetic material or device, whether placed by surgery or by catheter intervention, during the first 6 mo after the procedure.[†]
   - Repaired coronary heart disease with residual defects at the site or adjacent to the site of a prosthetic patch or prosthetic device (which inhibits endothelialization).
4. Hypertrophic cardiomyopathy, latent or resting obstruction (class 1C).
5. Mitral valve prolapse without mitral regurgitation or thickened leaflets (class 1C).

Dental procedures for which endocarditis prophylaxis is reasonable in these groups of patients: *All dental procedures* that involve manipulation of gingival tissue or the periapical region of teeth or perforation of the oral mucosa.

*Except for the conditions listed previously, antibiotic prophylaxis is no longer recommended for any other form of congenital heart disease.
†Prophylaxis is reasonable because endothelialization of prosthetic material occurs within 6 months after the procedure, per the American Heart Association recommendations (2007).[528]

Table 12-8

Revised American Regimens for Antibiotics for Dental Procedures[592]*

Situation	Agent	Regimen: Single Dose 30-60 min before Procedure	
		Adults	Children
Oral	Amoxicillin	2 g	50 mg/kg
Unable to take oral medication	Ampicillin *or*	2 g IM or IV	50 mg/kg IM or IV
	Cefazolin or ceftriaxone	1 g IM or IV	50 mg/kg IM or IV
Allergic to penicillins or ampicillin—oral	Cephalexin[††] *or*	2 g	50 mg/kg
	Clindamycin *or*	600 mg	20 mg/kg
	Azithromycin or clarithromycin	500 mg	15 mg/kg
Allergic to penicillins or ampicillin and unable to take oral medication	Cefazolin or ceftriaxone[†] *or*	1 g IM or IV	50 mg/kg IM or IV
	Clindamycin	600 mg IM or IV	20 mg/kg IM or IV

IM, Intramuscular; *IV,* intravenous.
*Only for those at risk (see Table 12-7).
†Or other first- or second-generation oral cephalosporin in equivalent adult or pediatric dosage.
†Cephalosporins should not be used in an individual with a history of anaphylaxis, angioedema, or urticaria with penicillins or ampicillin.

undergoing gastrointestinal or genitourinary procedures. No antibiotic coverage is suggested even for high-risk patients, but for those with existing gastrointestinal or genitourinary infections, an antienteroccocal agent is "reasonable" without, however, supporting trial data.

Primary prevention. Despite common perceptions, most infectious endocarditis is not preceded by medicosurgical or dental interventions, so the real answer lies in primary prevention.[518] Thus conditions

Table 12-9

European Recommended Prophylaxis for Adults for Dental Procedures at Risk[593]			
		Single Dose 30-60 Minutes Before Procedure	
Situation	Antibiotic	Adults	Children
No allergy to penicillin or ampicillin	Amoxicillin or ampicillin*	2 g PO or IV	50 mg/kg PO or IV
Allergy to penicillin or ampicillin	Clindamycin	600 mg PO or IV	20 mg/kg PO or IV

IV, Intravenous; *PO*, by mouth.
   Cephalosporins should not be used in patients with anaphylaxis, antiooedema, or urticaria after intake of penicillin and ampicillin.
   *Alternatively cephalexin 2 g IV, cefazolin or ceftriaxone 1 g IV.

predisposing to infective endocarditis, such as poor dental hygiene or genitourinary tract pathologic conditions, must be eliminated.

Peripheral Vascular Disease

Burns et al. write, "Peripheral vascular disease is a marker for systemic atherosclerosis; the risk to limb is low, but the risk to life is high."[529] The basis of therapy is medical treatment focused on aggressive risk-factor modification, including control of lipids, diabetes, and BP; smoking cessation; and exercise. Revascularization, either percutaneous or surgical, is indicated for patients with refractory symptoms causing significant disability or the presence of limb-threatening ischemia.[522,529,530] Large vessel disease is usually treated surgically but catheter-based therapy using stents and endovascular grafts are increasingly used alternatives.[531,532] In the area of critical limb ischemia, both endovascular and surgical revascularization (with a vein conduit) are reasonable initial procedures for critical limb ischemia —Class IIA.

Prophylaxis of cardiovascular complications. The basis of medical therapy lies in risk-factor modification, exercise training, and aspirin.[529] A supervised exercise program can result in a major improvement in motivated patients, but the benefits are lost if the patient stops exercising. Class I recommendations include a statement that all smokers or former smokers should be asked about their smoking status at every visit, and smokers should be assisted with counseling and the development of a quit-smoking treatment plan that includes pharmacologic therapy with varenicline, bupropion, or nicotine-replacement therapy.[533] To what extent smoking cessation improves symptoms is unclear, but its effect on the progression of disease and amputation rates is well documented.[534] Decreased amputation and rest ischemia are well documented, and in any event, the logic is irrefutable. In addition, ACE inhibitors, clopidogrel, and a statin can all be given with large trial justification.[535-537] Although without formal proof that clopidogrel, aspirin, statin, and an ACE inhibitor give additive protection and do not adversely interfere with each other, each agent acts by a different mechanism so that we recommend this combination. In the CHARISMA trial, a subset of patients with prior MI, stroke, or symptomatic peripheral arterial disease appeared to benefit from clopidogrel added to aspirin.[530] Antiplatelet therapy may be useful in patients with an abnormal ankle-brachial index who are currently asymptomatic with a level of evidence C. Ongoing major trials of statins, antiplatelet agents, recombinant growth factors, and immune modulators may result in clinically relevant new advances in the medical management of peripheral vascular disease in the future, but trials of gene therapy for therapeutic angiogenesis have been disappointing.[538] A randomized placebo-controlled trial of more than 500 patients with critical ischemia demonstrated no difference between fibroblastic growth factor (NV1FGF) on amputation and death.[539] On the other hand, autologous bone-marrow mononuclear stem cells appear to be safe and promising in preliminary trials.[540,541]

Cilostazol. Cilostazol, a phosphodiesterase-3 inhibitor, was approved in 2000 in the United States for intermittent claudication. It suppresses platelet aggregation and is a direct vasodilator. Increased walking distance was shown in a metaanalysis of 2702 patients.[542] The usual dose is 100 mg twice daily. It is metabolized by the cytochrome P-450 3A4 system, and hence open to interaction with ketoconazole, erythromycin, and diltiazem, as well as grapefruit juice, which should all be avoided.

Pentoxifylline. Pentoxifylline (*Trental*) decreases blood viscosity and maintains red cell flexibility of the erythrocytes as they are squeezed through the capillary bed. It is licensed for use in intermittent claudication in the United States. Yet in a randomized trial of pentoxifylline and cilostazol, only cilostazol improved both functional status and the walking impairment questionnaire.[543] ACC-AHA guidelines conclude that any benefits of pentoxifylline are marginal and not well established.[544]

Naftidrofuryl. Naftidrofuryl is a 5-hydroxytriptamine-2 receptor antagonist available in Europe. Mechanisms of action are unclear, but a recent consensus statement recommended its addition to cilostazol.[545] In a Cochrane metaanalysis of four trials an improvement in time to initial pain on treadmill walking over a 3- to 6-month period was noted.[546]

Other agents. Levocarnitine and L-propionyl-carnitine favorably improve the metabolic status of skeletal muscle to lengthen the walking distance. Neither preparation is licensed in the United States. Gingko biloba gives modest success but the mechanisms are unclear.[547] Buflomedil is an α-adrenergic blocker with vasoactive and rheologic properties licensed in Europe but not in the United States.

Ineffective therapies that should be discouraged include estrogen replacement, chelation therapy, and vitamin E supplementation. Ginkgo biloba has been shown to be moderately successful but problems with the studies have been identified and ACC-AHA guidelines concluded that benefit has not been established.[544] Other agents under investigation include verapamil, ACE inhibitors, anticlamydophila therapy, L-propionyl-carntine, prostaglandins, defibrotide (an agent stimulating fibrinolysis), and glutathione, among others.[548] Other potentially effective agents include prostaglandin, indirect vasodilators such as serotonin uptake inhibitors, phosphodiesterase inhibitors, sympatholytic agents, and toxofilin.

Claudication plus hypertension or angina. β-Blockers are still generally held to be relatively contraindicated in the presence of active peripheral vascular disease, although a metaanalysis of 11 pooled trials showed no adverse effects on the walking distance in mild to moderate disease.[549] Verapamil increases pain-free walking time[550] and is preferred to β-blockers, although without strict comparative studies.

Raynaud's Phenomenon

Once a secondary cause has been excluded (e.g., vasculitis, scleroderma, or lupus erythematosus), then calcium channel antagonists are logical. Nifedipine is best tested, and one 10-mg capsule may be taken intermittently at the start of an attack. β-Blockers are traditionally contraindicated, although the evidence is not good. Sustained-release glycerol trinitrate patches may be effective in Raynaud's phenomenon, but are limited by the frequency of headaches. Several reports attest to the efficacy of topical glycerol trinitrate in this condition.[551] Common-sense measures such as avoidance of exposure to cold and rapidly changing temperatures; keeping the digits warm; avoidance of sympathomimetic drugs such as decongestants, amphetamines, and over-the-counter drugs containing ephedrine; and, above all, smoking cessation are extremely important.[552] For intractable disease, spinal cord stimulation or thoracic or localized digital sympathectomy may provide relief.[553,554]

Beriberi Heart Disease

Beriberi heart disease is characterized by high-output CHF caused by thiamine deficiency. Common in Africa and Asia, in Western countries it is underdiagnosed especially in alcoholics and in those on "fad diets" or occasionally in patients receiving parenteral nutrition.[555] The basis of treatment is thiamine 100 mg parenterally followed by 50 to 100 mg daily with vitamin supplements, a balanced diet, and abstinence from alcohol. Even in Shoshin beriberi with peripheral circulatory shock and severe metabolic acidosis, thiamine remains the mainstay of treatment because the acidosis responds poorly to treatment. Diuretics are needed when diuresis is delayed beyond 48 hours of thiamine therapy (Professor DP Naidoo, University of Natal, South Africa, personal communication).

Cardiovascular Drugs in Pregnancy

Most cardiovascular drugs are not well studied for safety in pregnancy. ACE inhibitors, ARBs, warfarin, and the statins are all clearly contraindicated (Table 12-10). For pregnancy hypertension, methyldopa is best validated, and the diuretics are not as bad as often thought.

Cardiopulmonary Resuscitation*

In 2010 the AHA published new guidelines for cardiopulmonary resuscitation (CPR) and emergency cardiac care (Fig. 12-10).[556] The key issues and major changes addressed include:

- A simplified universal adult basic life support algorithm
- A change in sequence from airway-breathing-compression to compression-airway-breathing for *lone rescuers,* and use of compression-only rescue for rescuers untrained in CPR
- Continued emphasis on teaching rescuers to deliver chest compressions of adequate rate (at least 100 per minute) and depth to at least 2 inches (5 cm).[556]

   It is important to emphasize that the 2010 guidelines recommend omission of mouth-to-mouth "rescue" breathing for lay rescuers and witnessed cardiac arrest, based on evidence that adequate oxygenation can be provided by chest compressions only for several minutes following cardiac arrest. In addition, lay rescuers typically have difficulty attempting to establish an airway and ventilation of the lungs, consuming needed time to establish blood flow with chest compressions. Thus CPR, although still valid for trained healthcare providers, should for bystanders be replaced by continuous chest compression. The phrase "push hard and push fast" encourages rescuers to compress

---

*Section cowritten with Roger D. White, MD.

Table 12-10

Cardiovascular Drugs in Pregnancy			
Drug Category	Potential Adverse Effect on Fetus	Safety in Pregnancy (Classification)*	Trimester Risk (1, 2, 3)
β-Blockers	Intrauterine growth retardation; neonatal hypoglycemia, bradycardia	C or D	1, 3
Nitrates	None; may benefit by delaying premature labor	C	None
CCBs	None; may delay labor; experimentally embryopathic	C	None
Diuretics			
Thiazides	May impair uterine blood flow; usually regarded as C/I, yet metaanalysis suggests safety[†]	B or C	3
Furosemide	Experimentally embryopathic	C	(1)
Torsemide	None	B	None
Indapamide	None	B	None
ACE inhibitors; ARBs	Embryopathic in all semesters[†]; may be lethal	D or X	1, 2, 3
Digoxin	None	C	None
Antihypertensives			
Methyldopa	Well tested in pregnancy	B	None
Others as shown	Generally no adverse effects	C	None
Antiarrhythmics			
Amiodarone	Altered thyroid function	D	2, 3
Sotalol	None	B	None
Statins	Serious	X	1,2,3
Antithrombotics			
Warfarin	Embryopathic; crosses placenta with risk of fetal hemorrhage	X	1, 3
Heparin	None; does not cross placental barrier	C[‡]	None
Enoxaparin	No trials in humans	B	Not known
GpIIa/IIIb blockers			
Abciximab	No data in humans	C	? None
Eptifibatide	No data in humans	B	? None
Tirofiban	No data in humans	B	? None
Aspirin	High dose: risk of premature closure of patent ductus	None	3

ACE, Angiotensin-converting enzyme; *ARB,* angiotensin receptor blocker; *CCB,* calcium channel blocker; *C/I,* contraindication; *Gp,* glycoprotein.

*US Food and Drug Administration Pregnancy Categories range from A (completely safe) to D (considerable risk) and X (contraindicated).

[†]Data from Cooper et al. *N Engl J Med* 2006;354:2443.

[‡]For heparin, see p. 369.

ADULT CARDIAC ARREST

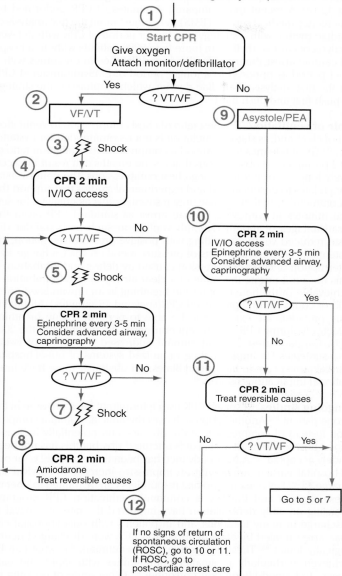

Figure 12-10 Algorithm for cardiopulmonary resuscitation (CPR) for adult cardiac arrest, when there is ventricular tachycardia (VT) or ventricular fibrillation (VF) or pulseless electrical activity (PEA), based on the recommendations of the American Heart Association.[556,588] *IO,* Intraoral; *IV,* intravenous; *ROSC,* return of spontaneous circulation.

at a rate of at least 100 compressions per minute and at a depth of at least 2 inches.

The first step. *The first step is to shout for help and to start chest compressions urgently.* As soon as an AED is available, it should be attached and a shock delivered if a shockable rhythm is detected. Following a shock, chest compressions are immediately resumed unless the victim quickly regains consciousness following the shock. If monomorphic wave form defibrillators are used, 360-Joule shocks are recommended. For biphasic wave forms, this is device specific ranging from 120-200 Joules with subsequent shocks at the same or higher energy levels (see Fig. 12-10). A recent trial compared 2 minutes of CPR performed by emergency medical service (EMS) personnel before the first analysis of cardiac rhythm with a strategy of a longer period of CPR with delayed analysis of cardiac rhythm. In more than 9000 patients without a hospital cardiac arrest, the trial identified no difference in outcomes with a brief period as opposed to a longer period of EMS-administered CPR for the first analysis of cardiac rhythm, which emphasizes the strategy of push first and push hard.[557]

Role of ventilation. The best ratio of chest compression to ventilation is not clear and, as stated, ventilation is not recommended for bystanders.[558] The guidelines recommend a compression-to-ventilation ratio of 30:2 prompted by observations that rescue breaths can result in excessively long interruptions during chest compressions. The controversial area relates to observational and experimental studies that support the recommendation that cardiac-only resuscitation is as effective for several minutes in witnessed cardiac arrest as standard CPR given the disadvantages of mouth-to-mouth ventilation such as bystander distaste, reduced ventricular filling with positive pressure ventilation, the potentially deleterious effects of pressure recoil on gas exchange, and interruption of chest compression caused by delays and intubation.[559] This does not negate the value of a clear airway or rapid intubation if achievable, or the benefit of rescue breathing in an unwitnessed arrest and of course during prolonged CPR (beyond 15 minutes). All healthcare providers are expected to be able to perform rescue breathing effectively during CPR.[560] A recent consensus document from the 2009 AHA Cardiac Arrest Survival Summit addressed a number of issues and strategies for implementing optimized systems of out-of-hospital cardiac arrest care in the United States, but obviously these have international implications as well.[561]

Ongoing studies. Reversed CPR uses intermittent back pressure in the prone patient.[562] Another approach uses rhythmic abdominal compression instead of compression of the rib cage and potentially increases blood flow to the heart and avoids fractured ribs, but this has not been widely accepted.[563] A major advance has been the use of AEDs for out-of-hospital cardiac arrest with an impressive increase in survival discharge.[564,565] Lay persons and first responders can be trained to operate these devices and the key is community education. CPR programs focusing on early defibrillation have improved the rate of survival to discharge in many locations, and in patients with out-of-hospital cardiac arrest treated by early defibrillation, 46% were discharged neurologically intact.[566] These data serve as a benchmark for what can be achieved, particularly in smaller communities with rapid and easy access to trained life-support personnel.[567] Other areas of ongoing investigation include whether to proceed shock delivery in VF arrest with a period of CPR or to shock immediately, and whether chest compressions delivered immediately after a shock can induce resumption of VF. The role of automated electronic analysis of the cardiac rhythm as a determinant as to whether to shock first or provide CPR first is under active investigation.[568-571]

Adjunctive pharmacotherapy. In patients with shockable rhythms (see Fig. 12-10), if the second shock fails to restore a hemodynamically effective spontaneous rhythm, either epinephrine 1 mg every 3 to 5 minutes or vasopressin 40 IU to replace the second dose of epinephrine should be administered, either intravenously or intraosseously in the event that venous access, either peripheral or via a central venous line (jugular, femoral, or subclavian) is not obtained. Comparisons of epinephrine versus vasopressin have not shown any differences in regard to survival to discharge.[572] Do not interrupt CPR to administer medications. After the third shock, amiodarone should be considered. The efficacy of amiodarone has been established by two clinical trials in patients with out-of-hospital cardiac arrest.[573,574] Lidocaine is logical but without evidence to support its efficacy and should not be used as the sole first-line antiarrhythmic drug. For polymorphic VT associated with a long QT interval (torsades de pointes), magnesium in a 1- to 2-g loading dose should be given.[575] Sodium bicarbonate is only used in prolonged resuscitation when respiration is controlled because carbon dioxide formed from bicarbonate permeates into cells to increase intracellular acidosis.

Asystole or pulseless electrical activity. Asystole and pulseless electrical activity account for up to 70% of all out-of-hospital cardiac arrests encountered by EMS[576,577] and has a dreadful prognosis.[578] A decline in the incidence of VF in out-of-hospital cardiac arrest has been accompanied by an increase in the incidence of asystole and pulseless electrical activity.[579] The focus is to perform resuscitation with CPR while attempting to identify reversible causes or complicating factors. AHA guidelines recommend epinephrine every 3 to 5 minutes with a single dose of vasopressin substituted for the first or second epinephrine dose.[580] No study has demonstrated that atropine administered in 1-mg doses every 3 to 5 minutes for asystole or slow pulseless electrical activity has had any effect on outcomes. CPR should not be discontinued during the administration of medications. During CPR the rhythm should be checked and shocks delivered for persistent or recurrent VF or VT followed by resumption of CPR after each shock.

Other interventions. Interventions not supported by outcome evidence include routine use of fibrinolysis, attempted pacing for asystole, administration of procainamide for VF or pulseless VT, and routine fluid loading. No recommendations for or against precordial thumps have been made, which in some studies led to a deterioration in cardiac rhythm.

When to call it off. The ethics of when to stop the "loops" and when not to resuscitate are becoming increasingly complex. The 2010 guidelines address the situation in detail. The increasing use of capnography during cardiac arrest provides readily measurable and objective data to guide decision making.[581]

Self-help by coughing. Those persons who are alone when having a heart attack and begin to feel faint should cough repeatedly and very vigorously, which might save them from fatal VF.[582]

Care of cardiac arrest survivors. The patient will have been urgently hospitalized and central nervous injury and cardiogenic shock are the major risks. Amiodarone is the most commonly used antiarrhythmic drug following a VF arrest or for ongoing ventricular arrhythmias. In unconscious patients with spontaneous circulation after recovery from cardiac arrest caused by VF, mild therapeutic hypothermia of 32° C to 34° C improves the neurologic outcome and long-term survival.[583-586] In a retrospective analysis of cardiac arrest survivors at the Mayo Clinic, survival was 64% in those treated with induced hypothermia versus 24% in patients not treated with hypotheramia.[587] Once the patient is stabilized, a full cardiac evaluation is required, including echocardiography and coronary angiography.

Long-term care. The substrate for sustained monomorphic VT is seldom abolished by bypass grafting, so that the indications for cardiac surgery must be decided in their own right. Nevertheless, it makes sense to consider an ischemic cause in such patients, and aggressively to treat coronary heart disease and LV failure aggressively both medically and, where indicated, surgically. Empirical β-blockade is the prime long-term antiarrhythmic treatment unless contraindicated, whereupon empirical amiodarone is the next choice. The ICD is widely regarded as the ultimate treatment, and it undoubtedly reduces SCD. The ICD has irrevocably altered the landscape for patients with malignant ventricular tachyarrhythmias, yet there are reservations. In patients with a cardiac arrest in the setting of decompensated heart failure, an ICD may simply replace SCD by delayed death resulting from heart failure. Thus ICDs should be selectively applied, specifically to patients at serious risk of SCD yet otherwise having a reasonable expected overall cardiac prognosis.

Acknowledgments

We wish to acknowledge the very major contributions from Professor Irene Lang at the University of Vienna (pulmonary hypertension), Dr. Larry Baddour at the Mayo Clinic (infective endocarditis), and Dr. Roger White, also at Mayo Clinic (cardiopulmonary resuscitation).

References*

*The complete reference list is available online at www.expertconsult.com.

6. Boden WE. Niacin in patients with low HDL cholesterol levels receiving intensive statin therapy. AIM-HIGH Investigators. *N Engl J Med* 2011;365:2255–2267.
7. Voight BF, et al. Plasma HDL cholesterol and risk of myocardial infarction: a mendelian randomisation study. *Lancet* 2012;380:572–580.
9. Cushman WC, et al. Effects of intensive blood-pressure control in type 2 diabetes mellitus. *N Engl J Med* 2010;362:1575–1585.
27. Fox K, et al. Ivabradine for patients with stable coronary artery disease and left-ventricular systolic dysfunction (beautiful): a randomised, double-blind, placebo-controlled trial. *Lancet* 2008;372:807–816.
28. Swedberg K, et al. Ivabradine and outcomes in chronic heart failure (shift): a randomised placebo-controlled study. *Lancet* 2010;376:875–885.
29. Noman A, et al. Effect of high-dose allopurinol on exercise in patients with chronic stable angina: a randomised, placebo controlled crossover trial. *Lancet* 2010;375:2161–2167.
30. Rajendra NS, et al. Mechanistic insights into the therapeutic use of high-dose allopurinol in angina pectoris. *J Am Coll Cardiol* 2011;58:820–828.
34. Frye RL, et al. A randomized trial of therapies for type 2 diabetes and coronary artery disease. *N Engl J Med* 2009;360:2503–2515.
35. Cassar A, et al. Chronic coronary artery disease: diagnosis and management. *Mayo Clin Proc* 2009;84:1130–1146.
36. Tonino PA, et al. Fractional flow reserve versus angiography for guiding percutaneous coronary intervention. *N Engl J Med* 2009;360:213–224.
39. Mauri L, et al. Drug-eluting or bare-metal stents for acute myocardial infarction. *N Engl J Med* 2008;359:1330–1342.
41. Stone GW, et al. Paclitaxel-eluting stents versus bare-metal stents in acute myocardial infarction. *N Engl J Med* 2009;360:1946–1959.
42. Marroquin OC, et al. A comparison of bare-metal and drug-eluting stents for off-label indications. *N Engl J Med* 2008;358:342–352.
52. Brener SJ, et al. Comparison of percutaneous versus surgical revascularization of severe unprotected left main coronary stenosis in matched patients. *Am J Cardiol* 2008;101: 169–172.
54. Serruys PW, et al. Percutaneous coronary intervention versus coronary-artery bypass grafting for severe coronary artery disease. *N Engl J Med* 2009;360:961–972.
61. Losordo DW, et al. Intramyocardial, autologous cd34+ cell therapy for refractory angina. *Circ Res* 2011;109:428–436.
66. Anderson JL, et al. 2011 ACCF/AHA FOCUSED UPDATE incorporated into the ACC/AHA 2007 Guidelines for the Management of Patients with Unstable Angina/Non-ST-Elevation Myocardial Infarction: a report of the American College of Cardiology Foundation/ American Heart Association Task Force on Practice Guidelines. *Circulation* 2011; 123:e426–579.
67. Mehran R, et al. Standardized bleeding definitions for cardiovascular clinical trials: a consensus report from the bleeding academic research consortium. *Circulation* 2011; 123:2736–2747.
68. Steg PG, et al. Bleeding in acute coronary syndromes and percutaneous coronary interventions: position paper by the working group on thrombosis of the European Society of Cardiology. *Eur Heart J* 2011;32:1854–1864.

69. Burls A, et al. Oxygen therapy for acute myocardial infarction: a systematic review and meta-analysis. *Emerg Med J* 2011;28:917–923.

72. Antman EM, et al. 2007 focused update of the ACC/AHA 2004 guidelines for the management of patients with ST-elevation myocardial infarction: a report of the American College of Cardiology/American Heart Association Task Force on Practice Guidelines: developed in collaboration with the Canadian Cardiovascular Society endorsed by the American Academy of Family Physicians: 2007 writing group to review new evidence and update the ACC/AHA 2004 Guidelines for the Management of Patients with ST-Elevation Myocardial Infarction, writing on behalf of the 2004 Writing Committee. *Circulation* 2008;117:296–329.

73. Bhatt DL, et al. Clopidogrel with or without omeprazole in coronary artery disease. *N Engl J Med* 2010;363:1909–1917.

74. Pare G, et al. Effects of CYP2C19 genotype on outcomes of clopidogrel treatment. *N Engl J Med* 2010;363:1704–1714.

75. Price MJ, et al. Standard- vs high-dose clopidogrel based on platelet function testing after percutaneous coronary intervention: the gravitas randomized trial. *JAMA* 2011;305: 1097–1105.

76. Wiviott SD, et al. Intensive oral antiplatelet therapy for reduction of ischaemic events including stent thrombosis in patients with acute coronary syndromes treated with percutaneous coronary intervention and stenting in the triton-timi 38 trial: a subanalysis of a randomised trial. *Lancet* 2008;371:1353–1363.

77. Schomig A. Ticagrelor—is there need for a new player in the antiplatelet-therapy field? *N Engl J Med* 2009;361:1108–1111.

78. James SK, et al. Ticagrelor versus clopidogrel in patients with acute coronary syndromes intended for non-invasive management: substudy from prospective randomised platelet inhibition and patient outcomes (PLATO) trial. *Brit Med J* 2011;342:d3527.

79. Hamm CW, et al. ESC guidelines for the management of acute coronary syndromes in patients presenting without persistent ST-segment elevation: the task force for the management of acute coronary syndromes (ACS) in patients presenting without persistent ST-segment elevation of the European Society of Cardiology (ESC). *Eur Heart J* 2011; 32:2999–3054.

80. Bhatt DL, et al. Intravenous platelet blockade with cangrelor during PCI. *N Engl J Med* 2009;361:2330–2341.

81. O'Donoghue ML, et al. Safety and tolerability of atopaxar in the treatment of patients with acute coronary syndromes: the lessons from antagonizing the cellular effects of thrombin-acute coronary syndromes trial. *Circulation* 2011;123:1843–1853.

96. Mega JL, et al. Rivaroxaban in patients with a recent acute coronary syndrome. *N Engl J Med* 2012;366:9–19.

97. Alexander JH, et al. Apixaban with antiplatelet therapy after acute coronary syndrome. *N Engl J Med* 2011;365:699–708.

98. Goodman SG, et al. Association of proton pump inhibitor use on cardiovascular outcomes with clopidogrel and ticagrelor: insights from the platelet inhibition and patient outcomes trial. *Circulation* 2012;125:978–986.

101. Scirica BM, et al. Relationship between nonsustained ventricular tachycardia after non-ST-elevation acute coronary syndrome and sudden cardiac death: observations from the metabolic efficiency with ranolazine for less ischemia in non-ST-elevation acute coronary syndrome-thrombolysis in myocardial infarction 36 (MERLIN-TIMI 36) randomized controlled trial. *Circulation* 2010;122:455–462.

103. Morrow DA, et al. Evaluation of the glycometabolic effects of ranolazine in patients with and without diabetes mellitus in the MERLIN-TIMI 36 randomized controlled trial. *Circulation* 2009;119:2032–2039.

105. Fox KA, et al. Long-term outcome of a routine versus selective invasive strategy in patients with non-ST-segment elevation acute coronary syndrome a meta-analysis of individual patient data. *J Am Coll Cardiol* 2010;55:2435–2445.

115. Dattilo PB, et al. Beta-blockers are associated with reduced risk of myocardial infarction after cocaine use. *Ann Emerg Med* 2008;51:117–125.

118. Jernberg T, et al. Association between adoption of evidence-based treatment and survival for patients with ST-elevation myocardial infarction. *JAMA* 2011;305: 1677–1684.

122. Silvain J, et al. Composition of coronary thrombus in acute myocardial infarction. *J Am Coll Cardiol* 2011;57:1359–1367.

129. Stone GW, et al. Heparin plus a glycoprotein IIb/IIIa inhibitor versus bivalirudin monotherapy and paclitaxel-eluting stents versus bare-metal stents in acute myocardial infarction (HORIZONS-AMI): final 3-year results from a multicentre, randomised controlled trial. *Lancet* 2011;377:2193–2204.

136. Le May MR, et al. A citywide protocol for primary PCI in ST-segment elevation myocardial infarction. *N Engl J Med* 2008;358:231–240.

137. Flynn A, et al. Trends in door-to-balloon time and mortality in patients with ST-elevation myocardial infarction undergoing primary percutaneous coronary intervention. *Arch Intern Med* 2010;170:1842–1849.

138. Glickman SW, et al. Care processes associated with quicker door-in-door-out times for patients with ST-elevation-myocardial infarction requiring transfer: results from a statewide regionalization program. *Circ Cardiovasc Qual Outcomes* 2011;4:382–388.

140. Terkelsen CJ, et al. System delay and mortality among patients with STEMI treated with primary percutaneous coronary intervention. *JAMA* 2010;304:763–771.

141. Wang TY, et al. Association of door-in to door-out time with reperfusion delays and outcomes among patients transferred for primary percutaneous coronary intervention. *JAMA* 2011;305:2540–2547.

142. Holmes Jr DR, et al. Systems of care to improve timeliness of reperfusion therapy for ST-segment elevation myocardial infarction during off hours: the Mayo Clinic STEMI protocol. *JACC Cardiovasc Interv* 2008;1:88–96.

143. Jollis JG. Moving care forward: prehospital emergency cardiac systems. *Circulation* 2010;122:1443–1445.

145. Danchin N. Systems of care for ST-segment elevation myocardial infarction: impact of different models on clinical outcomes. *JACC Cardiovasc Interv* 2009;2:901–908.

147. Henry TD, et al. The ideal reperfusion strategy for the ST-segment elevation myocardial infarction patient with expected delay to percutaneous coronary intervention: paradise lost or paradise renamed? *JACC Cardiovasc Interv* 2009;2:931–933.

148. Danchin N. Comparison of thrombolysis followed by broad use of percutaneous coronary intervention with primary percutaneous coronary intervention for ST-segment-elevation acute myocardial infarction: data from the French registry on acute ST-elevation myocardial infarction (FAST-MI). *Circulation* 2008;118:268–276.

149. McMullan JT, et al. Reperfusion is delayed beyond guideline recommendations in patients requiring interhospital helicopter transfer for treatment of ST-segment elevation myocardial infarction. *Ann Emerg Med* 2011;57:213–20, e211.

152. Van de Werf F, et al. Management of acute myocardial infarction in patients presenting with persistent ST-segment elevation: the task force on the management of ST-segment elevation acute myocardial infarction of the European Society of Cardiology. *Eur Heart J* 2008;29:2909–2945.

153. Ellis SG, et al. Facilitated PCI in patients with ST-elevation myocardial infarction. *N Engl J Med* 2008;358:2205–2217.

155. Gersh BJ, et al. Pharmacological facilitation of coronary intervention in ST-segment elevation myocardial infarction: time is of the essence. *JACC Cardiovasc Interv* 2010;3:1292–1294.

163. Stone GW, et al. Bivalirudin during primary PCI in acute myocardial infarction. *N Engl J Med* 2008;358:2218–2230.

171. Burzotta F, et al. Clinical impact of thrombectomy in acute ST-elevation myocardial infarction: an individual patient-data pooled analysis of 11 trials. *Eur Heart J* 2009; 30:2193–2203.

173. Thibault H, et al. Long-term benefit of postconditioning. *Circulation* 2008;117:1037–1044.

176. Piot C, et al. Effect of cyclosporine on reperfusion injury in acute myocardial infarction. *N Engl J Med* 2008;359:473–481.

177. Botker HE, et al. Remote ischaemic conditioning before hospital admission, as a complement to angioplasty, and effect on myocardial salvage in patients with acute myocardial infarction: a randomised trial. *Lancet* 2010;375:727–734.

178. Hausenloy DJ, et al. GLP-1 therapy: beyond glucose control. *Circ Heart Fail* 2008;1: 147–149.

179. Lonborg J, et al. Exenatide reduces reperfusion injury in patients with ST-segment elevation myocardial infarction. *Eur Heart J* 2012;33:1491–1499.

181. Berger JS, et al. Initial aspirin dose and outcome among ST-elevation myocardial infarction patients treated with fibrinolytic therapy. *Circulation* 2008;117:192–199.

182. Goodman SG, et al. Acute ST-segment elevation myocardial infarction: American College of Chest Physicians evidence-based clinical practice guidelines (8th ed.). *Chest* 2008; 133:708S–775S.

183. Antman EM, et al. 2007 focused update of the ACC/AHA 2004 guidelines for the management of patients with ST-elevation myocardial infarction: a report of the American College of Cardiology/American Heart Association task force on practice guidelines. *J Am Coll Cardiol* 2008;51:210–247.

184. Dangas G, et al. Role of clopidogrel loading dose in patients with ST-segment elevation myocardial infarction undergoing primary angioplasty: results from the HORIZONS-AMI (Harmonizing Outcomes with Revascularization and Stents in Acute Myocardial Infarction) trial. *J Am Coll Cardiol* 2009;54:1438–1446.

185. Patti G, et al. Outcome comparison of 600- and 300-mg loading doses of clopidogrel in patients undergoing primary percutaneous coronary intervention for ST-segment elevation myocardial infarction: results from the ARMYDA-6 MI (Antiplatelet Therapy for Reduction of Myocardial Damage during Angioplasty-Myocardial Infarction) randomized study. *J Am Coll Cardiol* 2011;58:1592–1599

186. Wijns W, et al. Guidelines on myocardial revascularization. *Eur Heart J* 2010;31:2501–2555

187. Montalescot G, et al. Prasugrel compared with clopidogrel in patients undergoing percutaneous coronary intervention for ST-elevation myocardial infarction (TRITON-TIMI 38): double-blind, randomised controlled trial. *Lancet* 2009;373:723–731.

188. Wiviott SD, et al. Greater clinical benefit of more intensive oral antiplatelet therapy with prasugrel in patients with diabetes mellitus in the trial to assess improvement in therapeutic outcomes by optimizing platelet inhibition with prasugrel-thrombolysis in myocardial infarction 38. *Circulation* 2008;118:1626–1636.

190. Montalescot G, et al. Intravenous enoxaparin or unfractionated heparin in primary percutaneous coronary intervention for ST-elevation myocardial infarction: the international randomised open-label ATOLL trial. *Lancet* 2011;378:693–703.

202. Wright RS, et al. 2011 ACCF/AHA focused update incorporated into the ACC/AHA 2007 guidelines for the management of patients with unstable angina/non-ST-elevation myocardial infarction: a report of the American College of Cardiology Foundation/American Heart Association Task Force on Practice Guidelines developed in collaboration with the American Academy of Family Physicians, Society for Cardiovascular Angiography and Interventions, and the Society of Thoracic Surgeons. *J Am Coll Cardiol* 2011;57:e215–367.

204. Lønborg J, et al. Exenatide reduces final infarct size in patients with ST-segment-elevation myocardial infarction and short-duration of ischemia. *Circ Cardiovasc Interv* 2012;5:288–295.

205. Selker HP, et al. Out-of-hospital administration of intravenous glucose-insulin-potassium in patients with suspected acute coronary syndromes: the IMMEDIATE randomized controlled trial. *JAMA* 2012;307:1925–1933.
206. Bøtker HE, et al. Remote ischaemic conditioning before hospital admission, as a complement to angioplasty, and effect on myocardial salvage in patients with acute myocardial infarction: a randomised trial. *Lancet* 2010;375:727–734.
207. Zhao YT, et al. Comparison of glucose-insulin-potassium and insulin-glucose as adjunctive therapy in acute myocardial infarction: a contemporary meta-analysis of randomised controlled trials. *Heart* 2010;96:1622–1626.
208. Najjar SS, et al. Intravenous erythropoietin in patients with ST-segment elevation myocardial infarction: REVEAL: a randomized controlled trial. *JAMA* 2011;305: 1863–1872.
211. Schmitt J, et al. Atrial fibrillation in acute myocardial infarction: a systematic review of the incidence, clinical features and prognostic implications. *Eur Heart J* 2009;30: 1038–1045.
218. Vlaar PJ, et al. Culprit vessel only versus multivessel and staged percutaneous coronary intervention for multivessel disease in patients presenting with ST-segment elevation myocardial infarction: a pairwise and network meta-analysis. *J Am Coll Cardiol* 2011; 58:692–703.
227. Lavie CJ, et al. Exercise training and cardiac rehabilitation in primary and secondary prevention of coronary heart disease. *Mayo Clin Proc* 2009;84:373–383.
246. Kushner FG, et al. 2009 focused updates: ACC/AHA guidelines for the management of patients with ST-elevation myocardial infarction (updating the 2004 guideline and 2007 focused update) and ACC/AHA/SCAI guidelines on percutaneous coronary intervention (updating the 2005 guideline and 2007 focused update): a report of the American College of Cardiology Foundation/American Heart Association Task Force On Practice Guidelines. *Circulation* 2009;120:2271–2306.
266. Camm AJ, et al. A randomized active-controlled study comparing the efficacy and safety of vernakalant to amiodarone in recent-onset atrial fibrillation. *J Am Coll Cardiol* 2011;57:313–321.
267. Camm AJ, et al. Guidelines for the management of atrial fibrillation: the Task Force for the Management of Atrial Fibrillation of the European Society of Cardiology (ESC) identifying patients at high risk for stroke despite anticoagulation: a comparison of contemporary stroke risk stratification schemes in an anticoagulated atrial fibrillation cohort. *Eur Heart J* 2010;31:2369–2429.
268. Kowey PR, et al. Vernakalant hydrochloride for the rapid conversion of atrial fibrillation after cardiac surgery: a randomized, double-blind, placebo-controlled trial. *Circ Arrhythm Electrophysiol* 2009;2:652–659.
275. Imazio M, et al. Colchicine reduces postoperative atrial fibrillation: results of the colchicine for the prevention of the postpericardiotomy syndrome (COPPS) atrial fibrillation substudy. *Circulation* 2011;124:2290–2295.
283. Van Gelder IC, et al. Lenient versus strict rate control in patients with atrial fibrillation. *N Engl J Med* 2010;362:1363–1373.
288. Kumar S, et al. Long-term omega-3 polyunsaturated fatty acid supplementation reduces the recurrence of persistent atrial fibrillation after electrical cardioversion. *Heart Rhythm* 2012;9:483–491.
289. Nodari S, et al. ω-3 polyunsaturated fatty acids in the prevention of atrial fibrillation recurrences after electrical cardioversion: a prospective, randomized study. *Circulation* 2011;124:1100–1106.
290. Le Heuzey JY, et al. A short-term, randomized, double-blind, parallel-group study to evaluate the efficacy and safety of dronedarone versus amiodarone in patients with persistent atrial fibrillation: the DIONYSOS study. *J Cardiovasc Electrophysiol* 2010;21:597–605.
291. Hohnloser SH, et al. Effect of dronedarone on cardiovascular events in atrial fibrillation. *N Engl J Med* 2009;360:668–678.
292. Kober L, et al. Increased mortality after dronedarone therapy for severe heart failure. *N Engl J Med* 2008;358:2678–2687.
293. Administration FDA. FDA drug safety communication. Multaq (dronedarone): an increased risk of death and serious cardiovascular adverse events. European Medicines Agency updates on ongoing benefit-risk review of multaq. 2011.
296. Dobrev D, et al. New antiarrhythmic drugs for treatment of atrial fibrillation. *Lancet* 2010;375:1212–1223.
298. Lip GY, et al. Identifying patients at high risk for stroke despite anticoagulation: a comparison of contemporary stroke risk stratification schemes in an anticoagulated atrial fibrillation cohort. *Stroke* 2010;41:2731–2738.
300. Stroke Risk in Atrial Fibrillation Working Group. Comparison of 12 risk stratification schemes to predict stroke in patients with nonvalvular atrial fibrillation. *Stroke* 2008; 39:1901–1910.
301. Lip GY. Identifying patients at high risk for stroke despite anticoagulation: a comparison of contemporary stroke risk stratification schemes in an anticoagulated atrial fibrillation cohort. *Stroke* 2010;41:2731–2738.
302. Lip GY, et al. Comparative validation of a novel risk score for predicting bleeding risk in anticoagulated patients with atrial fibrillation: the HAS-BLED (Hypertension, Abnormal Renal/Liver Function, Stroke, Bleeding History or Predisposition, Labile INR, Elderly, Drugs/Alcohol Concomitantly) score. *J Am Coll Cardiol* 2011;57:173–180.
303. Broderick JP, et al. Withdrawal of antithrombotic agents and its impact on ischemic stroke occurrence. *Stroke* 2011;42:2509–2514.
304. Connolly SJ, et al. Effect of clopidogrel added to aspirin in patients with atrial fibrillation. *N Engl J Med* 2009;360:2066–2078.

307. Gersh BJ, et al. Antiplatelet and anticoagulant therapy for stroke prevention in patients with non-valvular atrial fibrillation: evidence based strategies and new developments. *Rev ESP Cardiol* 2011;64:260–268.

308. Connolly SJ, et al. Dabigatran versus warfarin in patients with atrial fibrillation. *N Engl J Med* 2009;361:1139–1151.

309. Eikelboom JW, et al. Risk of bleeding with 2 doses of dabigatran compared with warfarin in older and younger patients with atrial fibrillation: an analysis of the randomized evaluation of long-term anticoagulant therapy (RE-LY) trial. *Circulation* 2011;123: 2363–2372.

310. Patel MR, et al. Rivaroxaban versus warfarin in nonvalvular atrial fibrillation. *N Engl J Med* 2011;365:883–891.

312. Holmes DR, et al. Percutaneous closure of the left atrial appendage versus warfarin therapy for prevention of stroke in patients with atrial fibrillation: a randomised non-inferiority trial. *Lancet* 2009;374:534–542.

314. Holmes Jr DR, et al. Left atrial appendage occlusion eliminates the need for warfarin. *Circulation* 2009;120:1919–1926; discussion 1926.

315. Whitlock RP, et al. Left atrial appendage occlusion does not eliminate the need for warfarin. *Circulation* 2009;120:1927–1932; discussion 1932.

317. Herrera Siklody C, et al. Incidence of asymptomatic intracranial embolic events after pulmonary vein isolation: comparison of different atrial fibrillation ablation technologies in a multicenter study. *J Am Coll Cardiol* 2011;58:681–688.

318. Calkins H, et al. Treatment of atrial fibrillation with antiarrhythmic drugs or radiofrequency ablation: two systematic literature reviews and meta-analyses. *Circ Arrhythm Electrophysiol* 2009;2:349–361.

319. Jais P, et al. Catheter ablation versus antiarrhythmic drugs for atrial fibrillation: the A4 study. *Circulation* 2008;118:2498–2505.

321. ClinicalTrials.gov Identifier: NCT00911508 Catheter Ablation vs. Anti-arrhythmic Drug therapy for Atrial Fibrillation Trial (CABANA) is ongoing.

322. Weerasooriya R, et al. Catheter ablation for atrial fibrillation: are results maintained at 5 years of follow-up? *J Am Coll Cardiol* 2011;57:160–166.

323. Wokhlu A, et al. Long-term outcome of atrial fibrillation ablation: impact and predictors of very late recurrence. *J Cardiovasc Electrophysiol* 2010;21:1071–1078.

325. Cha YM, et al. Success of ablation for atrial fibrillation in isolated left ventricular diastolic dysfunction: a comparison to systolic dysfunction and normal ventricular function. *Circ Arrhythm Electrophysiol* 2011;4:724–732.

337. Stevenson WG, et al. Irrigated radiofrequency catheter ablation guided by electroanatomic mapping for recurrent ventricular tachycardia after myocardial infarction: the multicenter thermocool ventricular tachycardia ablation trial. *Circulation* 2008;118: 2773–2782.

338. Kuck KH, et al. Catheter ablation of stable ventricular tachycardia before defibrillator implantation in patients with coronary heart disease (vtach): a multicentre randomised controlled trial. *Lancet* 2010;375:31–40.

341. Dickstein K, et al. ESC guidelines for the diagnosis and treatment of acute and chronic heart failure 2008: the task force for the diagnosis and treatment of acute and chronic heart failure 2008 of the European Society of Cardiology. Developed in collaboration with the heart failure association of the ESC (HFA) and endorsed by the European Society of Intensive Care Medicine (ESICM). *Eur Heart J* 2008;29: 2388–2442.

342. Hunt SA, et al. 2009 focused update incorporated into the ACC/AHA 2005 guidelines for the diagnosis and management of heart failure in adults: a report of the American College of Cardiology Foundation/American Heart Association task force on practice guidelines: developed in collaboration with the International Society for Heart and Lung Transplantation. *Circulation* 2009;119:e391–479.

343. Lindenfeld J, et al. HFSA 2010 comprehensive heart failure practice guideline. *J Card Fail* 2010;16:e1–194.

348. O'Connor CM, et al. Influence of global region on outcomes in heart failure beta-blocker trials. *J Am Coll Cardiol* 2011;58:915–922.

350. Zannad F, et al. Eplerenone in patients with systolic heart failure and mild symptoms. *N Engl J Med* 2011;364:11–21.

356. McNamara DM. Emerging role of pharmacogenomics in heart failure. *Curr Opin Cardiol* 2008;23:261–268.

357. Bardy GH, et al. Home use of automated external defibrillators for sudden cardiac arrest. *N Engl J Med* 2008;358:1793–1804.

360. Roy D, et al. Rhythm control versus rate control for atrial fibrillation and heart failure. *N Engl J Med* 2008;358:2667–2677.

361. Wilton SB, et al. Outcomes of cardiac resynchronization therapy in patients with versus those without atrial fibrillation: a systematic review and meta-analysis. *Heart Rhythm* 2011;8:1088–1094.

362. Becker RC, et al. The primary and secondary prevention of coronary artery disease: American College of Chest Physicians evidence-based clinical practice guidelines (8th edition). *Chest* 2008;133:776S–814S.

363. Massie BM, et al. Randomized trial of warfarin, aspirin, and clopidogrel in patients with chronic heart failure: the warfarin and antiplatelet therapy in chronic heart failure (WATCH) trial. *Circulation* 2009;119:1616–1624.

364. Homma S, et al. Warfarin and aspirin in patients with heart failure and sinus rhythm. *N Engl J Med* 2012 366:1859–1869.

367. Felker GM, et al. Diuretic strategies in patients with acute decompensated heart failure. *N Engl J Med* 2011;364:797–805.

370. O'Connor CM, et al. Effect of nesiritide in patients with acute decompensated heart failure. *N Engl J Med* 2011;365:32–43.

375. Jones RH, et al. Coronary bypass surgery with or without surgical ventricular reconstruction. *N Engl J Med* 2009;360:1705–1717.

377. Rouleau JL. New and emerging drugs and device therapies for chronic heart failure in patients with systolic ventricular dysfunction. *Can J Cardiol* 2011;27:296–301.

378. Gao R, et al. A phase II, randomized, double-blind, multicenter, based on standard therapy, placebo-controlled study of the efficacy and safety of recombinant human neuregulin-1 in patients with chronic heart failure. *J Am Coll Cardiol* 2010;55:1907–1914.

379. Cleland JG, et al. The effects of the cardiac myosin activator, omecamtiv mecarbil, on cardiac function in systolic heart failure: a double-blind, placebo-controlled, crossover, dose-ranging phase 2 trial. *Lancet* 2011;378:676–683.

383. Steinbeck G, et al. Defibrillator implantation early after myocardial infarction. *N Engl J Med* 2009;361:1427–1436.

385. Adabag AS, et al. Sudden death after myocardial infarction. *JAMA* 2008;300:2022–2029.

388. Sipahi I, et al. Impact of QRS duration on clinical event reduction with cardiac resynchronization therapy: meta-analysis of randomized controlled trials. *Arch Intern Med* 2011;171:1454–1462.

389. Stevenson LW. "A little learning is a dangerous thing." *Arch Intern Med* 2011;171: 1494–1495.

390. Camici PG, et al. Stunning, hibernation, and assessment of myocardial viability. *Circulation* 2008;117:103–114.

392. Velazquez EJ, et al. Coronary-artery bypass surgery in patients with left ventricular dysfunction. *N Engl J Med* 2011;364:1607–1616.

397. Slaughter MS, et al. Advanced heart failure treated with continuous-flow left ventricular assist device. *N Engl J Med* 2009;361:2241–2251.

398. Acker MA, et al. Mitral valve repair in heart failure: five-year follow-up from the mitral valve replacement stratum of the acorn randomized trial. *J Thorac Cardiovasc Surg* 2011;142:569–574, e561.

399. Siegel RJ, et al. The acute hemodynamic effects of mitraclip therapy. *J Am Coll Cardiol* 2011;57:1658–1665.

400. Powell LH, et al. Self-management counseling in patients with heart failure: the heart failure adherence and retention randomized behavioral trial. *JAMA* 2010;304:1331–1338.

401. Stevenson LW. Counting performance with therapies for heart failure: aiming for quality or quantity? *Circulation* 2010;122:561–566.

404. McMurray JJ, et al. Design of the reduction of events with darbepoetin alpha in heart failure (RED-HF): a phase III, anaemia correction, morbidity-mortality trial. *Eur J Heart Fail* 2009;11:795–801.

405. Anker SD, et al. Ferric carboxymaltose in patients with heart failure and iron deficiency. *N Engl J Med* 2009;361:2436–2448.

408. Peacock WF, et al. National Heart, Lung, and Blood Institute Working Group on Emergency Department Management of Acute Heart Failure: research challenges and opportunities. *J Am Coll Cardiol* 2010;56:343–351.

409. Borlaug BA, et al. Diastolic and systolic heart failure are distinct phenotypes within the heart failure spectrum. *Circulation* 2011;123:2006–2013; discussion 2014.

412. Mak GJ, et al. Natural history of markers of collagen turnover in patients with early diastolic dysfunction and impact of eplerenone. *J Am Coll Cardiol* 2009;54:1674–1682.

421. Gray A, et al. Noninvasive-ventilation in acute cardiogenic pulmonary edema. *N Engl J Med* 2008;359:142–151.

422. Gersh BJ, et al. 2011 ACCF/AHA guideline for the diagnosis and treatment of hypertrophic cardiomyopathy: a report of the American College of Cardiology Foundation/American Heart Association Task Force on Practice Guidelines. Developed in collaboration with the American Association for Thoracic Surgery, American Society of Echocardiography, American Society of Nuclear Cardiology, Heart Failure Society of America, Heart Rhythm Society, Society for Cardiovascular Angiography and Interventions, and Society of Thoracic Surgeons. *J Am Coll Cardiol* 2011;58:e212–260.

423. Abozguia K, et al. Metabolic modulator perhexiline corrects energy deficiency and improves exercise capacity in symptomatic hypertrophic cardiomyopathy. *Circulation* 2010;122:1562–1569.

428. Sorajja P, et al. Outcome of alcohol septal ablation for obstructive hypertrophic cardiomyopathy. *Circulation* 2008;118:131–139.

436. Bos JM, et al. Role of family history of sudden death in risk stratification and prevention of sudden death with implantable defibrillators in hypertrophic cardiomyopathy. *Am J Cardiol* 2010;106:1481–1486.

441. Cooper Jr LT. Clinical manifestations and diagnosis of myocarditis in adults. Rose, BD (Ed), UpToDate, Waltham, MA, 2007.

443. Frustaci A, et al. Randomized study on the efficacy of immunosuppressive therapy in patients with virus-negative inflammatory cardiomyopathy: the TIMIC study. *Eur Heart J* 2009;30:1995–2002.

446. Cooper Jr LT, et al. Usefulness of immunosuppression for giant cell myocarditis. *Am J Cardiol* 2008;102:1535–1539.

463. Rossebo AB, et al. Intensive lipid lowering with simvastatin and ezetimibe in aortic stenosis. *N Engl J Med* 2008;359:1343–1356.

466. Hannan EL, et al. Aortic valve replacement for patients with severe aortic stenosis: risk factors and their impact on 30-month mortality. *Ann Thorac Surg* 2009;87:1741–1749.

468. Vahanian A, et al. Transcatheter valve implantation for patients with aortic stenosis: a position statement from the European Association of Cardio-Thoracic Surgery (EACTS) and the European Society of Cardiology (ESC), in collaboration with the European

Association of Percutaneous Cardiovascular Interventions (EAPCI). *Eur Heart J* 2008;29:1463–1470.

469. Thomas M, et al. One-year outcomes of cohort 1 in the Edwards Sapien Aortic Bioprosthesis European Outcome (SOURCE) registry: the European registry of transcatheter aortic valve implantation using the Edwards Sapien valve. *Circulation* 2011;124:425–433.

470. Leon MB, et al. Transcatheter aortic-valve implantation for aortic stenosis in patients who cannot undergo surgery. *N Engl J Med* 2010;363:1597–1607.

471. Smith CR, et al. Transcatheter versus surgical aortic-valve replacement in high-risk patients. *N Engl J Med* 2011;364:2187–2198.

472. Bauer F, et al. Immediate and long-term echocardiographic findings after transcatheter aortic valve implantation for the treatment of aortic stenosis: the Cribier-Edwards/Edwards-Sapien valve experience. *J Am Soc Echocardiogr* 2010;23:370–376.

473. Kahlert P, et al. Silent and apparent cerebral ischemia after percutaneous transfemoral aortic valve implantation: a diffusion-weighted magnetic resonance imaging study. *Circulation* 2010;121:870–878.

474. Piazza N, et al. Procedural and 30-day outcomes following transcatheter aortic valve implantation using the third generation (18 fr) Corevalve Revalving System: results from the multicentre, expanded evaluation registry 1-year following ce mark approval. *EuroIntervention* 2008;4:242–249.

475. Kodali SK, et al. Two-year outcomes after transcatheter or surgical aortic-valve replacement. *N Engl J Med* 2012;366:1686–1695.

476. Makkar RR, et al. Transcatheter aortic-valve replacement for inoperable severe aortic stenosis. *N Engl J Med* 2012;366:1696–1704.

479. Rahimtoola SH. The year in valvular heart disease. *J Am Coll Cardiol* 2010;55:1729–1742.

481. Hilliard AA, et al. The interventional cardiologist and structural heart disease: the need for a team approach. *JACC Cardiovasc Imaging* 2009;2:8–10.

482. Messika-Zeitoun D, et al. Impact of degree of commissural opening after percutaneous mitral commissurotomy on long-term outcome. *JACC Cardiovasc Imaging* 2009;2:1–7.

492. Bhindi R, et al. Surgery insight: percutaneous treatment of prosthetic paravalvular leaks. *Nat Clin Pract Cardiovasc Med* 2008;5:140–147.

494. Gammie JS, et al. Trends in mitral valve surgery in the United States: results from the Society of Thoracic Surgeons adult cardiac surgery database. *Ann Thorac Surg* 2009;87:1431–1437; discussion 1437–1439.

495. Flameng W, et al. Durability of mitral valve repair in Barlow disease versus fibroelastic deficiency. *J Thorac Cardiovasc Surg* 2008;135:274–282.

496. Gillinov AM, et al. Valve repair versus valve replacement for degenerative mitral valve disease. *J Thorac Cardiovasc Surg* 2008;135:885-893, e881–882.

497. Feldman T, et al. Percutaneous repair or surgery for mitral regurgitation. *N Engl J Med* 2011;364:1395–1406.

501. Klings E. Cor pulmonale. In: Rose B, editor. *Uptodate*. Waltham, Mass; 2011.

505. Galie N, et al. A meta-analysis of randomized controlled trials in pulmonary arterial hypertension. *Eur Heart J* 2009;30:394–403.

506. Mayer E, et al. Surgical management and outcome of patients with chronic thromboembolic pulmonary hypertension: results from an international prospective registry. *J Thorac Cardiovasc Surg* 2011;141:702–710.

517. Sakao S, et al. Reversible or irreversible remodeling in pulmonary arterial hypertension. *Am J Respir Cell Mol Biol* 2010;43:629–634.

523. Bannay A, et al. The impact of valve surgery on short- and long-term mortality in left-sided infective endocarditis: do differences in methodological approaches explain previous conflicting results? *Eur Heart J* 2011;32:2003–2015.

524. Thuny F, et al. The timing of surgery influences mortality and morbidity in adults with severe complicated infective endocarditis: a propensity analysis. *Eur Heart J* 2011; 32:2027–2033.

525. Kim DH, et al. Impact of early surgery on embolic events in patients with infective endocarditis. *Circulation* 2010;122:S17–22.

533. Rooke TW, et al. 2011 ACCF/AHA focused update of the Guideline for the Management of Patients with Peripheral Artery Disease (updating the 2005 guideline): a report of the American College of Cardiology Foundation/American Heart Association Task Force on Practice Guidelines. *J Am Coll Cardiol* 2011;58:2020–2045.

539. Belch J, et al. Effect of fibroblast growth factor NV1FGF on amputation and death: a randomised placebo-controlled trial of gene therapy in critical limb ischaemia. *Lancet* 2011;377:1929–1937.

540. Gupta R, et al. Cell therapy for critical limb ischemia: moving forward one step at a time. *Circ Cardiovasc Interv* 2011;4:2–5.

541. Idei N, et al. Autologous bone-marrow mononuclear cell implantation reduces long-term major amputation risk in patients with critical limb ischemia: a comparison of atherosclerotic peripheral arterial disease and buerger disease. *Circ Cardiovasc Interv* 2011;4:15–25.

546. De Backer T, et al. Naftidrofuryl for intermittent claudication: meta-analysis based on individual patient data. *Brit Med J* 2009;338:b603.

548. Mohler E. Medical management of claudication. In: Rose B, editor. *Uptodate*. Waltham, Mass; 2011.

552. Wigley F. Pharmacologic and surgical treatment of the Raynaud's phenomenon. In: Rose B, editor. *Uptodate*. Waltham, Mass; 2011.

555. Wooley JA. Characteristics of thiamin and its relevance to the management of heart failure. *Nutr Clin Pract* 2008;23:487–493.

556. Field JM, et al. Part 1: Executive summary: 2010 American Heart Association Guidelines for Cardiopulmonary Resuscitation and Emergency Cardiovascular Care. *Circulation* 2010;122:S640–656.

557. Stiell IG, et al. Early versus later rhythm analysis in patients with out-of-hospital cardiac arrest. *N Engl J Med* 2011;365:787–797.
561. Neumar RW, et al. Implementation strategies for improving survival after out-of-hospital cardiac arrest in the United States: consensus recommendations from the 2009 American Heart Association Cardiac Arrest Survival Summit. *Circulation* 2011;123: 2898–2910.
566. Agarwal DA, et al. Ventricular fibrillation in Rochester, Minnesota: experience over 18 years. *Resuscitation* 2009;80:1253–1258.
568. Berdowski J, et al. Chest compressions cause recurrence of ventricular fibrillation after the first successful conversion by defibrillation in out-of-hospital cardiac arrest. *Circ Arrhythm Electrophysiol* 2010;3:72–78.
570. Simpson PM, et al. Delayed versus immediate defibrillation for out-of-hospital cardiac arrest due to ventricular fibrillation: a systematic review and meta-analysis of ran- domised controlled trials. *Resuscitation* 2010;81:925–931.
576. Lloyd-Jones D, et al. Executive summary: heart disease and stroke statistics—2010 update: a report from the American Heart Association. *Circulation* 2010;121:948–954.
577. Nichol G, et al. Regional variation in out-of-hospital cardiac arrest incidence and outcome. *JAMA* 2008;300:1423–1431.
581. Bakris GL. Recognition, pathogenesis, and treatment of different stages of nephropathy in patients with type 2 diabetes mellitus. *Mayo Clin Proc* 2011;86:444–456.
583. Dumas F, et al. Is hypothermia after cardiac arrest effective in both shockable and non- shockable patients? Insights from a large registry. *Circulation* 2011;123:877–886.
584. Lampe JW, et al. State of the art in therapeutic hypothermia. *Annu Rev Med* 2011;62: 79–93.
586. Sunde K, et al. Therapeutic hypothermia after cardiac arrest: where are we now? *Curr Opin Crit Care* 2011;17:247–253.
587. Fugate JE, et al. Does therapeutic hypothermia affect time to awakening in cardiac arrest survivors? *Neurology* 2011;77:1346–1350.
588. Sayre MR, et al. On behalf of the Adult Basic Life Support Chapter Collaborators. Part 5: adult basic life support: 2010 international consensus on cardiopulmonary resuscita- tion and emergency cardiovascular care science with treatment recommendations. *Circulation* 2010;122(Suppl. 2):S298–S324.
589. Anderson JL, et al. 2011 ACCF/AHA focused update incorporated into the ACC/AHA 2007 guidelines for the management of patients with unstable angina/non-ST-elevation myocardial infarction: a report of the American College of Cardiology Foundation/ American Heart Association Task Force on Practice Guidelines. *Circulation* 2011; 123:e426–579.
592. Nishimura RA, et al. ACC/AHA 2008 guideline update on valvular heart disease: focused update on infective endocarditis: a report of the American College of Cardiology/ American Heart Association Task Force on Practice Guidelines: endorsed by the Society of Cardiovascular Anesthesiologists, Society for Cardiovascular Angiography and Inter- ventions, and Society of Thoracic Surgeons. *Circulation* 2008;118:887–896.
593. Habib G, et al. ESC Committee for Practice Guidelines. Guidelines on the prevention, diagnosis, and treatment of infective endocarditis (new version 2009): the Task Force on the Prevention, Diagnosis, and Treatment of Infective Endocarditis of the European Society of Cardiology (ESC). Endorsed by the European Society of Clinical Microbiol- ogy and Infectious Diseases (ESCMID) and the International Society of Chemotherapy (ISC) for Infection and Cancer. *Eur Heart J* 2009;30:2369–2413.
595. You JJ, et al. Antithrombotic therapy for atrial fibrillation: antithrombotic therapy and prevention of thrombosis, 9th ed: American College of Chest Physicians evidence- based clinical practice guidelines. *Chest* 2012;141(Suppl. 2):e531S–575S.
596. Granger CB, et al. Apixaban versus warfarin in patients with atrial fibrillation. *N Engl J Med* 2011;365:981–992.

Index